Science

D0918229

Social System Perspectives

in Residential Institutions

SOCIAL SYSTEM PERSPECTIVES IN RESIDENTIAL INSTITUTIONS

EDITED BY

HOWARD·W·POLSKY

DANIEL·S·CLASTER

CARL GOLDBERG

. .

.

EAST LANSING

Michigan State University Press

1970

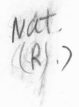

Nat.
(RI.)

12.50

CONTENTS

[v]

Section II: The Institution in Society

Section III: Internal Structure and Processes of Institutions

Social System Perspectives

in Residential Institutions

૪◆

INTRODUCTION

THE PURPOSE of this book of readings is to present, within a cohesive theoretical framework, an accumulating base of theory and treatment in residential institutions. Since the end of World War II, residential treatment has undergone radical changes. The observations and experiences of practitioners are becoming integrated with social science research theory. As major postulates of applied behavioral science emerge, the meaning of treatment and intervention is transformed. Perspectives of institutional reality are modified so that the practitioner becomes more discriminating of significant forces in the social field of patients and personnel. The individual and his social systems enter the purview of treatment in a new and dynamic way.

For both practitioners and social scientists, the residential institution serves as a human laboratory. The theorist-researcher can make his special contribution to practice by analytically probing the underlying assumptions of practice, teasing out significant variables for research, and from the research, deriving sounder principles for incorporation in a theoretical framework. The danger for the theorist is a too dogmatic application of theory to reality; the danger for the practitioner is an overly narrow view of his client's problems, their causes, and the avenues of treatment.

The readings in this collection demonstrate that contemporary social science does have an overarching theory which is useful for practitioners. The concepts developed in this book are general orientations and guidelines. They will be refined and recast in years to come; practical experience of treatment personnel will verify what is correct, amend what is incorrect, and provide direction for extending the theory. The practitioner is therefore an essential contributor to the development of applied behavioral science in residential centers.

While there is presently a need in social science for middle-range propositions and concepts, eventually they will have to be interconnected by a more comprehensive theoretical perspective. Social system theory represents, in our opinion, the best current synthesis. This theory rests on the familiar premise that the complex affairs of any social entity cannot be conducted unless they are organized in a systematic way. Social system theory grows out of a small set of fundamental organizing principles—centering about the system's maintenance and adaptation and impact upon its environmental situation—which are shared by all durable human social groups. To be sure, in more complex configurations these principles undergo considerable elaboration. The aim of behavioral sciences is to discover the operation of these principles in different social fields.

This book emphasizes the interlinking of theory, research, and treatment within residential institutions. According to Parsons,[1] theory is defined as "a body of logically interrelated *general concepts* of empirical reference." Concepts enable us to uncover uniformities underlying differences in social phenomena of varying scope and levels of complexity; the assumptions underlying the concepts make up the theoretical framework. Concepts can never encompass the totality of concrete social phenomena; in fact conceptualization implies selection of significant components in the social situation. Every social scientist, be he theorist or practitioner, exercises selection when he adopts any implicit or explicit symbolic system to define the scope of a social entity. Precise denotation limits the social phenomenon under study, yet enables the investigator to probe intensively its significant processes.

The days of muck-raking exposés of institutional problems are coming to an end; the behavioral scientist is now confronted with the task of coming up with reliable and valid statements about the components of the institutional system and systematic evaluation of individual functioning, institutional processes and social change. The operation of these social processes in institutions can be viewed as a special case of contemporary action theory. Our undertaking in this book is to treat institutional dynamics as an aspect of the general theory of social action, to link up a critical field of treatment with the modern behavioral science of social-system analysis.

Those of us in the rapidly maturing field of residential treatment have noted the increasing self-consciousness of all personnel with the total ongoing life of their rehabilitation communities. It is no longer assumed that in residential treatment, therapy is a special province of the professional psychotherapist treating a single resident. All inhabitants of the community contribute to an emergent social system that decisively influences the rehabilitative outcome of its residents. Hence, the recurrent focus upon the total therapeutic milieu presents practitioners, theorists, and researchers with the continuing challenge of conceptualizing, operationalizing, diagnosing and intervening into social system units within the institution, and between it and the community.

[1] Talcott Parsons, *The Structure of Social Action* (Second Edition), Glencoe, Ill.: The Free Press, 1949, p. 6.

This volume seeks to point the next stage of institutional development toward utilizing social system perspectives in the entire residential milieu. Staff and residents at all levels within institutions are experimenting with new scenarios created by their own hand. The readings in this book point to the urgency of this need and offer guidelines toward its fulfillment.

Section I

SOCIAL SYSTEM THEORY

INTRODUCTION

THE contemporary social science model of conceptualizing behavior as incorporated within social systems offers intriguing possibilities for intervention by the practitioner. The simple notion that a change in one part reverberates throughout the whole system offers new possibilities for discriminating the strategic components which will be most influential in treating individuals. By changing the entire system of forces impinging on actors within the system, practitioners may experiment with hitherto unforeseen possibilities for rehabilitation.

All of contemporary social theory is obviously not amenable to practical application by sociotherapists. An important consideration in selection of the articles which comprise this section is the usefulness of the concepts they discuss for situations in which residents and institutional personnel find themselves today.

In undertaking to link up this critical field of treatment with the modern behavioral science of social-system analysis, we shall treat institutional dynamics as an aspect of the general theory of social action. This section clarifies and spells out the theoretical dimensions of the social system perspective and its applications to various aspects of residential structures and processes.

In the first article, Fallding carefully probes the basic assumptions of structural-functional theory. The theory holds that individuals act the way they do because of the way they are related: human action eventuates in outcomes or functions, which Fallding defines as the product "secured through the bridges and bonds" established among the members of any social system. Social system analysis concerns itself with these products of a system and the extent to which it is functional for its members and the group as a whole.

Inevitably, members within and without a system evaluate the degree of function or disfunction of the system through implied comparisons with alternative possible outcomes. Fallding suggests several major criteria for evaluating social systems as functional, which he equates with normality and pathology.

[9]

We have no choice except to take as normal, healthy or functional those arrangements which exhibit both stability and adaptive change in the combination demanded by the time and place, and as abnormal, pathological or disfunctional in some degree those which do not (and it is of course a matter of degree.)

To the criteria of stability and adaptive change he adds a third important internal social imperative of every social system—integration. The various activities within a social system have to be "so *deployed* that they do not interfere with one another." These three formal criteria for social system functioning—stability, adaptive change, and integration—do not exempt the investigator from spelling out the manifest and latent functions of the social system that men create. Ultimately we can say that social systems function because they produce products that are needed by man. Two of the most difficult tasks in functional analysis are those of specifying the human needs that a given social system meets and evaluating its degree of success.

In "Small-Scale System Analysis: Three Models for Social Work," Polsky analyzes therapist-client *transactions* in the perspectives of social system, culture and personality. A comparison of theorists representing these three approaches reveals contrasting assumptions about man and his social relationships. The psychoanalyst stresses the transformation of intra-psychic disturbance into interpersonal struggles; the cultural anthropologist views conflict as an emergent of value differences; the sociologist conceptualizes disfunctioning as resulting primarily from role strains and intergroup competition for material and symbolic resources.

Scott employs social system theory to analyze residential centers ranging from mental hospitals to prisons in society. From the point of view of society, the twin functions of custody and resocialization of the residents have resulted in internal contradictions within residential systems that reflect the power relationships among external organizations such as state legislatures, courts, professional associations and private philanthropic groups. Residential institutions, moreover, must recruit personnel in a competitive labor market, which leads to difficulties in financing and staffing. Furthermore, the attitudes and values of the people in the community are critical in influencing the reincorporation of former inmates into the societal system. Finally, Scott points to the anomalous role within institutions of attendants and guards, who are closest to the residents and are often given authority for custody and control, but have no direct responsibilities for therapy and resocialization. This results in anti-social or asocial accommodation patterns between attendants and residents; together they generate considerable resentment against the administration.

In his article on the organizational "character" of corrective institutions for juvenile offenders, Zald carefully traces the interrelationship of the external environment and the structured relationships of staff, and the effects of this upon client behavior. Zald points out that many of these institutions are "resource-deprived," because they must function in a critical external climate of opinion. They have not sufficiently concretized realistic rehabilitative goals, nor have they demonstrated the efficacy of one technique over another.

Stainbrook presents a more optimistic outlook of the significant impact that social science is having upon treatment within residential institutions. He traces the impact of the small group system upon the physiological and psychic functioning of patients in the hospital setting. He shows how communication can be improved in a hospital by better understanding of its organizational structure. The dispersion and concentration of power in the hospital is correlated with the degree of hostility generated among the staff, which in turn is related to the degree of commitment of the staff to the organizational tasks of the hospital. Clarification of the roles of both the patient and diverse staff members in the hospital can serve as an important aid to the patients' therapeutic outcome.

Most important of all is redefining the patient role so that he can become a more active participant in the helping process. This of course in turn has repercussions throughout the entire hospital social structure. Stainbrook states: "The organizational structure and dynamics of the hospital society are significant determinants of the expression and destiny of behavioral disease." The efficacy of the psychotherapy system is considerably enhanced by recognition of the needs and perceptions engendered in the patient *and* therapist by other parts of the hospital system.

In their theoretical paper "The Structure and Functions of Adult-Youth Systems," Polsky and Claster attempt to formulate a practical middle-range scheme for analyzing counselor-resident transaction. A model derived from Parsons' functional imperatives specifies the child-care worker in the cottage as fulfilling four key role-segments: custodian (adaptation), counselor (goal attainment), nurturer (pattern-maintenance and tension management), and judge-friend (integration). The authors maintain that contrasting distinctive styles of cottage life emerge according to the ways these functions are fulfilled by counselors.

L. J. Henderson's article has achieved the status of a classic over the past thirty years. He was the first writer to conceptualize physician and patient as a social system, pointing out the crucial fact that patients receive doctor's messages quite differently, depending upon their backgrounds and history of experiences. The way in which patient and physician interact is largely conditioned by the way in which each member selects, according to his own system of sentiments, from what the other is saying.

In a more recent analysis of the doctor-patient relationship, Szasz and Hollender see three modalities of interaction embedded in the doctor-patient relationship. Each is based upon technical and medical procedures, the social setting, and the attitudes of the participants. In the model of activity-passivity, the physician is active and the patient is passive. Extremely disturbed psychotic patients or severely physically disabled patients assume a very passive role vis-a-vis the doctor. In the model of guidance-cooperation, both parties contribute more actively to the on-going relationship. The patient is still subordinate, but more like a student receiving guidance from a teacher, while the doctor expects more active cooperation from the patient. In the model of mutual participation, the patient takes most care of himself and casts the doctor in a less over-powering position. At the same time, the physician helps the patient to help himself. The authors discuss the complementarities and conflicts in each of these paired systems of relationships. They conclude that ". . . each of the three types of therapeutic relationships is entirely appropriate under certain circumstances and each is inappropriate under others."

In an important critique of cases in which organizational theory has been applied to the study of mental hospitals, Etzioni uncovers several critical gaps and distortions. Such studies generally employ a "human relations" approach. Etzioni suggests a conflict-theory orientation to call attention to differences among staff in ideological stances, economic positions and commitment to organizational tasks. Most studies, he says, fail to specify the conflicting interests within the hospital system, and between the hospital and the community—a failure which results in illusions about therapeutic milieu engineering within the hospital. Viewing the hospital system as strata with conflicts of interest would alert investigators to the actual bargaining and compromises which go on within hospitals. Many hospital problems cannot be solved simply by improving communication, for they are the results of objective conditions, such as inadequate or scarce budgetary structures.

Another major distortion is that of conceptualizing the hospital system as a "society." This orientation obscures such important factors as trade unions and professional associations, communal ties, governing boards, political interests in the hospital, and other external structures which affect hospital processes. Furthermore, attempts to change staff roles within the hospital run up against professional and semi-professional associations' images of the roles their members are expected to play within the hospital. Etzioni criticizes the use of human relations techniques—democratization, permissiveness, group therapy, and community meetings—as forms of manipulation for maintaining controls over subordinate staff members and patients. Various forms of therapeutic milieu meetings that call upon "participation" by lower echelon staff members often are turned into manipulative techniques.

The therapeutic community is often an illusion, because the staff and patients revert to their formal statuses outside of the community meeting, and the formal structure is threatened by exposés that have taken place within the meeting. Etzioni calls for a more balanced orientation to hospital systems, employing both the "communication" human relations point of view and conflict theory.

219

CHAPTER 1   Functional Analysis in Sociology*

HAROLD FALLDING

LIKE other statements which have appeared in recent years,[1] the papers on functional analysis by Kingsley Davis[2] and Ronald Philip Dore[3] illustrate the amount of spadework that remains to be done here. While the contributions of Talcott Parsons[4] and Robert Merton[5] have been epoch-making, we have not yet the common code which Merton sought. Yet more than ever there is need for a code that would serve as scaffolding for diverse workers to build in unison. The scaffolding could always be dismembered mentally by anyone looking into basic questions,[6] but for anyone interpreting data it needs to stay provisionally fixed. The following is not the code called for but a rally to persevere in winning through to it.

The paper states in synoptic form only some of the set of assumptions which, if assembled, might orient sociologists more uniformly to their task. As it is the tradesman's last that is being fashioned, the writer does not follow into the assumptions behind the assumptions as the philosopher would—yet an exercise like this makes it easier to see what some of these postulates are. The writer is aware, moreover, that what he proposes as definite will still prove controversial. His main purpose is to represent functional analysis in sociology not as part of explanation but as a form of measurement which belongs to the natural history phase of the science. And an attempt is made to elicit some of the specific dimensions of measurement, of the kind Hempel[7] has asked for. As this proceeds, the way in which disorganization is implicated in dysfunction begins to appear plainer. The kinship connection of these two chief mourners has scarcely yet been traced.

1. Functional analysis involves evaluation. Sociology treats behavior in situations which pose a problem of regulation, rather than dealing solely with situations where regulation is achieved. But before we ever speak of

* Reprinted from the *American Sociological Review*, 28 (1963), 5–13, by permission of the author and the American Sociological Association.

social events, a system of regulated interpersonal contact either exists in some degree, or the participants are aware that one is called for and have adumbrated it—or, having lost what was won, have abrogated it. To designate the realized desideratum we can speak of "a group" or, alternatively, of "social arrangements," "social organization," "social structure," "social system." While if we speak of the function of a social system as a whole it is simply to specify what product is secured through the bridges and bonds thus established between man and man. It may be bread or bullion, music or medicine, sympathy or salvation. Then if we speak in addition of the function of any activity *contained within* a social system we refer to the effect it has in strengthening (or weakening) these productive bonds. For instance, conflict itself has been analyzed by Coser[8] as having positive functions in some social structures, and by this he simply aims to show that it can strengthen existing productive bonds by sealing their corrosions—e.g., when a hampering grievance is aired and removed and everyone is "able to get on with the job." Contained within a casket of existing bonds conflict may work like fire to purge them of imperfections; but, without these, it would presumably not even constitute a social phenomenon, much less a functional one.

The notion of function in connection with societies and their component groups has been variously employed, as Merton[9] showed. But the usage that has come to prevail takes as the function of an activity *within a system* the contribution it makes to the whole. We have therefore come to see the importance of specifying precisely both the part and the whole to which a functional statement refers. A practice which is functional within one social region need not be functional in one which is more (or less) inclusive. Other things also have to be specified if functional statements are to mean anything. As Nagel[10] stressed, we should say to what state of the whole the practice in question is contributory. But, more important than any of this, should we not bear in mind all the time what the product of the whole system is, since this itself may or may not be functional for those who bear the cost of the system and so expect to benefit? Very frequently in sociology it is whole, bounded action-systems that are being judged to be functional or dysfunctional *for man* and, only by transference, any parts within them which may make them so. And this is because social action is prompted by human need.

The examination of the properties of the "functional system" that has been undertaken by Nagel[11] seems to concentrate on the penultimate question of the sustained functioning of the system of action and does not ask whether, when functioning, it is functional for those who operate it. Nagel's formalization greatly facilitates our analysis of the internal process of change and compensatory counter-change by which a system achieves equilibrium. But this has to be linked to the more ultimate question of whether the system itself is functional or dysfunctional in yielding products matched to human need. In the writer's view, asking this ultimate question is what makes it worth while to ask the penultimate one.[12] Malinowski's[13] insistence on this is one of his enduring contributions to the discussion.

Furthermore, there is a teleological residue in functional thinking that is scarcely disposed of by Nagel's[14] demonstration that the explanatory element in functionalism is simply causal explanation put in a roundabout way. Where a need-satisfaction stands at the end of a process of human endeavour it exercises some directive power over the efforts taken to achieve it. Here we have a case, then, of the kind of process for which Braithwaite[15] has striven to preserve recognition, wherein the anticipated future goal controls the present movement towards it, so that the end achieved is not the passive effect of a causal chain but, to some extent at least, the cause of its own causes. Braithwaite[16] points out that the field of study explored by cybernetics is largely concerned with teleological mechanisms like this. Such processes, once launched, may achieve the end in view—or may fail and so be "in vain." Does not the anticipation of an end to be achieved underlie all our judgments of function or dysfunction, when those judgments are made in such a way as to imply a comparison with the alternative possible outcome? In the writer's view, what we are interested in *when we make this comparison* is not explanation but evaluation.

2. *The evaluation involved in functional analysis is objective and needs no apology.* To ask the function of any social arrangement is to call for its justification—or alternatively for its condemnation. The positive and negative polarity inherent in the terms (eu)functional and dysfunctional should betray at once that evaluation is afoot. A great deal of unnecessary hedging in sociological work would be obviated if this could be frankly admitted. At the same time, sociological work could be more easily purged of covert, private evaluations, if it were allowed that evaluation of this objective kind is intrinsic in sociological analysis, and altogether honorable. Yet, in saying this, we have to distinguish the two meanings given to "subjective" when that state of mind is unfavorably contrasted with the "objective." It can mean biased *or* intuitive. When it has the former meaning subjectivity is to be deplored, because by it the person's perception is distorted. When it has the latter meaning it is simply to be regretted, since the person is not yet able to share his vision of what may well be the truth. The first kind of subjectivity has to be expunged from science altogether, but the second kind is the anlage of science and has to be protected and fostered till its testimony can be objectified. In saying that the evaluation in functional analysis is objective, freedom from subjectivity of the first kind is mainly what is being claimed of course. Yet this gives us grounds for believing that freedom from subjectivity of the second kind can also be achieved with time.

We imply objective evaluation of two kinds, in fact, whenever we give a function. Basically, we are making a judgment as to whether the expenditure that goes into the creation and maintenance of the arrangement is worthwhile; but we determine this worthwhileness by both a backward and a forward look, as it were. The backward look tries to sum up the efficiency of the arrangement in producing its effects. To the extent that it is inefficient, wasteful, it is dysfunctional in a way. The forward look examines whether the effects themselves are valuable in terms of some schedule of needs which we postulate for the life of man in society. Some instances will make this plainer.

We may say, as Gluckman[17] has done, that the function of rituals of rebellion in Africa is to channel off the resentment that the natives feel for their chiefs and so preserve stability in the existing authority arrangements—thereby ensuring the continuing supply of everything those arrangements guarantee. We would then be implying (i) that these ritual expressions of aggression are efficient means of dissipating resentment and (ii) that it is desirable to maintain an uninterrupted need-satisfaction, and hence social stability. We may say, with Davis,[18] that the function of social stratification is to "insure that the most important positions are conscientiously filled by the most qualified persons."[19] We would then be implying (i) that a grading of rewards is an efficient means of motivating suitable persons to accept greater responsibilities, while a division of labor into tasks of unequal importance is an efficient means of securing common needs, and (ii) that it is desirable to satisfy common needs continuously. We may say, with Merton,[20] that the function of the political boss in the U.S.A. is "to organize, centralize and maintain in good working condition 'the scattered fragments of power' which are at present dispersed."[21] We would then be implying (i) that buying political support from diversified groups by dispensing help to them is an efficient means of concentrating power and (ii) that all such groups need some access to power and that the power secured by them needs to be concentrated to some degree. Or finally we may say, with Parsons,[22] that two functions of institutionalizing a "collectivity-orientation" in the professional role of the scientist are (a) to protect the public from arbitrary interference by men whose special knowledge gives them an advantage and (b) to expose the ideas of any scientist to the critical scrutiny of his fellows. We would then be implying (i) that role-institutionalization is an efficient means of restraining individuals who, in an intellectual sense, handle dynamite, and (ii) that society needs their contribution to knowledge.

But it would save misunderstanding if it could be appreciated that evaluation made in ways like the above is sociological evaluation only. *So far as present society is concerned*, X is functional, Y dysfunctional— that is always the implicit stipulation. There may well be supernal heights or historical perspectives from which a socially functional arrangement can be judged bad and a dysfunctional one good—just as ill-health is sometimes recalled with gratitude because it brought spiritual blessing, or poverty because it put one in the way of great fortune at a later time— but that would not be incompatible with recognizing the arrangements as *socially* functional or dysfunctional.[23] Furthermore, this helps us to see that intellectual judgments about function and dysfunction contain no ethical imperative. We cannot pass from "The instruction of children is functional" to "Thou shalt instruct children." As sociologists we hold no whip. (Fortunately, though, our sociology is redeemed from the final futility by the fact that men exist who are not sociologists merely.)

3. *Evaluating social arrangements as functional or dysfunctional is equivalent to classifying them as normal or pathological. This is a necessary preliminary to the search for causal explanation.* A physiologist cannot arrive at the function of the liver by generalizing directly from a random collection of livers which contains some diseased specimens. He distinguishes between the diseased and healthy organs at the outset and, setting the diseased ones aside, generalizes from the healthy ones. Certainly, *by contrast,* he gains some understanding of healthy functioning from an examination of the diseased cases, but can only do so if he first sets them in opposition by classifying them apart. His account of the liver would be altogether confounded if it simply averaged the properties of the whole collection. Distinguishing normal from pathological cases is one of his first assignments, and precedes causal knowledge of the conditions of normal or pathological functioning. Social systems are more complex than livers, of course, but the two things are alike in this respect. The instance will therefore serve to show what confusion can invade an intellectual discipline if, being concerned with things that have system-properties, it fails to recognize that character in them and evaluate them accordingly. It should show, further, that evaluation, forced upon us in this way, is simply *scientific measurement.* It amounts to quantification of those dynamic properties, possession of which defines the class of things in question. To evaluate systems is to have appropriated the dimensions for measuring them. In what follows, the three major dimensions for the significant measurement of social systems are proposed, as well as some of the minor dimensions implied in them.

It may require a titanic effort to overcome the clinging prejudice that *any* view about social desiderata will be ideologically colored and therefore suspect, but the effort has to be made. Through the whole of modern sociology two principal objective social imperatives have been fulminating, forcing recognition for themselves. Adaptive change (which implies rationality) and stability have *both* had to be assumed necessary in the social arrangements men make. These are the two main components of efficiency which, it was said, we gauge by a kind of backward look. They are the states of the social system (Nagel's G's) without which it cannot be properly productive of anything. They are, as such, nobody's political ideology; and there is no sense in calling a sociologist conservative or radical because his work illustrates the necessity of the one or the other—and as likely as not it will illustrate the necessity of both. Man, an anxious creature who looks before and after, works for his satisfactions over time and has therefore to bind time, and social organization and culture take their origin from this and must develop a certain conservatism to be of service to him. Yet, even in its most colloquial usage, stability has never meant fixity. We must not suppose that stable social arrangements mean arrangements that are fixed forever. They are simply arrangements that materialize as expected for as long as they are wanted. In no sense, either, is stability an *opposite* of change, so it would be wrong to think that combining them necessarily meant striking some mean of moderation or gradualism. Commitment to stability still leaves men free to adapt to a world which changes, or of which their knowledge changes, by various means. But to be of service stable social arrangements must yield—have a certain plasticity.

We have no choice except to take as normal, healthy or functional those social arrangements which exhibit both stability and adaptive change in the combination demanded by the time and place, and as abnormal, pathological or dysfunctional in some degree those which do not (and it is of course a matter of degree). It is admittedly a delicate calculation to make and often still largely beyond us, so we make it in a rough, rule-of-thumb way (perhaps in a way which is subjective in the second of the above senses.) Yet we have no choice but to make it—and very early in our sorting of the data. To do this does not imply that the abnormal or pathological phenomenon is being pronounced "evil" in some ultimate sense. It simply means it is being classified sociologically, given a negative sociological valency so that it will not be confused with the positive counterpart which in other respects will deceptively resemble it. The well-organized family is thus not to be taken for the same sociological phenomenon as the disorganized one, the high morale department store for the same thing as the low morale store, the nation riddled with suicide and homicide for the same thing as the one where these are rare, the church or school which moves with the times for the same thing as the one made redundant through its archaisms. It is only after we have set such contrasting phenomena in classes apart that we can sample the cases in each class and arrive at causal laws about functional and dysfunctional systems. It would be a pity if the attention that has been given to functionalism were taken for an invitation to make functional analysis the end of sociological inquiry—for then it would be still-born. It is rather the end of sociology to explain—"explained" functions: to show what things have a constant association with various functional or dysfunctional operations.

4. The stabilization of rational arrangements is what we mean by social organization (social cohesion or solidarity being roughly synonymous.) The stability requirement presents an internal challenge, the rationality requirement an external challenge. The internal challenge to social organization is to motivate lasting support. Stability is only secured in social arrangements if everyone involved in them is "satisfied with them"—at the very least "prepared to put up with them." Everyone must have his reward or the guarantee of it. Thus the maintenance of stability is essentially a matter of the enlistment of motives. While every person's reward will not be the same, everyone will have the same expectation of a certain reward and hence share a positive regard for, or valuation of, the arrangements. We probably claim too much if we mean more than this when we say that value-consensus is the basis of social order. But where this is lacking in even a single individual there will be disorganization in some degree, however localized. His guarantee of reward is the individual's security, and conformity to the arrangements of the group is what he will give in return for the security gained. In this lies the group's power of control over him, and the insurance of its own organization at the same time. A consensus (of the kind specified) and security and control for individuals, are therefore further indices of social normality. We can also say that communication of a certain effectiveness will be necessary if everyone involved is to know what the arrangements are and if consensus is to be reached in upholding them. Stability implies all this.

But we can say more. Whether individuals are satisfied with their rewards depends largely on whether they think them fair in comparison with the rewards of others. Any social system at all is in danger of being convulsed if a supposed injustice is unearthed—although the convulsion does not necessarily occur. The victim may grin and bear it if he thinks rebellion will prove more costly of justice still. Or there may be sanctioned channels through which he will work for a change. But, on the other hand, he may harbor resentment and be uncooperative, or take the law into his own hands and fight for his rights. Whatever the eventuality, the basement beneath every social system is piled with inflammatory tinder. Justice is the thing that damps it, although it is essentially subjective justice. It is justice which is seen and felt to be sufficient ("fair enough") by those concerned. And what is accepted as sufficient today may appear in a different light tomorrow—even without the situation changing.

This is the craving in the elementary social nature of man which has to be appeased by the institutions man makes if it is not to devour them. Homans,[24] having explored this "subinstitutional" level of behavior, points out how men face a problem perennially of reconciling their institutions with it. The social processes of Park and Burgess[25] could be regarded as stages on the way to the reconciliation. As a condition of stability, then, "sufficing justice" must be added to the indices of social normality. Some

people's misgivings about functionalism stem from a suspicion that the
positive regard it pays to stability implies a condemnation of just revolt.
But this is a misreading of functionalism's case; and it is unfortunate if,
because of it, lovers of justice have failed to take functionalists for their
friends. Actually, functionalism implies that a *system is deficient* in respect
of stability, if anyone under it withdraws support through being denied
justice.

5. *The external challenge to social organization is to cope with "present
and foreseeable circumstances."* Change in their external situation may
force a group to "make rearrangements," but a change in their knowledge
of the same situation can have the same effect. (A changed view of the
justice of existing arrangements is but an instance of the latter.) The ultimate source of the external impulse to change, therefore, is new knowledge—or probably more correct still, novel experience. Washburne[26] has
proposed the overwhelming event as the source of all social change, and
thereby simplifies our thinking about it considerably. But there seems no
reason why an event should be overwhelming in its proportions in order
to force social change, so long as it is overwhelming in its novelty. Man's
intelligence and sensibility impose on him a growing burden of new
knowledge; to accommodate, he must change his ways continually. He
has no option but to be put at a loss through having one day's practice
made unequal to the next day's knowledge.

He does have some option, though, in his reaction to this. This state is
essentially the one of *anomie* where procedures and norms for dealing
with perceived realities are lacking. Individuals can be torpedoed by this
experience or seek recovery: a negative and positive reaction are both
possible. One instance of the negative reaction is the anomic suicide which
Durkheim[27] identified. Other instances, which do not require going out
of life altogether, are the various forms of pseudo-conformity commonly
styled "hypocrisy." Such are the "bohemian" and "philistine" stances described by Thomas and Znaniecki[28]—and are the "other-directedness" and
"tradition-directedness" of Riesman[29] identical with them? But the positive
reaction to *anomie*, whereby recovery is achieved, is one of reorganization.
And this is not infrequently (perhaps always) approached by a denoue-
ment of collective behavior and ideology. By collective behavior in some
form men make a primitive communication of sharing in a predicament,
and then, in resurgent ideology they re-affirm their responsibility to one
another *as men*. This tides them over the break-down in their actual role
obligations, and prepares them for a different definition of duties. The
resiliency or adaptability we look for in social systems when making functional analysis requires them to meet novelties by absorbing them in this
way, rather than be themselves shattered by shock. Once again, it shows
misunderstanding when critics of functionalism represent it as opposed
to change. It is not opposed to change in social systems but to their death

when they have still a work to do. If some novelty should leave men unable to cope completely, that would not be social change but social extinction. It is from knowing that human life is impossible without society and society impossible without adaptive change that the functionalist deprecates this bleak alternative. The writer wonders, though, whether attempts to defend the usefulness of functional analysis for the study of change have sufficiently exploited the fact that an adaptation requirement implies that readiness to change is itself one of the properties of the system which has to be maintained.[30]

As well as large-scale changes, changes have constantly to be made within the minutiae of life. Even in those safe places of society where norms are firmly established, the norms rarely fit the case exactly. So it is required that the actors themselves supply an informal, on-the-spot structure like an inner lining to the formal. Both for these minor adaptations and for major ones the recruits to any social system need to come equipped in advance to do both more and different things than the rules prescribe. Here is a critical instance of the past laying its hand on the present. For what re-asserts itself here is nurture, not biological nature. It is the *human* nature which is fashioned in the primary group which constitutes this re-generative capacity, and if any man has been denied this group he will be denied this nature and capacity also. If ideology is the theory of recovery, the imprint of primary group involvements is the empirical basis of the theory. In the primary group men will have experienced the unrestricted mutuality, the universal love, which acts like embryonic tissue for the secondary structures that can grow anew between them wherever their ways drift into chaos.[31]

6. *If a diversity of arrangements is made by the one set of individuals, it is required that the arrangements be integrated among themselves.* A third objective social imperative appears in modern sociology, whenever the system to be analyzed has more than one side to it. This is integration. Just as a discourse needs to be coherent and consistent to be convincing, a social system needs to be integrated to be productive. For just as a discourse draws separate facts together, a social system may be compounded of a number of sets of arrangements. Food production, say, as well as the maintenance of health and the taking of recreation, may all be undertaken by one set of people. These various activities must be so *deployed* that they do not interfere with one another. If they are all scheduled for one time, for instance, they will. If the product of one is an obstacle to the achievement of another, they will—as when some food which is harmful to health is produced and used. The compatibility of their ends has always ultimately to be faced by a group if they are not to leave themselves open to self-defeat. This forces them to settle on some hierarchy for their preferences, so that they will know which to further when the ends come into competition with one another. It will force them

further. They will have to settle whether any of their aims are to be pursued for their own sake and without limit (and perhaps these alone should be called their "values"). All questions of the compatibility of ends are really economic questions, in the most generic sense of that term. For these considerations are forced on us by scarcity—by how far the material will stretch. Included in "the material" in this case is that of which man himself is made. Being in a state of contradiction, for example, can be intellectually, emotionally or morally insupportable by man because of the way he is made—just as it is impossible for a cake to be both actual and eaten because of the nature of cakes.

While all co-ordinating efforts contribute to social integration, legislation and adjudication are two of its most deliberate expressions. But the sanctifying or sacralizing operations of religion probably provide the prototypical instance of it. This is the group's radical approach to integration, in that it is the object here not to deny any normal activity, but to deny autonomy of aim to every activity. All activities, and the society itself, are recalled to the service of an overmastering end, and thereby integrated among themselves.

7. *It is because the demand for need-satisfaction through them is unrelenting, that social arrangements much achieve stability, adaptive change and integration. For this reason, making judgments of function or dysfunction, normality or pathology, presupposes a whole catalogue of assumptions about human needs.* It was said that part of our judgment that an operation is functional rests on our assumption that the product of the operation is needed by man. This must be one of the main reasons why functional thinking seems unsatisfactory to many people—for who shall say what the things are that man *must have under all circumstances?* And who shall so disentangle the inherited need from its cultural modification as to evaluate the latter as a means of supplying the former? Yet, unsatisfactory though this admittedly seems, such assumptions must be made if sociological work is to have depth and significance. These assumptions make a back-drop of our own providing to all the empirical observations we make. But the back-drop is not itself non-empirical for all that. It has been woven from the cumulative experience of mankind, as we have each been able to absorb this. We accept as human needs all those satisfactions which men have striven to repeat at many different times and places and by many different means. We assume that men need food, for example, because, under so many varied circumstances, we know they have acted *as though* they needed it. It is not for any different reason that we assume they need shelter, mutual protection, status, skillfulness, explanations of natural phenomena and the consolations of religion. What any sociologist assumes here should hardly be that minimum range of needs to which all his colleagues will give ready assent, but that whole spectrum to which his own vision has admitted him. It is precisely here that the social sci-

entist is served by his explorations of the arts and humanities, as well as by the diversity of his experience and his range of sympathy and imagination. Perhaps it is by exceptional endowment here that the great sociologist is marked out. If he lends us his eyes for a time we may devise instruments which will compensate other men for their partial blindness.

NOTES TO CHAPTER 1

1. See Harry C. Bredemeier, "The Methodology of Functionalism," *American Sociological Review*, 20 (April, 1955), pp. 173-180; Bernard Barber, "Structural-Functional Analysis: Some Problems and Misunderstandings," *American Sociological Review*, 21 (April, 1956), pp. 129-135; Walter Buckley, "Structural-Functional Analysis in Modern Sociology," in Howard Becker and Alvin Boskoff (eds.), *Modern Sociological Theory in Continuity and Change*, New York: The Dryden Press, 1957, pp. 236-259; Francesca Cancian, "Functional Analysis of Change," *American Sociological Review*, 25 (December, 1960), pp. 818-827.
2. Kingsley Davis, "The Myth of Functional Analysis as a Special Method in Sociology and Anthropology," *American Sociological Review*, 24 (December, 1959), pp. 752-772.
3. Ronald Philip Dore, "Function and Cause," *American Sociological Review*, 26 (December, 1961), pp. 843-853.
4. See especially, Talcott Parsons, *The Social System*, Glencoe, Ill.: The Free Press, 1951; Talcott Parsons, R. F. Bales, and E. A. Shils, *Working Papers in the Theory of Action*, Glencoe, Ill.: The Free Press, 1953; Talcott Parsons and Neil J. Smelser, *Economy and Society*, Glencoe, Ill.: The Free Press, 1956; Talcott Parsons, "An Outline of the Social System," in Talcott Parsons, Edward Shils, Kaspar D. Naegele and Jesse R. Pitts (eds.), *Theories of Society: Foundations of Modern Sociological Theory*, Glencoe, Ill.: The Free Press, 1961, pp. 30-79.
5. See Robert K. Merton, *Social Theory and Social Structure*, Glencoe, Ill.: The Free Press, 1957; Robert K. Merton, "Social Problems and Sociological Theory," in Robert K. Merton and Robert A. Nisbet (eds.), *Contemporary Social Problems, An Introduction to the Sociology of Deviant Behavior and Social Disorganization*, New York: Harcourt, Brace and World, 1961.
6. An analysis at this basic level has been undertaken by a number of authors. See, e.g., S. F. Nadel, *The Foundations of Social Anthropology*, London: Cohen and West, 1953, pp. 368-408; Ernest Nagel, "A Formalization of Functionalism," *Logic Without Metaphysics*, Glencoe, Ill.: The Free Press, 1956, pp. 247-283; Dorothy Emmet, *Function, Purpose and Powers: Some Concepts in the Study of Individuals and Societies*, London: Macmillan, 1958; Carl G. Hempel, "The Logic of Functional Analysis," in Llewellyn Gross (ed.), *Symposium on Sociological Theory*, Evanston, Ill.: Row, Peterson and Co., 1959, pp. 271-307; Richard Bevan Braithwaite, *Scientific Explanation, a Study of the Function of Theory, Probability and Law in Science*, Cambridge: The University Press, 1959, pp. 319-341.

7. Hempel writes: "For the sake of objective testability of functionalist hypotheses, it is essential, therefore, that definitions of needs or functional prerequisites be supplemented by reasonably clear and objectively applicable criteria of what is to be considered a healthy state or a normal working order of the systems under consideration; and that the vague and sweeping notion of survival then be construed in the relativized sense of survival in a healthy state as specified." Carl G. Hempel, *op. cit.*, p. 294.

8. Lewis A. Coser, *The Functions of Social Conflict*, Glencoe, Ill.: The Free Press, 1956.

9. Robert K. Merton, "Manifest and Latent Functions," *Social Theory and Social Structure*, Glencoe, Ill.: The Free Press, 1957, pp. 19-84.

10. Ernest Nagel, *op. cit.*

11. *Ibid.*

12. Bredemeier suggests that functional analysis loses its point if it fails to hold in view at least the needs which are induced in the actors by the normative definitions of the dominant culture. Harry C. Bredemeier, *op. cit.*, p. 179. Cancian, on the other hand, passes over the idea that "functional" might mean "fulfilling a basic need" for no reason save that such a view is "inappropriate according to Nagel's concept of a functional system." Francesca Cancian, *op. cit.*, p. 820. Even so, one wonders whether it would be as inappropriate as Cancian says. For we would scarcely ask, as Cancian suggests, what keeps need constant but would make *need-satisfaction* our G, and ask whether or not this is maintained.

13. B. Malinowski, *A Scientific Theory of Culture, and Other Essays*, New York: Oxford University Press, 1960.

14. Ernest Nagel, "Teleological Explanation and Teleological Systems," in Herbert Feigl and May Brodbeck (eds.), *Readings in the Philosophy of Science*, New York: Appleton-Century-Crofts, Inc., 1953, pp. 537-558.

15. Richard Bevan Braithwaite, *op. cit.*, pp. 328-336.

16. *Ibid.*, p. 328.

17. Max Gluckman, *Rituals of Rebellion in South-East Africa*, Manchester: University of Manchester Press, 1954.

18. Kingsley Davis and Wilbert E. Moore, "Some Principles of Stratification," *American Sociological Review*, 10 (April, 1945), pp. 242-249; Kingsley Davis, *Human Society*, New York: Macmillan, 1959, pp. 364-389.

19. *Ibid.*, p. 367.

20. Robert K. Merton, *op. cit.*, pp. 70-82.

21. *Ibid.*, p. 72.

22. Talcott Parsons, *The Social System*, London: Tavistock, 1952, pp. 335-345.

23. Merton makes the same point as this when he stresses that judgments about social disorganization are not moralizing judgments but technical judgments about the working of social systems. Robert K. Merton, "Social Problems and Sociological Theory," in Robert K. Merton and Robert A. Nisbet (eds.), *Contemporary Social Problems, An Introduction to the Sociology of Deviant Behavior and Social Disorganization*, New York: Harcourt, Brace and World, 1961, pp. 719-723. Although he is referring to the notion of social disorganization, Merton attempts in this same essay to relate social disorganization to social dysfunction. He suggests that disorganization may be

viewed as the resultant of multiple dysfunctions. *Ibid.,* pp. 731-737. Martindale states that all the critics of the notion of social disorganization base their objection at least partly on the fact that valuations are inherent in it. See Don Martindale, "Social Disorganization: The Conflict of Normative and Empirical Approaches," in Howard Becker and Alvin Boskoff (eds.), *Modern Sociological Theory in Continuity and Change,* New York: The Dryden Press, 1957, pp. 340-367; E. M. Lemert, *Social Pathology,* New York: McGraw-Hill Book Co., 1951, pp. 3-26; C. Wright Mills, "The Professional Ideology of Social Pathologists," *American Journal of Sociology,* 49 (Sept., 1943), pp. 165-180; Louis Wirth, "Ideological Aspects of Social Disorganization," *American Sociological Review,* 5 (Aug., 1940), pp. 472-482. But could the critics see that the need for evaluations orginates from the data and not the evaluators the practice might seem less objectionable to them.

24. George Caspar Homans, *Social Behavior: Its Elementary Forms,* New York: Harcourt, Brace and World, 1961, pp. 378-398.

25. Robert E. Park and Ernest W. Burgess, *Introduction to the Science of Sociology,* Chicago: Univ. of Chicago Press, 1924.

26. Norman Foster Washburne, *Interpreting Social Change in America,* New York: Random House, 1954.

27. Emile Durkheim, *Suicide,* edited by George Simpson, Glencoe, Ill.: The Free Press, 1951.

28. William I. Thomas and Florian Znaniecki, *The Polish Peasant in Europe and America,* New York: Dover Publications, 1958.

29. David Riesman, in collaboration with Reuel Denney and Nathan Glazer, *The Lonely Crowd,* New Haven: Yale University Press, 1950.

30. Cancian, in replying to critics of functionalism, and to Dahrendorf and Hield especially, comes close to doing so when she states that examining a stable rate of change is one of the four possible ways in which change can be incorporated in functional analysis. See Francesca Cancian, *op. cit.,* pp. 823-826; Ralf Dahrendorf, "Out of Utopia," *American Journal of Sociology,* 64 (September, 1958), pp. 115-127; Wayne Hield, "The Study of Change in Social Science," *British Journal of Sociology,* 5 (March, 1954), pp. 1-10. But this hardly suffices. It is not a stable rate of change that the normal society must exhibit, but a stable capacity to change at variable rates according to the challenge of the times.

31. Students of disaster draw attention to the way in which primary group solidarity reasserts itself when secondary structures collapse, thus supplying evidence for Cooley's idea that the primary group is the nucleus from which all social organization grows. See Charles E. Fritz, "Disaster," in Robert K. Merton and Robert A. Nisbet, *op. cit.,* p. 689; Charles H. Cooley, *Social Organization,* New York: Scribner, 1909.

ξ❧

Chapter 2   Small-Scale System Analysis:
Three Models for Social Work*

HOWARD W. POLSKY

A MATURE profession abjures ad hoc explanations and grand theories of social problems and intervention. It toils rather at creating a crescive body of middle-range principles, techniques and concepts that is receptive to its experience and its guide.[1]

Social work is deeply committed to the practicality of social theory. It evaluates and uses the relevant formulated experience of all disciplines. More than any other social force, theory shapes the practitioner's intervention into the complex interplay of social and psychic realities. Theory is the means by which the profession understands itself, its clientele and the treatment process.

But what is social work to do when social theory itself is in crisis? The only recourse is continuous discussion about alternative theories. The various approaches between and within social science and psychiatry constitute an opportunity for creative upsets and reconstructions. In this spirit I have undertaken a review of contemporary theories of elementary behavior.

The impetus to a new look at primary social exchange has two sources: (1) studies of the small group as a social system are surgent in natural and experimental situations. (2) psychoanalysis not only revolutionized our concept of personality, but is significantly infiltrating small group theory as well, now by the psychiatrists themselves. The key fact of our time is this: *the client-worker's cultural and social field rather than the insular client is emerging in the foreground as the dual focus of diagnosis and intervention.*

The overall direction is quite clear. As long ago as 1927 Sir Arthur Eddington[2] highlighted the scientific reaction away from microscopic analy-

* Revised version of paper read at Field Supervisors' Conference, Columbia University School of Social Work, March 23, 1964.

sis. "Science," he noted, has shifted from the "entities reached by the customary analysis (atoms, electric potentials, etc.) to the qualities possessed by the system as a whole, which cannot be split up and located, a little bit here and a little bit there." He continued, "We often think that we have completed our study of one, when we know all about two, because 'two' is one and one. We forget that we still have to make a study of 'and.'" The study of "and" in social behavior is termed "transaction": reciprocal, reverberating processes of social exchange.[3]

My thesis is that current theory and research into social transaction can be captured by three models: culture exchange, social system and "transference." In general I have in mind the superordinate-subordinate "tutorial" relationship: child care worker-resident, teacher-student, social work-client, parent-child, supervisor-supervisee.

THE THREE MODELS OF SOCIAL TRANSACTION

THE CULTURE-EXCHANGE MODEL

THE culture exchange model can be pictured as follows:

CULTURE-EXCHANGE MODEL

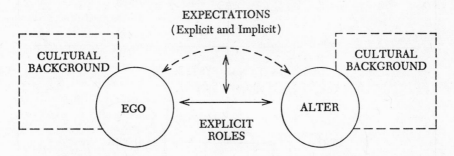

Ego and alter have explicit roles, e.g., social worker-client and each member has expectations about how he and his exchange partner *should* act. Should or ought—expectation—is the key term in all culture exchange paradigms. Social work is greatly influenced by the culture concept. We are fully aware that clients enter transaction with quite different sets.

Culture exchange derives from man conceived as a symbolic animal. He reacts to the exigencies of the social situation with an ensemble of beliefs, ideas, attitudes, outlook, in short, a culture. This *weltanschauung* interacts with alter's influence in the exchange: ". . . what persons *are* can only be understood in terms of a set of beliefs and sentiments which define what they *ought to* be."[4]

Florence Kluckhohn's value orientation paradigm points up in a systematic way the differences in outlook among people stemming from diverse cultures.[5] Orientations vary in emphasis toward time, nature, work, the nature of man, the supernatural, and relationship to the group. Other theories about culture exchange emphasize psychological motives and the exchange structure itself and will be reviewed below.

The social system model is fundamentally different from the culture exchange paradigm and derives from quite a different set of assumptions. Now instead of looking at differences generated by varying expectations in ego and alter, we place them together in a social system and examine independently problems of joint goal-attainment and group maintenance:[6]

THE SOCIAL SYSTEM MODEL

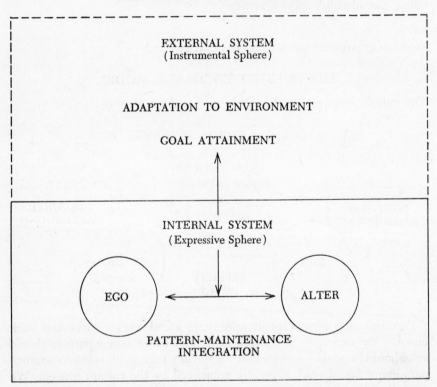

EXTERNAL SYSTEM
(Instrumental Sphere)

ADAPTATION TO ENVIRONMENT

GOAL ATTAINMENT

INTERNAL SYSTEM
(Expressive Sphere)

EGO   ALTER

PATTERN-MAINTENANCE
INTEGRATION

Ego and alter now confront each other as they confront together their environment. People in a relationship evolve not only common goals but adaptations[7] to the organizational framework in which they are functioning. Another set of problems arises in their internal relationship: maintenance of "loyalty" to the relationship and the integration of ego and alter.

The social system approach derives from the "functional imperatives" that flow from the nature of the system. Over many years of laboratory experiments, Bales observed in a variety of problem-solving groups, the emergence of two *system roles*.[8] The instrumental role consisted of taking initiative and leadership in formulating goals and coordinating tasks to solve the problem efficiently. The instrumental leader was frequently not the best-liked person in the group. Another individual, the expressive leader, excelled in giving support to members and mediating intra-group differences. This role was not directly important to the tasks (instrumental) sphere, but was crucial in building group morale. These two system roles, the instrumental and expressive, underlie social system theory. Their discovery indicates that stable group achievement and gratification in relationships depend largely upon how these specific functions are carried out.

In agencies this distinction is found between the executive and the "key man." The latter, often high up in the hierarchy, is accessible to rank and file, and serves as an important outlet for differences among the members in the organization. The social worker too performs functions that can be derived from client and worker conceptualized as a social system. I will sketch these functional roles below and indicate how they are shaped by the agency structure.

THE TRANSFERENCE MODEL

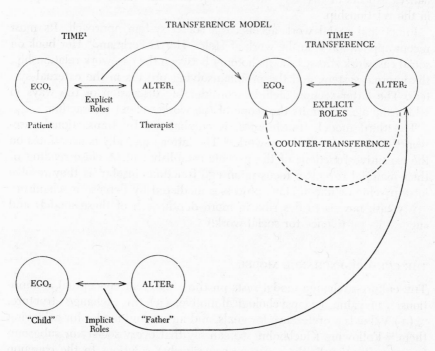

Whereas in the first two models we concentrate upon the exchange process as it is derived from culture and the social system, in the transference model we turn to the inner psychic world of the individual. We ask ourselves how patterns of behavior ingrained in the person's earlier life history become articulated with the social structure. How is psychopathology re-enforced by the group organization? Or, how does a pathological group system become internalized within the individual?

The key concept in this model is a slightly extended definition of transference: transferring to the superordinate person feelings, thoughts and implicit roles relating to parental or other significant figures of an earlier period of life.

A synthesis is required of work by psychiatrists familiar with field concepts. They include John Spiegel, Gregory Bateson, and Lyman Wynne. I will articulate their work below.

Social work, primarily casework, falls into these three models. A line of evolution can be traced from Mary Richmond and Gordon Hamilton to Lucille Austin and Florence Hollis,[9] all of whom emphasize the first model, culture exchange. They concentrate on the relationship. To be sure they discuss transference, the client's social environment and the agency framework in which the relationship evolves; but the main thrust of their work is built on culture exchange: How the client is influenced by the interactive process and his use of the relationship to the point where he internalizes aspects of the very methodology that the social worker employs in the relationship.

Functional social work accents the social system approach. Its most recent application is in the work of Helen Harris Perlman.[10] Her book on social casework stresses the dichotomy between the casework relationship, the internal system, and the problem-solving process in the external system. The latter section includes considerable discussion of the ways in which the agency limits the scope of the worker-client transaction.

The third model, transference, is emphasized by transactional casework[11] and ego-oriented casework.[12] The latter especially concentrates on the executive functions of the psychic establishment. A close reading of their material reveals a focus upon ego functions insofar as they resolve intra-psychic or unconscious processes mediated by defense mechanisms.

My task now is to describe in more depth each of these models and suggest its pertinence for social work.

THE CULTURE-EXCHANGE MODEL

THE culture-exchange model rests on three different conceptual assumptions: (1) value, (2) psychological-motive, (3) the exchange structure.

(1) Value is a preference for goals, and means and modes for achieving them.[13] Following Kluckhohn, we can say that every society or subgroup favors (often implicitly, not very consciously) solutions to the common human situation, for example a past, present or future time orientation. These orientations are the precipitates of an individual's experience within the cultural group in which he lives.

Leshan[14] has shown that individuals from different class backgrounds tend to emphasize past, present or future orientations. The upper class (traditional) person sees his life as continuous with several or more generations. He eats at traditional hours and enacts in general traditions set up in the past. Middle class individuals emphasize the future, create long tension-relief sequences and enact plans that terminate far in the future. Low income groups favor the present, quick sequences of tension and relief and regard the future as an indefinite, vague and diffuse region with highly uncertain rewards.

The cultural approach was of special importance during the large foreign immigration to this country. As the native born children of different ethnic stocks have become somewhat homogenized, the cultural perspective shifted to class differences. Anomie theory[15] contends that substantial numbers of the lower class have the same goals of the middle and upper classes, but because of their class disadvantage in achieving these goals, evolve disproportionately certain kinds of deviant modes of behavior.

By and large, social workers are sensitive to the differences in value orientations among their clientele and strive to suspend judgments about the superiority of their own class value system. The social worker realizes that he must become cognizant of the culture of his client so that his help will be appropriate to the cultural perspective which guides his client's behavior. This avoids unnecessary conflicts which may stem from misguided attempts to force the client to adopt the generally middle-class values of the social worker. The only systematic cultural-orientation scheme available to us is being developed by Florence Kluckhohn and John Spiegel.[16]

A second approach to culture-exchange rests on assumptions of universal psychological motivation. Zetterberg phrases a central sociological assumption about motivation as follows:[17]

A person tends to engage in actions that help him maintain the evaluations he receives from his associates at or above a given level considered favorable by him in the given situation.

Favorable evaluations are gained either by achieving goals highly esteemed by society or directly building relationships through winning friends and influencing people. This approach ties in with the central interest of sociologists in problems of social status and "impression-management." The pertinence to social work lies in the obvious observation that all clients do not have the same need to maintain favorable evaluations from their workers. Adopting the social worker and his agency as a positive or negative source of influence is an issue that lies at the heart of reference group theory.[17a]

Underlying George C. Homans' approach to culture exchange is the concept of man as a cost-plus accountant.[18] In social inter-action each party is making a contract not only between himself and Other, but within himself in assessing the cost and profits of maintaining the trans-action.

A brief example illustrates this process. An office worker, Person, does not want to go to his supervisor for help that he needs on his job so he approaches a colleague. Person needs help with his work which is the profit that he is seeking. The cost is the loss of prestige or pride in asking for help. Other also is functioning with a profit and cost calculus; his profit is gaining recognition and approval by Person approaching him for help. His loss is taking time from his own work to help Person. This inter-change process is complicated when Third Party enters the situation and competes with Person for Other's help.

The upshot is a concept of distributive justice, a consensus of what is fair, in the minds of all the participants. Each party has an idea of what is fair to ask for and what is fair for Other to give. This intriguing theory is built purely on utilitarian and rational assumptions that man essen-tially knows what he wants and goes after it. Transaction is a bargaining process not only between Person and Other, but within Person, and many intervening factors change or frustrate each party's expectations.

Postulations about universal psychological motives are always in danger of being culture-bound. It is implied that Person and Other are exchanging values *because* it is profitable and desirable to be ahead of the game, not because of the inherent joy in attaining worthwhile goals. The calcula-tion of exchange becomes the raison d'être for interaction. This is a small step to an assumption of social exchange as essentially manipulation of self and others.

Schelling[19] has developed a fascinating variation of Homans' economic orientation to social exchange. He sees the essence of exchange tactics in indeterminate situations as the adoption of a voluntary irreversible sacri-fice of freedom of choice. Overcoming an adversary depends upon the power of the individual to bind himself. Weakness becomes strength and freedom, paradoxically, capitulation. By burning bridges behind oneself, the opponent is undone.

A simple example illustrates this approach. If a buyer can pay no more than $16,000 for a home and the seller wants $19,000, he can convince the seller of his maximum price by making an irrevocable commitment that he can pay only $16,000 and unambiguously communicate this decision to the seller. Thus he can squeeze the range of indeterminacy down to a point that is favorable to him. For example, by making a bet with a third party that he can pay no more than $16,000 for the house, the buyer need only communicate this ultimatum to the seller and he has "lost." This theme, by the way, underlies the film *Dr. Strangelove*.

This variation of economic theory of psychological motivation is useful in social work. In therapy it is essentially to build up the bargaining strength of the patient so that he cannot employ his weakness as a club to threaten the therapist. In institutions the poorest risks are residents who have no bargaining strength at all. The boy who refuses to abide by institutional routines and does not respond to punishment or deprivation is daring the authority to "ship him." The boy with little ties to the institution has great power to make the institution do what he wants, namely, release him.

The only recourse the institution has, if it wants to keep him, is to relax its controls in a step-wise way so that the boy can gain strength by making ties to the institution with which it can barter to treat him. Patients with the least strength are the most trouble because they have so little to barter.

Obviously, increasing the strength of the residents adds to the problem of institutional control because their new found strength can become a potential threat against the institution.

A third approach to culture exchange concentrates on the exchange structure itself. Herbert C. Kelman[20] has isolated three structures of social influence: compliance, identification and internalization. He focuses upon the nature of the exchange structure in relationship to the meaning of the superordinate's influence upon the subordinate.

Compliance is acceptance of influence by the subordinate because he hopes to achieve a favorable reaction from the other person. He may be concerned with attaining specific rewards or in avoiding punishment that the superordinate controls. The critical factor is the authority which induces him to behave and evinces attitudes that the superordinate wants him to adopt.

Identification in contrast is acceptance of new behavior by the subordinate because the relationship is of a satisfying self-defining character. The subordinate's role in the relationship is an important part of his self-image and he accepts influence because he wants to maintain the relationship to the superordinate person. The subordinate adopts new behavior and attitudes not because he is compelled to but because of a genuine liking and comfortableness in wanting to be with the superordinate person and to be liked by him. This is close to identification in the classical psychoanalytic sense.

Internalization is influence acceptance by the subordinate because it is congruent with his own value system. It is intrinsically rewarding and he adopts it because he finds it useful for the solution of a problem, congenial to his orientation or demanded by his own value perspective. In internalization the subordinate perceives new attitudes and behavior as inherently conducive to the maximization of his own goals and values. The influencing agent plays an important role in internalization but the crucial dimension is the partner's credibility, i.e., his influence is regarded by the subordinate as intimately tied in with his own goals.

Kelman has carefully analyzed the antecedent, intervening and consequent characteristics of each structure of influence. Effective social work may very well go through these processes in stages; I believe that our field can profit from a careful consideration of Kelman's contribution.

THE SOCIAL SYSTEM MODEL

IN THE social system approach, the social context is critical. The social relationship is conceptualized in interaction with the larger system in which it is embedded. Perhaps this is seen more cogently in total institutions and other authoritarian settings that are severely circumscribed by time, space and function, but it is also true in other agencies.

The best way to gain insight into social system theory is to grasp the internal and external axis discussed above with the means-ends axis. The individual and the group are purposive organisms that formulate goals and experiment with methodologies for attaining them. This results in the following four-fold paradigm of social roles, functions and phases.

	MEANS (INSTRUMENTAL)	ENDS (CONSUMMATORY)
EXTERNAL	ADAPTATION	GOAL-ATTAINMENT
INTERNAL	PATTERN-MAINTENANCE AND TENSION MANAGEMENT	INTEGRATION

The above paradigm can be used for systems ranging from the doctor-patient relationship to society. At the societal level, the four sub-systems are the economic (adaptation): manufacture and distribution of goods; government (goal-attainment): internal and international policy-making; the family (pattern-maintenance): inculcating loyalty to our culture and mores; and, religion, mass media, law (integration): unite people internally.

In the social worker-client relationship conceptualized as a social system, four key functions can be derived that the worker assumes at various stages. I call these functions role-segments which relate to the system imperatives as follows:

System function	*Role-segment*
Adaptation	Custodian
Goal attainment	Counselor
Pattern-maintenance	Nurturer
Integration	Judge

The custodial role indicates that the worker and the client must adapt to the regulations of the agency. But the social worker and client are not merely adapting to the agency, for they are also formulating and attaining goals that emanate from the client but which are compatible with the worker's and the agency's value-system. Counselor is the role the worker assumes to help the "student" to formulate and attain goals.

Correspondingly, two role segments relate to the maintenance of the internal system. In the nurturer role the social worker directly supports the client when he is immobilized by anxiety or emotional disturbance. The integration function is fulfilled by assuming a judge-like, monitoring, or friend role (depending on the state of the internal system) in which the worker evaluates, mediates and enjoys the client's activity vis-a-vis himself, the agency and society.

I believe the analytical breakdown of these various functions enables us to make more effective use of the total functioning of different socializing agents in our society. The mother-infant transaction characterizes nurturance; the counselor role is institutionalized by the teacher in our society; the integration role is assumed by judge; and, the custodial function is performed in its purest form by the policeman or guard in institutions.

I am arguing, however, that in each of the above institutionalized roles, the superordinate plays at various stages in the relationship all four role-segments. The most important principle of social system theory is that the larger organization in which the transaction of social worker-client is being enacted determines how the four functions will be deployed and performed.

This can be illustrated by the changing role of the probation officer and welfare department investigator.[21] The agency determines the major function. The parole officer, for example, initially, was a punitive officer, custodian in our terms, who supervised the parolee by insuring his adaptation to society by not breaking any law. Next, he became a protective officer who balanced the community's need for protection with the client's protection from the community. He assumed more of a judge-like (or better, conciliator) role in which he balanced community need with his knowledge of the client and his life history. A third stage evolved when the parole officer took a more active role in rehabilitating the parolee (counseling) by helping him attain training, education and work, recreation, and general social adjustment to family and community. Finally, with the increased education and gradual adoption of social work ideology, the parole officer and welfare department worker increased attention to psychological and emotional factors influencing the client's behavior.[22]

My main point is that the social worker must utilize all four role-segments in the successful performance of parole officer in this authoritarian agency-setting. Not only does each of the role-segments contain inherent dilemmas but also the problem of appropriate assumption of each role-segment to the situation which the client and agency present the worker.

Most important of all, the agency is modifying the parole officer role. This change of role is not a one-way street which stems from the agency, but is actively influenced by the worker, social work schools, the profession and the community.

Here I will not take time to outline the interrelationships between the build-up of the internal system and the adaptation and attainment of goals in the external system. This dialectic has been discussed for the client-therapist by Talcott Parsons in *Working Papers in the Theory of Action.*[23]

This analysis of the helping and socializing role in diverse settings should enable us to improve the total functioning of the social worker role. Total institutions and repressive authoritarian agencies are undergoing transformations from custody to counselling and therapy. However, in this transformation, custodial functions remain and the dilemmas, contradictions and conflicts inherent within each role-segment and the allocation among them are critical issues which have to be worked out theoretically and practically in order to increase the social worker's potentiality for effectively helping the client.[24]

THE TRANSFERENCE MODEL

THE psychiatrist's Man is a multi-layered personality with intense inner conflict that has to be brought under control. Whereas in the sociological orientation, goal achievement and social acceptance occupy the center of the stage, for the psychiatrist the unconscious is the most important force in social interaction.

In recent years, psychiatry has turned attention to the reinforcement of psycho-pathology in the patient's social field. Their approach adds a fresh dimension to social exchange which will have to be integrated with social system theory. Here I will synthesize three approaches to the interrelationship of individual and social pathology based upon the transference model.

John Spiegel[25] conceptualizes human interaction as serving two major purposes: attainment of culturally valued goals, and maintenance of personal integrity. This is illustrated in a brief example. Joanne, a preadolescent girl, repeatedly made demands on her father for gifts. The original desire was gratification achieved through enjoyment of the gifts. Gradually the behavior fused with the defensive need to test whether she was being rejected or not. The original desire is gratification, the latter, a defense goal.

Although human interaction is organized primarily to pursue external goals, it often becomes enmeshed with mutual testing for love, approval and acceptance. When affectional needs are unmet, interaction eventuates in powerful implicit roles which dominate the interpersonal transactions. By "altercasting,"[25a] inducing the partner to take a role complementary to the individual's pathological distortions, ego and alter are caught up in an implicit role structure. In the case above, the father at first gratified Joanne's demands inconsistently by bestowing and withholding gifts. The daughter defined withholding as confirmation of her fear of rejection and pestered her father by increasing her demands.

Eventually, the father defined the daughter's motivation as coercive and assigned to her the role of pest and selected for himself the victim role. This relationship was stabilized with the aid of this implicit role structure, but also covered up underlying unmet defensive needs of love and acceptance.

In another article[26] Spiegel suggests how the implicit (or "character") role relationship (described in the example of Joanne and her father) is transferred to later relationships. A bright 23 year old Ph.D. in mathematics undertakes psychotherapy. The first sessions proceed with the girl in the patient role seeking help and the doctor in his appropriate role. In the fourth session, the girl launches into a brilliant analysis of a play she had seen the evening before. After twenty minutes or so, the doctor interrupts to enquire why she is telling him all this. She covers up by calling herself an "idle gossiper."

In the ensuing moments the doctor penetrated the evolving implicit role structure by pointing out to the girl that she was assuming a critic role and casting him into an admiring appreciator in a role relationship similar to the way she always gained the attention of her detached professor-father. The girl reacted with shame and the doctor quickly gave her support. The transference model can now be rediagrammed more accurately for the client as follows:

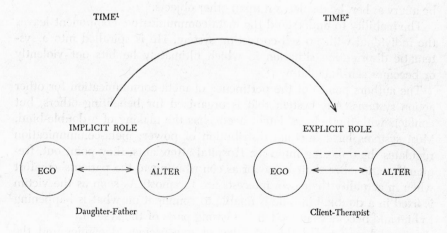

TIME¹   TIME²

IMPLICIT ROLE   EXPLICIT ROLE

EGO ⟷ ALTER   EGO ⟷ ALTER

Daughter-Father   Client-Therapist

Spiegel is non-pareil in specifying the induction techniques by which ego casts alter into complementary implicit role positions that re-enforce defenses. Every social worker should be fully familiar with these inter-personal strategies and techniques.[27]

The thrust of Spiegel's contribution lies in a subtle analysis of the intermeshing of intra-psychic conflicts and their conversion into implicit roles which intermesh with the explicit role-system. Transference and counter-transference lurk in every exchange relationship and in every transference we search now for structural re-enforcement in the social exchange structure, in the subtle inter-play of explicit and implicit roles.[28]

Whereas Spiegel has specified the structuring of unconscious forces in their interaction with the explicit role-structure, Bateson and his collab-orators[29] have developed important insights into the operation of un-conscious forces in communication.

Every message is not only an explicit statement but also a meta-communication, an emotional message about the communication. If I say to someone, "close the door" my tone conveys my feeling about alter. I can say "close the door!" in such a peremptoral way that I am implicitly at-tacking alter as if to append, "you idiot!" In pathological groups, the victim is caught in a double bind in the interplay of manifest and latent communication.

An example. A psychotic boy approaches his anxious and insecure mother visiting him in the hospital. He puts his arm around her and she stiffens. He senses rejection and withdraws, whereupon the mother says, "But why are you withdrawing from me, dear?" The boy is in a bind. If he approaches he senses rejection, if he withdraws, he is accused of rejecting her. He cannot approach, withdraw, or make a comment about his action: "Mother, when I approach you, I have the feeling that you do not want me to." His mother can comment on his withdrawal. Since he is unable to be angry at her, he displaces it upon other objects.

The inability to understand the meta-communicative component leaves the individual with no self-correcting system. He is spiralled into a sys-tematic disorienting situation in which ultimately he hits out violently or becomes self-immolating.

The authors point out the pertinence of meta-communication for other action systems. Any system that is organized for benefiting others, but conflicts with the helpers' latent needs, has the making of a double-bind. Most systems have unequal distribution of power; meta-communication regulates the opposing interests. Hospital attendants, they point out, fre-quently rationalize their behavior as contributing to the patients' comfort when in actuality their own interests are foremost. As soon as the victim is fixed in a double-bind, he is unable to comment on what is happening to him and becomes enraged at the wrong parts of the system.

Spiegel has detailed the interplay of unconscious dynamics and the group role-structure; Bateson has delineated how this operates in communication interchange; Wynne and his collaborators have turned attention to the theory of personal identity and group organization.[30]

The relationship can be posed as a dilemma: how can the individual be a *whole* person and yet a *part* of a larger whole like a family or peer group? The answer lies in the individual maintaining the line between himself and the group, yet relinquishing appropriately his sovereignty for the group. The dilemma is a false dilemma. Angyal[30] uses the inelegant term, "intermediate whole," as a working philosophical concept by which the individual can accept the responsibility for himself and relinquish his sovereignty to be part of a group.

The theorists of pseudo-mutuality[31] have picked up this theme and employ it as a central organizing concept. Genuine mutuality tolerates divergence of self interests, indeed, thrives upon the recognition of inevitable individual differences. Pseudo-mutuality is a miscarried solution for the deviant group members being only a *sense* of relationship which ultimately becomes the raison d'être of its members. In pseudo-mutuality real divergence is a threat to the whole group and avoided at all costs. However, when divergence is suppressed or avoided, growth of the relationship and individual identities are severely aborted.

Small groups with high pseudo-mutuality exhibit the following characteristics: (1) an unvarying role structure despite external and internal change; (2) a group norm that insists on the desirability of the role-structure; (3) intense concern over divergence from the group; (4) absence of spontaneity. The undefined group boundaries become a "rubber fence" which engulfs each member and prevents autonomous differentiation. Members conceal important experiences and feelings from each other which threaten group solidarity. Outside persons are often inducted as pseudo-intermediaries into a very plausible group togetherness.

The pseudo-mutual organization has a special impact upon its most inadequate member. He is pervaded with the distorted group modes of perception and communication. His responses become tenuous and unreliable and markedly inconsistent in understanding what to expect of himself or others. A flood of anxiety accompanies every individualizing movement away from the group. The rubber fence of the family becomes an internalized rubber fence and results in what Erikson calls "identity diffusion."[32]

The key to pseudo-mutuality is a member striving for a sense of relationship and the compulsive need to fit into the group. These engulfing roles are matched by a culture of myths and legends which accentuate the dire consequences of divergence from the group. This pseudo-mutual role-structure is assimilated into the personality structure of group members, particularly the least adequate individual.

The above orientation focuses upon the interplay of individual identity and group relational needs. Mere focus upon the social system without delving into the meaning of the individual's role for his personality structure, blurs the quality of the subjective experiences of real people. Man's struggle for identity and his needs for relationship become a critical axis for understanding social transaction.

CONCLUSION

TELL me your assumptions and I will tell you your lies. The strategy of social exchange theory demands simplification. The limited conclusions always require future research; nevertheless, the bolder investigators leap across the boundaries and challenge self-evident concepts about social behavior, postulate connections, construct models and build theory.

Each of the above approaches is favored by the academician and practitioner. The sociologist's man is rational, competitive, achievement-minded, status-seeking, goal-formulating and in general a shrewd bargainer. The psychotherapists are impressed with man's weaknesses, his irrationality, insecurity, and his elaborate defense maneuvers to maintain integrity; the over-riding importance of emotional support and solidarity to the point where elaborate pseudo-mutual structures are created.

Whereas sociology is impressed with the ability of man to communicate ideas and the binding force of consensual norms, the psychotherapists are impressed with the diverse strategies of disguise unconsciously elaborated by individuals in interaction with each other. The psychoanalyst stresses the transformation of intra-psychic conflict into interpersonal struggles; the sociologist emphasizes the reverse: intra-group struggles eventuate in intra-psychic conflict.

Theory and practice are conditioned by the institutional context in which sociologists and therapists function. Educational institutions are examination centers with a high value placed upon competition and achievement. In psychotherapy a high premium is placed upon cooperation and uninhibited talk, and the elicitation of subtle and intense anxieties. In academia, stress is placed on symbolic skills, goal-formulation, and methodologies for achieving them. In therapy, high values are placed on empathy, listening with the third ear, relatedness.

The decisive difference among the three models is the relative focus upon individual, social system and culture. The sociologist and anthropologist are environmentalists who look primarily at hostility and aggression in society and culture. The psychiatrist is more concerned with the internalized touchiness of the individual group member.

From this mountain, it looks like the sociologist's social system will have to confront the psychiatrist's Man. If this is so, social system theory will be radically modified to show how the rich inner fantasy (creative and pathological), life of individuals interlocks with the social roles men adopt by virtue of being members of society and imbibers of a culture.[33]

NOTES TO CHAPTER 2

1. The clearest expression of this viewpoint in sociology can be found in Robert K. Merton, in "Introduction" and Part I. "Sociological Theory," *Social Theory and Social Structure*, The Free Press of Glencoe, New York, 1962, pp. 3-102.
2. Sir Arthur Eddington, *The Nature of the Physical World*. Ann Arbor Paperback, The University of Michigan, 1958, pp. 103-104.
3. See for example, John Dewey and Arthur F. Bentley, "Knowing and the Known," Beacon Press, Boston, 1949; Paul W. Kurz, "Human Nature, Homeostasis and Value," *Philosophical and Phenomenological Res.*, XVII, No. 1, Sept., 36-55; John P. Spiegel, "A Model for Relationships Among Systems" in Roy R. Grinker, ed., *Toward a Unified Theory of Behavior*, Basic Books, N.Y. 1956, pp. 16-26.
4. Talcott Parsons, Chapter 1, "The Superego and the Theory of Social Systems," in *Working Papers in the Theory of Action*. Talcott Parsons and Robert F. Bales and Edward A. Shils. The Free Press of Glencoe, Ill., 1953, p. 18.
5. Florence R. Kluckhohn, "Dominant and Variant Value Orientations," in Clyde Kluckhohn, Henry A. Murray and David M. Schneider, eds. *Personality in Nature, Society and Culture*, Alfred A. Knopf, Inc., New York, 1953, pp. 342-57. See also Florence R. Kluckhohn and Fred L. Strodtbeck, John M. Roberts, *Variations in Value Orientations*, Row, Peterson, Evanston, Ill., 1961.
6. This paradigm is adapted from Talcott Parsons, "General Theory in Sociology," *Sociology Today*, eds., Robert K. Merton, Leonard Broom, and Leonard S. Cottrell, Jr., Basic Books, New York, 1959. p. 7.
7. Restrictions on the superordinate can be as severe as upon the subordinate in the social system. In an otherwise positive report about New York City's Bronx High School of Science, an exchange teacher from England reported: "It was after I returned to New York from an Easter vacation spent with friends who teach at colleges that I suddenly realized how much of a depression I had been suffering . . . was due to one thing. I had been beginning to see myself in the way New York's educational administrators apparently want their teachers to see themselves: overburdened by officialdom, left little or no say in the planning of curricula and examinations, and even barely trustworthy enough to do an honest day's work without constant checks and supervisions." (*The New York Times*) "The News of the Week in Review," Sunday, April 5, 1964, p. E 7, Col. 6.
8. Robert F. Bales, "The Equilibrium Problem in Small Groups" in *Working Papers in the Theory of Action*, Talcott Parsons, Robert F. Bales and Edward A. Shils, The Free Press, Glencoe, Ill., 1953, pp. 112-161. Robert F.

Bales, "Task Status and Likeability as a Function of Talking and Listening in Decision-Making Groups" in L. D. Whyte, ed., *The State of the Social Science*, Chicago, 1956, pp. 148-161.

9. In her latest book, Florence Hollis emphasizes in direct treatment reflective discussion of: the nature of the current situation; dynamics of client's response patterns; and, genetic development of response patterns. Florence Hollis, *Case Work, a Psycho-social Therapy*, Random House, New York, 1964, p. 78.

10. Helen Harris Perlman, *Social Casework, a Problem-solving Process*, The University of Chicago Press, Chicago, 1957.

11. Roy R. Grinker and others, *Psychiatric Social Work: A Transactional Case Book*, Basic Books, New York, 1961.

12. Howard J. Parad and Roger R. Miller, eds., *Ego-Oriented Casework, Family Service Association of America*, New York, 1963.

13. Talcott Parsons and Edward A. Shils, *Toward a General Theory of Action*, Cambridge, Harvard University Press, 1959.

14. L. Leshan, "Time Orientation and Social Class," *Journal of Abnormal and Social Psychology*, Vol. 47, No. 3, July 1952, pp. 589-592.

15. Robert K. Merton, "Social Structure and Anomie," and "Continuities in the Theory of Social Structure and Anomie" in *Social Perspectives on Behavior*, eds. Herman D. Stein and Richard A. Cloward, The Free Press of Glencoe, Inc., New York, pp. 517-559.

16. Florence R. Kluckhohn and John P. Spiegel, "Integration and Conflict of Family Behavior," Report #27, Topeka, Kansas: Group for the Advancement of Psychiatry, 1954.

17. Hans L. Zetterberg, *Social Theory and Social Practice*, The Bedminister Press, New York, 1962, p. 86.

17A. Ch. VIII, "Contributions to the Theory of Reference Group Behavior" and Ch. IX, "Continuities in the Theory of Reference Groups and Social Structure," in *Social Theory and Social Structure*, Robert K. Merton, The Free Press of Glencoe, 1963.

18. George C. Homans, *Social Behavior, Its Elementary Forms*, Harcourt Brace and World, Inc., New York, 1961.

19. Thomas C. Schelling, "An Essay on Bargaining," *The American Economic Review*, Vol. XLVI, June 1956.

20. Herbert C. Kelman, "Processes of Opinion Change," *Public Opinion Quarterly*, Spring 1961.

21. Here I draw on two fine studies: Lloyd E. Ohlin, Herman Pevin and Donnell M. Pappenfort, "Major Dilemmas of the Social Worker in Probation and Parole," in *Social Perspectives on Behavior*, eds., Herman D. Stein and Richard A. Cloward, The Free Press of Glencoe, Inc. New York, pp. 251-260; Edwin Thomas, Donna L. McLeod, Pauline Bushey, Lydia F. Hylton, *In-Service Training and Reduced Workloads*, Russell Sage Foundation, New York, 1960.

22. I discovered that the nursery school movement underwent a somewhat similar development: "Once it was a custodial center, then a pre-kindergarten school for habit-training, then a guidance center for children and their parents . . . now it is my feeling that one function of the nursery

school should be to take greater initiative in recognizing when and where emotional conflict is interfering with the normal process of growth." Sylvia Brody, "Theory and Research in Child Development. Implications for Nursery School Teachers." Paper read at Conference of Early Childhood Education Council, April 26, 1958, pp. 12-13.

23. Talcott Parsons, *Working Papers in the Theory of Action*, The Free Press of Glencoe, Ill., 1953, pp. 232-245.

24. Howard W. Polsky, Daniel S. Claster and Robert A. Falcier, "The Child Care Worker's Role in Residential Treatment," mimeographed.

25. John P. Spiegel, "The Resolution of Role-Conflict within the Family" in *The Family*, Norman W. Bell and Ezra F. Vogel, The Free Press of Glencoe, Ill., 1960, pp. 361-381.

25A. "Altercasting is Defined as projecting an identity, to be assumed by Other(s) with whom one is in interaction, which is congruent with one's own goals." Eugene A. Weinstein and Paul Deutsch Berger, "Some Dimensions of Altercasting," *Sociometry*, Vol. 26, No. 4, Dec., 1963, pp. 454-467.

26. John P. Spiegel, "The Social Roles of Doctor and Patient in Psychoanalysis and Psychotherapy" in *Personality and Social Systems*, eds. Neil K. Smelser and William T. Smelser, John Wiley & Sons, Inc., New York, 1963, pp. 600-607.

27. ————, op. cit.

28. Many illustrations of this viewpoint can be found in *The American College*, edited by Nevitt Sanford, Wiley, N.Y., 1962.

29. Gregory Bateson, Don D. Jackson, J. Haley and John Weakland, "Toward a Theory of Schizophrenia" in *Personality and Social Systems*, eds. Neil K. Smelser and William T. Smelser, John Wiley & Sons, Inc., New York, 1963, pp. 172-187.

30. Andras Angyal, "A Theoretical Model for Personality Studies" in *Theoretical Models and Personality Theory*, eds., David Krech and George S. Klein, Duke University Press, Durham, 1952.

31. Lyman C. Wynne, Irving M. Ryckoff, Juliana Day, and Stanley I. Hirsch, "Pseudo-mutuality in the Family Relations of Schizophrenics," in *The Family*, Norman W. Bell and Ezra F. Vogel, The Free Press of Glencoe, Ill., 1960, pp. 572-594.

32. Erik Erikson, "The Problem of Ego Identity," *Journal of The American Psychoanalytic Association*, IV, 1956, pp. 56-121.

33. A modest attempt at utilizing the transference model as described above can be found in Howard W. Polsky, Irving Karp and Irwin Berman, "The Triple Bind: Toward a Unified Theory of Individual and Social Deviancy," *Journal of Human Relations*, Vol. 11, No. 1. In this volume Section III, Chapter 21.

CHAPTER 3   Action Theory and Research
in Social Organization[*]

FRANCES GILLESPIE SCOTT[1]

THE general theory of action as put forth in the writings of Talcott
Parsons and his associates[2] and in two recent articles by Parsons[3] provides a theoretical framework for research on social organization which
offers an alternative to *ad hoc* studies. Of theoretical and methodological
importance is its conception of the organization as a social system in its
own right, related in stated ways to other social systems, all operating
within the society, which in its turn is seen as the most inclusive system.

An organization is defined as "a social system which is organized for
the attainment of a particular type of goal; the attainment of that goal is at
the same time the performance of a type of function on behalf of a more
inclusive system, the society."[4] The society, acting on the basis of its
values, evaluates, ranks, and rewards an organization according to the
latter's contribution to the society's functioning. The result is the differential distribution of power to organizations performing different functions.[5]
Continued access to and exercise of power is, to be sure, directly related
to the organization's ability to operate successfully, that is, to its continuing performance of socially valued functions. It would follow that, if
the functions are highly valued and so the prestige of the organization is
high, the requisite power will be allocated sooner or later, and, if the
functions are obsolete, unnecessary, or ill performed, the organization will
either acquire new ones or cease to exist. An analysis of the allocation of
power and its exercise is crucial to an analysis of the structure and function of the organization.[6]

Organizational types.   On the most general level organizations may be
classified according to the *primacy* of the type of function as assessed by

[*] Reprinted from the *American Journal of Sociology*, 64 (1959), 386–395, by permission of The University of Chicago Press. Copyright © 1958, 1959 by The University of Chicago. All rights reserved.

[44]

the society. It is with reference to the function in the *society* as a system that we now view organizations. Parsons' conception of the four basic problems of any action system is of central interest.[7] An "action system" is composed of a number of units (which are, observably, role behaviors in a *social* system); this action system is confronted with a series of basic problems which must be solved if it is to continue operating as a system. These are: (1) *adaptive problems*, the adapting of behavior to the physical and social environment of the system and the manipulation of objects, including persons, so as to make for more favorable relations; (2) *gratificatory problems*, activity connected with the attainment and enjoyment of the goals of the system; (3) *integrative problems*, activity directed to the "adjustment" of the relations of system members to each other; and (4) *pattern-maintenance problems*, activity directed toward the maintenance of the identity of the system as a system, renewal and reaffirmation of its own values and existence.

In a social system some of the members have primarily adaptive roles, some primarily integrative, and so on. The system is conceived as directing attention, by virtue of the interaction of its members among themselves or with members of other systems, to first one and then another problem. Normally, the direction of activity or movement is from the solution of pattern-maintenance problems to either the solution of adaptive or integrative problems and thence to the solution of goal-attainment problems. A "phase" of a social system is considered as the interval of time when one of the four is being given primacy.[8]

This paradigm is, first of all, applied to the society as a social system to determine the predominant system problem of the society at any given time toward the solution of which a given organization is functioning and thus the type of goal of the organization. An indication of the power allocated to it is given by the type of function, or goal, and by its relationships to other organizations. The paradigm is also applied to the organization itself as a social system with problems of its own system maintenance. Indeed, the paradigm is applicable not only on these two levels of analysis but further in investigating smaller divisions of the organization, such as departments, as social systems in their own right, thus establishing for each role the primacy of the problem of the organizational system toward which behavior in the role is directed.[9]

In relationships between a system and its component subsystems, the subsystems perform functions that are primarily, but not exclusively, directed to one or another of the system problems. For example, the economy as a subsystem of society functions to produce goods valued by the society; these goods may be used to solve the adaptive system problem of the larger society by "adding value" to the society's ability to control and manipulate its environment. The functions of any subsystem may contribute to the solution of more than one system problem, just as any given action of a role incumbent within the subsystem may contribute to the solution of more than one problem for the subsystem. However, the relative primacy of the function for solution of one of the four system problems of the larger system is the basis for classification of the organization.

Methodological usefulness of organizational types. While it may be extremely enlightening to contrast the internal structure of organizations which perform different and perhaps differentially evaluated functions for the society, and hence belong to different primary types on the most general level, it is methodologically important to compare the structure of organizations which function with respect to the same problems of the society, in order to derive generalizations valid for this type. When such preliminary work has been accomplished, comparisons of organizations belonging to different primary types would provide generalizations valid for all organizations, as well as statements of special variables which affect the organizational structure and the interaction processes in organizations performing different and differently valued functions. If this work were undertaken systematically with the theory of action as the explicit theoretical frame of reference, prediction in terms of action theory would then be possible.

The empirical work on bureaucracy, industrial organizations, and the social organization of various specialized institutions such as mental hospitals yields hypotheses which can be stated in systematic terms and which future studies can utilize and attempt to test. We shall examine investigations of mental hospitals and penal institutions, classified as integrative organizations which operate to solve integrative problems for the society.

Similar theoretical formulations and research hypotheses can eventually be constructed for organizations having different functions, for example, churches and schools as pattern-maintenance organizations, business and manufacturing organizations as functioning to solve adaptive problems, and some governmental agencies and fiduciary firms as oriented to goal-attainment. Systematic relationships thus established can lead to valid generalizations about social organizations.

RELATIONS OF INTEGRATIVE ORGANIZATIONS TO SOCIETY

ALTHOUGH there are other organizations which perform integrative functions, mental hospitals and penal institutions have been chosen for two principal reasons. First, there apparently has been no systematic linking of studies of these organizations, although the fruitfulness of such a comparison has been suggested by several writers. This may be due to a division of labor whereby social psychologists study mental hospitals and criminologists study penal institutions in an attempt to solve practical problems which have been considered entirely different. Second, as yet there have been few published structural studies of either of these, especially of prisons.[10] Their philosophies of administration and their public expectations are undergoing considerable change at present; hence they offer opportunities for experimental studies in the processes of organizational change and accompanying structural transformations.

In the activity of these organizations directed to solution of society's integrative problem, the emphasis is upon identifying and determining the relationships between and among the units in such a way that the system is enabled to maintain itself. A distinction is made between members and nonmembers on the basis of their particular relationship to the system, and the release of emotionally toned activity toward them is permitted. However, the system's interest in the individual member is not in terms of his specific performances in a given role but in his diffuse quality as system member. He must demonstrate that he shares the same values, that he has the same expectations, that he "likes the same things," as the other members, or at least that he is trying to come to this state of affairs. The integrative organization functions to see to it that members of society *do* in fact manifest the same values and expectations within allowable limits and, if they do not, to win them over or to expel them. Classified with mental hospitals and prisons as integrative are organizations concerned with "the adjustment of conflicts and the direction of motivation to the fulfillment of institutionalized expectations."[11] Interest groups, the courts, the legal profession, and jails, parole agencies, reformatories, and general hospitals also belong in this category. The last are included because the ill person is considered as temporarily relieved of his social responsibilities but is expected to help cure himself as soon as possible so he may return to the full status of societal member.[12]

Both the criminal and the madman are viewed as non-system-members in all respects. The madman is committed to a mental hospital and the criminal is sentenced to prison without their consent and against their will.

The goals of integrative organizations. The primary goal of these organizations is protection of society from former members who have been designated as feared and dangerous by the courts. In varying degrees punishment is also an aim. However, a relatively new course of action has been gaining acceptance, that is, "treatment" or resocialization. It was extended first to madmen, who were redefined as mentally ill; eventually, it was applied to the criminal, who in many circles is also considered either as mentally ill or as socially maladjusted and in need of treatment rather than punishment. There has been a shift from the protective closing of ranks as a technique of integration to the re-forming, in a literal sense, of the offending member and then readmitting him to the system. The re-forming has become a new goal of these organizations.

Relations to other organizations in society. The complications which arise from the often co-existing goals of protecting society by safe custody and of resocialization are reflected in the relationships of the organizations to others as diverse as state legislatures, newspapers, courts, research agencies, professional associations, and private philanthropic and "social action" interest groups. Frequently, appropriations of public money or the operation of the mental hospital or prison are foci of contention with these outside groups.[13] These power relationships between and among organizations affect the attainment of goals and can and do result in their redefinition.

Power is allocated by society to organizations in a proportion roughly correlative to the importance of their functions. The one considered most important in American society today is the solution of the adaptive problem (e.g., economic production, technical competence), although this may be in the process of change.[14] Probably next is pattern maintenance (e.g., science, education), on the one hand, and the maintaining of personal motivation on the other (e.g., family, personal health). Integrative problems come third. This consideration, when combined with the fact that state mental hospitals and penal institutions are thought of as non-profit organizations and yet must recruit personnel in a competitive labor market, leads to difficulties in financing and staffing.

That budgeting for both organizations is usually done by state legislatures[15] distinguishes organizations such as prisons and mental hospitals from the privately financed or general hospital. Public schools, highway construction and maintenance, military and defense activities, of course, compete with integrative organizations for tax appropriations, possibly at the expense of mental hospitals and prisons. Such deprivation of financial resources has apparently led, in part, to the production by inmates (prisoners or patients) of goods and services necessary to their own maintenance, so that the "output" of the organization is used as human resources for the upkeep of the organization. The system necessity for this particular kind of work has important implications for internal structure.

Several considerations enter into the problem of personnel recruitment: the existence of a free labor market, the inability to pay a fair wage, and the generally low prestige of workers who perform personal services, unless they are professionals. The professional personnel—physicians, nurses, psychiatrists, psychologists, sociologists—create further problems of recruitment; such persons have professional standards and ethics which are often violated in the day-to-day operation of large-scale mental hospitals and prisons. They often have professional standards of success which have little or nothing to do with their formal position in the organization but are related to the outside. However, many mental hospitals and prisons have been able to provide intern or in-service training. Thus a relatively constant stream of medical interns, junior psychiatrists and psychologists, student psychiatric social workers and nurses, and prospective parole and probation officers pours in and out; few of them remain.

Furthermore, mental hospitals have historically been administered by medical doctors, on the commonly held assumption that physical and mental diseases are closely related; penal institutions have been administered by untrained political appointees, on the assumption that little professional skill is necessary to keep men safely confined. Neither organization has had trained administrators; the experience neither of a doctor nor of a politician necessarily equips one to attain the two goals of the organizations simultaneously; yet, if these organizations do not enjoy a traditional method of recruitment which guarantees effective personnel, it is because society has not granted the requisite power.

State mental hospitals and prisons usually have little to say about the assignment of inmates, which further distinguishes them from other organizations performing similar integrative functions. For example, private hospitals may require that patients be cared for by specified physicians and so on; "interest groups" have varying conditions of membership; private psychiatric hospitals almost always select patients on financial and sometimes symptomatic grounds. In private general or psychiatric hospitals as contrasted with state mental hospitals or prisons, we should expect to find different points of strain which would to a large degree stem from their very different relationships to the larger society and other organizations with respect to financing and admittance of patients.

Problems created by the value system of society. The value system of society must be taken into account when considering exchange across the boundaries of the organizational system with other units of society, for example, the occupations as exemplified by specific employers; here the social worker in the mental hospital and the guidance or welfare officer in the prison (who may also be a social worker) play crucial roles.

One job of the social worker is to see to it that the society, or at least the local community, accepts the "cured" inmate as a system member. This usually means that the prospective "readmitted" member must accept society's values in making his own living and in his behavior in general. Society is reluctant to take back those it has defined as non-members, especially since diffuse, affectively toned actions have been taken against them. On the individual level we might profitably analyze this reluctance as guilt or fear; in the social system it involves receiving a member who is thought likely to disrupt the system. This consideration, combined with the inability of experts to effect reliable cure or resocialization in any given case, makes the problem of exchange across the boundaries of the organizations as systems unlike the problems of exchange, for example, of pattern-maintenance organizations, like universities, which also "produce" socialized and trained human beings. The larger social system does not *want* the products of the mental hospital or the prison. But the social worker, or to some extent, the administrator is expected to find a market for these products. Here the social worker is faced with revising the value system of society, a difficult and sometimes impossible task. When it can be accomplished locally, the problems of exchange are solved;[16] otherwise, frustration results both for the organization and for the social worker, whose loyalty to the organization may be jeopardized.[17]

Certain aspects of the operation of prisons, and to some extent of mental hospitals, have traditionally put strains upon the loyalty of employees, in addition to those strains brought about by low-prestige, low-salaried employment. Few are motivated by personal or professional ethics to remain in positions simply to help other people when better-paying positions carrying higher prestige are available. Added to this is the frequent requirement that employees live in the institution or be on call at all hours or the further restrictions on personal life which conflict with society's conception of a contract of employment as based principally upon technical or productive efficiency and not upon one's way of life.

That change is taking place in the value system of the society with respect to integrative organizations is evident from public concern with "cure," therapy, rehabilitation, resocialization, or whatever name is given to the process by which outcaste members are expected to be transformed into responsible persons who can be reincorporated into the societal system. It is this very concern which presents dilemmas and misunderstandings within the internal system of the mental hospital and the prison, for the staff of these organizations are also members of the larger society.

STRUCTURAL PROBLEMS IN INTEGRATIVE ORGANIZATIONS

THE operative code of an organization, its mechanisms of achieving its goal, is a problem of internal structure; it is this area which has been the focus of most empirical studies. Strains arise not only from power relations with other subsystems, from conflicts and changes in social values, but also from the structure of the organization itself. We shall examine some of these strains, especially as they become manifest through the role of the attendant in the mental hospital and the guard in the prison and of the professional "treatment" officers of both organizations, always assuming that both organizations explicitly hold to the equally valued goals of custody and of resocialization and that the relative emphasis given either goal varies considerably from one concrete organization to the next.

Mechanisms of goal attainment may be seen in the structure of authority through which processes having to do with policy decisions, allocative decisions, and integration of the organization take place. If the only goal of the prison, for example, were custody and/or punishment, a rigidly hierarchical structure, resembling as closely as possible the prototype of the military organization, would be ideal. In fact, prisons have traditionally been organized along much these lines. In such an organization the inmate population is to be "kept in its place," quiet and confined. There is little need for communication from guards to warden, for decisions are made by the warden and transmitted downward. The prison is run "by the book," and rules for the behavior of inmates, as well as guards, theoretically are universally applied and swiftly enforced. There is likely some division of labor, for example, a recognition of the "business" part of the prison, the "medical," and the "custody" divisions. Policy and allocative decisions, however, place the emphasis upon the custodial division and assign it primacy not only with respect to facilities and personnel but with respect to implementation of its goal—secure confinement.[18] The structure of mental hospitals has been of this nature, with separation of the custodial from the medical-psychiatric functions and emphasis upon the goals of the former, owing to whatever exigencies of operation. Although the goal of the mental hospital has from the beginning been resocialization or cure to a greater extent than has that of the prison, in actual fact the two organizations have traditionally achieved virtually the same goal, namely, custody.

Goal implementation and the "inmate subsystem." We have outlined above the conception of an action system, the maintenance of which requires the solution of the four system problems of adaptation, goal-attainment, integration, and pattern-maintenance. Our postulate is that solution of the integrative problem of the organizational system of the mental hospital or prison and the structural problems connected with it require primacy in order that the goal of resocialization be carried out successfully.

Here we must consider not only the subsystems within the organization, such as the "professional subsystem" composed of physicians, psychiatric "experts," social workers, and nurses, and the "attendant subsystems" in the mental hospital, and their organizational parallels in prisons, but the very important fact that goal implementation for the organization is predicated upon the existence of an "inmate subsystem," with which the whole of the organizational staff must come to terms.[19] This inmate subsystem is both raw material and product to the staff. However, resocialization requires it to be intimately associated with the staff subsystems, to adopt their values and goals, and to help with their goal implementation. Hence the staff system must, as a functional prerequisite to goal attainment, integrate the inmate system into its own system. This is a more formal way of stating what has been attempted in organizations where "twenty-four-hour therapy," the "therapeutic community," and "total push" emphasis has been introduced. It is, on the organizational level, what is implied by Sutherland's "differential association" theory.[20]

The traditional conception of therapy is individualistic: the doctor and patient form a microscopic social system wherein the rules of the game of the outside world are suspended. This is a one-to-one relationship; it is time-consuming, requires highly skilled professional services, and in the present shortage of professional personnel is obviously unattainable in state mental hospitals and penal institutions. In the latter, indeed, it is doubtful whether such therapy can ever be completely successful because of the workings of the inmate system. However, systematic theoretical consideration provides us with a key; resocialization can be realized by "integrative therapy." By this, we do not mean group therapy as practiced by one psychiatrist and a group of patients but a common effort by the entire staff of the mental hospital or prison to integrate individuals and groups belonging to the inmate system into its own social system; only when this has been done can the resocialization goal be accomplished. This requires a reorientation of the values of the employees, and especially of non-professional staff, so that they accept, as system members, persons stigmatized by social expulsion. And it requires supreme integrative efforts within the organization to keep the system together in the face of these unusual requirements. The very structure of both mental hospitals and prisons has resulted in the most strenuous requirements being placed upon those persons least likely to be able to accept and deal with them from the standpoint either of training or of professional ethics, namely, the attendant and the guard. Upon them, too, fall custodial and housekeeping duties; they are responsible for preventing escapes, for preventing inmates from injuring each other, and for seeing that the wards are clean.

The consequences of incomplete integrative processes, both on the level of the integration of inmate with guard subsystems and of the integration of guard with professional subsystems, can hinder goal attainment. In a prison which recently became treatment-oriented, the professional staff mistrusts the ability of the guards to accept the deviations of prisoners (i.e., to accept them as members of the guard's own system) and hence withholds information which would be important to the guard in dealing with the inmate, except from some guards who are considered more responsible. There is incomplete integration of the professional subsystem with the guard subsystem, as well as lack of integration of the guard subsystem with the inmate subsystem. The result has been a testing and challenging of the skill, authority, and knowledge of the professionals by the guards, which sometimes is observed by inmates, before whom the professional cannot easily defend himself, with ensuing defeat and degradation of the professional. The extent to which fear of the inmates, either as a group or as individuals, prevents integration of the attendant-guard system and the inmate system is indeterminate; the discussion of fear of inmates is taboo, at least in prisons. This is an aspect of the integrative process which warrants further research.

Interesting parallels may be seen in the use made of the inmate system in the mental hospital and in the prison. For example, both systems give rise to a classification of inmates which is not in accordance with the professional classification but is custodial. In mental hospitals patients are classified by attendants as "privileged patients, limited privilege patients, and patients without privileges." In prisons, the guards classify prisoners as "minimum, medium, or maximum security risks." Every new patient or prisoner must undergo classification; his actions for the first few days or weeks of his confinement play a large part in establishing his category, and assignment ultimately affects his chances for treatment, for work and recreation—indeed, for his entire experience there. The classification is essentially the basis of a status hierarchy, made mandatory by the demands placed upon the attendant-guard for custody and for housekeeping. The attendant must rely upon some of the patients not only to keep the wards clean and tidy but to control other patients; the guard in a parallel manner must rely upon some of the prisoners. The effect of the structure of informal authority is to emphasize custody or housekeeping at the expense of resocialization. Even more subversive results arise: patients in actual fact are put in the position of controlling the chances of other patients for treatment and privileges. There are indications that prisoners control the accumulation of "good time" by other prisoners through the ability to "frame," "mess up," or "bring heat to" a fellow prisoner, leading to punishment, solitary confinement, and loss of parole chances. The privileged inmates are those most useful to the attendant-guard system and, to some extent, those most nearly integrated with it. But, instead of this leading to prompt readmission into society when the inmate is cured, it may lead to the inmate's being kept on to do custodial work and housekeeping, especially in mental hospitals.

The integrative situation in prisons is different in at least one important respect: the relative strength, hostility, and rationality of the inmate subsystem. Each new prisoner not only must be subjected to classification by the guards but also must come to terms with the inmate subsystem and be assigned a status there. The values of the "prisoner's code" are inimical to those of the guard; hence the problem of integration becomes even more difficult of solution and crucial to resocialization. McCorkle suggests that the chief value in the inmate system is the possession and exercise of coercive power, a condition which disorganizes the system, where, indeed, many controls are not internal but are supplied by the external coercion of the guard's system.[21] However, this shaky inmate system is not further undermined and exploited for resocialization purposes because the guards need it to keep order in the prison. Moreover, the custodial officer is likely to look upon the psychiatrist or other treatment officer as obstructing discipline, while the latter regards the former as obstructing treatment. This is, in fact, precisely what is occurring, because of the lack of system integration of the two arms of the organization's staff.

We can now see why a change from custodial to "therapeutic" structure may result in prison riots. If the administration permits the allocative and integrative decisions necessary to implementing resocialization, this means a change in the established relationship between the guard's system and the inmate system and a breakdown of the inmate system as an effective means of coercing inmates and guards. The old relationship in which the guard had to grant privileges to powerful inmates in order to perform his own custodial and housekeeping duties gives way to a situation where the need for and preferred response to treatment determines the relationship between guard and prisoner and between guard and professional as well. Resocialization is given equal or preferential value with custody, and a concomitant breakdown of the old basis of guard-inmate interaction results.[22]

The result of the interrelationships between the attendant-guard subsystem and the inmate subsystem, and of the relative paucity of professional personnel and the prestige and authority differentials between them and the attendant-guard subsystem, is a blocking and/or distortion of communication precisely at the point crucial to goal attainment. The attendant-guard is given authority for custody but not at all or only indirectly for resocialization. Yet he is expected to promote resocialization, although he neither knows how nor has he been assigned clear-cut authority to do so. Nevertheless, attendants feel that they know what is good for the patient and what his capacities with respect to resocialization are; guards feel that they know what the prisoner is "really" like and what steps must be taken to control him—because they are, in fact, the persons nearest him for the longest periods of time and because they are, in fact, in the position to implement or ignore directives.

In actual practice the professional who most highly values resocialization and is most capable of implementing it is separated from the inmate not only by the attendant-guard system but also by his administrative functions, such as supervision of personnel, record-keeping, and so on. What little time he has left for direct therapeutic work is likely to be confined to the few inmates who are already in a favorable position vis-à-vis the attendant-guard system; and these are not necessarily the inmates who can benefit most from therapy or who need it most in the light of the goals of the organization. This problem is particularly crucial in mental hospitals, where "back-ward" patients tend to accumulate over the years. In prisons, under the present system of sentencing for a minimum number of years, successful cure often could not hasten release. Whether the inmate subsystem can, under these conditions, ever contribute positively to resocialization is problematic. Certainly, it would have to be closely integrated with the attendant-guard system, and the attendant-guard system, in turn, would have to be closely integrated with the professional system.

The structure of an organization which gives primacy to integrative problems, under conditions where integration involves the dual problems of integration of an uninterested or hostile subsystem and of system members themselves, must of necessity be decentralized with respect to allocative decisions, insofar as is possible within the limits of its total resources and facilities. In the mental hospital the attendant must be able to requisition whatever supplies he needs on the ward without bureaucratic delays and inconveniences; he must be able to ask for and receive additional personnel during critical periods when such personnel might very well enable members of the attendant system to interact more frequently and intimately with the members of the inmate system and hence prevent overt outbreaks.[23] It is the attendant who is most likely to be able to anticipate the day-to-day needs, both physical and emotional, of the ward.

But this does not mean that decentralized decision-making must necessarily lead to unclearness and confusion of the lines of authority. The decision to assign allocative decisions to the attendant is itself a policy decision and can be made only when both the attendant-guard and the professional subsystems are agreeable to relinquishing some of their former authority. Such agreement is closely linked with decisions related to integration of the organization; if allocative decisions are to be decentralized to facilitate goal implementation, the professional and the attendant-guard subsystems must be in agreement, and the attendant-guard must be so integrated into the professional system as to be motivated toward implementing the resocialization of the inmate. It is known that attendants and guards have a conception of mental illness and of crime different from that of the professional staff. Furthermore, it does not seem possible to set forth specific "rules of treatment." The professional must work through the attendant-guard subsystem to reach the inmate system which is the object of resocialization; apparently, the only way is through a conscious decision to concentrate upon integration of the attendant system with the professional system on one level, and, through it, integration of the inmate system with the attendant system, as the means of goal attainment.

Structural restrictions unfavorable to goal implementation. It is suggested that indeterminate sentences, the length of which would be determined by professionals such as psychiatrists, psychiatric social workers, or sociologists, based upon the inmates' progress toward resocialization or incorporation of conventional social values, would overcome some of the hindrances to therapy of fixed sentences. On the one hand, this involves the relationship of the prison as an organization to the courts; we would have here the commutation of legitimately imposed sentences by an unauthorized organization; profound changes must take place in values to legitimize such procedure. An important practical obstacle, at the moment, is the inability of social scientists to measure such variables as degree of resocialization or of incorporation of values. On the other hand, even with indeterminate sentences, the "prisoner's code" will not permit

special privilege based on treatment criteria, for it is extremely difficult, as
we have seen, to state just what are the rules for treatment because of
their individualistic nature. Release would be considered by other inmates
as special privilege, with resulting disturbances and further alienation
from the guard subsystem. Theoretically, effective integration could overcome these disturbances; empirically, since such procedures have never
been tried, the result is problematic.

NOTES TO CHAPTER 3

1. Expansion of a paper read to the American Sociological Society, Seattle,
   August, 1958.
2. Talcott Parsons, *The Social System* (Glencoe: Free Press, 1951); Talcott
   Parsons and Edward A. Shils (eds.), *Toward a General Theory of Action*
   (Cambridge, Mass.: Harvard University Press, 1952); Talcott Parsons, Rob-
   ert F. Bales, and Edward A. Shils, *Working Papers in the Theory of Action*
   (Glencoe: Free Press, 1953).
3. Talcott Parsons, "Suggestions for a Sociological Approach to the Theory of
   Organizations—I and II," *Administrative Science Quarterly*, I (June and
   September, 1956), 63-85 and 255-39.
4. *Ibid.*, p. 238.
5. See Talcott Parsons, "A Revised Analytic Approach to the Theory of Social
   Stratification," in Reinhard Bendix and S. M. Lipset (eds.), *Class, Status
   and Power* (Glencoe: Free Press, 1953), pp. 92-128.
6. For a more detailed discussion see *ibid.;* also Parsons *et al., Working
   Papers,* esp. chap. v.
7. See Parsons *et al., Working Papers,* esp. pp. 179-90.
8. *Ibid.*, chaps. iii and v.
9. The application of the paradigm on different levels of analysis is suggested
   by Parsons, "A Revised Analytic Approach to the Theory of Social Stratification," *op. cit.*, esp. pp. 108-11.
10. A notable exception is Donald Clemmer, *The Prison Community* (Boston:
    Christopher Publishing House, 1940). Several studies by other American
    social scientists are nearing completion.
11. Parsons, "Suggestions for a Sociological Approach to the Theory of Organi-
    zation," *op. cit.*, p. 229.
12. Parsons, *The Social System,* chap. x, "The Case of Modern Medical Prac-
    tice," esp. pp. 439-47.
13. See Lloyd E. Ohlin, "Interest Group Conflict and Correctional Change,"
    unpublished paper read before the Social Science Research Council Confer-
    ference Group on Research in Social Organization of Correctional Agencies,
    April, 1957.
14. Parsons, "A Revised Analytic Approach to the Theory of Social Stratifica-
    tion," *op. cit.*, p. 106.
15. See Ivan Belknap, *Human Problems of a State Mental Hospital* (New York:
    McGraw-Hill Book Co., 1956), pp. 31-36; M. Greenblatt, R. H. York, and
    E. L. Brown, *From Custodial to Therapeutic Patient Care in Mental Hospi-*

tals (New York: Russell Sage Foundation, 1955), pp. 38-39; Clemmer, *op. cit.*, p. 274.

16. See Maxwell Jones, *The Therapeutic Community* (New York: Basic Books, 1953).
17. L. E. Ohlin, Herman Piven, and D. M. Pappenfort, "Major Dilemmas of the Social Worker in Probation and Parole," *National Probation and Parole Association Journal*, II (July, 1956), 211-25.
18. For a discussion of the difficulties this causes for the professional subsystem see Harvey Powelson and Reinhard Bendix, "Psychiatry in Prison," *Psychiatry*, XIV (February, 1951), 73-86.
19. For a discussion of the "inmate system" in prisons see Lloyd W. McCorkle and Richard Korn, "Resocialization within Walls," *Annals of the American Academy of Political and Social Science*, CCXCIII (May, 1954), 88-98; McCleery, *op. cit.*
20. Donald R. Cressey, "Changing Criminals: The Application of the Theory of Differential Association," *American Journal of Sociology*, LXI (September, 1955), 116-20.
21. McCorkle and Korn, *op. cit.*, p. 90.
22. See Greenblatt *et al., op. cit.*, chap. xv, pp. 295-321.
23. That such additional personnel can be effective in preventing ward disturbances and that attendants can sense when such disturbances are about to erupt is shown by A. H. Stanton and M. S. Schwartz, *The Mental Hospital* (New York: Basic Books, 1954), pp. 394-400.

꒰ꔛ

CHAPTER 4   The Correctional Institution for Juvenile Offenders: An Analysis of Organizational "Character"*

MAYER N. ZALD

INTRODUCTION

DURING the last decade the sociological study of large organizations has emphasized the limitations of Weber's ideal-type of bureaucracy as a model of organizational behavior. Moving away from a focus on bureaucracy and its pathologies, organizational research has begun to examine the variety of factors that affect and limit different types of organizations. The purpose of this paper is to describe the juvenile correctional institution as one type of large-scale social organization.[1]

First of all, institutions for delinquents share with other organizations, such as hospitals, certain attributes usually associated with communities. Secondly, they belong to a class of large-scale social organizations that have multiple goals, and thus have functional problems like these organizations. Thirdly, correctional institutions are of interest because of their critical role in our society's attempt to minimize anti-social behavior.

In this paper the major patterns of similarity and dissimilarity between correctional institutions and other types of organizations will be delineated and explained. Further, some of the dimensions along which correctional institutions vary among themselves will be indicated. A "charac-

* This paper was written as part of an on-going project supported by research grant M-2104, from the National Institute of Mental Health, Public Health Service. Morris Janowitz and Robert Vinter, directors of the project at the University of Michigan, have greatly aided the author by their critical comments on earlier drafts of the paper. The conceptual framework of the project is included here. The general hypotheses which the project attempts to test are stated in a previous publication by Vinter and Janowitz (35).

Reprinted from *Social Problems*, 8 (1960), 57–67, by permission of the author and the Society for the Study of Social Problems.

ter analysis" of these organizations, as systems of action, may make it possible (a) to summarize and integrate a scattered body of knowledge; (b) to specify areas where research is needed; and (c) to set forth some concepts and dimensions that may be useful in such research.

The concept of organizational "character," most fully developed by Philip Selznick (30), stresses interdependencies, commitments, fixed limitations and capacities of different types of organizations. Using the concept of organizational "character" the present analysis aims at a middle range level of theoretical abstraction.[2]

To describe the "character" of correctional institutions we will discuss their goals, their relationships to the larger community, and, finally, their internal structures.[3]

THE GOALS OF CORRECTIONAL INSTITUTIONS

LIKE universities, mental hospitals and some other large-scale social organizations, correctional institutions can be said to have multiple goals. Their prime functions are to incarcerate—that is, establish custody over—the offender *and* to rehabilitate the delinquent. These goals may be incompatible because maximization of one may lead to inadequate fulfillment of the other. Business firms, in contrast, typically have one primary goal and several secondary goals or "functions" that are usually evaluated in relation to the primary goal.

It is often said that mental hospitals and, to a lesser extent, prisons are moving from an emphasis on incarceration and punishment to an emphasis on treatment and rehabilitation. Institutions for delinquents have had a goal of rehabilitation from the beginning. Bowler and Bloodgood (2, p. 9) point out that the first Houses of Refuge in Boston, New York, and Philadelphia were quite clear in their emphasis upon rehabilitation as the primary goal of the organization. The earliest state institutions combined emphasis on rehabilitation with a covert goal of custody. Advocates of military training, of farming, of vocational programs all visualized their programs as rehabilitative. Society has become more humanitarian and less repressive in its concepts of social control. As social welfare, mental hygiene, and social science concepts have spread, the general public and the expanding mental health professions have pressed for the implementation of treatment goals, even though the details of treatment techniques have in themselves been subject to considerable debate among contending professional groups.

In many states physical punishment and repressive controls have been legally denied the juvenile institution, and rehabilitative goals have been formally established. Yet it is rarely the case that correctional institutions can also abandon custodial goals. A variety of legal statutes govern the admission and retention of the offender by the institution, and assignment of the delinquent is often intended to protect the community. Rehabilitative goals have not been substituted for custodial goals in most cases; rather they have been added to organizational goals. It is possible, therefore, to place a given institution on a continuum whose poles are defined by goal ratios in which custody or rehabilitation predominate. Most institutions may be characterized by the degree of dominance of one goal over the other. However, knowledge of the goal ratio alone is insufficient for understanding the structures of the institutions. Institutions with similar goal ratios may stress differing means. Thus one treatment-oriented institution may stress the casework relationship as the primary means while another might stress the utilization of the milieu. One custodial institution might stress negative sanctions for running away while another might not allow opportunities for escape.

All of the diverse functions associated with these two goals are not inherently in conflict. A custodially-oriented institution, for example, could use techniques usually associated with treatment to achieve discipline and control (36; 23). Conversely, custodial control may be a prerequisite in some cases for effective rehabilitation. In certain situations custodial needs and therapeutic needs might dictate similar policies or decisions. But it is also true that they might dictate divergent solutions. If the multiple goals of the organization have not been clearly delineated and their relationship defined, the potentiality of organizational conflict is raised. That is, consensual validation of the norms and rules and of their relative importance will be absent.

In a formal sense an organization may be said to have split or multiple goals when the goal-setting agents—those who charter the organization and to whom the highest organizational authorities are responsible—conceive of the organization as having multiple purposes or functions. However, the actual degree of dominance of one goal over another is not wholly determined by the chartering agents. Even if they were to specify quite precisely the relative emphasis upon goals that were to be expected, the organization might not be able to realize this goal ratio. Depending upon its resources, structure, personnel, and clientele, the institution might be more or less successful in attaining its goals. Moreover, in many cases there may be a large degree of indeterminancy in the charter. Internal and external pressure groups may argue for one or another interpretation of the goals at various times and for policies which support their interpretations (7). The existence of the two major goals of custody and rehabilitation heighten the possibility of conflicting occupational role groups and the development of conflicting policies. The manner in which multiple goals affect the relation of the institution to the larger society and how they affect the structure and effectiveness of the organization will be discussed in later sections.

THE ORGANIZATION AND THE EXTERNAL ENVIRONMENT

THE relation of an organization to its environment may profitably be discussed in terms of (1) external factors that affect the input of facilities and legitimation, (2) the process of evaluation of the output of the organization, and (3) factors that affect the demographic characteristics of staff and clientele.

Sources of Legitimation and Facilities. Resource inputs to an organization are of several different kinds and effect the autonomy or independence of an organization. The designation of organizations as autonomous is largely a matter of degree. Any organization exists in a matrix of intricate relations with the larger society and must meet certain standards in order to exist. One organization may be said to be more autonomous than another to the extent that it has greater control over its environment, has more freedom in determining its own goals, judging its own effectiveness, and perpetuating its own personnel. An organization may have a narrowly limited area of operation and yet be largely autonomous in its operation. The converse may also be true. A correctional institution organized under a department of corrections is ordinarily less autonomous than is an institution less directly related to a department of government. The more a private institution depends on a limited number of sources for facilities, the more its autonomy is limited.

Public institutions receive facilities—money and capital investment— from legislative and judicial units of government or their administrative agents, while private institutions are primarily dependent upon charitable organizations or fund raising drives. Both public and private institutions receive legitimation from the state and from professional and lay associations. As sources of facilities, legislatures operate primarily with reference to two criteria: the tenor of the times and the pressure of the budget. The variability of both of these factors is conducive to organizational instability.

Facilities for public institutions are often channeled through a state agency responsible for all organizations of a similar type. Operating through a state department has both advantages and disadvantages for an organization. On the one hand it allows all of the correctional institutions to be treated as a single power unit rather than as fragmented institutions. It is a further advantage to give the job of organizational defense into a separate department of government with prestige and a staff of civil servants. However, this arrangement necessitates meeting standards set by an external agency directly responsible for the institution's continual effectiveness. Since the agency is more likely to accept rehabilitative goals, is not in direct contact with the clients, is more often in contact with standard-setting national welfare agencies, such as the Children's Bureau, we would expect the operating organizations to develop defensive patterns of relating to the parent agency. This should be especially true of the more custodially oriented organizations.

There is little research in this area. The literature on public administration treats of somewhat similar situations in its discussion of central office-field office relations, but there are no systematic studies of the relationship of correctional institutions to their administrative departments.

Private institutions, although relatively more autonomous in establishing organizational policy and acquiring personnel, have the complex problem of insuring the receipt of facilities through fund raising associations and foundations.

Etzioni (9) has recently traced the implications, for both society and organizations, of receiving financial support from a source different from the payment of clients for services received. Almost all public and many private organizations fall into this category. As compared with business organizations, such organizations should have problems in harmonizing the possibly conflicting interests of clients and sponsors. First, there is not a necessary relationship between the quality of service rendered to clients and the input of resources. Secondly, clients sent to these organizations are usually involuntary participants.

Evaluation of Output. It is obvious that any large-scale organization must satisfy the needs of others in the society by its output if it is to continue in existence. Organizational stability is dependent upon how successful it is in fulfilling its custodial and rehabilitative tasks with the allotted resources. Unlike a private business which may go into bankruptcy if it fails to offer a satisfactory product, correctional institutions monopolistically meet a continuing need of our society. Thus, lack of organizational success in satisfying this need is more likely to lead to a turnover of executive personnel.

The output of the correctional organization is evaluated by the agencies directly in contact with it, and, more diffusely, by the general public. The broader public usually becomes involved in the organization only when: (1) the organization does not maintain control over those committed to it, as reflected in riots or escapes; (2) some level of care dictated by the standards of the times is not maintained; (3) public norms of humanitarian treatment are violated. Public officials, professional associations, and crusading journalists may bring pressure to bear when the second and third conditions occur as judged by professional criteria. Ohlin and Pappenfort have pointed out that there are many possible incidents which could be used to threaten organizational stability. Only a few of these are actually turned into crises, sometimes by external organizations or associations (22).

The rehabilitative output of the organization can be judged in terms of several criteria. It can be judged by evaluating the recidivism rate of released clients, by evaluating the "personality" changes occurring while in the institution, or by evaluating the degree to which the organization meets standards (empirical or theoretical) which are supposed to insure success. At best, however, rehabilitation seems to "pay off" to the society at large only in the long run. However, when there are either runaways or other "incidents" the larger public is quick to apply pressure. Since control and rehabilitation are not always compatible and since rehabilitation is a vague and difficult to establish criterion, a continuous pressure for emphasizing control instead of rehabilitation is implied, if an institution is to be free of demands for reorganization.

In addition to official agencies directly related to the institution, various professional associations influence operations by establishing standards for their members and for organizations utilizing the members' services. Social work, psychiatric, correctional, medical, and educational associations all formulate standards which can be utilized in defense of their functions, and which are related to their "professional images." Sociologists have, unfortunately, rarely studied the relationships *between* organizations. As Levine, White, and Pierson note, sociologists make many assumptions about the interaction of organizations, but few study it directly (14). Ohlin's paper "Interest Group Conflict and Correctional Objectives," is one of the few exceptions to this generalization (20).

An institution may attempt to create sources of support by coopting elements of the local community (29). Cooptation may involve the formation of citizens' advisory committees or the encouragement of volunteer activities for the institution. Such devices, while helping to create a stable relationship with the community, may also lead to lessened organizational autonomy, problems of internal coordination, and others.

Demographic Characteristics of Staff and Clients. The external environment effects not only the type and amount of resources allocated to the institution but also affects its personnel and clientele. The state of the local labor market may markedly affect the character of institutional personnel. For instance, a college community can provide staff at the lower levels quite different from an industrial community in terms of their orientation toward juvenile offenders. This does not imply that college students *per se* are more desirable as rehabilitative employees. Rather, a college community provides a large number of potential employees whose ideologies may be more compatible with the rehabilitative philosophy, but whose student status precludes high salary demands. However, use of college students leads to high turnover and other instabilities (15, p. 23). Further, the opportunity for various types of activities, for both clients and staff, will vary from community to community. The size of the local community may also determine the off-the-job social relations of the staff. The isolation of some institutions increases the dependence of the staff upon each other for social activity, heightening the communal aspects of the institution.

The charatceristics of the clients are to an even greater extent affected by the environment of the institution. Clients are provided the organization by the courts. Operating under mandates from the legal system, the courts must determine who among their clientele are to be sent to correctional institutions and how the clients are to be treated. This complex decision involves a variety of factors, such as the available capacity of institutions in the area, the nature of the offense and the available ways of dealing with the offender. The nature of this decision may be systematic apart from the requirements for admission formally set by an institution. For example, offenders may be sent to the institution in the absence of a reasonable alternative and not with the intention of thereby protecting society or rehabilitating delinquents. If this were a constant practice, it would affect organizational operation at several points including, among others, its discharge policy and process, its training program, its distribution of facilities, and the nature of its clientele. Some of these problems have been dealt with in social work research concerning the intake and referral systems of agencies. However, this research tends to be administrative rather than sociological.

The type of community from which the delinquent comes may also influence his values and orientations. The physical isolation of the correctional institution also contributes to the degree of deprivation that the delinquent feels; e.g., he may be deprived of contacts with family and peers.

Client characteristics together with the input of facilities largely determine the degree to which various organizational goals can be pursued. If, as workers in the field claim (13, p. 34) delinquents have become more aggressive, brutal, and acting-out in their anti-social acts, more organizational activity may have to be devoted to meeting custodial requirements in order to placate the surrounding community.

THE INTERNAL SYSTEM

WITHIN an institution power and resources are distributed to maintain stability and attain goals. However, depending upon the distribution of power and the ideology of key personnel goals may be redefined and reshaped to differing specifications than those held by the governing board of the institution. The translation of goals into organizational practice can be shown by discussing three sets of interpersonal relationships; (1) staff relationships with other staff, (2) staff relationships with clients, and (3) client relationships with clients.

Staff-staff relations. The formal table of organization of the correctional institution defines the positions and the authority relations among positions that are supposed to characterize the institution. At a minimum, the table indicates a superintendent and an assistant superintendent; teachers, a nurse; a business and maintenance staff; and a staff variously called cottage parents, attendants, or supervisors. Even the most custodial institution for delinquents must have teachers, for in most states the law requires that children under sixteen years of age go to school. As institutions adopt contemporary modes of differentiating and treating delinquents, psychologists, psychiatrists, and social workers are added to the staff. The formal organization is not synonymous with the actual organization, nor is it complete. Any discussion of the internal structure of a correctional institution must include an analysis of the informal structure of the staff—as well as the social organization of the clientele. McCleery (16, 17), John and Elaine Cummings (11, pp. 50-72) and Novick (19) have shown that even on the formal level, however, the correctional institutions with different goal orientations will differ sharply in their authority structures; decentralization of power tending to be greater in rehabilitative institutions.

The existence in the organization of more than one goal raises the probability of role behavior having to meet diverse criteria. It allows conflict to develop between position occupants whose individual tasks are associated with the divergent goals. Thus, cottage parents and counselors whose performances largely are judged, respectively, in terms of their contributions to custodial and rehabilitative goals and whose perspectives are largely shaped by these goals, will often find themselves in conflict (37). "Interest groups" may form in any organization. But the value of their effects on the organization can usually be determined by reference to the dominant goal. In correctional institutions a group may develop an ideology, defenses, and norms which further its goal and its power and prestige at the expense of another group's goals and power (1, pp. 123-144; 23; 36).

Correctional institutions with marked custodial orientations are characterized by the relatively high actual power of the cottage parent and custodial staff, while institutions with predominantly rehabilitative orientations raise the power level of rehabilitative positions, defining custodial roles in relation to the rehabilitative function and lowering the power of the cottage staff. In many cases, where the definition of goals is in flux and unstable, inter-group conflict may be chronic or the external and internal necessities of control will emphasize custodial goals by default. For example, eligibility for discharge, in theory a rehabilitative decision, may be manipulated by the custodial staff as a control sanction.

Even if inter-group conflict is minimal, conflicting role expectations of the administration may lead to intra-role conflict. Thus the cottage counselors at one of the schools described in the MacIver report on institutions for delinquents seem to be subject to extreme role strain (16, p. 23).

Cressey (8) and Grusky (13) have described such conflicts in a prison setting and in the setting of a minimum security camp. In less custodial institutions the cottage parent is generally asked to maintain control but is not, from his point of view, given the sanctions to do his job right.

Since correctional institutions are often in an unstable relation to their environment, superintendents typically find a good deal of their time taken up with organizational defense; that is, with protecting the organization and maximizing the receipt of facilities and legitimation (36). The superintendent may be led to abrogate his authority to personnel that insure organizational stability. The combination of chronic pressure to economize, the inherent difficulty of evaluating the efficacy of rehabilitative policy, and the need to maintain organizational stability and control create recurring pressures that minimize the rehabilitative orientation. However, there is evidence that various organizations of personnel and policy are compatible with a given budget, and, furthermore, that adequate funds do not insure rehabilitative organization (21).

A typical bifurcation occurs along professional–non-professional lines. Part of the staff is highly educated, trained, middle class, and professionally oriented, while another part tends to be poorly trained, have little education and is of lower class origin. Status distinctions may lead to restricted communication between groups, turning each into a closed social unit similar to the status-linked groupings in hospitals.

Adult members of lower status groups have difficulty gaining access to higher status groups. In contrast, many organizations provide defined channels of mobility by which members can rise in the organization. Blocked upward mobility increases the individual's dependence on his own status group for support and solidifies the group as a unit for social control. This tends to raise the power of key custodial personnel through their ability to reward or punish individuals dependent on them. Thus effective institutionalization of rehabilitative policy is further blocked. Barriers to communication and interaction are probably lowest between the maintenance staff and the custodial staff, allowing informal patterns of cooperation to develop. Some institutions have developed committee mechanisms to help bridge this gap (5, 19).

Staff-client relations. As compared with most organizations in our society, staff-client relationships differ significantly in the juvenile correctional institution. Basic to this difference are four characteristics: (1) clientele and staff form a community; (2) the clients typically are drawn from a low social class and are social deviants; (3) staff are in a clearly superordinate position in relation to clients; and (4) adult and adolescent cultures are markedly divergent in our society. The fact that the staff associate almost continuously with the clients means that relationships tend to diffuseness, particularism, and affectivity; staff may easily develop warm relationships with some boys and none at all with others. This is in contrast with most bureaucratic organizations in which the relationships with clients tend towards specificity, universalism, and affective-neutrality. In most correctional institutions the cottage personnel tend to interact on a more intimate, diffuse, and personalized basis with the delinquents than do the rehabilitative, professional staff. The professional staff tend to interact on a segmented and specific basis with the clients (12). Thus, in many ways, lower level staff have more chance to establish warm, supportive relationships than anyone else, which according to current theory, are necessary for changing identifications and values. Yet, the demands of the role of the cottage parent and his own attitudes may only reinforce the boys' estrangement from society. Cottage staff find themselves confronted with the problem of managing from 15 to 70 boys. They must accomplish routine housekeeping, keep order, and prevent escapes. Unlike prisons, juvenile institutions usually do not even provide a wall to contain the delinquents. Few sanctions are available to the cottage staff; they have little training, often get little positive support from the professionals or the administration, and are most readily evaluated in terms of the visible criteria of control and cleanliness.

The correctional institution must maintain discipline and minimize violence in a population that has demonstrated its own lack of personal controls. The difficulty of maintaining control will vary with the age, sex, and traits of the delinquents that the institution serves. Since rewards may be largely controlled by staff, they have the opportunity to develop a variety of reward structures to achieve ends. However, the reward structure is a reflection not only of the ends sought but also of staff perspectives on what means will achieve these ends. This entails a view of the nature of the clientele and how they will respond (an implicit learning and behavior theory).

As stated by Gilbert and Levinson (11, pp. 20-36), the custodial orientation gives rise to an ideology that focuses upon the inherent nature of the client's difficulty and his lack of maleability. The ideology stresses rigid distinctions between types of people and the use of authoritarian techniques of interpersonal control. In contrast, the ideology of rehabilitation and therapy focuses on the socio-psychological causes of deviancy, on maleability and on permissiveness in interpersonal relations.

The utilization of sanction structures and interpersonal relationships congruent with these ideologies may have great effect upon client attitudes and upon client informal organization (12; 27). Client attitudes may be hostile to the organization, or docile but distant, or cooperative and cynical, or cooperative and personally involved in the institution's program. An instructive comparison of attitudes can be made from the description of attitudes reported by Clemmer (4, p. 152) and McCorkle, Elias and Bixby (18, pp. 109-157). Our knowledge in this area has been gained predominantly with prison populations. We would expect anti-social and anti-organizational attitudes to be less crystallized for juvenile offenders than for adult criminals. Therefore, the institution should be able to have a greater effect upon the former.

Staff-client relations in an institution with custodial goals tend to be more restrictive than in a rehabilitative institution. They are more "rule-oriented" and work to maintain social distance between staff and client. In ideal form they serve to maintain an objective fairness. At worst, favoritism and individual bargaining take place (32).

Client-client relations. Rehabilitation implies a substitution of positive social values for anti-social values. Yet it has long been said that the major product of penal institutions is the teaching of criminal values. If it is assumed that the juvenile delinquent is more amenable to change than the adult offender and is less committed to anti-social patterns, then the values esteemed by the client informal organization may be crucial in negating or supporting delinquent behavior patterns.

The incoming delinquent is completely dependent upon other offenders and upon staff for all social gratifications and deprivations, and for many definitions of cognitive reality. Thus, other clients serve as a major socialization agent to organizational practices and perspectives. As in any social system, clients rank actors and behave towards them in terms of a set of relevant criteria. The new client must, if he or she is to gain status and its rewards, adequately meet these criteria.

To a certain extent status criteria are imported into the organization. Instrumental and socio-emotional leadership have a degree of similarity in both delinquent and nondelinquent peer groups. Sophistication, athletic ability, personal appearance, strength, personality characteristics are all brought with the boy into the organization. However, the criteria that may be most affected by institutional practices are also those that are most relevant to rehabilitative goals. For instance, client organization may stress "con" values—the unfairness of society and staff, and the necessity of proving one's worth by anti-social behavior; or it may stress the necessity of facing reality, being fair, and proving one's worth by socially approved means.

Like the mental hospital which must accommodate the hospital to the patient, correctional institutions with rehabilitative aims cannot merely force the offender to accommodate to it. They require voluntaristic participation and identification. We would expect client organization to favor attitudes that support goals of rehabilitation the more the clients perceive the staff as working for the interests of the clients.[4] When there is not this perception overt compliance may take place, but covertly rehabilitative goals are sabotaged. Professional staff working in predominantly custodial institutions have often found themselves being "used" by the other staff and by the clients.

Some kind of *modus vivendi* must be reached between client leadership and staff in any institution if perpetual crisis is to be avoided. Staff in an institution have something to bargain with. They can "sell" prerogatives, positions, and psychological rewards. And what they "sell" influences not only the ranking criteria but also the structure of client organization. Structures can be found ranging from those that are hierarchically organized around the control of violence and communication to those that are less rigid and decentralized (16; 38). The multiple goals of most institutions affect client structure by: (1) introducing inconsistencies into the relationships between staff and clients; (2) allowing clients to play off one staff group against the other; and (3) by presenting client organization with an unstable situation. The existence of conflicting staff groups contributes to the breakdown of a rigid client structure by giving access to facilities to clients who are not among the more influential of the clients, thus breaching the monolithic client system of more custodial institutions or prisons.

The ability of the institution to affect client organization is also dependent upon the personality structure of the offender. Reiss's investigations would imply that the "Relatively Integrated" delinquent should be more adaptive than either the "Defective Super-Ego" or the "Weak Ego" offender (25; 26). Since the delinquent sub-culture supports the values of the peer group, the problem of the correctional institution is to structure the situation so that the anti-social values of the primary group are replaced by more positive ones (6). Rehabilitation of the "Defective Super-Ego" and the "Weak Ego" offender may well require both extinction of delinquent values and development of socially approved values by therapeutic techniques.

CONCLUSIONS

WE have attempted to delineate the character of correctional institutions for delinquents. Reflecting a growing body of literature, the analysis has stressed the fact, that, like other large-scale organizations, these dependent institutions are involved in a web of relationships with the external environment.

Strategically, the analysis has proceeded from the characteristics of the goals and the external environment to the structured relationships of the staff and their effects upon client behavior. Some of the characteristics which are most striking about correctional institutions are (a) the critical climate of opinion in which they operate; (b) the fact that they are resource-deprived institutions; (c) the abstract quality of rehabilitative goals and the difficulty of proving one technique to be more successful than another; (d) the multiplicity of functions assigned the institutions; and finally (e) the fact that these are "total institutions."

Correctional institutions will vary along many of the dimensions discussed. For example, we should not expect all local communities to have equal tolerance of escapees. The size of the community, its history, and other factors will condition its reaction to the institution. Similarly we should not expect all guards or cottage parents to develop ideologies congruent with the goals of the organization. Future research must be directed at ascertaining the conditions under which the phenomena herein described occur.

NOTES TO CHAPTER 4

1. The terms large-scale organization and organization are used interchangeably in this paper.
2. Frances Scott has recently discussed mental hospitals and prisons within a Parsonian framework (27). The analysis presented here will be less inclusive.
3. On occasion this analysis uses studies of mental hospitals as well as prisons. Paucity of organizational research on juvenile correctional institutions, as well as similarities among these organizations justifies this extension. Pertinent recent studies include those of McCleery (16; 17) and Sykes (33) for prisons, Belknap (1), Caudill (3), Stanton and Schwartz (31), and the book edited by Greenblatt, Levinson, and Williams (11) on mental hospitals.
4. In many ways delinquents stand in a relation to the organization similar to the primary members of military or industrial organizations. Their identification with the organization seems to be a crucial determinant of their organizational behavior.

REFERENCES

1. Belknap, Ivan, *Human Problems of a State Mental Hospital* (New York: McGraw-Hill, 1956).
2. Bowler, Alida C., and Bloodgood, Ruth S., *Institutional Treatment of Delinquent Boys, Part I. Treatment Programs of Five State Institutions* (Washington, Children's Bureau Publication No. 228, 1935).
3. Caudill, William, *The Psychiatric Hospital as a Small Society* (Cambridge: Harvard, 1958).
4. Clemmer, Donald, *The Prison Community* (Boston: Christopher, 1940).
5. Craig, Leita P., "Reaching Delinquents Through Cottage Committees," *Children*, 6 (July-August, 1959), 129-134.
6. Cressey, Donald R., "Contradictory Theories in Correctional Group Therapy Programs," *Federal Probation*, 18 (June, 1954), 20-25.
7. ———, "The Nature and Effectiveness of Correctional Techniques," *Law and Contemporary Problems*, 23 (Autumn, 1958), 754-771.
8. ———, "Contradictory Directives in Complex Organization: The Case of the Prisons," *Administrative Science Quarterly*, 4 (June, 1959), 1-19.
9. Etzioni, Amitai, "Administration and the Consumer," *Administrative Science Quarterly*, 3 (September, 1958), 251-264.

10. Goffman, Erving, "The Characteristics of Total Institutions," in *Symposium on Preventive and Social Psychiatry* (Washington: Government Printing Office, 1957), 43-84.
11. Greenblatt, Milton, Daniel G. Levinson, and Richard Williams, eds., *The Patient and the Mental Hospital* (Glencoe, Ill.: Free Press, 1957).
12. Grusky, Oscar, *Treatment Goals and Organizational Behavior: A Study of an Experimental Prison Camp*, unpublished Ph.D. dissertation (Ann Arbor, The University of Michigan, 1957).
13. "Juvenile Delinquency," *Interim Report of the Committee on the Judiciary, U.S. Senate* (Washington: Government Printing Office, 1954).
14. Levine, Sol, Paul E. White, and Carol L. Pierson, "Interaction Among Organizations," (paper delivered at the 1959 meetings of the American Sociological Society).
15. MacIver, Robert M., director, "Three Residential Treatment Centers," *Interim Report No. IX of the Juvenile Delinquency Evaluation Project of the City of New York* (March, 1958).
16. McCleery, Richard H., *Policy Change in Prison Management* (Lansing: Governmental Research Bureau, Michigan State University, 1957).
17. ———, "Communication Patterns as a Basis for a System of Authority and Power" (paper prepared for the SSRC seminar on corrections, undated).
18. McCorkle, Lloyd W., Albert Elias, and F. Lovell Bisby, *The Highfields Story* (New York: Henry Holt, 1958).
19. Novick, A. G., "Training School Organization for Treatment," *The Proceedings of the National Association of Training Schools and Juvenile Agencies*, 54 (Chicago, 1958), 72-80.
20. Ohlin, Lloyd E., "Interest Group Conflict and Correctional Objectives," (paper prepared for the Ad Hoc Committee on Correctional Organization of the SSRC, April, 1957).
21. ———, "The Reduction of Role Conflict in Institutional Staff," *Children*, 5 (March-April, 1958), 65-69.
22. Ohlin, Lloyd E., and Donnell Pappenfort, "Crisis, Succession and Organizational Change," (mimeographed paper, 1956).
23. Powelson, Harvey, and Reinhard Bendix, "Psychiatry in Prisons," *Psychiatry*, 14 (February, 1951), 73-86.
24. Redl, Fritz, "The Meaning of Therapeutic Milieu," symposium in Greenblatt, Milton, Daniel G. Levinson, and Richard Williams, eds., *The Patient and the Mental Hospital* (Glencoe, Ill.: Free Press, 1957), 503-516.
25. Reiss, Albert, "Social Correlates of Psychological Types of Delinquency," *American Sociological Review*, 17 (December, 1952), 710-718.
26. ———, "Delinquency as the Failure of Personal and Social Control," *American Sociological Review*, 16 (April, 1951), 196-207.
27. Schrag, Clarence, "Leadership Among Prison Inmates," *American Sociological Review*, 19 (February, 1954), 37-42.
28. Scott, Frances G., "Action Theory and Research in Social Organization," *American Journal of Sociology*, 64 (January, 1959), 386-96.
29. Selznick, Philip, *TVA And the Grass Roots* (Berkeley: University of California Press, 1949).

30. ———, *Leadership and Administration: a Sociological Interpretation* (Evanston: Row Peterson, 1957).
31. Stanton, Alfred H., and Morris Schwartz, *The Mental Hospital* (New York: Basic Books, 1954).
32. Sykes, Gresham, "The Corruption of Authority and Rehabilitation," *Social Forces,* 34 (March, 1956), 257-62.
33. ———, *The Society of Captives: A Study of a Maximum Security Prison,* (Princeton: Princeton University Press, 1958).
34. Vinter, Robert D., "Juvenile Correctional Institution Executives: A Role Analysis" (mimeographed paper, 1958).
35. Vinter, Robert D., and Morris Janowitz, "Effective Institutions for Juvenile Delinquents: A Research Statement," *Social Service Review,* 33 (June, 1959), 118-131.
36. Vinter, Robert D., and Roger Lind, *Staff Relationships and Attitudes in a Juvenile Correctional Institution* (Ann Arbor: School of Social Work, 1958).
37. Webber, George H., "Conflicts Between Professional and Non-Professional Persons in Institutional Delinquency Treatment," *Journal of Criminal Law, Criminology, and Police Science,* 48 (June, 1957), 26-43.
38. Weeks, H. Ashley, and Oscar W. Ritchie, *An Evaluation of the Services of the State of Ohio to its Delinquent Children and Youth* (Columbus: Bureau of Educational Research, Ohio State University, 1956).
39. Wells, Fred L., Milton Greenblatt, and Robert W. Hyde, "As the Psychiatric Aide Sees His Work and Problems," *Genetic Psychology Monographs,* 53 (February, 1956), 3-75.

ৡৡ

CHAPTER 5   The Hospital as a
Therapeutic Community*
EDWARD STAINBROOK

As A PRELUDE to the sharing of our understanding of the idea of the
psychiatric hospital as a healing community, we need a conceptual
model to represent the structure and functions of the hospital society. That
is to say, we have to be able to set up in words and syntax what is going on
in the hospital, both in terms of the human transactions and of the social
structure in which the process dynamics of human behavior occur as the
hospital endures through time.

At the present time we are in the very interesting position of inheriting
two distinct and yet allied trends in the theories of human behavior. We
might say, if we like to make dichotomies, that one of these concerns is
oriented towards the study of the intra-psychic person and another is
oriented towards the study of the extra-psychic. On the one hand, human
behavior is being considered in terms of the development of individual
perception, the conscious and unconscious aspects of the perceptions of
others and the perceptions of self, the learning integration of experiences,
and the constant generalization from original learning to subsequent
learning. There is agreement that an individual's responses are not to be
stated exclusively in terms of an objective consensus by others of what the
environment means but also in terms of the person's own learning about
what the environment has meant and means. So far as much of our
psychological investigation is concerned, we have turned our attention
from the external situation and the attendant hope that if it was completely specified we would thereby have the prediction of the inevitable
response to the understanding that one has to know the phenomenal
world of the other.

One of the most important channels into the world of another is

* Reprinted from *Neuropsychiatry*, 3 (1955), 69–87 by permission of the author
and the journal.

through communication, mostly verbal, many times non-verbal. We know that the interpersonal communication process is fraught with all sorts of possibilities of distortion, of change, of untruth, and that in order to know the internal perception of another, we first have to deal with a lot of operational maneuvers which individuals have learned in order to protect themselves and their world from scrutiny by others. Out of this intimate communicative interaction which became part of psychiatry largely through the psychoanalytic psychotherapeutic process, we are more and more aware of the essential nature of man. We have more understanding of even the vague and distorted kinds of non-logical processes of communication. What before was considered an unintelligible communication, either verbal or non-verbal, now even in the market place is assumed to have communication value. This change in psychiatry in the understanding of another has been a very important determinant of our present relationships to all sorts of people but particularly to those who, because they have come into despair or anxiety or too much hostility about their relationships to other people, have chosen to protect themselves by distorting communication.

In general, the emphasis on the intra-psychic life of man is the imprint which psychoanalysis has given to the present order of understanding of the human being. We have seen also in our recent century a great development in the social sciences. These are the sciences which are directed to the understanding of man and his interaction with other men, to the understanding of how men structure their interaction with each other, to the question of how optional and necessary values and meanings change behavior and become part of the total field of the determination of human action.

The social sciences no longer need to apologize for being called sciences, but within medicine we still have certain prejudices about the adequacy of social science research. There is yet some difficulty in asking the medical sciences to accept the behavioral sciences on an equal basis with all of the sciences in medicine. Nevertheless, the task of the physician at the present time is to stand as the integrator for the application of behavioral science knowledge to the problems of health and disease. Just as he must relate to all the basic sciences commonly accepted as being the basic sciences of medicine, so, too, he must now add the area of the basic behavioral sciences, that is to say, psychology, anthropology and sociology.

The utilization of social science theory and methods is essential to extend the range of intellectual visibility and of the intelligibility of human behavior in the hospital. When we think about what it is profitable to borrow from the social scientists, first of all we might speculate about the meaning of the physical structure of the hospital. Architects habitually start out by making some sort of model of the hospital. Sometimes it's an actual miniature of the building itself; sometimes it's much more abstract.

But this, I think, is where we ought to start. Too frequently we haven't started with the consideration of what is in the structure of the building itself which is going to determine the behavior of the people and their task performance or living interaction within the building.

Buildings and houses affect personal interaction. The Eskimo igloo, for example, is designed to have the family live as an interacting unit within one room. Contrast this to a Moslem middle- or upper-class where there is actually built into the house difficulties of making transactions between the female quarters and the rest of the house. Some small but significant part of the contribution to the disorganization of the Kikuyu society arose from limitations on the earlier homestead creation of several houses for the successive wives of a Kikuyu male and the consequent complications of a polygamous family interacting in one house.

In the history of the psychiatric hospital movement, in 1844 when the American Association of Medical Superintendent of Institutions for the Insane was formed (the forerunner of the American Psychiatric Association) by actual vote the members decided they never wanted to be superintendents of hospitals which included more than 250 patients in their confines. Then, progressively throughout the 19th century, every time they met that figure was revised upwards until now we have the situation of the Pilgrim State Hospital on Long Island with 15,000 patients. Here, again, the question of size, of structure, of communication, of cohesiveness in terms of inter-relationships between all of the people in the hospital is a function directly, to a very large extent, of the physical space in which the life space is imbedded. Problems of architecture are important.

I would like to illustrate in respect to architecture and physical building Robert Merton's excellent phrase, the "self-fulfilling prophecy." Three architects, who were interested in building a new state hospital came in consultation to discuss their plans. They told me that they were conceiving a three-story building for convalescent patients on the ground floor, semi-disturbed patients on the second floor, and disturbed patients on the third floor. They had a different kind of architectural style and different kinds of materials from below upwards. The third floor was designed as a very barren, uninteresting architectural situation because it was their insistence that they were going to get disturbed patients and they had to prepare for them. Under the self-fulfilling prophecy, if the very physical space of the hospital anticipates disturbed behavior in the people who are going to inhabit it, it will inevitably tend to produce stereotypic expectancies that this kind of behavior is going to happen, both on the part of the patient, who has to learn how to be a patient in this environment, and on the part of the personnel, who also have expectancies about how patients are going to behave in a disturbed ward.

While, therefore, we tend not to begin our discussions about the hospital as a therapeutic community with the architecture, I think, that it is very important that we start there, because it is the physical space which determines a good deal of the possibilities of interaction in the life space. In these days, incidentally, when we are so pressured about social inter-action, we mustn't forget that although there is a great deal of corrective communication in participant interaction with others, there is also a great deal of necessity in everyone, and particularly in the person who has become disturbed in his living, to have also considerable self-communica-tion, or privacy. How one provides in the psychiatric hospital for the time to be alone as well as for the time to be together is not only an administra-tive problem, it is also an architectural problem. The provision for privacy where self-communication can go on and behavioral alteration may take place may be fully as important as communication with others.

In summary, it is obvious that many specific ways in which communica-tion between people and communication with self is blocked or facilitated is inherent in the very internal physical planning of the hospital structure.

In his *The Social System,* Talcott Parsons remarks that a theory of sys-tems is a necessary requisite for a systematic theory of human action. In our consideration of the hospital as a therapeutic community, we shall find a theory of systems very helpful in understanding the interrelations of physiology, personality, and the social systems of the hospital. You can think of systems as either closed or open systems. A system can have heavy boundaries, and all of the activity that goes on within the system may be confined within the walls of the system. There are some systems like that. They are not associated, however, with living, breathing, biolog-ically active and psychologically sensitive people. The systems which we have to use to describe organic transaction are open systems—systems which are in reciprocal transactions with other systems. By postulating open-ended, interactional systems as conceptual models for the interrela-tions of physiology, personality, society and culture, you can easily see that stress applied in the community may, by way of some organization and some sub-group within the organization get into the personality sys-tems of the people who compose the sub-group formation and ultimately into the physiology of persons. It is no breach of logical thinking to see that community pathology or community stress may ultimately result in physiopathology. The physiological system has certain transactions with the personality system. Sometimes these are neurophysiological transac-tions; sometimes they feed into changes in the need-tension systems of the person; sometimes they condition ego functions and so lead to changes in the personality system. The personality system similarly feeds back into the physiological system and outwards into the small group system. Tensions evoked in one individual carry over into his small group formation, create tensions among other people in the sub-group and the rising sub-group tensions may pour out into wider ramifications in either the community or within the organization itself.

One provocative consideration that might very well flow out of this kind of conception is to think of the current impress in American society of the conjugal family, the small family which has to maintain also its isolation from other parts of the family to maintain self-esteem and status. One can't go home to mother or go back to father in order to get sustenance and succorance when one is in distress. There is a high need in terms of the self-esteem values to want to work it out on one's own, to be independent. The stress induced by cultural values and meanings impinging upon the small group of the family may induce tensions in the people who compose the family group, and the tensions in the individual personality may also be reflected in the individual physiology. The relationship between such psychosomatic conditions as peptic ulcer and certain cultural values and family structure is certainly presumptive.

The hospital society may also be described from the standpoint of its communication structure. More basic to that, of course, would be the organizational structure itself. Many of you have seen, I hope, Jules Henry's recent paper about the whole problem of organizational structure (1). It is important to know whether you have vertical line formation in the organization or whether you have many situations in which people are in multiple subordination to several sources of authority and control and power in the organization and to be aware of what this means in terms of organizational behavior. In many of our psychiatric and general hospitals the problem is one of multiple subordination. Nurses get caught most particularly in this kind of stress position where in-coming communications sometimes inconsistent with past communications, sometimes not really authentic or true, or sometimes not even intelligible, may come from several sources. The nurse has the task of executing some act of behavior as the result of deciphering, comprising, integrating all of these different communications. This doesn't necessarily mean that a multiple subordinate kind of organization is pathogenic. It does mean that if you do have a multiple subordination established, then you must have communication between the various communicating sources to the multiple subordinate so that a high consensus of agreement is achieved by everybody who feeds messages into this multiple subordinate position.

When we consider the communications from below upwards as well as those from above downwards, then the nurse, who is in a conflictful position because of conflicting messages from above, may be working with patients with whom the meaning of communication is not clear and where one may not know what the communication is intended to convey, either verbally or non-verbally. The nurse is, therefore, in a very crucial position in the psychiatric hospital in terms of her position in gathering information from below upwards as well as taking it from above downwards and issuing actions and directions as a reaction to this heavy bombardment of various kinds of communication upon her.

Other things being equal, communication channels will follow organizational lines. Therefore, one can make a model of a psychiatric hospital by making a chart of its organization. The chart of organization will also be a chart of communication. It is possible to further extend this by making a chart and putting every single person, including the patients, into some position in this communication structure as outlined for any one particular hospital.

What conceivably would be the advantage of doing this? First of all, certain hypotheses might be proposed about situations obtaining in this communication structure. For example, if we have individuals who are peripheral to the group and with whom there is little communication and who do not participate in the communication consensus of the organization, then we can expect certain things almost inevitably to happen. These people will tend to be less committed to the organizational tasks and goals. If there is no very intense hostility, then perhaps there will only occur a kind of goal-less, deviant behavior where the work patterns which should be done and the interactions with people which should go on will tend to get a little more deviant without correction. If hostility is high, and hostility is rather likely to be high in the peripheral isolated positions, then there may occur all sorts of projective attributions to the sources of power and control within the society. Particularly for patients in a psychiatric hospital these projective attributions to the central figures may be very autistic and regressive and tend to become more and more unreal because they are uncorrected by adequate communication. Even for non-patients in the psychiatric hospital system, however, the central figures in the hospital may become threatening omnipotent, and conceived as evil and mysterious figures. Paying attention, therefore, to communication channels is important.

Many people, of course, are in a very favorable communication position within the structure. They know a good deal of what goes on everywhere because of their position in this communication network. Patients, particularly, in hospital are many times in a much more favorable communication situation than many of the employees or the doctors or nurses. The patient occupies several different roles in hospital sub-groups and out of these positions gets communication sometimes that he shouldn't have, true, but many times the patient knows a great deal more about what is going on within the hospital than any of the staff.

The relationship of psychotherapy or of any treatment to the communication process is a very important one. As a matter of fact, if psychotherapy did not do any more than provide constant, intelligible and authentic communication about the hospital society to the patient and made possible intelligible communication from the patient to the hospital society, it would already have performed an adequate function within the organization. Group therapy performs a very definite repetitive pattern of communication in the hospital and so insures that the whole society is in much better cohesiveness than if this opportunity for communication did not exist.

The problem of communication fluidity is not only restricted to the psychiatric hospital. One of the problems that exists in government relating to security and morale is precisely that of the organizational character of communication. If people in government do not know how much information and of what sort there is about them and who has it in the system, then very interesting individual security maneuvers are set up. First of all, if you are unsure about who knows what about you and where in the system, you will increase your vigilance of listening and you will try to find out who knows what and about whom and where. The result of your increased efforts to listen will also mean that more of your verbal transactions with others will be around the problem of who knows what. You will be feeding back into the communication system, therefore, more and more information which otherwise you would not put into that system. At the same time, because of your heightened vigilance about listening, you will pick up more communication than you would ordinarily pick up in the system. When the communication system begins to go awry, when one doesn't know who knows what about whom or where the information is, or realizes with guilt and anxiety that one has said too much or has heard too much, then you have a pathology of organizational behavior. Security in such an organization is a function of administration and can be achieved by an awareness of the individual psychological implications of the structure and functions of the organization. We talk a good deal these days, incidentally, about loyalty oaths, which are usually conceived as being from below upwards. We don't hear very much about the loyalty oath from above downwards. In any kind of organization, however, the problems of communication and of the possibility of the psychopathology of communication is an important subject for constant administrative awareness.

One may analyze also the social structure of the hospital in terms of the power structure. Power is related to control and the characteristics of control also determine how much psychopathology or increased tensions you will get in a system. I think you can make the proposition that the more demands for conformity there are upon the people within an organization the more you are apt to engender hostility and the more you will have to constantly work to maintain the system in equilibrium. This is a restatement of the problem of the so-called authoritarian administration. The more one has the system heavily loaded up with *musts* rather than *mays*, the more the administrator will have to exercise vigilant control, and out of these transactions more counter-hostility will be invoked in the individuals who are in the organization. Moreover, when hostility is high, we can make the proposition that identifications with the organizational tasks and values are likely to be less involved; so, similarly, when anxiety in personnel is high, commitment to organizational tasks is apt to be low. Wherever communication in an organization is inadequate, motivation for the organizational task is also apt to be less intense. The hospital can be analyzed, therefore, in terms of power structure and of control, and of who controls, and under what emotional atmosphere, and with what communication pattern.

We may now turn to considerations of role behavior. Role can be described as the set of consistent expectations that one has learned about how one shall act and about how others are to act within the organizational context of the hospital. It is a definition of work and of other interactional patterns. Explicit and unambiguous definitions of role patterns of action are difficult to establish in organizations that are changing as rapidly in their theory of function as are our psychiatric hospitals. There is conflict even within one psychiatric hospital about what shall be the theory and modes of treatment or even about what shall be the theory of disease. Hence conflicts about what values shall obtain and about what interaction shall go on are constantly occurring in the psychiatric hospital. Nevertheless, there must be constant attempts to keep as explicit as possible the characteristics of the action role of people in the hospital.

This has particular relevance to the interactions between the psychiatric resident and patients. Residents enter psychiatry ordinarily with certain expectations of how they are going to play the doctor role. To oversimplify, we may say that they are motivated by needs to know and to help. Nevertheless, the resident has to learn how he is going to be permitted to be a psychiatrist in the particular hospital in which he finds himself. If the system of the hospital induces needs in the resident psychiatrist which contravene the needs of the patient, then conflict may be produced in both resident and patient about their reciprocal anticipations in relation to each other.

When a patient comes into a hospital, he can turn either to the nurses and attendant staff, he can turn to the physicians, he can turn to other patients, he can turn to the physical space of the hospital or he can turn to himself for his need gratification. The psychiatrist may, if his needs to help are in conflict with his needs to know because of his anxiety about an administration who will punish him in some way if he does not know quickly or adequately enough, begin to try to know the patient completely before he tries to help him. The patient, in such a circumstance, may be defeated or disappointed in his seeking for help from the physician and turn from the psychiatrist to other possible sources of help in the hospital.

Similarly if we attend to the nursing situation you have the problem of the nurse passing from one society into another hospital society. This may be particularly true in the Veterans Administration, incidentally, where the rotation plan for nurses is in practice. The nurse may be in conflict about the theory and practices of the hospital sub-group into which she is coming. She barely learns what the theory of one sub-group is before she is plunged into another sub-group and has to relearn all over again with all the attendant difficulty and maybe with a lack of specification which might go into the learning. I think one other incidental difficulty here is that in psychiatry, by and large, we prefer to proceed on the assumption that people ought to discover how it is with them or what they should do. But there is also a real need to teach by structuring the task and situation and making sure that the nurse very quickly and easily learns what the expectancies are. The constant specification of roles of interaction which must go on around individual patients is a sharing of values of the hospital society. Frequently, we try to get by without enunciating our values. I suppose that values are the most difficult things about which to really become specific and articulate. Whatever values the hospital is operating on for the moment, whether or not they may be the ideal values, ought to be specified, even if in the specification one has to admit that we are not doing what we think we ought to do. The defense against really knowing what one is doing is high, not only in the individual but in the group.

If we are not aware of how we are going to behave in a conscious expectant way, we cannot expect the patient to learn what sort of patient role he should have in relationship to us. The ability to share ambiguities in a non-threatening atmosphere, to talk out what one is really doing, to agree upon the same methods and the same goals becomes essential.

There are other important social science concepts that I think we have to look at for just a moment. I have used the term "patient role" and "sick role." Every man, anywhere, any time, can define himself as ill, but a social process of recognition of the illness must occur, followed by an initiation into a process of helping. In other words, an institutionalization of illness must obtain before the patient is socially recognized as ill and before he becomes a patient. The conception of how the hospital society should function with reference to the patient role and the sick role begins before the patient gets to the hospital. The patient may have voluntarily assumed the sick role, he may have had the sick role impressed upon him, he may be in resistance and rebellion against acceptance of the sick role. These are important things to know before one inducts him into a hospital society where you want him to learn to be a patient with the maximum productive utilization of the helping process.

The difficulties of acceptance of the sick role, of course, are complicated by many factors. There are shameful sick roles, and mental disease is still in many ways a shameful sick role. The struggle by the patient over the acceptance of a shameful sick role may create the first therapeutic task for the physician.

In the field of law and psychiatry, too, we are asking people who are deviants, in terms of their social behavior which has been detected by a process of law, to accept a sick role. The problem here is not whether or not they should be sick—that is a matter for legal and medical decision. The problem is that if the prisoner role is changed into a patient role and the prisoner is sent to the psychiatric hospital, then it ought to be very clear that the psychiatric hospital conceives of itself as having a meaningful kind of patient role in process for this person. Too frequently, however, you will find that the patient who comes as a patient when he might have been a prisoner is not perceived by the psychiatric hospital as being sick. The result of this is that such a person becomes, from the standpoint of social personal interaction in the hospital system, worse off than if he were a prisoner—he becomes an anonymous figure in the hospital society. In the Durkheim sense, he is in a position of anomie. Closer collaboration is called for between the psychiatric hospital and the law about deciding in the beginning whether we want this patient to occupy a sick role or a penitent role. Let's decide before we select the organization to which he should go. This decision should, I think, best be accomplished by a group of physicians and legal representatives who assess the situation from the standpoint of what kind of role we want the deviant person to occupy as a consequence of his deviance. It seems to me that it is only in this way that we can approach the understanding and the successful treatment of crime.

All of us in the psychiatric hospital have certain stereotyped expectations about the sick role. We use such terms habitually as a deteriorated or a dilapidated patient, or we say this patient is out of contact, or we employ various other kinds of phrases which to us imply a certain anticipation about how a patient with a specific diagnosis is going to behave. In other words, the diagnosis is not only many times a "knowing," it is also a prophecy of expectation about behavior, and if the situation sets itself up with certain expectancies that people are going to behave in a certain way, then inevitably many times people will begin to behave in that particular way. Every patient has to learn how to be a patient and he will learn how to be a patient differently, depending upon the social society, upon the hospital in which he is. This is true not only for the psychiatric hospital, it is also true for a three-day or a five-day stay in a general hospital. You have to learn how they are going to allow you to be sick in that particular hospital. This doesn't seem to be so significant in terms of the short stay of acute illness, but in terms of the longer run, "How shall I re-find my meaning and how shall I be in the world in this particular hospital" becomes determined by the particular organizational characteristics of the patient role. How the patient learns to be a patient is going to be of the utmost significance in terms of how he, too, relates to the task that he should perform in the organization.

One of our great difficulties in this respect is that in our psychotherapeutic efforts we try to turn the patient into an active participant in the helping process, whereas the stereotyped expectancy of being in a hospital is that you shall be in bed, passive, dependent and taken care of. This poses very often a crucial decision as to what needs shall be met in the initial phase of hospital residence and how soon one shall begin to represent to the patient that there is a meaningful participation which implies certain activity on his part as his contribution to the sick role within the helping situation. The destiny of disease is conditioned, therefore, by the characteristics of the sick role as well as by the psychopathology of the disease. It is also meaningful to talk about the reinforcement or the extinction of psychopathology by the interaction in the hospital society.

In summary, then, people come to the hospital with certain expectations. They come either gladly or reluctantly accepting the sick role or completely disowning it. If patients are blocked in finding expression of their needs in one area of the hospital, they will seek to find this expression in other areas of the hospital or become more autistically concerned with themselves. There is no meaning, therefore, in describing the natural history of schizophrenia unless you consider the situational context in which the schizophrenic individual is behaving. We know now that extraordinarily sick and disorganized patients under certain hospital conditions may not manifest the excitement and destructiveness that were ordinarily associated in Kraepelin's time with the concept of catatonic schizophrenia. The organizational structure and dynamics of the hospital society are significant determinants of the expression and destiny of behavioral disease.

If we turn to considerations of psychotherapy in the hospital, it is obvious that for a long time we behaved as if there was very little difference between the psychotherapeutic transactions within the hospital and those without the hospital. We talk uncritically about transference and counter-transference problems in the hospital as if they related only to the goings-on in the two-person system of the therapist and the patient, whereas actually that two-person system, to take individual psychotherapy, is a task-performing sub-group within the total hospital society. The total hospital society will pour its tensions into that two-person system. There may be an interference with the task of the psychotherapeutic transactions because of the therapist's organizationally induced tensions. The patient, too, is a great transmitter of tensions from other sub-groups of the hospital system.

People are carriers of stimuli, and they may transmit tension from one social system to another. In a little study we did in our own hospital, we found that it was precisely those nurses who were having difficulties in their own family who were having difficulties with the patients on the floor. The tensions induced in the small group of the family were transmitted into the society of the therapeutic community and so the input into the therapeutic society was definitely affected by tensions arising and derived from another social system.

Transference and the counter-transference always has to be thought about not only in terms of what are the unreal perceptions which the patient projects upon the physician or the physician onto the patient but about the very real perceptions patient and therapist have of each other within the context of the hospital system. In order to make this clear, I think you could think about a continuum of psychotherapeutic treatment from the analytic kind of treatment where the patient is on a couch and the analyst sits behind the patient, to that of face-to-face psychotherapy in the hospital in which both patient and therapist reside. In the ordinary analytic situation not only do you have relative "not knowing" about the therapist, but you have the facilitation of the subjective phantasies projected onto the therapist because there is no constant correction by visual cues of the actual reactions of the therapist. The patient leaves at the end of the hour and ordinarily is not seen again until the next day, so there is minimal face-to-face contact and a rather complete isolation of the analyst and the patient. If still within the ambulatory situation the patient and the therapist sit face-to-face with each other, then you have the next phase in the gradient toward the introduction of other real situations within the transference situation. There is the play of response constantly seen on the face and the other non-verbal communications that provide for more adequate reality testing. Then, as you proceed from this face-to-face contact by changing from the ambulatory consulting room to a hospital society, both the therapist and the patient almost inevitably encounter each other in many different roles throughout the day and night. Such a change significantly extends and changes the perception of the therapist. For example, how the therapist actually behaves, maybe without saying anything at all as he makes ward rounds or as he passes inadvertently through the ward, will either reinforce or tend to extinguish the distorted projective perceptions that the patient has of the therapist, even without direct overt transaction between them. Or the therapist may, as he passes on ward rounds in the evening, quite inadvertently enforce some acting out behavior on the part of a character disorder which would immediately change the perception of the therapist to somebody who might covertly approve, aid, and abet those aspects of the patient's behavior which in therapy we are trying to get him to renounce. The psychotherapeutic process has all of this feed-in and I think the way you have to understand it is in terms of how the two-party system of psychotherapy is conditioned by the needs and perceptions engendered in the patient and in the therapist by other parts of the system.

It seems to me that our contemporary concern about knowing the whole hospital society in terms of its impingement upon all the personnel and in terms of how finally this means something in the facilitation or inhibition of the experiences the patient has to have in order to heal means a renascence of exciting clinical administration. We are seeing administration restored in the psychiatric hospital to its basic medical dignity. I say this with every good feeling about administrators in the past. Now, however, administration has to add to itself the social science knowledge which aids in the integration of treatment within the functions of the whole hospital. This is a big job. Someone has to undertake the direction of the whole hospital society, particularly in terms of communication transactions and of detecting where tensions are and how those tensions are going to be resolved. Someone has to be in almost constant observation of the interactional processes in the hospital, or by extending roles that are already existing, we must develop the informational channels we need in order to do this kind of administration. This kind of administrative information can only grow out of something like participant observation within the hospital society itself.

What the psychiatric hospital needs for the immediate future is to become an organization-studying organization.

BIBLIOGRAPHY

1. Henry, J.: The Formal Structure of a Psychiatric Hospital, *Psychiatry*, 1954, 17: 139-151.

ॐ

Chapter 6 The Structure and Functions
of Adult-Youth Systems[*]

HOWARD W. POLSKY AND DANIEL S. CLASTER

"Nothing we ever do is, in the strict scientific literalness, wiped out. Of course, this has its good side as well as its bad one. As we become permanent drunkards by so many separate drinks, so we become saints in the moral, and authorities and experts in the practical and scientific spheres, by so many separate acts and hours of work."[1]

IN THE last few decades behavioral science has been profoundly influenced by structural-functional theory.[2] Unfortunately, all the social scientists who are working in this tradition are not agreed upon the precise denotations of these concepts. By "structure" we refer to a set of relatively stable and patterned relationships of individuals and groups: "function," we define as the consequences of the social activity for the adaptation or maintenance of the structure and its components. Structure refers to relatively enduring patterns, and, function, shorter-range processes growing out of and creating the social structure.

Structural-functional theory is the native-born son of gestalt theory.[3] It dominates behavioral science today because social scientists require a theoretical orientation that is adequate for analyzing the transactions of individuals in social systems. Structural-functional theory seeks to overcome the atomistic, uni-dimensional interaction perspective by emphasizing the impact of environment upon individuals via social systems in which they are actors.

Structural-functional theory is used increasingly as an orientation for analyzing transactions within and between systems in equilibrium, but it

[*] Paper presented at the University of Oklahoma Fifth Social Psychology Symposium: "Problems of Youth: Transition to Adulthood in a Changing World" organized by the Institute of Group Relations, May 6-7, 1964. This paper is based on a demonstration project supported by the National Institute of Mental Health. MH-993-03.
Reprinted from *Problems of Youth: Transition to Adulthood in a Changing World*, edited by Muzafer and Carolyn Sherif (Chicago: Aldine, 1965), pp. 189–211.

is equally useful in studying deviant behavior and social disorganization. It is possible to consider American society as a comprehensive system, and focus on the worlds of the adult and the adolescent as subsystems. Then we look at both functional and dysfunctional consequences of the transactions between adolescents and adults in terms of the socialization function of the larger system.[4]

In our fast-changing society, many adolescents are not lagging behind. James Coleman, who has conducted intensive research into adolescent societies, has commented on their increasing social sophistication, their discontent with a passive role, and passionate involvement in activities which they can call their *own*.[5]

Much of the problem of "lagging adolescents," however, arises in their lack of concern and involvement in activities which adults believe would be most beneficial for their development and functioning as responsible citizens in society, for example, the lack of passionate devotion to scholarly work. In fact the norms of the adolescent community often counterpose them. It has been pointed out many times that organized athletics represents one area for positive action by adolescents which carries its own rigorous discipline. Undoubtedly, athletics absorbs energy which would be directed against society in violence and other forms of deviancy.

We find missing in contemporary studies of adolescents a probing analysis of the interpersonal structure of adult-youth systems. The central issue is how the structure of adult-youth relationships free, inhibit or frustrate the abundant energy that can potentially be released by adolescents for mutually furthering society's and their interests. What do we know about the structure of adult-youth relationships which we can use to reenforce the fulfillment of constructive and creative aims of our society rather than impeding them?

Getzels and Jackson[6] compared students high in scores on creativity tests, but not especially high in scores of I.Q. tests with students high in I.Q., but not especially high in scores on creativity tests. The performance of both groups on standardized achievement tests were nearly identical. They differed markedly however in their attitudes and relationships with the teachers. The highly creative were far less concerned with conforming to teachers' demands and much more imaginative and wide-ranging in their interests. The personal traits they preferred were negatively correlated with what they felt the teachers preferred. The personal traits of high I.Q. students were highly correlated with what they felt the teachers preferred. The teachers preferred the high I.Q. students to the highly creative ones.

What underlies the suggestion in this study that the teacher's role inhibits and under-selects creativity? The answer to this complex problem lies in the direction of conceptualizing the interrelationship of teacher-student transaction as a system with the institutional and societal

contexts to which it is interrelated. A British exchange teacher, who spent
a year in New York City's Bronx High School of Science, probably put
his finger on the central problem. He had high praise for both the students' obvious liveliness and intelligence, and the superbly equipped
physical facilities. But he made this shrewd negative criticism: "It was
after I returned to New York from an Easter vacation spent with friends
who teach at colleges that I suddenly realized how much of the depression I had been suffering . . . was due to one thing. I had been beginning
to see myself in the way New York's educational administrators apparently want their teachers to see themselves: over-burdened by officialdom,
left little or no say in the planning of curricula and examinations, and
even barely trustworthy enough to do an honest day's work without
constant checks and supervisions."[7]

A full discussion of the adult-youth transaction in any social system
requires an analysis of all the critical social systems in which the adult
functions because they impinge upon his relationship with the younger
generation. Excellent examples of how the press within the economic
sphere can reverberate through the family system are given in *Five
Families*[8] and *Family Worlds*:[9] I quote briefly from a description of one
family in the latter study:

> The Littleton family is scarcely in a position to organize time to serve the
> group's needs or to assist the family in its pursuit of overt individual or group
> objectives. The emotional separateness of the members is augmented by the
> daily routine that they have established for themselves. A summary of these
> routines is provided as each member described the activities of an average day:
> Mr. Littleton: Work, work, work from five until two every day; five until three
> on Saturdays, home, bed, and up.
> Interviewer: Can you tell me generally what the family usually does on other
> days?
> Mr. Littleton: I couldn't tell you. I know what they do and where they go, but I
> don't know just when they have the activities. Now Bobby is beginning Cub
> Scouts.
> The emotional tone, echoing fatigue and despair, with which Mr. Littleton
> speaks of his day, reveals his distaste for his own routine and his uninterest in
> the family's daily schedule. His description shows a diffuse view of the day,
> anchored by the beginning and end points of his work schedule. He has little
> sense of being able to order his day, and he feels bound by a routine from which
> he sees no way of escape.

In the ensuing discussion, we hope to make clear the multiple roles
adults attend to in the superordinate-subordinate relationships formed
with adolescents in diverse social systems. We will then exemplify the
conceptual framework with a research project into child care worker-
resident transactions currently being conducted in a residential treatment
center for emotionally disturbed and delinquent adolescents.

A CONCEPTUAL FRAMEWORK FOR ADULT-YOUTH TRANSACTIONS

OUR main task is to formulate a practical middle-range scheme for analyzing adult-youth systems. By social system we mean an interdependence of parts so that a change in one will have repercussions for the entire system. The concept of social system emphasizes the relations between the units rather than the individual characteristics of the actors. The social system is open and in active interchange with the larger organization in which it is embedded.

Generally, a system is conceptualized by boundarying the amount of energy transacted with it. The internal parts are in close and dense interaction with each other and together form a functional relationship with the environment.

In the social system model we place the adult and youth together within it and examine independently problems of joint adaptation and goal-attainment in the external system and group support and integration in the internal system. This is simply diagrammed as follows:

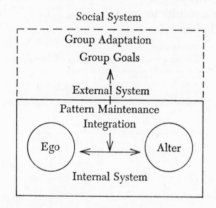

The social system approach derives from the functional imperatives that flow from the nature of the system. This type of analysis was pioneered by Robert Bales at Harvard.[10] Over many years of laboratory experiments, he observed in a variety of groups confronted with problems to work out together the emergence of *system roles.*

The instrumental role consisted of taking initiative and leadership in formulating goals and coordinating tasks presented to the group. The instrumental leader was frequently not the best-liked person in the group. Another person, the expressive leader, excelled in supporting individual members and mediating intra-group tensions and differences. This role was not directly important in the task or instrumental sphere, but was critical in building group morale. These two system roles, the instrumental and expressive, underlie all social system theory. Their discovery is important because they indicate that group achievement and gratification out of relationships depend largely upon how these specific functions are carried out.

In agencies, this distinction is between the executive, the instrumental leader, and the expressive "key man"; the latter, often high in the hierarchy, is accessible to the rank and file and serves as an important outlet for differences among the members in the organization. The same distinction can be seen in the system roles performed by adults in interaction with adolescents. Perhaps the example taken from our current research in a total institution for youths reflects the differentiation most cogently because the system is more circumscribed by time, space and function; but it should also be generalizable for less boundaried systems in communities.

The other major distinction among functional roles, according to our system theory adaptation, can be visualized by crisscrossing the internal and external axis above with the instrumental-consummatory (expressive) axis. The individual and the group are conceived as purposive, i.e., organisms which formulate goals and experiment with diverse means for attaining them. This results in the following four-fold paradigm of social roles, functions and phases:[11]

	Instrumental	Consummatory (expressive)
Internal	Adaptation	Goal-attainment
External	Pattern-Maintenance and Tension-Management	Integration

The above paradigm can be used for adult-youth interaction conceptualized as a system with foci ranging from the teacher-student relationship to the child care worker-resident transaction. In the adult-youth relationship, four key functions are derived that the adult assumes at various stages. We call these functions role-segments and they are related to the system imperatives as follows:

System Function	Role-Segment Range
adaptation	protector-custodian
goal-attainment	advisor-counselor
pattern-maintenance	consoler-nurturer
integration	friend-judge

The custodial role indicates an orientation by the adult with reference to the youth adapting to the regulations of the agency or the society in which the transaction is enacted. Goal-attainment reflects not mere adaptation to externally imposed standards but formulation and attainment of goals emanating from the youth's needs and which are at the same time compatible with the adults' and the society's value system. Counselor is the role in which the superordinate enables the subordinate to formulate and attain such goals.

Correspondingly, two functions contribute to the maintenance of the internal system. "Nurturer" characterizes the supporting role of the adult, in which he enables youths who are immobilized (e.g. psychologically disturbed) and unable to function at an adequate level within the system. Finally, the integrative function is fulfilled by assuming a friend, judge-like, or monitor role; here the adult evaluates the youth's activity vis-a-vis peers and himself, the agency and society.

The analytical breakdown of these various functions enables us to analyze more effectively the total functioning of the various socializing agencies in our society. The mother-infant transaction is essentially characterized by nurturance; the counselor role is institutionalized by the teacher in our society; the integrative role is assumed in one extreme fashion by the judge, especially at a time when the youngster has violated the rules of society; finally, the custodial function is assumed in its purest form by the policeman or guard in a reformatory.

We argue, however, that in each of the above institutionalized roles, the superordinate in the adult-youth relationship performs each of the four role-segments at various stages. Now the most important implication of conceptualizing the adult-youth relationship as part of a larger social system is that it sensitizes us to the constraint exercised on the interpersonal transactions by the more inclusive system. In other words, the larger more powerful organization determines which function should be stressed and how it should be performed. This results in an intermediate or emergent adult-youth structure which directly determines the on-going interaction between adult and youth.

How the agency structures the function of its workers can be briefly illustrated by the changing role of the probation officer.[13] Initially, he was defined as a "punitive officer," a custodian who supervised the parolee by insuring his adaptation to society and nonviolation of law. Next the parole officer became a protective officer, a balancer of the community's need for protection and the youngster's protection from the community. He assumed a judge-like role in which he balanced community need with a knowledge of the client and his life history. A third stage evolved when the parole officer took a more active role in rehabilitating the parolee by helping him attain work, recreation, and assistance in general social adjustment to family and society. This rehabilitative role is similar to the counselor function. Finally, with increased education and gradual adoption of social work philosophy, the parole officer increased his attention to psychological and emotional factors influencing the client's behavior and was much more sensitive to giving reassurance and support (the nurturance role).

Our main point is that the superordinate socializing agent performs effectively to the extent that he utilizes all four role-segments of his central enabling function. He must first decide on the appropriate role-segment for the presenting situation, and then adopt a specific pattern of behavior within the rubric of each role segment. He may choose to enact one role segment at a time, or several simultaneously; within each role segment, conduct may be rigidly or diffusely defined. All of this must be seen in the context of the relevant social system. In the example of the parole officer's changing role, it is important to emphasize that it is not the legal agency alone which is chiefly responsible for modification. This change of role is not a one-way street which stems alone from the courts, but the change is actively influenced by recruitment practices, social work schools, the stature of profession and the community.

The adult and youth should be conceptualized as a system in whatever setting they are articulated. Four indispensable functions can be derived from the conceptualization of their relationship as a social system. But this is only a point of departure. We want to use the above framework now to analyze the diverse structures that emerge out of the interaction of adult and youth as their system functioning is related to the larger field in which it is embedded.

Total institutions and repressive authoritarian reformatories are undergoing a transformation from custody to therapy. However, in this transformation, custodial functions remain and the dilemmas, contradictions and conflicts inherent within each role-segment as well as how they impinge upon each other are critical theoretical and research problems which have to be probed in depth in order to increase adults' potential for effectively socializing youngsters. We turn now to a comparison of cottage adult-youth systems in a progressive, psychotherapeutically-oriented residential treatment center.

THE COTTAGE SYSTEM IN THE RESIDENTIAL INSTITUTION

THE most obvious perceptual context of the cottage is a separate building occupied by 19 youngsters and four staff members (two are normally on at a time). Our focus consists of the recurrent internal patterns and the interchanges of three senior cottages (boys' ages from 15 to 18) with the institution. The cottage staff is given a set of implicit prescriptions of how the cottage should function. Staff have some autonomy within this structure to develop their own procedures, in effect, to evolve distinctive subcultures. In this treatment center, much more attention and prestige is conferred upon the psychiatrists and psychiatric case workers, who see individual youngsters throughout the week in a clinic removed from the cottage, than upon the staff in the cottages.

The chief function worked out in detail for cottage workers is the custodial: as supervisors of the cottage, they maintain constant track of the children. They wake them in the morning and put them to bed at night. Their numerous responsibilities include preparing snacks during the evening, mending and laundering clothes, and supervision of canteen and allowance.

In order to manage the cottage, the staff evolves a structure super-imposed upon the routines and sanctions prescribed by the institution. However, we would be seriously amiss to abridge the total functioning of the cottage system by concentrating solely on the custodial or adaptive function. We have adopted a four-fold functional sphere for the manifold activities differentially performed by staff with youngsters in the three cottages. This can be pictured as follows:

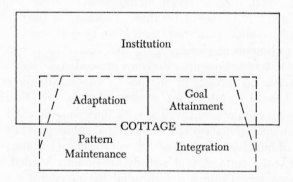

Adaptation and goal attainment refer to the activities that the cottage performs in what Homans calls the "external system." Adaptation refers to all activities and routines incumbent upon the cottage to perform by virtue of membership in the institution: cleaning-up, wearing appropriate dress, adherence to the time schedules, general conformity with institutional regulations. We also include in this category the punishment or deprivation of youngsters who have violated institution rules.

The cottage, however, does not merely respond to institutional rules. In addition to being molded by the institution through all of its adaptive adjustments, there are many activities which emanate from youngsters and cottage staff. All activities not directly sponsored by the institution which are generated from within the cottage we place in the goal-attainment sphere. This includes activities such as ping pong and chess, a singing group, an auction, a camera club, card-playing, record groups, etc. Needless to say, the cottages vary in the kind and complexity of group activities and autonomous goals formulated, participated in and attained.

In addition to the two external functions are two internal functions.

Pattern-maintenance (tension management and latency) is any activity in which the staff member is giving direct emotional or psychological support to a youngster or group. This ranges from the expression of sympathy for a youngster with a sprain to the structured individualized private sessions carried on in two cottages by the two professional head counselors. By pattern maintenance we mean direct assistance to the individual which is of a bucking-up character. Mostly it is directed at youngsters who are in a temporary state of depression, rebellion, or general confusion.

The final function we concentrate upon is the integrative: the informal relationships of staff with youngsters not especially goal-oriented, related to fulfilling an adaptive task, or, directly psychologically-supportive. By integrative function, we mean the informal interplay of staff and youngsters in general conversations and bull sessions. We call this *integrative* because we think that the major function of this kind of interchange is cementing internal relationships along specific values and themes.[14]

Before presenting concrete examples of how each of these four functions is performed, a word about methodology.* Three senior cottages have been intensely observed by three members of the research team. Systematic observation consists of half-hour time samples during which the observer observes at close range a staff member's interaction with a resident. These transactions are rated on a pre-coded observation schedule. General observation consists of one hour contact with the cottage after which the observer dictates a less structured summary of staff members' interaction with each other as well as with the youngsters. All observation is based upon operationalism of the functional spheres outlined above.

As a part of our research demonstration project on cottage systems, two of the three senior cottages under study are directly headed by two professional counselors. Cottage 1 is headed by an educator who stresses stable, orderly routines; cottage 2 is directed by an old-line non-professional who is concerned about orderly routines, but in addition has developed an easy-going, joking relationship based upon an implicit contract that the cottage have "no trouble"; cottage 3 is headed by a professional social group worker who has considerable influence with the administration. In order to simplify the analysis of the cottage system, we will focus primarily upon the head counselor in each cottage, and later advance tentative propositions of how they are supported by their assistants.

In cottage 1, the head counselor is preoccupied with cottage routines which he supervises in a prep-school fashion. During regular checkups, he may run his finger across cabinet edges and behind radiators to see

---

* For a full discussion of theoretical orientation, methodology and findings of the research summarized below see Howard W. Polsky and Daniel S. Claster, *A Comparative Analysis of Three Cottage Systems*, Hawthorne Cedar Knolls School, Hawthorne, N.Y., mimeographed.

that every bit of dust is collected. Once seeing that a bed was loosely made, he pulled out the covers and stripped it of its blankets and sheets. These activities seem to be carried out not only during the specific time allotted for general room-cleanup but pervade the cottage during the entire week. The head counselor's assistant also has assumed this supervisory custodial role; both undertake joint inspections to rate the youngsters' cleanup according to a merit scheme.

The other major activity the head counselor-educator performs is private sessions with individuals in his office. These last from ten to twenty minutes and cover different subjects but are mostly concerned with the current upset of the youngster in the cottage. This activity is carried out only by the head counselor in cottage 1. In addition, the head counselor plays games with the youngsters but always to win; he plays hard and generally beats all the boys in ping pong and in chess. This is the general level of complexity of goal attainment in the cottage, although recently there has been an attempt to form a committee of boys to plan a party. Finally, we find relatively little initiation by this head counselor of informal integrative activity with groups of youngsters. Representing the cottage to the institution, maintaining stable orderly routines, and conducting individual sessions leave little time for informal lengthy interpersonal contacts with the youngsters.

In contrast to the "prep school" atmosphere in cottage 1, in cottage 2 we have the classic accommodation picture between old-line non-professional staff and youngsters which was described in detail in *Cottage Six*.[15] In contrast to that study, however, cottage 2 has less open physical aggression among the youngsters. The head counselor carries out the adaptive function in an arbitrary, dictatorial manner. Whenever any youngster has a job to do and falls down on it, the counselor will yell at him until he does it right. However, the counselor is not too sticky about how thoroughly the job is done. He wants it done in conformity with institutional expectations, but does not go beyond them as in cottage 1.

The other major activity the head counselor performs is general bull sessions with the youngsters. Often this has a delinquent undertone. The counselor initiates discussions of past exploits such as the boys' excessive drinking of diluted wine during the last Passover holiday. He discussed in detail a boy's attempt to go AWOL. The other negative feature of his extensive informal contact with the youngsters is the denigration of their ambitions. One boy is intent upon attending college and has been poring over college catalogues. He is the butt of considerable wry joking by the counselor who casts great doubt upon his ability to achieve this important goal. Much of this informal transaction is in good fun, but its denigrating repetitiveness has the earmarks of considerable hostility. It appears that the counselor gains superiority by belittling both the boys' ambitions and accomplishments, especially in the intellectual sphere. In this cottage there is little "alter-therapy" that the counselor performs in any formal sense and relatively less informal personal support of the youngsters. Finally, the counselor does little to help the youngsters plan and execute autonomous goals. A singing group receives scant attention. This cottage has little purposeful autonomous group activity.

The other non-professional counselors in this cottage take their clues from the head counselor and support his orientation and prevailing mode of operation. Communication among the counselors is centered about practical problems and routines. The female staff person is new and is taking over some of the nurturing aspects of staff work but it is too early yet to clearly delineate her role in the total emergent staff pattern.

In cottage 3, headed by a skilled group worker, the prevailing atmosphere is quite different from that in cottages 1 and 2. First of all the adaptive sphere is unusually self-regulating with much less active cottage direction than in the other two cottages. The boys routinely take care of their various daily tasks without much prompting by the staff, especially the group worker. He operates in a unique way. Often he will suggest to boys standing around, to take advantage of the time to get some cottage task completed. After a discussion with the youngsters, he generally leaves it up to them to decide if they want to do it now or later. This is in marked contrast to the head counselor's persistent needling in cottages 1 and 2.

The non-professional assistants in cottage 3 are somewhat more insistent upon pressing the youngsters to do the adaptive tasks adequately, but the head counselor does not spend much time with this functional sphere. The head counselor's preoccupation is enabling the youngsters to formulate and execute cottage goals. They have had overnight hikes, dinners at restaurants, planning a huge auction sale, and remodelling of each bedroom after a college with its pennant, picture and colors. The cottage is a buzz of activity; at this writing over 90% of the boys are intensely involved in painting and repairing auction wares for a big sale.

Another important role the head counselor plays in this cottage is alter-therapist. He conducts group therapy sessions with the youngsters and also speaks to them individually in closed sessions in his office. This counselor has little informal interaction with the youngsters; much of his general contact seems to be organized around enabling the youngsters to formulate and attain the cottage goals discussed above. However, his two female assistants do spend a considerable amount of time in informal integrative transactions. The counselor has so organized his staff, however, that they too have been increasingly participating in enabling the youngsters to execute various cottage goals.

* * * *

In cottages 1 (the prep-school headed by the educator) and 2 (the old-line non-professional) we find most activity directed toward adaptive routines. These routines are pursued throughout the day and week rather than limited to specific time periods. The important difference between cottage 1 and 2 lies in the other functional spheres. Cottage 1 in addition has developed an elaborate alter-therapy system whereby individual youngsters are counseled in the office of the head counselor. A peculiar conflict emerges in cottage 1 where the educator is both "therapist" and chief custodian. I quote from our general observation log:

Two boys burst into the cottage in a high vocal state of elation. The head counselor immediately challenged them pointedly about their leaving the cottage when he had told them not to. One boy said: "I told you I was going. I had an appointment with the social worker and you can't keep me from seeing my social worker when I was supposed to go."

The counselor repeated that they were not supposed to go anywhere unless they had his permission. The upshot was a vehement argument between the boys and the counselor. During the dialogue the counselor stressed that the boy had first obligations to the cottage and to him as his cottage parent irrespective of obligations elsewhere.

During the discussion the boy insisted that he wanted to see his social worker because the head director had denied him a "session." The counselor's retort was that he would have to give it at a time when he had time.

This is a conflict between the head counselor in his custodial-disciplinarian role and alter-therapist role. This role conflict rarely occurs in cottage 2 where individuals and groups are addressed privately only when they have violated institutional regulations. In 2 the head counselor reinforces his authoritarian adaptational procedures with a great deal of kidding and joking in bull sessions much of which has a delinquent flavor. In contrast, in cottage 3 we find the adaptive routines are limited to specific time periods. The group worker uses himself and the other staff people to develop multiple group activities. The "basic work," i.e., the routines have been worked out to the extent where the cottage is much more peer-regulated without intensive staff supervision. In cottages 1 and 2 the staff are used primarily to back-stop supervising cottage routines. The educator's assistants take "orders" from him in carrying out custodial functions. The other staff participate with the youngsters in games but do not help the boys organize complex group goals. In cottage 2, the head counselor gives very little direction to the other staff, all of whom work together in a laissez faire fashion. In cottage 3, the group worker-director has consciously assigned manifold functions to his counselors. Each of them has a task to do in the custodial sphere, but is also assigned a group activity which is carried out with his guidance.

Among the most important differences among the three staff directors is that the group worker in cottage 3 has considerable influence with the administration. In addition to his group work skills, and a group-process perspective for utilizing his staff, he, more than the others, develops in the external environment opportunities which his youngsters can exploit.

As for internal regulation, the staff work as if a minimum of dictation of routines is best for everyone. In fact the group worker joined a cottage that was very stable in carrying out routines. The female housekeeper remained in the cottage after the group worker entered and continued to be chiefly responsible for cottage routines.

THE EMERGENT COTTAGE STRUCTURE

THE cottage staff role, especially the head counselor, can be seen as dovetailing institutional administrative tasks with the needs and social order of the residents. Like the foreman, his marginal position subjects him to varying pressures compounded by the juxtaposition of an authoritarian structure and living together with rebellious youngsters. Just as the foreman carries the essential function of bridging the gap between management and the workers, so the head counselor is crucial in bridging the administrative structure with a developmental program in the cottage.

The point of departure of comparing the different adjustment patterns of cottage systems stems primarily from how each counselor conceived his custodial role, that is the handling of problems imposed by the institutional structure. Our case materials point to three emergent structural patterns. The head counselors' centers of gravity in the cottage system can be best summarized in the following diagrams:

THREE HEAD COUNSELORS' CENTERS OF GRAVITY

(IMPRESSIONISTIC Estimate of Time and Effort Directed at Four Functional Spheres:

(A) Adaptation, (G) Goal-Attainment, (L) Latency and Pattern-Maintenance, (I) Integration)

HEAD COUNSELORS' ACTIVITY IN THREE COTTAGES

Head Counselors' Activity in Three Cottages

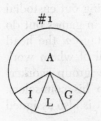 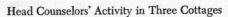 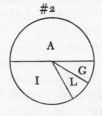 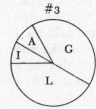

In Cottage 1, the educator has gone far beyond the institutional requirements for maintaining clean and orderly routines in the cottage. He is also developing a growing opposition among the youngsters who see his carrying out of this sphere as unduly extreme. The educator meets this opposition by many individual sessions with the youngsters. He realizes that he must develop more fully autonomous goals, but has not been able to acquire staff to carry out this function.

In cottage 2, an extreme split prevails between two major functions carried out by the head counselor. He is very dominant and dictatorial in supervising the boys' fulfillment of cottage and institutional tasks. However, he moderates this role with an attempt to be a "buddy" of the boys and enters into considerable "horse play" with them, much of which has a semi-delinquent flavor. He is not trained to help the youngsters attain autonomous goals and he does not use much of his time for individual alter-therapy sessions. He is able to mediate the extreme custodial role with his joking relationship.

In cottage 3, the center of gravity is in marked contrast to cottages 1 and 2. The attainment of autonomous goals has become the head counselor's main preoccupation and the youngsters and the other staff are caught up in a considerable amount of autonomous planning, coordinating and executing of goals. Individual boys gain prestige by their ability to perform maintenance tasks: plumbing, electrical repairing, painting, gardening, etc. A "big brother-apprentice" system has been established; new boys are attached to the more skilled youngsters and are slated to take over their jobs when they leave the institution. Thus in the third cottage, the activity around attaining goals sharply conditions how all the other functions in the cottage are performed.

The counselors in the first two cottages are not challenging the institutional structure. In cottage 1, the heavy emphasis is placed upon identification with administrative superiors and even going further in institutionalizing rigid adaptive routines. This strategy is in danger of increasing the opposition of the residents to the staff in the cottage. In cottage 2, the administration is conciliated by impressing upon the youngsters the need to conform to the regulations of the institution. This is tempered with an easy-going, semi-delinquent, orientation to the youngsters in which the impression is conveyed that they together must see to it that there is little trouble and maximum conformity.

The old-line counselor in the second cottage uses himself to allay the tension that arises from adaptation to institutional regulations. Instead of communication upward to the institution, the counselor and the resident build up a cumulative joint suspicion of the institution. There is joint resentment at administrative rules. Popularity with the youngsters is purchased at the cost of united opposition to administrative rigidity or ignorance.

Our multiple functional analysis of the cottage care worker's role and the emergent social structure become crucial to the potentiality of autonomous developmental goals that can emerge among the residents. We must give close attention to how functions are originally carried out and how they eventuate in a particular type of cottage social organization. Effective counselors cannot be expected among staff who are surrounded by pressures which undermine their counselor function. In order to inaugurate resident programs and goals, the social forces to which the counselor and the residents must adapt have to be carefully engineered.

In cottage 1, for example, the feedback to the staff is qualitatively different than in the group worker's cottage 3. When the head counselor-educator is not present, his assistants have their hands full maintaining order in the cottage in the way he does. A staff member will not give a boy canteen until he has finished his job and will closely check whether the job has been completed. This results often in a struggle over how well the job has been done. When it is not, the counselor will not give the canteen and hence a bitter struggle emerges between the residents and the staff. One counselor has, in effect, become an "enforcer," to force his will upon the boys when they are not conforming. The whole cottage seems to be struggling around the fulfillment of cottage tasks in a manner appropriate to the high standards established by the head counselor. Not only the residents, but the staff too have their hands full in regulating the cottage according to this prep-school mode. This results in the residents looking upon staff members as "power hungry." Staff-resident integration is on a quid pro-quo basis so that canteens are traded for conformity of the youngsters to the adaptive tasks of the cottage and institution. A recent analysis of attitude and behavior change as related to the exchange structure of superordinate and subordinate is pertinent here.

Herbert C. Kelman has isolated three structures of social influence: compliance, identification and internalization.[16] He focuses upon the nature of the exchange structure in relationship to the meaning of the superordinate's influence upon the subordinate.

Compliance is acceptance of influence by the subordinate because he hopes to achieve a favorable reaction to the other person. He is concerned with attaining specific rewards or in avoiding punishment that the superordinate controls. The critical factor is the superordinate's authority which induces him to behave and evince attitudes that the superordinate wants him to adopt.

Identification, in contrast, is the acceptance of new behavior by the subordinate because the relationship is of a satisfying self-defining character. The subordinate's role vis-a-vis the superordinate is an important part of his self-image and he accepts influence because he wants to maintain the relationship to the superordinate person. The subordinate adopts new behavior and attitudes not because he is compelled to but because of a genuine liking and comfortableness in wanting to be with the superordinate person and to be liked by him. This is close to identification in the classical psychoanalytic sense.

Internalization is influence accepted by the subordinate because it is congruent with his own value system. It is intrinsically rewarding and he adopts it because he finds it useful for the solution of a problem that is congenial to his orientation or demanded by his value perspective. In internalization the subordinate perceives new attitudes and behavior as inherently conducive to the maximization of his own goals and values. The influencing agent plays an important role in internalization but the crucial dimension is the partner's credibility, i.e. his influence is regarded by the subordinate as intimately tied in with his own goals.

Kelman has carefully analyzed the antecedent, intervening and consequent characteristics of each structure of influence. Effective work with youngsters may very well go through these processes in stages. However, our research indicates that the superordinate can create a structure in which one or another of these kinds of influences will predominate by stressing certain functions in his transactions with the youngsters.

In cottages 1 and 2, the head counselor is compelled to adopt an extreme custodial position in order to induce the youngsters to carry out cottage and institutional tasks. The functioning of this role-segment conflicts with the counselor's ability to carry out the other functions in an effective manner. This is quite in contrast to cottage 3, in which the adaptive sphere is of considerably less importance because the head counselor has defined his primary role as counselor: the planning and development of autonomous cottage goals. Thus he uses himself to induce the youngsters to promote their own group goals and methodologies compatible with their needs.

The cottage care worker's role as a man in the middle is analogous to the factory foreman described in sociological literature. A typology of "middle man" roles that the village level worker plays in India has been described by Dubey and Sutton.[17] In their study they found four types of accommodating, conflicting pressures from the powerful administrative hierarchy and the Villagers whose needs they are presumed to serve. These constellations are (1) the link pattern, (2) the block pawn, (3) the Village idol and (4) escape.

The link pattern describes a man who can work with both the Village and the "block" (next higher administrative unit) in such a way as to accomplish his basic function of effectively communicating administrative policy to the Village and Village needs to the administration. The block pawn identifies primarily with administrative superiors and becomes enmeshed in the bureaucratic organization to an extent which keeps him from being sensitive to the welfare of the Village for whose needs he is responsible. The Village idol takes sides with the villagers and is suspicious and even resistant to the administrative program. Finally the escapist resigns or escapes psychologically by acting minimally on behalf of either the block or the village.

These ideal types provide a framework in which to view the counselors in the three senior cottages. The educationally oriented head counselor in cottage 1, who imposes a set of requirements on the boys and devotes a great deal of energy to seeing that they are lived up to, approaches the block pawn in that his major identification is with the upper administrative echelon. This counselor is a model of identification by the boys; he has built up his image with individual talks with the residents—and relating to them by playing ping pong, etc. His goal in forming these attachments is subservient to achievement of greater control. His expressive patterns of relationships are directed toward the ultimate goal of meeting the demands of superior authorities in the institution.

In cottage 2, the non-professional head counselor is a combination of the village idol and escapist. On the one hand he does relate to the boys on the basis of many delinquent values, on the other, he appears not really to side with either the boys or the institution but rather aims toward a mutual adjustment. He is not idolized by the boys nor on the other hand is he awarded much recognition by his administrative superiors. He has been able to work out a pattern of not rocking the boat which is not so unsatisfactory as to cause him to be completely rejected either by the administration or by the boys.

The counselor in cottage 3 has been known to capture the boys by virtue of his demonstration of skills with which they identify—athletic skills, knowledge about jazz music, etc. In addition, the boys are aware that he can fulfill needs because of his connection with the higher administration for physical and other resources. On the other side, administrative recognition that this young man embodies the approach to cottage care which has high prestige in the institution makes these greater resources available to him.

THE NEXT STAGE OF DEVELOPMENT IN INSTITUTIONS

THE total institution constitutes a network of sub-systems designed to bring about effective collaboration among the staff and rehabilitation of the youngsters. Contemporary efforts to design a therapeutic milieu today are focused on the role of the cottage care worker. Paradoxically, for many years, he was the forgotten man in the institution. But he is the only adult in day-to-day direct contact with the youngsters and his functioning conditions the boys' total living situation. The cottage care worker is crucial in bridging the distance between the institution and the youngsters.

The main definition of the cottage care worker's role stems from the institutional structure. He was for many years conceived as a custodian who had a special skill for regulating a controlled integrated life but also had a "feel" for children. The amount of specific training designed for the cottage care worker varied in institutions but in most is still unsystematic. The fact of the matter is that he is often "trained" by professionals who have no intimate contact with cottage life. Since he cottage care worker is directly dependent upon administrative superiors, the pressures stemming from the administration for controlling the youngsters are of crucial importance.

Today his role is conceived as multi-functional. He must perform the custodial dimension. He must be sensitive to the emotional disturbances of individual youngsters. He is now becoming trained to think through the atmosphere in the cottage which is most conducive to enabling the youngsters to constructively cooperate. He also must be skilled in enabling the youngsters to formulate goals, to become motivated toward attaining them and to helping them coordinate their efforts to achieve them.[18] Any efforts designed to help the cottage attain autonomous goals must flow from an understanding of the felt needs and interests of the residents. Needless to say, he can help the cottage achieve goals only by gaining ample "back-stopping" by other personnel. The most important tendency he must overcome both within himself and among the residents is the expectation that the institution provides everything and that the residents are essentially passive, conforming dependents.

How can the institution imbue the cottage care workers with goals and methods of working with residents in a grass-roots manner? His low subordinate status in the administrative hierarchy is geared toward emphasis of control. A wide-spread acceptance of the multifunctional definition of his role may facilitate his effort to organize his tasks within a more coherent and effective pattern. Thus he must learn how to implement his function within the cottage of helping it attain autonomous goals by more effective communication upward to administrators in the institution.

Hence, he must think through the following issues: how much obedience is expected from the administrative bureaucracy; how does he resolve difficulties of enabling the group to attain goals and the rigid structure in which the cottage must function; how does he work out a balance among his multiple functions; and how does he resolve the conflict in influencing the cottage toward autonomous goals and changing the expectations of the institution?

It is clear in our analysis of the different adjustment patterns of cottage care workers that each emphasis derives from the strengths the head counselor develops to handle adaptive and goal problems that are imposed by the marginality of his position. The cottage worker must strive to match the level of interest and motivation and resources in the cottage with opportunities to exploit new patterns in the institution. This involves calculated risks. In Appendix I two documents are presented from our files which illustrate (A) the ambitious desires of a small group of senior boys to radically extend their areas of decision-making in the institution and (B) the administration's determination to sharply curb both cottage staff and residents' autonomous functioning.

The next stage of institutional development lies in the direction of developing a perspective of residential treatment in which the resident groups are afforded an opportunity to plan and execute goals stemming from their own interests and needs. In several total institution settings, this program is being advanced. Two outstanding examples are Jones' therapeutic milieu[19] and the program of sociotherapy initiated by Paul Daniel Sivadon in France.[20] The latter is especially perceptive about the need to promote autonomous goals by resident groups.

Sivadon asserts that one of the main problems of residents in institutions is the great amount of time that lays heavily on their hands. Furthermore, there are always gripes and complaints that the residents have about the restrictions of their freedom and their ability to plan and attain goals. The basic need of overcoming passivity within the controlled authoritarian environment is attained by provoking the residents into meeting their gripes by positive and constructive group activity. In fact, he has asserted that the most important function of the resident-counselor is to incite the residents to work out their complaints in positive programs of group action. If it is boring for the residents, they should be helped to voice their complaints, but also encouraged to take the next step in planning a program which can overcome the ennui. This has the advantage of using group process not only for developing programs but also for enabling the residents to work more effectively with each other. Through these activities they learn from their own errors and instead of projecting their impotency onto the institution and an enervating intra-institutional conflict, they are forced to look more at their own individual and joint functioning, to locate their inadequacies and develop strategies for overcoming them.

Sivadon's program essentially guides the group worker's activity in cottage 3. He is very familiar with Sivadon's work and spends most of his time thinking through programs which he and his assistants can enable the youngsters to follow through.

Cottages 1 and 2 cannot attain new orbits because they are stuck in the adaptational sphere. The imposition upon the youngsters of carrying out the cottage tasks influences the entire social functioning of the cottage system. There is an over-emphasis upon the institutional value of maintaining a stable and orderly cottage and a corresponding de-emphasis of the counselor-role enabling the youngsters to promote autonomous goals.

The crystallization of the adaptive function results in a spiralling effect in which imposition upon the youngsters results in resentment which further rigidifies the counselor's attempts to make the youngsters conform. The primary emphasis upon adaptive tasks results in the cottage orbiting about the problem of maintaining order. They try to offset this through an informal easy-going, joking relationship with semi-delinquent overtones in one cottage, and, individual alter-therapy sessions in the other. What is overlooked in these two cottages is the possibility of enabling the youngsters to formulate and carry through on autonomous cottage and sub-group goals which are related to their individual and collective needs. Thus each head counselor institutes a regime which has a multiplier effect upon certain kinds of investments. The growth and crystallization of a significant function is the degree to which that activity is channelled from the receivers, the residents, back to the formulators, the counselors. But in cottage 3, the process has been reversed. Instead of the counselors imposing upon the youngsters the execution of cottage tasks, the youngsters themselves are urged to formulate and carry through goals and the counselors use themselves to enable the youngsters to meet these goals.

The differences in the cottages are revealed in how the counselor's assistants are deployed. In cottages 1 and 2, the difficulties emerging around maintaining a stable cottage have so grown and multiplied that the assistants are also utilized to maintain this basic order. This only increases the feeling of constraint that the youngsters have and the attitude of being surrounded, controlled and/or attacked by the counselors. In cottage 3, on the other hand, the assistants have been increasingly used as assistant group workers who enable the youngsters to meet autonomous cottage goals. Thus, as the goal-attainment sphere grows in importance, the staff members are increasingly utilized to increase the potency of this functional sphere. Our general observation seems to support the view that this is the most effective way to induce youngsters to adopt more positive values and behavior. It is in line with a conclusion stated by Sherif after extensive research with adolescent groups:[21]

The crux of the matter for effective policy and action is not the busy-work as such, not the programmed activities *as such*, or even the end-products of training to exhibit for public display. The cardinal point is to insure throughout (whatever the activities) the youth's feeling of having a *function* in their initiation, development, and execution.

What we do not take part in initiating and developing and producing, what we engage in without our own choosing and aspiring, is not felt as ours. What we do not feel as ours lacks in the experience of inner-urgency and in sense of responsibility. The important thing to actualize at the very start is not immediate technical proficiency, but the feeling of participation, the feeling that we have functions of a larger scale of things, the feeling that we have indispensable roles with others in things that all feel should be done.

Thus we see in the third pattern of adjustment the social group worker's main function is to link the youth's needs with a dynamic reciprocal impact upon the institution. This means that his function is not merely having the cottage adapt to institutional regulations, but the creation with youths of goals that they can attain within the authoritarian setting. This means that the worker must have influence with the administration to carry on within and outside of the cottage a variety of goals that are primarily planned and executed by the youngsters for themselves.

APPENDIX

H.R.S.

Hollymede Resistance Society
Aims and Purposes:

Our primary purpose is, simply, the resistance of authority.

We will resist authority whenever and wherever we feel that power to be abused.

We will publish articles and other thought pieces aimed at stimulating thought and debate among our fellow HRS students.

Our Aims and Purposes:

An end to compulsory religious observance.

Greater freedom to achieve intellectual stimulation, i.e. access to books, lectures, theatre, etc.

An end to compulsory education.

An end to the school-cottage conflict, which leaves students little or no time for academic pursuits.

An end to the unnatural separation of males and females.

An end to student pressure on other students and the molestation of aforesaid students.

An end to campus fighting and instigating.

An end to regimentation and unfair group punishment.

An end to all student discrimination.

The allowance of students to dress and comport themselves according to the limitations of society, not the unnatural regulations imposed by Hollymede.

In order to facilitate the accomplishment of these ends, we purpose to establish a forum for student discussion of common problems and ideas to be reviewed by staff. We also intend to nominate and support an H.R.S. candidate in the next student council election.

APPENDIX

HOLLYMEDE SCHOOL
Hollymede, New York

April 23, 1964

To: All Staff and Student

From: Assistant Director

I wish to share my observations and feelings about conditions in this school at this time. I note with dismay an untherapeutic atmosphere. Students are impudent, disrespectful, and many of them behave as if they were ignorant of the philosophy and structure of this institution. Many staff members permit students to act in an undisciplined and disrespectful manner. The response of the adult to the student has been inadequate. There is a failure on the part of the adult to recognize or respond to the seriousness of these situations. This failure on the part of the adult reflects a neglect of parental responsibility. Where children violate school rules and the adults do not respond nor do they take action in these situations—we have in effect neglected children. It is our responsibility to teach children right from wrong. It is wrong to be non-judgmental in the treatment of children. We should teach good manners.

What we teach is accomplished within a framework of routines and regulations which we accept as helpful. There is neglect of many of these routines by many staff members. For example, the pass system is being neglected. We do not fill out line up slips correctly. The system of accountability is not taken seriously.

To correct some of these defects I will repeat in this note some of the rules and regulations to be followed:

1. No child is permitted to go from one place to another without a pass, unless supervised directly by a staff member.
2. Line up slips are to be filled out correctly, and the child care person responsible for that slip shall record only those students who are physically present. These line up slips are to be made out in the morning when students are transferred from the responsibility of child care people to school personnel. A slip is to be made out at 3 p.m., and given to the O.D.

It has been brought to my attention that there is neglect of accountability. In some situations students have run away and it has taken two or three hours for child care people to report such incidents. I will ask that the O.D. call in the evening and that we have cottage checks at unannounced times.

The student population has misinterpreted the recreation program philosophy. At this time we have a very full program, and hope to add to it. However, students have abused the privileges granted to them. There is much wandering in the evening and violation of our trust to the point that I feel that something drastic must be done. If the student population continues to abuse the privileges I will cancel all after-school activities, all off-grounds recreation trips, and will assign staff directly to the cottages. I am informing the Unit Supervisors that all violations of rules and of common decency are to be reported to me. I will review the punishments given by the Unit Administrators. I will also order appropriate personnel at this school to bring to the attention of Courts such behavior as absconding, out of place, disrespect, and use of abusive language. Students at this school are to obey lawful, reasonable orders of the adults. It is within the realm of possibility that I will bring a complaint to a judge and ask that children who do not obey such requests and orders be considered as persons who committed delinquent acts.

The students not only misinterpret rules but make their own. There is no unwritten law that says a new student has a right to run away once or twice. Every runaway is a serious offense and is against the law of the state of New York. It is to be dealt with by the staff of this school in a most serious manner and there is to be a consequence. The consequence preferred by me is dismissal from the school and return to Court. There are certain rules at this school which I feel are most important, and I will not compromise with the consequences that are to be meted out for the following offences:

1. Assault of a staff member.
2. Illicit boy-girl relationships, boys going to girls' cottages and girls going to boys' cottages.
3. Students bringing pills or other drugs and alcohol to the school and giving them to other students.

I consider the above offences reasons for expulsion from this school and return to Court.

The looseness, lack of control I see is alarming. Our failure to listen to children and their requests for controls is equal to parental neglect and is also a rejection of children. We cannot be ignorant of the movements and whereabouts of our students. We all have different responsibilities, but some are common to all staff members. One of these is acceptance of the importance of accountability.

XX:zz

NOTES TO CHAPTER 6

1. William James, *The Principles of Psychology,* quoted in *Human Behavior,* Bernard Berelson and Gary A. Steiner, Harcourt, Brace & World, Inc., New York, 1964, p. 132.
2. For recent descriptions of structural-functional theory see the following: Bernard Barber, "Structual-Functional Analysis: Problems of Misunderstanding," *American Sociological Review,* Vol. 21, No. 2, April 1956, p. 131; Harold Fallding, "Functional Analysis in Sociology," *American Sociological Review,* Vol. 28, No. 1, February 1963; Walter Buckley, "Structural-Functional Analysis in Modern Sociology" in *Modern Sociological Theory,* ed., Howard Becker and Alvin Boskoff, The Dryden Press, New York, 1957; Ernest Nagel, Chapter 10, "A Formalization of Functionalism," *Logic Without Metaphysics,* Free Press, Glencoe, Ill., 1956, pp. 247-287; Carl G. Hempel, Chapter 9, *"The Logic of Functional Analysis,"* Symposium on Sociological Theory, ed., Llewellyn Gross, Roe, Peterson and Co., New York, 1959, pp. 271-311; Howard W. Polsky, "Structural-Functional Theory: Guide Line to Group Work," Group Work Section Meetings, 1962-1963, Group Work Section, New York City Chapter, National Association of Social Workers.
3. Paul W. Kurtz, "Human Nature, Homeostasis and Value," *Philosophical and Phenomenological Res.,* XVII, No. 1, Sept. 36-55.
4. Robert K. Merton, "Social Problems and Sociological Theory," in Robert K. Merton and Robert A. Nesbet, *Contemporary Social Problems.* N.Y.: Harcourt Brace and World, 1961, pp. 697-737.
5. See for example *The Adolescent Society,* James S. Coleman, The Free Press of Glencoe, New York, 1961, pp. 311-329.
6. J. W. Getzels and P. W. Jackson, "The Study of Giftedness: a Multi-dimensional Approach," in *The Gifted Student,* Cooperative Research Monograph #2, U.S. Department of Health, Education and Welfare, U.S. Government Printing Office, Washington, 1960, pp. 1-18.
7. Writer unidentified, quote taken from *The New York Times,* "The News of the Week in Review," Sunday, April 5, 1964, E 7, column 6.

8. Oscar Lewis, *Five Families*, Science Editions, Inc., New York, 1962.
9. Robert D. Hess and Gerald Handel, *Family Worlds*, The University of Chicago Press, 1959, p. 141.
10. Robert F. Bales and Philip E. Slater, "Role Differentiation in Small De-cision-Making Groups" in Talcott Parsons and Robert F. Bales, *Family, Socialization and Interaction Process*, Free Press, Glencoe, Ill., 1955; Robert F. Bales, "The Equilibrium Problem in Small Groups" in *Working Papers in the Theory of Action*. Talcott Parsons, Robert F. Bales and Edward A. Shils. The Free Press, Glencoe, Illinois, 1953, pp. 112-161. Robert F. Bales, "Task Status and Likeability as a Function of Talking and Listening in Decision-Making Groups," in L. D. Whyte, ed., *The State of the Social Sciences*, Chicago, 1956, pp. 148-161.
11. Talcott Parsons, "General Theory in Sociology," *Sociology Today*, eds., Robert K. Merton, Leonard Bromm and Leonard S. Cottrell, Jr., Basic Books, New York, 1959.
12. Howard W. Polsky, "Three Models of Transaction for Social Work," paper read at Field Supervisors Conference, Columbia University School of Social Work, March 1964, mimeographed.
13. Lloyd E. Ohlin, Herman Pevin and Donnell M. Pappenfort, "Major Dilem-mas of the Social Worker in Probation and Parole," in *Social Perspectives on Behavior*, eds., Herman D. Stein and Richard A. Cloward, The Free Press of Glencoe, Inc., New York, pp. 251-260.
14. For an excellent discussion on the concept of *theme*, see Robert D. Hess and Gerald Handel, *Family Worlds*, The University of Chicago Press, 1959, pp. 11, ff; see also Henry A. Murray et al., *Explorations in Personality*, New York, Oxford University Press, 1938, and Morris Opler, "Themes as Dy-namic Forces in Culture," *American Journal of Sociology*, LI, 198-206.
15. Howard W. Polsky, *Cottage Six*, Russell Sage Foundation, New York, 1962.
16. Herbert C. Kelman, "Processes of Opinion Change," *Public Opinion Quarterly*, Spring 1961.
17. D. C. Dubey and Willis A. Sutton, Jr., "A Rural Man-in-the-Middle: the Indian Village Level Worker in Community Development," paper read at the August 1962 Meeting of the Rural Sociological Society.
18. Howard W. Polsky, "A Social System Approach to Residential Treatment," to be published in *Group Work in Institutions*, ed. Henry Maier.
19. Maxwell Jones, *The Therapeutic Community*, Basic Books, New York.
20. Paul Daniel Sivadon, "Techniques of Sociotherapy," *Psychiatry*, Vol. 20, No. 3, August 1957.
21. Muzafer Sherif and Carolyn W. Sherif, *Reference Groups*, Harper & Row, New York, 1964, pp. 314-315.

ह≈

CHAPTER 7   The Physician and Patient
as a Social System*

L. J. HENDERSON

MEDICINE is to-day in part an applied science. Mathematics, physics, chemistry, and many departments of biology find applications in this hospital and in the practice of all skillful physicians. Meanwhile, the personal relations between the physician and the patient remain nearly what they have always been. To these relations, as yet, science has been little applied, and it is unlikely that the men in this room are upon the whole as much concerned about their personal relations with patients as a similar group of Boston doctors must have been in the days of James Jackson. A multitude of important new facts and theories, of new methods and routines, so far absorb the physician's attention and arouse his interest that the personal relations seem to have become less important, if not absolutely, at least relatively to the new and powerful technology of medical practice. This condition, for which nobody is to blame, might perhaps be modified if it were possible to apply to practice a science of human relations. But such a science is barely growing into the stage where applications are possible.

The psychologists and sociologists are the professional custodians of what little scientific knowledge we possess that is conversant with personal relations. But from them we have, as yet, little to learn, for they are in general little aware of the problem of practicing what they know in the affairs of everyday life. Indeed, skill in managing one's relations with others is probably less common among professional psychologists and sociologists than among the ablest men of affairs or the wisest physicians. So the personal relations of the physician with his patients and with their

* An address delivered at the Harvard Medical School Colloquium, Vanderbilt Hall, December 20, 1934, and at a Medical Staff Meeting, Massachusetts General Hospital, January 21, 1935.

Reprinted from the *New England Journal of Medicine*, 222 (1935), 819–823, by permission of the *Journal*.

families are still understood, when they are understood, at the empirical level, as they were in the days of Hippocrates. Such skill is not only empirical but it is also, as we vaguely say, intuitive. Sometimes in those favored persons whose perceptions and sensibilities are well suited to the task, it results in patterns of behavior that are among the most interesting and, if I may use the word, beautiful that I know. As I came into this room, I was saying that if Dr. Frederick Shattuck could only be here he, who knew so much more about my subject than I shall ever know, would have been able after I had finished to say many things to you and to me. Doctors like him have always existed and will always exist, but their skill dies with them except when their apprentices have learned in some measure to imitate them.

The necessary condition for the effective transmission of acquired knowledge seems to be scientific formulation, and for this purpose some kind of theory, working hypothesis, or conceptual scheme is necessary. In this way the natural sciences are preserved and transmitted, and the rôle of scientific laws and generalizations is seen to be not merely economy of thought, as Mach said, but also the effective remembering of the successful and economical thought of the past. A well learned theory is remembered in the right place at the right time, and this is a necessary condition for its use. Accordingly my first subject is the theory of the relation between physician and patient.

* * * *

Four centuries ago, Machiavelli was thinking of certain great problems of human society and writing two famous books. In so doing, he reached scientific generalizations about the influence of the sentiments upon the actions of men and, through these actions, upon the fate of human societies. As a whole, these conclusions stand; but from this great and ingenious work of Machiavelli's almost no developments have followed. The science of statecraft and of the influence of the sentiments upon human behavior is little different to-day from what it was in Florence in the 16th century.

In the following century, another Florentine, Galileo, published his "Dialogues on Two New Sciences." From this work a great part of modern science has grown out. The two men were perhaps equal in ability and in originality. Why has the influence of one been small and that of the other inestimably great?

In seeking a partial answer to this question, I ask you to consider the names of the subjects that are taught in modern universities, and to divide them, so far as may be, into two classes: first, history, politics, economics, sociology, law, literature, etc.; secondly, logic, mathematics, physics, chemistry, biology, grammar, harmony, etc. Most subjects will fall well enough into one or the other of these two classes. Next I ask you to consider the behavior of the professors who cultivate the two classes of subjects. Those who are adepts of subjects of the second class, when they differ, commonly do so at the frontiers of knowledge, where growth occurs. Moreover, their differences are ordinarily settled by observation, experiment, mathematical calculation, and logical analysis. But in the subjects of the first class differences of opinion occur at all points, and frequently they cannot be resolved. The differences and the disputes seem to be interminable, and there is often no accepted method of reaching a conclusion.

Such a contrast between the behavior of the skilful devotees of the two classes of subjects must depend in part upon differences in the nature of the two classes of subjects, for we cannot admit that a natural selection of professors so nearly perfect as to produce this striking result should occur. Now there is, in fact, one difference between the two classes of subjects which, as I think, is sufficient in a rough approximation to explain the phenomenon. The subjects of the second class do not, in general, consider the interrelations of two or more persons. The subjects of the first class always consider the interrelations of two or more persons. Thus in history, politics, economics, sociology, law, literature, etc., the interrelations and interactions of people are always concerned, but in logic, mathematics, physics, chemistry, biology, grammar, harmony, etc., except perhaps in certain subjects on the borders of biology, they are ruled out. Perhaps this distinction also goes far to explain the curious condition of psychology in our own time. At any rate I am persuaded that it goes far to explain why we have little more than empirical knowledge about the relations of physician and patient.

* * * *

Willard Gibbs's generalized physico-chemical system is possibly the most famous piece of scientific work that has been done by an American. According to Gibbs, any arbitrarily isolated portion of the material universe may be regarded as a physico-chemical system. In a first approximation, it may be characterized as follows: A physico-chemical system is made up of components. Components are individual chemical substances such as water, salt, etc. They exist in phases. Phases are physically homogeneous parts of the system, either solid, or liquid, or gaseous such as ice, a salt solution, or air. The system is further distinguished by the concentration of the components in the phases, by its temperature, and by its pressure. For many purposes no other factors need be considered.

The Italian sociologist, Pareto, formerly professor at the University of Lausanne, has described a generalized social system which may be usefully compared with Gibbs's physico-chemical system. Pareto's social system is made up of individuals. They are perhaps analogous to the components of Gibbs's system. The individuals are heterogeneous, that is, unequal. They are unequal in size and in age. There are two sexes. They have different educations. They belong to different social and economic classes, to different institutions, to different social structures. They suffer from different pathological conditions, and their mental differences are different far beyond our computation and description. This heterogeneity suggests the heterogeneity of solid, liquid, and gaseous phases in the physico-chemical system.

These individuals possess, or at least manifest, sentiments. I implore you not to ask me to define the word sentiment, but to permit me to use it without definition to include in its meaning a variety of mental states. For example, I desire to solve a problem; that is a sentiment. You have a feeling that the constitution of the United States should be preserved; that is a sentiment. Affection for the members of your family is a sentiment. The feeling of personal integrity is a sentiment. The desire to express your gratitude for a kindness is a sentiment. The sexual complexes of psychoanalysts, even though they may be unconscious, are for my purpose sentiments.

The individuals who make up social systems also have economic interests, and they have and use language. This use of language is sometimes a non-logical manifestation of sentiments. For example, I read the other day the following title of a sermon, posted up in front of a church in a New England town, "One on God's side is a majority." Language is also sometimes used, though less often than we fondly suppose, to perform logical operations and to express their results.

A physician and a patient make up a social system. And that is my first point.

Many of you, I fear, will think this introduction singularly irrelevant to the subject of my discourse, and so vague and general that it can hardly be of any use in the premises. To them I venture to suggest that it is possible that they may be mistaken, and I ask them to try to follow what I now have to say receptively, postponing criticism until they have received my whole statement.

* * * *

Two persons, if no more are present, make up a social system. These individuals are heterogeneous. They have and are moved by sentiments and interests. They talk and reason. That is a definition. I shall now state a theorem. In any social system the sentiments and the interactions of the sentiments are likely to be the most important phenomena. And that is my second point. Sometimes the interaction of the sentiments of the individuals making up a social system is hardly less important than gravitational attraction in the solar system.

In the eighteenth century, before a wave of sentimentality swept over the western world, some people saw human relations pretty clearly. They had not been brought up on Rousseau and others whose writings have continued down almost to the present time to influence the intellectual atmosphere in which men have formed this habit of thought. Among the more successful eighteenth century observers of the mechanism of human behavior was Lord Chesterfield. From one of his letters to his son I venture to quote:

"I acquainted you in a former letter, that I had brought a bill into the House of Lords for correcting and reforming our present calendar, which is the Julian; and for adopting the Gregorian. I will now give you a more particular account of that affair; from which reflections will naturally occur to you, that I hope may be useful, and which I fear you have not made. It was notorious, that the Julian calendar was erroneous, and had overcharged the solar year with eleven days. Pope Gregory the Thirteenth corrected this error; his reformed calendar was immediately received by all the Catholic Powers in Europe, and afterwards adopted by all the Protestant ones, except Russia, Sweden, and England. It was not, in my opinion, very honourable for England to remain in a gross and avowed error, especially in such company; the inconveniency of it was likewise felt by all those who had foreign correspondences, whether political or mercantile. I determined, therefore, to attempt the reformation; I consulted the best lawyers and the most skilful astronomers, and we cooked up a bill for that purpose. But then my difficulty began: I was to bring in this bill, which was necessarily composed of law jargon and astronomical calculations, to both which I am an utter stranger. However, it was absolutely necessary to make the House of Lords think that I knew something of the matter; and also to make them believe that they knew something of it themselves, which they do not. For my own part, I could just as soon have talked Celtic or Sclavonian to them, as astronomy, and they would have understood me full as well: so I resolved to do better than speak to the purpose, and to please instead of informing them. I gave them, therefore, only an historical account of calendars, from the Egyptian down to the Gregorian, amusing them now and then with little episodes; but I was particularly attentive to the choice of my words, to the harmony and roundness of my periods, to my elocution, to my action. This succeeded, and ever will succeed; they thought I informed, because I pleased them; and many of them said, that I had made the whole very clear to them; when, God knows, I had not even attempted it. Lord Macclesfield, who had the greatest share in forming the bill, and who is one of the greatest mathematicians and astronomers in Europe, spoke afterwards with infinite knowledge, and all the clearness that so intricate a matter would admit of: but as his words, his periods, and his utterance, were not near so good as mine, the preference was most unanimously, though most unjustly, given to me. This will ever be the case; every numerous assembly is *mob*, let the individuals who compose it be what they will. Mere reason and good sense is never to be talked to a mob; their passions, their sentiments, their senses, and their seeming interests, are alone to be appealed to. Understanding they have collectively none, but they have ears and eyes, which must be flattered and seduced; and this can only be done by eloquence, tuneful periods, graceful action, and all the various parts of oratory."

It is not only to a mob that reason and good sense cannot effectively be talked. A patient sitting in your office, facing you, is rarely in a favorable state of mind to appreciate the precise significance of a logical statement, and it is in general not merely difficult but quite impossible for him to perceive the precise meaning of a train of thought. It is also out of the question that the physician should convey what he desires to convey to the patient, if he follows the practice of blurting out just what comes into his mind. The patient is moved by fears and by many other sentiments, and these, together with reason, are being modified by the doctor's words and phrases, by his manner and expression. This generalization appears to me to be as well founded as the generalizations of physical science.

If so far I am right, I think it is fair to set up a precept that follows from all this as a rule of conduct: The physician should see to it that the patient's sentiments do not act upon his sentiments and, above all, do not thereby modify his behavior, and he should endeavor to act upon the patient's sentiments according to a well-considered plan. And that is my third point.

I believe that this assertion may be regarded as an application of science to the practice of medicine, and that as such it will bear comparison with the applications of physics, chemistry, and biology to practice. However, in this case the application of science to practice is peculiarly difficult. If I am to speak about it, I must in the first place beg explicitly to disclaim any skill of my own. It is not my business to deal with patients, nor has it been my business to perform that kind of operation that Chesterfield so well describes in his letter. Accordingly, what I am now to say to you is, in the main, second-hand knowledge that I have cribbed from others.[1] It represents, so far as I can understand what I have seen and heard, the soundest judgment based upon experience, skillful performance and clear analysis in this field. In order to be brief and clear, I shall permit myself the luxury of plain assertion.

In talking with the patient, the doctor must not only appear to be, but must be, really interested in what the patient says. He must not suggest or imply judgments of value or of morals concerning the patient's report to him or concerning the patient's behavior. (To this there is one exception: When the patient successfully presents a difficult objective report of his experiences, it is useful to praise him for doing well what it is necessary that he should do in order to help the physician to help him.) In all those matters that concern the psychological aspects of the patient's experience few questions should be asked and, above all, no leading questions. There should be no argument about the prejudices of the patient, for, at any stage, when you are endeavoring to evoke the subjective aspect of the patient's experience or to modify his sentiments, logic will not avail. In order to modify the sentiments of the patient, your logical analysis must somehow be transformed into the appropriate change of the patient's sentiments. But sentiments are resistant to change. For this reason, you must so far as possible utilize some part of the sentiments that the patient has in order to modify his subjective attitude.

When you talk with the patient, you should listen, first, for what he wants to tell, secondly, for what he does not want to tell, thirdly, for what he cannot tell. He does not want to tell the things the telling of which is shameful or painful. He cannot tell you his implicit assumptions that are unknown to him, such as the assumption that all action not perfectly good is bad, such as the assumption that everything that is not perfectly successful is failure, such as the assumption that everything that is not perfectly safe is dangerous. We are all of us subject to errors of this kind, to the assumption that quantitative differences are qualitative. Perhaps the commonest false dichotomy of the hypochondriac is the last of those that I have just mentioned: the assumption that everything not perfectly safe is dangerous.

When you listen for what the patient does not want to tell and for what he cannot tell you must take especial note of his omissions, for it is the things that he fails to say that correspond to what he does not want to say plus what he cannot say. In listening for these omissions, which is a difficult task, you must make use of every aid that is available. Among the available aids are the results of psychoanalysis. Many of them are well established; but if you wish to preserve a scientific point of view, you must beware of psychoanalytical theories. Use these theories, if you must use them, with skepticism, but do not believe them, for they are themselves in no small measure rationalizations built up by an eager group of enthusiastic students who are unquestionably seeking new knowledge, but whose attitude is strangely modified by a quasi-religious enthusiasm, and by a devotion to the corresponding quasi-theological dogmas. As a useful corrective for undue confidence in the importance of such theories, it is well to recall Henri Poincaré's judicious and skeptical remark: "These two propositions, 'the external world exists,' or, 'it is more convenient to suppose that it exists,' have one and the same meaning." In truth, all theories, but above all others those that refer to the sentiments of men, must be used with care and skepticism.

Therefore, beware of your own arbitrary assumptions. Beware of the expression of your own feelings. In general, both are likely to be harmful, or at least irrelevant, except as they are used to encourage and to cheer the patient. Beware of the expression of moral judgments. Beware of bare statements of bare truth or bare logic. Remember especially that the principal effect of a sentence of confinement or of death is an emotional effect, and that the patient will eagerly scrutinize and rationalize what you say, that he will carry it away with him, that he will turn your phrases over and over in his mind, seeking persistently for shades of meaning that you never thought of. Try to remember how as a very young man you have similarly scrutinized for non-existent meaning the casual phrases of those whom you have admired, or respected, or loved.

Above all, remember that it is meaningless to speak of telling the truth, the whole truth, and nothing but the truth, to a patient. It is meaningless because it is impossible;—a sheer impossibility. Since this assertion is likely to be subjected to both objective and subjective criticism, it will be well that I should try to explain it. I know of no other way to explain it than by means of an example. Let us scrutinize this example, so far as we may be able, objectively, putting aside all our habits of moralistic thought that we acquired in early years and that arise from the theological and metaphysical traditions of our civilization.

Consider the statement, "This is a carcinoma." Let us assume in the first place that the statement has been made by a skillful and experienced pathologist, that he has found a typical carcinoma—in short, that the diagnosis is as certain as it ever can be. Let us also put aside the consideration that no two carcinomas are alike, that no two patients are alike, and that, at one extreme, death may be rapid and painful or, at another extreme, there may be but a small prospect of death from cancer. In short, let us assume, putting aside all such considerations, that the statement has nearly the same validity as the assertions contained in the nautical almanac. If we now look at things, not from the standpoint of philosophers, moralists, or lawyers, but from the standpoint of biologists, we may regard the statement as a stimulus applied to the patient. This stimulus will produce a response and the response, together with the mechanism that is involved in its production, is an extremely complex one, at least in those cases where a not too vague cognition of the meaning of the four words is involved in the process. For instance, there are likely to be circulatory and respiratory changes accompanying many complex changes in the central and peripheral nervous system. With the cognition there is a correlated fear. There will probably be concern for the economic interests of others, for example, of wife and children. All these intricate processes constitute the response to the stimulus made up of the four words, "This is a carcinoma," in case the statement is addressed by the physician to the patient, and it is obviously impossible to produce in the patient cognition without the accompanying affective phenomena and without concern for the economic interests. I suggest, in view of these obvious facts, that, if you recognize the duty of telling the truth to the patient, you range yourself outside the class of biologists, with lawyers, and philosophers. The idea that the truth, the whole truth, and nothing but the truth can be conveyed to the patient is an example of false abstraction, of that fallacy called by Whitehead, "The fallacy of misplaced concreteness." It results from neglecting factors that cannot be excluded from the concrete situation and that have an effect that cannot be neglected. Another fallacy also is involved, the belief that it is not too difficult to know the truth; but of this I shall not speak further.

I beg that you will not suppose that I am recommending, for this reason, that you should always lie to your patients. Such a conclusion from what I have said would correspond roughly to a class of fallacies that I have already referred to above. Since telling the truth is impossible, there can be no sharp distinction between what is true and what is false. But surely that does not relieve the physician of his moral responsibility. On the contrary, the difficulties that arise from the immense complexity of the phenomena do not diminish, but rather increase, the moral responsibility of the physician, and one of my objects has been to describe the facts through which the nature of that moral responsibility is determined.

Far older than the precept, "the truth, the whole truth, and nothing but the truth," is another that originates within our profession, that has always been the guide of the best physicians, and, if I may venture a prophecy, will always remain so: So far as possible, "do no harm." You can do harm by the process that is quaintly called telling the truth. You can do harm by lying. In your relations with your patients you will inevitably do much harm, and this will be by no means confined to your strictly medical blunders. It will arise also from what you say and what you fail to say. But try to do as little harm as possible, not only in treatment with drugs, or with the knife, but also in treatment with words, with the expression of your sentiments and emotions. Try at all times to act upon the patient so as to modify his sentiments to his own advantage, and remember that, to this end, nothing is more effective than arousing in him the belief that you are concerned whole-heartedly and exclusively for *his* welfare.

What I have said does not conform in my manner of saying it to the rules that I have suggested for your relations with patients. I have tried to talk reason and good sense to you, following, so far as I have been able, the habits of a lecturer upon scientific subjects. With some of you I have surely failed to accomplish my object. To them I suggest that this failure is an excellent illustration of the phenomena that I have been describing, for, unless I am mistaken, if you dislike what I have said, it is chiefly because I have failed to appeal to and make use of your sentiments.

NOTE TO CHAPTER 7

1. I owe my information to my colleagues, Professors Elton Mayo, F. J. Roethlisberger, and their associates. The theory and practice of interviewing developed by Mayo were applied and adapted with the advice and collaboration of the Harvard Department of Industrial Research by the Western Electric Company in the course of an elaborate investigation at the Hawthorne Works of the Company. A valuable description of these Western Electric methods of interviewing may be found in Bingham and Moore's *How to Interview*, New York, 1931; Second Edition, 1935. In all this it is possible to discern more than traces of the methods of psychoanalysis, divested however of the usual theoretical and dogmatic accompaniments, and therefore considerably modified.

CHAPTER 8   The Basic Models of the

Doctor-Patient Relationship*

THOMAS S. SZASZ AND MARC H. HOLLENDER

INTRODUCTION

WHEN a person leaves the culture in which he was born and raised and migrates to another, he usually experiences his new social setting as something strange—and in some ways threatening—and he is stimulated to master it by conscious efforts at understanding. To some extent every immigrant to the United States reacts in this manner to the American scene. Similarly, the American tourist in Europe or South America "scrutinizes" the social setting which is taken for granted by the natives. To scrutinize—and criticize—the pattern of other peoples' lives is obviously both common and easy. It also happens, however, that people exposed to cross cultural experiences turn their attention to the very customs which formed the social matrix of their lives in the past. Lastly, to study the "customs" which shape and govern one's day-to-day life is most difficult of all.[1]

In many ways the psychoanalyst is like a person who has migrated from one culture to another. To him the relationship between physician and patient—which is like a custom that is taken for granted in medical practice and which he himself so treated in his early history—has become an object of study. While the precise nature and extent of the influence which psychoanalysis and so-called dynamic psychiatry have had on modern medicine are debatable, it seems to us that the most decisive effect has been that of making physicians explicitly aware of the possible significance of their relationship to patients.

The question naturally arises as to "What is a doctor-patient relationship?" It is our aim to discuss this question and to show that certain

* Reprinted from the *Archives of Internal Medicine*, May, 1956, Vol. 97, pp. 585–592 (copyright 1956, by American Medical Association), by permission of the authors and the journal.

philosophical preconceptions associated with the notions of "disease," "treatment," and "cure" have a profound bearing on both the theory and the practice of medicine.[2]

WHAT IS A HUMAN RELATIONSHIP?

THE concept of a relationship is a novel one in medicine. Traditionally, physicians have been concerned with "things," for example, anatomical structures, lesions, bacteria, and the like. In modern times the scope has been broadened to include the concept of "function." The phenomenon of a human relationship is often viewed as though it were a "thing" or a "function." It is, in fact, neither. Rather it is an abstraction, appropriate for the description and handling of certain observational facts. Moreover, it is an abstraction which presupposes concepts of both structure and function.

TABLE 1.
Three Basic Models of the Physician-Patient Relationship

MODEL	PHYSICIAN'S ROLE	PATIENT'S ROLE	CLINICAL APPLICATION OF MODEL	PROTOTYPE OF MODEL
1. Activity-passivity	Does something to patient	Recipient (unable to respond or inert)	Anesthesia, acute trauma, coma, delirium, etc.	Parent-infant
2. Guidance-cooperation	Tells patient what to do	Cooperator (obeys)	Acute infectious processes, etc.	Parent-child (adolescent)
3. Mutual participation	Helps patient to help himself	Participant in "partnership" (uses expert help)	Most chronic illnesses, psychoanalysis, etc.	Adult-adult

The foregoing comments may be clarified by concrete illustrations. Psychiatrists often suggest to their medical colleagues that the physician's relationship with his patient "per se" helps the latter. This creates the impression (whether so intended or not) that the relationship is a thing, which works not unlike the way that vitamins do in a case of vitamin deficiency. Another idea is that the doctor-patient relationship depends mainly on what the physician does (or thinks or feels). Then it is viewed not unlike a function.

When we consider a relationship in which there is joint participation of the two persons involved, "relationship" refers to neither a structure nor a function (such as the "personality" of the physician or patient). It is, rather, an abstraction embodying the activities of two interacting systems (persons).[3]

THREE BASIC MODELS OF THE DOCTOR-PATIENT RELATIONSHIP

THE three basic models of the doctor-patient relationship (see Table 1), which we will describe, embrace modes of interaction ubiquitous in human relationships and in no way specific for the contact between physician and patient. The specificity of the medical situation probably derives from a combination of these modes of interaction with certain technical procedures and social settings.

1. *The Model of Activity-Passivity.* Historically, this is the oldest conceptual model. Psychologically, it is not an interaction, because it is based on the effect of one person on another in such a way and under such circumstances that the person acted upon is unable to contribute actively, or is considered to be inanimate. This frame of reference (in which the physician does something to the patient) underlies the application of some of the outstanding advances of modern medicine (e.g., anesthesia and surgery, antibiotics, etc.). The physician is active; the patient, passive. This orientation has originated in—and is entirely appropriate for—the treatment of emergencies (e.g., for the patient who is severely injured, bleeding, delirious, or in coma). "Treatment" takes place irrespective of the patient's contribution and regardless of the outcome. There is a similarity here between the patient and a helpless infant, on the one hand, and between the physician and a parent, on the other. It may be recalled that psychoanalysis, too, evolved from a procedure (hypnosis) which was based on this model. Various physical measures to which psychotics are subjected today are another example of the activity-passivity frame of reference.

2. *The Model of Guidance-Cooperation.* This model underlies much of medical practice. It is employed in situations which are less desperate than those previously mentioned (e.g., acute infections). Although the patient is ill, he is conscious and has feelings and aspirations of his own. Since he suffers from pain, anxiety, and other distressing symptoms, he seeks help and is ready and willing to "cooperate." When he turns to a physician, he places the latter (even if only in some limited ways) in a position of power. This is due not only to a "transference reaction" (i.e., his regarding the physician as he did his father when he was a child) but also to the fact that the physician possesses knowledge of his bodily processes which he does not have. In some ways it may seem that this, like

the first model, is an active-passive phenomenon. Actually, this is more apparent than real. Both persons are "active" in that they contribute to the relationship and what ensues from it. The main difference between the two participants pertains to power, and to its actual or potential use. The more powerful of the two (parent, physician, employer, etc.) will speak of guidance or leadership and will expect cooperation of the other member of the pair (child, patient, employee, etc.). The patient is expected to "look up to" and to "obey" his doctor. Moreover, he is neither to question nor to argue or disagree with the orders he receives. This model has its prototype in the relationship of the parent and his (adolescent) child. Often, threats and other undisguised weapons of force are employed, even though presumably these are for the patient's "own good." It should be added that the possibility of the exploitation of the situation—as in any relationship between persons of unequal power—for the sole benefit of the physician, albeit under the guise of altruism, is ever present.

3. *The Model of Mutual Participation.* Philosophically, this model is predicated on the postulate that equality among human beings is desirable. It is fundamental to the social structure of democracy and has played a crucial role in occidental civilization for more than two hundred years. Psychologically, mutuality rests on complex processes of identification—which facilitate conceiving of others in terms of oneself—together with maintaining and tolerating the discrete individuality of the observer and the observed. It is crucial to this type of interaction that the participants (1) have approximately equal power, (2) be mutually interdependent (i.e., need each other), and (3) engage in activity that will be in some ways satisfying to both.

This model is favored by patients who, for various reasons, want to take care of themselves (at least in part). This may be an overcompensatory attempt at mastering anxieties associated with helplessness and passivity. It may also be "realistic" and necessary, as, for example, in the management of most chronic illnesses (e.g., diabetes mellitus, chronic heart disease, etc.). Here the patient's own experiences provide reliable and important clues for therapy. Moreover, the treatment program itself is principally carried out by the patient. Essentially, the physician helps the patient to help himself.

In an evolutionary sense, the pattern of mutual participation is more highly developed than the other two models of the doctor-patient relationship. It requires a more complex psychological and social organization on the part of both participants. Accordingly, it is rarely appropriate for children or for those persons who are mentally deficient, very poorly educated, or profoundly immature. On the other hand, the greater the intellectual, educational, and general experiential similarity between physician and patient the more appropriate and necessary this model of therapy becomes.

THE BASIC MODELS AND THE PSYCHOLOGY OF THE PHYSICIAN

CONSIDERATION of why physicians seek one or another type of relationship with patients (or seek patients who fit into a particular relationship) would carry us beyond the scope of this essay. Yet, it must be emphasized that as long as this subject is approached with the sentimental viewpoint that a physician is simply motivated by a wish to help others (not that we deny this wish), no scientific study of the subject can be undertaken. Scientific investigation is possible only if value judgment is subrogated, at least temporarily, to a candid scrutiny of the physician's actual behavior with his patients.

The activity-passivity model places the physician in absolute control of the situation. In this way it gratifies needs for mastery and contributes to feelings of superiority.[4] At the same time it requires that the physician disidentify with the patient as a person.

Somewhat similar is the guidance-cooperation model. The disidentification with the patient, however, is less complete. The physician, like the parent of a growing child, could be said to see in the patient a human being potentially (but not yet) like himself (or like he wishes to be). In addition to the gratifications already mentioned, this relationship provides an opportunity to recreate and to gratify the "Pygmalion Complex." Thus, the physician can mold others into his own image, as God is said to have created man (or he may mold them into his own image of what they should be like, as in Shaw's "Pygmalion"). This type of relationship is of importance in education, as the transmission of more or less stable cultural values (and of language itself) shows. It requires that the physician be convinced he is "right" in his notion of what is "best" for the patient. He will then try to induce the patient to accept his aims as the patient's own.

The model of mutual participation, as suggested earlier, is essentially foreign to medicine. This relationship, characterized by a high degree of empathy, has elements often associated with the notions of friendship and partnership and the imparting of expert advice. The physician may be said to help the patient to help himself. The physician's gratification cannot stem from power or from the control over someone else. His satisfactions are derived from more abstract kinds of mastery, which are as yet poorly understood.

It is evident that in each of the categories mentioned the satisfactions of physician and patient complement each other. This makes for stability in a paired system. Such stability, however, must be temporary, since the physician strives to alter the patient's state. The comatose patient, for example, either will recover to a more healthy, conscious condition or he will die. If he improves, the doctor-patient relationship must change. It is at this point that the physician's inner (usually unacknowledged) needs are most likely to interfere with what is "best" for the patient. At this juncture, the physician either changes his "attitude" (not a consciously or deliberately assumed role) to complement the patient's emergent needs or he foists upon the patient the same role of helpless passivity from which he (allegedly) tried to rescue him in the first place. Here we touch on a subject rich in psychological and sociological complexities. The process of change the physician must undergo to have a mutually constructive experience with the patient is similar to a very familiar process: namely, the need for the parent to behave ever differently toward his growing child.

WHAT IS "GOOD MEDICINE"?

LET us now consider the problem of "good medicine" from the viewpoint of human relationships. The function of sciences is not to tell us what is good or bad but rather to help us understand how things work. "Good" and "bad" are personal judgments, usually decided on the basis of whether or not the object under consideration satisfies us. In viewing the doctor-patient relationship we cannot conclude, however, that anything which satisfies—irrespective of other considerations—is "good." Further complications arise when the method is questioned by which we ascertain whether or not a particular need has been satisfied. Do we take the patient's word for it? Or do we place ourselves into the traditional parental role of "knowing what is best" for our patients (children)?

The shortcomings and dangers inherent in these and in other attempts to clarify some of the most basic aspects of our daily life are too well known to require documentation. It is this very complexity of the situation which has led, as is the rule in scientific work, to an essentially arbitrary simplification of the structure of our field of observation.[5]

Let us present an example. A patient consults a physician because of pain and other symptoms resulting from a duodenal ulcer. Both physician and patient assume that the latter would be better off without these discomforts. The situation now may be structured as follows: healing of the ulcer is "good," whereas its persistence is "bad." What we wish to emphasize is the fact that physician and patient agree (explicitly or otherwise) as to what is good and bad. Without such agreement it is meaningless to speak of a therapeutic relationship.

In other words, the notions of "normal," "abnormal," "symptom," "disease," and the like are social conventions. These definitions often are set by the medical world and are usually tacitly accepted by others. The fact that there is agreement renders it difficult to perceive their changing (and relativistic) character. A brief example will clarify this statement. Some years ago—and among the uneducated even today—fever was regarded as something "bad" ("abnormal," a "symptom"), to be combated. The current scientific opinion is that it is the organism's response to certain types of influences (e.g., infection) and that within limits the manifestation itself should not be "treated."

The issue of agreement is of interest because it has direct bearing on the three models of the doctor-patient relationship. In the first two models "agreement" between physician and patient is taken for granted. The comatose patient obviously can not disagree. According to the second model, the patient does not possess the knowledge to dispute the physician's word. The third category differs in that the physician does not profess to know exactly what is best for the patient. The search for this becomes the essence of the therapeutic interaction. The patient's own experiences furnish indispensable information for eventual agreement, under otherwise favorable circumstances, as to what "health" might be for him.

The characteristics of the different types of doctor-patient relationships are summarized in Table 2. In this connection, some comments will be made on a subject which essentially is philosophical but which continues to plague many medical discussions; namely, the problem of comparing the efficacy of different therapeutic measures. Such comparisons are implicitly based on the following conceptual scheme: We postulate disease "A," from which many patients suffer. Therapies "B," "C," and "D" are given to groups of patients suffering with disease "A," and the results are compared. It is usually overlooked that, for the results to be meaningful, significant conceptual similarities must exist between the operations which are compared. The three categories of the doctor-patient relationship are concretely useful in delineating areas within which meaningful comparisons can be made. Comparisons between therapies belonging to different categories are philosophically (and logically) meaningless and lead to fruitless controversy.

To illustrate this thesis let us consider some examples. A typical comparison, with which we can begin, is that of the various agents used in the treatment of lobar pneumonia: type-specific antisera, sulfonamides, and penicillin. Each superseded the other, as the increased efficacy of the newer preparations was demonstrated. This sort of comparison is meaningful because there is agreement as to what is being treated and as to what constitutes a "successful" result. There should be no need to belabor this point. What is important is that this conceptual model of therapeutic comparisons is constantly used in situations in which it does not apply; that is, in situations in which there is clear-cut disagreement as to what constitutes "cure." In this connection, the problem of peptic ulcer will exemplify a group of illnesses in which several therapeutic approaches are possible.

This question is often posed: Is surgical, medical or psychiatric treatment the "best" for peptic ulcer?[6] Unless we specify conditions, goals, and the "price" we are willing to pay (in the largest sense of the word), the question is meaningless. In the case of peptic ulcer, it is immediately apparent that each therapeutic approach implies a different conception of "disease" and correspondingly divergent notions of "cure." At the risk of slight overstatement, it can be said that according to the surgical viewpoint the disease is the "lesion," treatment aims at its eradication (by surgical means), and cure consists of its persistent absence (nonrecurrence). If a patient undergoes a vagotomy and all evidence of the lesion disappears, he is considered cured even if he develops another (apparently unrelated) illness six months later. It should be emphasized that no criticism of this frame of reference is intended. The foregoing (surgical) approach is entirely appropriate, and accusations of "narrowness" are no more (nor less) justified than they would be against any other specialized branch of knowledge.

To continue our analysis of therapeutic comparisons, let us consider the same patient (with peptic ulcer) in the hands of an internist. This specialist might have a somewhat different idea of what is wrong with him than did the surgeon. He might regard peptic ulcer as an essentially chronic disease (perhaps due to heredity and other "predispositions"), with which the patient probably will have to live as comfortably as possible for years. This point is emphasized to demonstrate that the surgeon and the internist do not treat the "same disease." How then can the two methods of treatment and their results be compared? The most that can be hoped for is to be able to determine to what extent each method is appropriate and successful within its own frame of reference.

If we take our hypothetical patient to a psychoanalyst, the situation is even more radically different. This specialist will state that he is not treating the "ulcer" and might even go so far as to say that he is not treating the patient for his ulcer. The psychoanalyst (or psychiatrist) has his own ideas about what constitutes "disease," "treatment," and "cure."[7]

CONCLUSIONS

COMMENTS have been made on some factors which provide satisfactions to both patient and physician in various therapeutic relationships. In conclusion, we call attention to two important considerations regarding the complementary situations described.

First, it might be thought that one of the three basic models of the doctor-patient relationship is in some fundamental (perhaps ethical) way "better" than another. In particular, it might be considered that it is better to identify with the patient than to treat him like a helplessly sick person. We have tried to avoid such an inference. In our opinion, each of the three types of therapeutic relationship is entirely appropriate under certain circumstances and each is inappropriate under others.

Secondly, we will comment on the therapeutic relationship as a situation (more or less fixed in time) and as a process (leading to change in one or both participants). Most of our previous comments have dealt with the relationship as a situation. It is, however, also a process in that the patient may change not only in terms of his symptoms but also in the way he wishes to relate to his doctor. A typical example is the patient with diabetes mellitus who, when first seen, is in coma. At this time, the relationship must be based on the activity-passivity model. Later, he has to be educated (guided) at the level of cooperation. Finally, ideally, he is treated as a full-fledged partner in the management of his own health (mutual participation). Confronted by a problem of this type, the physician is called upon to change through a corresponding spectrum of attitudes. If he cannot make these changes, he may interfere with the patient's progress and may promote an arrest at some intermediate stage in the evolution toward relative self-management. The other possibility in this situation is that both physician and patient will become dissatisfied with each other. This outcome, however unfortunate, is probably the commonest one. Most of us can probably verify it first-hand in the roles of both physician and patient.[8]

At such juncture, the physician usually feels that the patient is "uncooperative" and "difficult," whereas the patient regards the physician as "unsympathetic" and lacking in understanding of his personally unique needs. Both are correct. Both are confronted by the wish to induce changes in the other. As we well know, this is no easy task. The dilemma is usually resolved when the patient seeks another physician, one who is more attuned to his (new) needs. Conversely, the physician will "seek" a new patient, usually one who will benefit from the physician's (old) needs and corresponding attitudes. And so life goes on.

The pattern described accounts for the familiar fact that patients often choose physicians not solely, or even primarily, on the basis of technical skill. Considerable weight is given to the type of human relationship which they foster. Some patients prefer to be "unconscious" (figuratively speaking), irrespective of what ails them. Others go to the other extreme. The majority probably falls somewhere between these two polar opposites. Physicians, motivated by similar personal "conflicts" form a complementary series. Thus, there is an interlocking integration of the sick and his healer.

SUMMARY

THE introduction of the construct of "human relationship" represents an addition to the repertoire of fundamental medical concepts.

Three basic models of the doctor-patient relationship are described with examples. The models are (a) Activity-passivity. The comatose patient is completely helpless. The physician must take over and do some-

TABLE 2.

Analysis of the Concepts of "Disease," "Treatment," and "Therapeutic Result"

DOCTOR-PATIENT RELATIONSHIP	THE MEANING OF "TREATMENT"	THE "THERAPEUTIC RESULT"	THE NOTIONS OF DISEASE AND HEALTH	IN MEDICINE (ILLUSTRATIVE EXAMPLES)	IN PSYCHIATRY (ILLUSTRATIVE EXAMPLES)
1. Activity-passivity	Whatever the physician does; the actual operations (procedures) which he employs	Alteration in the structure and/or function of the patient's body (or behavior, as determined by the physician's judgment; the patient's judgment does not enter into the evaluation of results; e.g., T & A is "successful" irrespective of how patient feels afterward	The presence or absence of some unwanted structure or function. The actual state of affairs. The same state without the disability	1. Treatment of the unconscious patient; for example, the patient in diabetic coma; cerebral hemorrhage; shock due to acute injury; etc. 2. Major surgical operation under general anesthesia	1. Hypnosis 2. Convulsive treatments (electroshock, insulin, etc.) 3. Surgical treatments (lobotomy, etc.)

| 2. Guidance-cooperation | Whatever the physician does; similar to the above | Similar to the above, albeit patient's judgment is no longer completely irrelevant; success of therapy is still the physician's private decision; if patient agrees, he is a good patient, but if he disagrees he is bad or "uncooperative" | The presence or absence of "signs" and "symptoms"; the physician's particular concept of "Disease" "Health" (e.g., infection) (usually, no disease; e.g., no infection) | Most of general medicine and the postoperative care of surgical patients (e.g., prescription of drugs, "advice" to smoke less, etc.) | 1. "Suggestion," counseling, therapy based on "advice," etc.
2. Some modifications of psychoanalytic therapy
3. So-called psychotherapy "combined" with physical therapies (e.g., electric shock) |
| 3. Mutual participation | An abstraction of one aspect of the relationship, embodying the activities of both participants; "treatment" cannot be said to take place unless both participants orient themselves to the task ahead | Much more poorly defined than in the previous models: evaluation of the result will depend on both the physician's and the patient's judgments and is further complicated by the fact that these may change in the very process of treatment | The notions of disease and health lose most of their relevance in this context; the notions of more-or-less successful (for certain purposes) modes of behavior, adaptation, or integration take the place of the earlier, more categorical concepts | The treatment of patients with certain chronic diseases or structural defects; for example, the management of diabetes mellitus or of myasthenia gravis; "rehabilitation" of patients with orthopedic defects, such as learning the use of prostheses, etc. | 1. Psychoanalysis
2. Some modifications of psychoanalytic therapy |

thing to him. (*b*) Guidance-cooperation. The patient with an acute infectious process seeks help and is ready and willing to cooperate. He turns to the physician for guidance. (*c*) Mutual participation. The patient with a chronic disease is aided to help himself.

The physician's own inner needs (and satisfactions) form a complementary series with those of the patient.

The general problem usually referred to with the question "what is good medicine?" is briefly considered. Different types of doctor-patient relationships imply different concepts of "disease," "treatment," and "cure." This is of importance in comparing diverse therapeutic methods. Meaningful comparisons can be made only if interventions are based on the same frame of reference.

It has been emphasized that different types of doctor-patient relationships are necessary and appropriate for various circumstances. Problems in human contact between physician and patient often arise if in the course of treatment changes require an alteration in the pattern of the doctor-patient relationship. This may lead to a dissolution of the relationship.

NOTES TO CHAPTER 8

1. Ruesch, J., and Bateson, G.: Communication: The Social Matrix of Psychiatry, New York, W. W. Norton & Company, Inc., 1951.
2. In our approach to this subject we have been influenced by psychologic (psychoanalytic), sociologic, and philosophic considerations. See in this connection Dewey, J., and Bentley, A. F.: Knowing and the Known, Boston, Beacon Press, 1949; Russell, B.: Power: A New Social Analysis, New York, W. W. Norton & Company, Inc., 1938; Szasz, T. S.: Entropy, Organization, and the Problem of the Economy of Human Relationships, Internat. J. Psychoanal. 36:289, 1955; and Szasz, T. S.: On the Theory of Psychoanalytic Treatment, read before the Annual Meeting of the American Psychoanalytic Association, Atlantic City, N.J., May 7, 1955; Internat. J. Psychoanal., to be published.
3. Dubos, R. J.: Second Thoughts on the Germ Theory, Scient. Am. 192:31, 1955.
4. Jones, E.: The God Complex, in Jones, E.: Essays in Applied Psychoanalysis, London, Hogarth Press, 1951, Vol. 2, p. 244; and Marmor, J.: The Feeling of Superiority: An Occupational Hazard in the Practice of Psychotherapy, Am. J. Psychiat. 110:370, 1953.
5. We omit any discussion of the physician's technical skill, training, equipment, etc. These factors, of course, are of importance, and we do not minimize them. The problem of what is "good medicine" can be considered from a number of viewpoints (e.g., technical skill, economic considerations, social roles, human relationships, etc.). Our scope in this essay is limited to but one —sometimes quite unimportant—aspect of the contact between physician and patient.

6. Such a question is roughly comparable to asking, "Is an automobile or an airplane better?"—without specifying for what. See Rapoport, A.: Operational Philosophy, New York, Harper & Brothers, 1954.
7. Zilboorg, G.: A. History of Medical Psychology, New York, W. W. Norton & Company, Inc., 1941; and Bowman, K. M. and Rose, M.: Do Our Medical Colleagues Know What to Expect from Psychotherapy? Am. J. Psychiat. 111:401, 1954.
8. Pinner, M., and Miller, B. F., Editors: When Doctors Are Patients, New York, W. W. Norton & Company, Inc., 1952.

ॐ

CHAPTER 9   Interpersonal and Structural Factors

in the Study of Mental Hospitals*

AMITAI ETZIONI

THE youngest branch of organizational theory is the study of mental
hospitals. Twenty years ago, when Rowland pioneered in the field,
the major sources of information on the mental hospital were books
written by former patients.[1] Today there are a number of excellent studies
of the organizational structure of the mental hospital.[2] The new studies
follow in the steps of organizational research in other areas,[3] especially in
the area of industrial relations.[4] Such a transfer of ideas, concepts, and
perspectives from one area of study to another benefits both the new
studies and the theory of organization itself.[5] But there is a constant
danger that the analogy will be overdrawn. Moreover, in this particular
instance organizational studies had certain childhood diseases that tended
to be contagious when the earlier models were applied to the new areas of
research. This paper will discuss the consequences of transferring one set
of ideas—the human-relations approach—from industrial relations theory,
and applying those ideas to analysis of the structure of the mental hospital, without fully considering the implications of other aspects of the
theory.

The study of industrial relations is more or less split into two camps. On
one side are the advocates of the human-relations approach, including
disciples of Elton Mayo and Kurt Lewin.[6] On the other side are the
scholars who object to the human-relations school, which they name
"managerial sociology," and which they criticize for being manipulative,
biased in favor of management—for example, earlier studies ignored the
role of the trade unions—and unrealistic.[7] Another way of putting the
difference is to say that the human-relations school is for "peace in indus-

* Reprinted by special permission of The William Alanson White Psychiatric Foundation, Inc., and the author from Psychiatry, 23 (1960), 13–22 (copyright by the
Foundation).

try," harmony, and "understanding" between the employer and employees, while the opponents emphasize the objective significance and positive function of industrial conflict. The human-relations people emphasize two-way communication, while the opponents stress the role of the trade unions. The human-relations school suggests therapeutic interviews and participation in decision-making; the opponents point to economic, political, cultural, and other 'real' differences between workers and management.

Although it is difficult to integrate the two approaches on the ideological level, an unbiased examination of them reveals that in illuminating two aspects of industrial organization, *both schools are vital to a better understanding of the organizational process.* Interpersonal relations are better understood if structural factors are taken into account. The process of communication within small groups can be better analyzed when the outside communal and political ties of the workers and managers are considered. Structural analysis benefits from study of interpersonal relations, as shown, for example, by studies of informal relations. In short, a theoretical integration of the two approaches is possible.[8]

Where do the new studies of the mental hospital fit into this picture? In general, many of these studies are inclined to accept the human-relations approach. Many studies of mental hospitals focus on the communication system among the personnel, emphasizing the importance of "understanding" among the various members and ranks of the staff. They see the mental hospital as a "therapeutic community"[9] or "small society," rather than as a large-scale organization and a work place. Finally, they favor conferences and wide participation in the process of decision-making. I shall examine all these points in detail subsequently.

One of the reasons why the human-relations approach is so readily accepted in the study of the mental hospital is that there is a high congruence between the ideas and techniques of psychotherapy and those of the human-relations orientation.[10] Psychological insights in general and psychoanalysis in particular played an important role in the early development of the human-relations school.[11] The ideas of increasing self-understanding by communication with a trained professional, and of solving or accepting conflicts by becoming aware of their existence, are very close to the idea of increasing understanding between worker and management by increasing communication between them with the help of the human-relations expert. Increased communication is expected to reduce industrial conflict, if not to abolish it altogether. From this it is only one step to the suggestion that the mental hospital staff has to be made more aware of the organizational process. "Being aware" is considered an important therapeutic factor on the organizational level.[12]

Not all studies of mental hospitals follow this line. One of the outstanding exceptions is the Stanton and Schwartz study.[13] The authors combine an analysis of the communication system with an analysis of the power structure. Stanton and Schwartz, as well as a few other investigators, put much emphasis on the relation between formal and informal structures,[14] on the lines of authority,[15] and on the relation between "functional" and "scalar" status.[16] But even in these studies many of the other structural factors are neglected, or are acknowledged as important in one chapter and then overlooked as relevant to problems discussed in other chapters.

COMMUNICATION AND STRUCTURAL FACTORS

THE studies of mental hospitals examine two major channels of communication: between staff and patients, and among various staff members. The influence of objective factors on communication between staff and patients will not be discussed here because it would involve an evaluation of psychiatry which is far beyond the competence of the author.

Communication among various staff members is considered an essential mechanism for effective operation of the hospital. Cases of conflict and misunderstanding are attributed to lack of communication or to communication blocks among the staff.[17] It is suggested that when sufficient avenues of communication are supplied, the blocks are removed and, as Stanton and Schwartz said in describing one such instance, "Misunderstanding after misunderstanding disappeared like magic."[18] There is no doubt that some problems arise from communication blocks whose removal allows the problems to be solved. But it is necessary to specify more clearly which problems can be handled by increased communication and which cannot. In the case described by Stanton and Schwartz, the nurses complained that the soap supply was rationed and insufficient. In a conference with the administrator the nurses learned that no such rationing had been intended and that the amount of soap available was for all practical purposes unlimited. The nurses' complaint had resulted from an inquiry from the housekeeper about the amount of soap used, which had been misinterpreted to mean that soap would be rationed. There was no 'real' problem. Since the whole problem was created by distorted communication it is no wonder that it disappeared like magic once the block was removed. What would have happened if in the conference between the nurses and the administrator it had turned out that soap was really to be rationed because "too much" had been used? One wonders if communication would have been so helpful in such a situation.

Now soap is not of vital concern to the nurses—although it may, of course, acquire symbolic significance if it is seen as reflecting the attitude of the hospital toward patient health, or as expressing the money versus service conflict. But more vital conflicting interests may also be subject to similar exaggerated 'solutions.' For example, Caudill devotes a long analysis to the case of "the TV petition."[19] The patients petitioned to be allowed to watch TV every evening of the week instead of one evening,

When the petition was brought up in administrative conference, the nurses objected to the extension of TV "privileges." Actually they would have preferred to forbid watching TV altogether. The head of the hospital saw this as a problem of communication. First of all, he believed that there was insufficient information about the deeper, "psychodynamic" reasons which motivated the patients to hand in the petition. As the "meaning" of the petition was not clear, the head of the hospital felt that he was unable to decide how to react. Second, there seemed to him to be too little communication with the nurses about the therapeutic significance of the "other twenty-three hours," in which the social activities of the patients and presumably watching TV were included.

I doubt that the situation required so complicated an approach. The patients wanted to watch TV because they were bored and liked to watch fights. The nurses did not want the patients to watch TV because it meant that they would be late for the 11:15 bus and because it would interfere with the change of shifts. While "communication" brought these factors out during the administrative conference, it seems that the training of the hospital head prevented him from seeing the significance of these simple facts. Moreover, it seems that no additional communication about these factors could change them. The issue was solved, typically, after the session was over, by a simple bargaining process; it was decided in a discussion between the hospital head, who sided with the patients, and the nurse supervisor to enable the patients to watch TV two nights a week but not to serve food after the program so that the nurses could catch their buses. Like so many conflicts of interests, this one was solved by *bargaining* and *compromise* and not by a sheer increase of communication.[20]

If the nurses, who often have no special training for work in mental hospitals, do not feel free to establish "warm" personal relations with patients, it is not because the information that this is necessary has not reached them, but because it does not fit into their professional image, which is based on long training, and is reinforced by interaction among the nurses and by other mechanisms. This cannot be greatly changed by communication sessions any more than psychiatrists can be changed, in the same or similar ways, from, for example, psychoanalysts to group therapists.

Many of the problems discussed in studies of state mental hospitals seem to be the result of objective conditions which no communication can overcome—such as questions of budget. Some of the problems seem related to establishing and maintaining working and social conditions which will secure enough people who are willing to work in the mental hospital. Other problems might be decreased if personnel were trained more specifically in accordance with the needs of the mental hospital. Still others might be minimized if the objective organizational structure were adapted to the special needs of the mental hospital. If these basic needs were satisfied, some of the remaining problems might be solved by better communication.

But even within these limits, the importance of better communication is much less than some of the studies of mental hospitals seem to assume. "Being aware" might decrease the emotional tension involved in a conflict, but it might also draw more clearly the line between management of the hospital—especially in profit-making organizations—and the employees, thus increasing tensions and potential conflicts. There is also the danger of a utopian approach to communication. Even if it can be shown that some difficulties disappear when communication is increased, it does not follow that all problems yield to this technique. The effect and flow of communication are limited and influenced by structural conditions. The demands on psychiatrists' time limit communication. A psychiatrist devotes a limited number of hours to a hospital, of which a considerable part is devoted to nonprofessional activities.[21] An increase in communication, by writing and reading reports or by participating in administrative and "therapeutic team" conferences, would mean that even less time was available for therapy. Psychiatrists already seem to feel deprived because administration does not leave enough time for their professional activities, in which they do not usually include communication with lay personnel.

Increased communication is recommended for still another reason. It is advocated as a means of enhancing the identification of staff members with the organization. In order to feel that they are part of the "therapeutic community," everybody must know "all that is going on." It is easy to understand that certain information will give the personnel a feeling of participation and an increased understanding of their own roles and the roles of others. For example, staff members should understand the basic policy of the hospital, and should be informed about progress of the patients. Attempts to increase communication beyond that point means taking time from other activities, and arousing rather than satisfying an "inside-dopester" attitude which is harmful to the organization. Even with a daily orientation conference for each staff member, some people will be "uninformed," or at least will feel that they are, and thus will be left out of the group.

The assumption behind the suggestion that everybody should be informed about the organizational process in general is that the hospital staff constitutes *one* social group to which everyone wants to or should want to belong. This is obviously not the case. The hospital community is at best a group of groups. Most members can feel quite at home in the hospital if they are well-integrated members of one or two small groups and if they are informed about what their clique is doing. Only leaders of such groups usually have the interest and the need to be informed in greater detail about what is going on in the hospital community in general and in other and higher cliques in particular. This brings up the question, "What is the nature of the social structure of the mental hospital?"

THE HOSPITAL AS A "SMALL SOCIETY"

IF THE term *society* is used in a strictly sociological way, a hospital is not a small society, because societies have functional autonomy and hospitals do not. Functional autonomy means that all the basic functional needs of a social system are internally regulated.[22] Since the hospital secures staff, patients, and facilities from the outside, and only partially controls their recruitment, it cannot technically be seen as a society.

But even if the term is defined more loosely, the assumptions and associations that such terms as "small society" and "therapeutic community" bring to mind are quite misleading. Use of the terms often indicates a tendency to neglect the influence of external factors on the internal process of the mental hospital, and also to oversimplify some aspects of the internal process.

This limited perspective is not accidental. It is one of the most important trademarks of the human-relations approach to the study of industry. Historically, it follows from the application of anthropological techniques to the study of large-scale organizations. The anthropologist tends to see each social unit as an isolated society. This approach often overlooks such factors as trade unions and professional associations; communal ties such as social groups, governing boards, political institutions, and other structures and attitudes which affect the organizational process; and such internal factors as the influence of multigroup membership.

THE INFLUENCE OF PROFESSIONAL ASSOCIATIONS

THE various professional and semiprofessional groups which interact in the mental hospital have clear images of their respective roles.[23] Attempts to change these roles within a single hospital seem to be almost always doomed to failure because these role-images are created and reinforced by many factors which are external and beyond the control of each hospital. While the image is usually created during the training period, it is constantly reinforced by the professional associations and professional social groups.[24] The professional associations also act as interest groups which support their members in the struggle to maintain or improve their professional image and position. At the same time these associations serve as reference groups in terms of standards and professional ethics, as well as prestige systems.[25] One cannot expect basic changes in the techniques applied by hospital psychiatrists, for instance, or in the relationships between psychiatrists and clinical psychologists, without taking such factors into account.[26] With few exceptions, the influence of such associations is not analyzed. Often they are not even mentioned. I wonder if the scholars who have explored these issues have found those associations uninfluential, or have preferred to focus on other aspects of the material, or have been limited by their conceptual scheme to the study of what was going on in the "small society," to the neglect of influences on the behavior of the staff from outside the walls of the hospital.

THE INFLUENCE OF COMMUNAL TIES

THE mental hospital is usually a "total institution"[27] only for patients. The staff, as a rule, does not live on the premises. Even in cases where the lower-level staff lives in the hospital, most of the physicians and other professional personnel live outside. Studies of industries have found it fruitful to examine the social life and relationships of workers and various levels of management outside the factory.[28] Similar studies of the off-the-job social relations of and among various staff groups of mental hospitals would be of much interest. Some studies of the social background and social ties of the patients are of great help.[29] But if more were known about the social life of the physicians and nurses, better understanding might result of their conflicting aspirations and reference groups, and of the lack of common language, which have been described in several studies.[30] Such data reveal, for example, some of the mechanisms which reinforce the professional image of the nurse and are responsible for the fact that she quite often prefers to work on the closed rather than on the open ward, and prefers to increase the patient's assurance by wearing a stiff cap and handing the patient his medication rather than by smoking a cigarette and engaging in informal talk with him.

For a long time it was believed that the main primary relations of workers were based on on-the-job relationships. But some recent studies cast doubt on this generalization. One study, for instance, reports that only 10 percent of the workers stated that their main primary relationships were based on work relationships.[31] It seems now that other primary groups—such as families, neighbors, and so forth—have much influence on the aspirations and attitudes of the actors in organizational contexts.[32] A fuller understanding of aspirations and attitudes will be achieved only when the communal ties are taken into account.

There is another type of communal tie which seems to be of much importance but is only rarely analyzed by the scholars who study mental hospitals, perhaps because access to this aspect of the organizational structure is limited. Usually lower and middle levels of organizational authority are studied; sometimes the head of the organization is also covered. Almost no organizational study considers higher authorities—such as the board of trustees, the health department, the governor, and so forth—or such expressions of the communal structures as the press and the local chamber of commerce.[33] While higher and external authorities are of great significance in the study of all organizations, they are of special interest in the case of mental hospitals.[34] Most mental hospitals are state hospitals and therefore more dependent on external authority than many other organizations. Also, the functioning of the mental hospital is highly influenced by the community 'license'—that is, attitudes concerning what are right and wrong methods of care.[35]

Community pressure can affect what is already a built-in strain in the mental hospital, the conflict between the therapeutic and custodial functions. To some degree, custodial activities are means for therapeutic goals. If the patients cannot be kept in the hospital, they cannot benefit from its service. Some suicide-prone patients have to be controlled for their own safety. But community pressure sometimes results in considerable expansion of custodial activities beyond the therapeutic needs. The community often does not want to be bothered by patients or is afraid of them. On the other hand, the community may also be the source of initiative and pressure to introduce more humane methods of treatment into the mental hospital.[36] The internal conflict between custodial and therapeutic functions cannot be fully understood unless the community orientation and the channels of its expression are studied.

THE INFLUENCE OF MULTIGROUP MEMBERSHIP

ONE of the most important early discoveries of industrial sociology was that workers act as group members and not always on rational grounds. Studies of the mental hospital have rediscovered this tendency. "Recent literature shows a refreshing new point of view. There is an awareness of the fact of interaction, of the importance of the group. . . ."[37] But with the rediscovery of the significance of small groups, some of Mayo's early mistakes in applying the human-relations approach to industrial theory have also been repeated. The assumption is often made that the patient or staff member is a member of one group at a time. While this may be true in some marginal cases, people are usually members of more than one group at a time. Consequently, adjustment problems develop, especially when these groups are competing for the loyalties and resources of the members. One of the most important characteristics of a person in modern society is that he knows how to adjust to multigroup membership, to be at the same time a trade union member and a factory worker, a member of two families—orientation and procreation—or an obedient soldier and a good buddy.

The patients in the mental hospitals quite often seem to have difficulties along this line. They tend to become overinvolved in one group and to reject their obligations to other groups. Part of the therapeutic process is the reconstruction of the ability to participate in multigroup situations. Several hospital practices, often pursued quite unwittingly, either help to satisfy or interfere with the need of the patient to maintain or to reconstruct his ability for multigroup participation. The widespread practice of sending patients on furloughs instead of giving them simple, direct discharges, seems to have positive effects, such as supplying the patient with an exercise in multigroup activity. On the other hand, the ambivalent, if not hostile, attitude of the hospital staff toward a patient's relatives endangers any ties that the patient may have to the external social life[38] and tends to increase his investment in the hospital community. This may later make weaning from the hospital more difficult and block his recovery.[39] Similarly, the objection of some personnel to transferring patients from room to room and ward to ward on the basis that it will weaken their group ties[40] is not always justified. The patient may need these opportunities to become a member of two or more groups at the same time. Such movement might also provide the patient with more social permissiveness and some immunity from the group pressure to conformity. By learning to play his membership in one group against that in another group, the patient may gain some privacy and independence. Some patients seem to use various groups as a ladder on their way to convalescence. With improvement in their mental health, they climb to more 'advanced' patient groups.[41] The hospital, it seems, should encourage such mobility, and support and create opportunities for multigroup membership for patients who are ready for it.

CONFERENCES AND PARTICIPATION IN DECISION-MAKING

THE human-relations school is in favor of conferences and group discussions between the superior and his subordinates where information about future activity is given and a group decision is made. That support of the subordinates for a new activity is enhanced in this way has been proved in a number of important experiments conducted by Lewin and others.[42] These conferences, however, may be evaluated differently according to their purpose.[43] If they are used to spread information in a way which diminishes unnecessary anxiety, they can certainly be of great help. One human-relations training movie shows a case in which tension is created among workers when new machines, which they believe will create unemployment, are brought into the factory. Once management explains that the new machines will be used for expansion of the factory and that new workers will be hired, anxiety is completely dispelled. The film does not deal with a case in which anxiety would be justified because the new machines mean that some workers will have to be fired. A conference of the type shown in the movie is just another channel of communication, which, like those discussed previously, can function only under certain structural conditions.

But conferences are supposed to function not only as channels of downward or upward communication. They are also believed to offer an opportunity for the personnel, and even the patients,[44] to participate in the process of decision-making, thus increasing their commitments to the decisions made. Democracy is believed to be a more efficient way of management.[45]

A study by Caudill, in which verbatim notes of 63 administrative conferences were taken, gives a different evaluation of "conferences" with groups of patients and of their "self-government," as shown in a discussion by the heads of the hospital:

> *Miss Nugent* [nurse]: . . . Are you going to have a gripe session?
> *Dr. Scott:* I'm personally against these gripe sessions.
> *Dr. Shaw:* So am I, particularly if the patients feel that they are legislating at these sessions and find out later that they are not.
> *Dr. Scott:* The only good that these gripe sessions do is that if you can get the patients as a group to scrutinize what is going on in their behavior. . . .[46]

In other words, conferences with the patients, disguised as upward communication ("gripe sessions"), serve actually for downward communication and direction. Similarly, in some industries, human-relations techniques are applied to the extent that conferences with workers are used as the modern way of giving orders, but the direction of order-giving remains the same. Thus "participation" can be turned into a manipulative technique, not a way of sharing the power to decide.

What about the administrative conferences? Although patients are manipulated, does the staff really participate in the decision-making process? A detailed analysis of the material supplied by Caudill shows that these conferences are either manipulative or blocks to communication, and serve as a source of anxiety rather than as a positive influence. Stanton and Schwartz reach a similar conclusion in their discussion of staff conferences in another mental hospital. They state: "Conferences and discussions were regarded *as a means of rationalizing hospital interference,* and as discussions which might interfere with clear personal insight into the problem" (italics mine).[47]

In one sense, the administrative conferences of mental hospitals seem to have gone even further than similar conferences in industry. In industrial conferences, usually only two levels of authority confer and there is only one representative of the higher level. These are conferences between a superior and his subordinates—that is, the people he works with. Special attention is paid to arranging conferences in a way which will not confuse the lines of authority. In the administrative conferences described in the studies of mental hospitals, the heads of hospitals, nurse supervisors, charge nurses, staff nurses, senior and junior physicians, and others participate. This creates several peculiar and unnecessary tensions: (1) Conflicts among superiors are acted out in front of those who ordinarily have to accept their orders. (2) Conflicts of superiors with their superiors are discussed in front of subordinates. (3) Subordinates' actions, which have been based on orders or general directions from superiors, are scrutinized by the superiors' colleagues in front of the subordinates. (4) Subordinates attempt to undermine directions to which they object by by-passing their immediate superior and asking the opinion of the conference about the action which should be taken.

The implicit assumption on which these conferences seem to rest is that since "we are all part of the therapeutic community," things can be discussed freely with disregard of statuses and lines of authority. But this assumption is unrealistic, as indicated by the behavior of the participants in the conference. As Caudill shows, they tend to participate in the communication process according to their rank. Thus, the subordinates tend to be more passive. Also, much of the conference time is wasted on defensive behavior in response to the tensions described previously. Further, actors in the conference frequently do not transfer information upward, thus avoiding the possibility that it will be used against them. Subordinates in general tend not to pass upward information which is disadvantageous for them, but the conference aggravates this tendency.

Although the studies of mental hospitals indicate the helpfulness of transferring concepts and theorems from one area of organizational studies to another, they show that inappropriate and incomplete ideas can be transferred as well. In adopting the human-relations approach used in industrial theory, some studies of mental hospitals seem to overemphasize (1) the importance of communication, (2) the totality of the institution, and (3) the benefits of participation in decision-making conferences. In so doing, the studies neglect somewhat the study of structural factors, such as budget and time limitations; real differences in personnel; the influence of such external factors as professional associations, communal ties, and so forth; and the unchangeable locus of certain decisions. A balanced analysis of the influence of interpersonal and structural factors, of internal process and external ties, and of the origins of authority, will ensure a fruitful, realistic development of this young branch of organizational theory.

NOTES TO CHAPTER 9

1. Howard Rowland, "Interaction Processes in the State Mental Hospital," *Psychiatry* (1938) 1:323-337.
2. For example, William Caudill, Fredrick C. Redlich, Helen R. Gilmore, and Eugene B. Brody, "Social Structure and Interaction Processes on a Psychiatric Ward," *Amer. J. Orthopsychiatry* (1952) 22:314-334; and Alfred H. Stanton and Morris S. Schwartz, *The Mental Hospital*; New York, Basic Books, 1954.
3. For a recent outstanding review and analysis of organizational research, see James G. March and Herbert A. Simon, *Organizations*; New York, J. Wiley, 1958.
4. Charles K. Andrew, "Industrial Technics *Can* Be Used," *Modern Hospital* (No. 6, 1955) 84:67-72. Also, Caudill finds "a very direct parallel" to his

work in a study of a factory by Rice. William Caudill, *The Psychiatric Hospital As a Small Society;* Cambridge, Harvard Univ. Press, 1958. A. K. Rice, "The Use of Unrecognized Cultural Mechanisms in an Expanding Machine-Shop," *Human Relations* (1951) 4:143-160. See also Milton Greenblatt, Richard H. York, and Esther Lucile Brown, *From Custodial to Therapeutic Patient Care in Mental Hospitals;* New York, Russell Sage Foundation, 1955; p. 21, n. 1.

5. An elaborate discussion of a tentative model of organizational analysis, and the problems involved in its application to the study of organizations in particular industries, is included in the author's "Industrial Sociology: The Study of Economic Organizations," *Social Research* (1958) 25:303-324.

6. For a recent discussion and bibliography, see Conrad M. Arensberg, and others, editors, *Research in Industrial Human Relations;* New York, Harper, 1957.

7. For two outstanding criticisms, see Reinhard Bendix and Lloyd H. Fisher, "The Perspectives of Elton Mayo," *Review of Economics and Statistics* (1949) 31:312-321; and Clark Kerr and Lloyd H. Fisher, "Plant Sociology: The Elite and the Aborigines," pp. 281-309; in *Common Frontiers of the Social Sciences,* edited by Mirra Komarovsky; Glencoe, Ill., Free Press, 1957.

8. It is important to note that a leading scholar of the human-relations school pointed out that studies which apply the human-relations approach are increasingly often covering what are referred to here as "structural factors." William Foote Whyte, "Human Relations Theory—A Progress Report," *Harvard Business Review* (1956) 34:Sept.-Oct., 125-132. For further elaboration of this point see Etzioni, "Human Relations and the Foreman," *Pacific Sociological Review* (1958) 1:33-38.

9. For a discussion of this concept and the ideas associated with it, see Maxwell Jones, *The Therapeutic Community;* New York, Basic Books, 1953.

10. Especially as formulated by Harry Stack Sullivan, *The Interpersonal Theory of Psychiatry,* edited by Helen Swick Perry and Mary Ladd Gawel; New York, Norton, 1953.

11. See F. J. Roethlisberger and William J. Dickson, *Management and the Worker;* Cambridge, Harvard Univ. Press, 1939.

12. See Caudill, footnote 2, p. 323; and Caudill, footnote 4.

13. See footnote 2.

14. Ivan Belknap, *Human Problems of a State Mental Hospital;* New York, McGraw-Hill, 1956.

15. Jules Henry, "The Formal Social Structure of a Psychiatric Hospital," *Psychiatry* (1954) 17:139-151.

16. Harvey L. Smith and Daniel J. Levinson, "The Major Aims and Organizational Characteristics of Mental Hospitals," pp. 3-8; in *The Patient and the Mental Hospital,* edited by Milton Greenblatt, Daniel J. Levinson, and Richard H. Williams; Glencoe, Ill., Free Press, 1957.

17. "In many such instances, conflicting spheres of responsibility and interest, which in themselves sustained older intergroup tensions, necessitated requests and explanations going through long and often parallel lines of communication if problems were to be settled." Greenblatt, footnote 4; p. 269.

18. See footnote 2; p. 239.
19. Caudill, footnote 4; Ch. 4, pp. 68-86.
20. The settlement reached in each case depends to a considerable degree on the relative power of the interacting groups. It is important to keep in mind that power, defined as the ability of ego to affect the behavior of alter, is only in part based on communication. Other sources of power include command over means and rewards, such as force and material objects. The adherents of the human-relations approach—and also other scholars who do not identify with this approach—tend to see communication as the only source of power. For various discussions of this issue, see: Harold D. Lasswell and Abraham Kaplan, *Power and Society;* New Haven, Yale Univ. Press, 1950; Chester I. Barnard, *The Functions of the Executive;* Cambridge, Harvard Univ. Press, 1956; esp. Ch. 12, pp. 161-181; Robert E. Agger, "Power Attributions in the Local Community: Theoretical and Research Considerations," *Social Forces* (1956) 34:322-331. Richard H. McCleery focused on this issue in an empirical study of *Policy Change in Prison Management;* East Lansing, Governmental Research Bureau, Michigan State Univ., 1957.
21. According to Belknap, 60 percent of the time of physicians in South Mental Hospital is devoted to administrative work. See footnote 14; p. 108.
22. For a discussion of the concept, see Talcott Parsons, *The Social System;* Glencoe, Ill., Free Press, 1951; p. 19.
23. Two recent studies are devoted to this subject. Ivar E. Bery, Jr., studied the nurses from this viewpoint in *Role, Personality, and Social Structure: A Study of Nursing in a General Hospital;* unpublished Ph.D. dissertation, Harvard Univ., 1960. Charles Perrow studied doctors and administrators in *Authority, Goals, and Prestige in a General Hospital;* unpublished Ph.D. dissertation, Berkeley, Univ. of California, 1960.
24. The same problem comes up in other areas of interaction among various groups of professionals. See, for instance, William Caudill and Bertram H. Roberts, "Pitfalls in the Organization of Interdisciplinary Research," *Human Organization* (1951) 10:Winter, 12-15; Fredrick C. Redlich and Eugene B. Brody, "Emotional Problems of Interdisciplinary Research in Psychiatry," *Psychiatry* (1955) 18:233-239.
25. This is discussed and documented in a different context by Harold L. Wilensky, *Intellectuals in Labor Unions;* Glencoe, Ill., Free Press, 1956; pp. 134-136; Alvin W. Gouldner, "Cosmopolitans and Locals: Toward an Analysis of Latent Social Roles—I," *Administrative Science Quarterly* (1957) 2:281-306; esp. pp. 287-289; Leonard Reissman, "A Study of Role Conceptions in Bureaucracy," *Social Forces* (1949) 27:305-310.
26. See August B. Hollingshead and Fredrick C. Redlich, *Social Class and Mental Illness;* New York, Wiley, 1958; esp. pp. 370-390; Maurice H. Krout, editor, *Psychology, Psychiatry, and the Public Interest;* Minneapolis, Univ. of Minnesota Press, 1956; Edgar F. Borgatta, "The Certification of Academic Professions: The Case of Psychology," *Amer. Sociological Review* (1958) 23:302-306.
27. See Erving Goffman, "The Characteristics of Total Institutions," pp. 43-84; in *Symposium on Preventive and Social Psychiatry;* Washington, D.C., Walter Reed Army Institute of Research, 1957.

28. See, for example, W. Lloyd Warner and J. O. Low, *The Social System of the Modern Factory;* New Haven, Yale Univ. Press, 1947; Alvin Ward Gouldner, *Patterns of Industrial Bureaucracy;* Glencoe, Ill., Free Press, 1954.

29. Henry B. Richardson, *Patients Have Families;* New York, Commonwealth Fund, 1945; Greenblatt, footnote 16; pp. 501-608.

30. Alvin Zander, Arthur R. Cohen, and Ezra Stotland, *Role Relations in the Mental Health Professions;* Ann Arbor, Institute for Social Research, Univ. of Michigan, 1957; Mark Lefton, Simon Dinitz, and Benjamin Pasamanick, "Decision-Making in a Mental Hospital: Real, Perceived, and Ideal," *Amer. Sociological Review* (1959) 24:822-829.

31. Robert Dubin, "Industrial Workers' Worlds: A Study of the 'Central Life Interests' of Industrial Workers," *Social Problems* (1956) 3:131-142.

32. For an outstanding study, see Elizabeth Bott, *Family and Social Network;* London, Tavistock Publications, 1957.

33. For one of the few exceptions, see Cyril Sofer, "Reactions to Administrative Change," *Human Relations* (1955) 8:291-316. For an informative study of these relationships in a general hospital, see Temple Burling, Edith M. Lentz, Robert N. Wilson, *The Give and Take in Hospitals;* New York, Putnam, 1956; esp. pp. 39-50. For a systematic conceptual framework for analysis, see Talcott Parsons, "The Mental Hospital as a Type of Organization," pp. 108-129; in Greenblatt, footnote 16.

34. Some of the characteristics of top administration in organizations which have professional goals are analyzed in the author's "Authority Structure and Organizational Effectiveness," *Administrative Science Quarterly* (1959) 4:43-67. A model for the analysis of the relationship between external authorities and internal organizational processes is included in Amitai Etzioni and Paul F. Lazarsfeld, "Innovations in Universities," in *Historical Material on Innovations in Higher Education,* collected and interpreted by Bernhard J. Stern (unpublished monograph, Planning Project for Advanced Training in Social Research, Columbia Univ., 1952-53). Some of the methodological problems involved are analyzed by Allen H. Barton and B. Anderson, "A Change in an Organizational System"; in *Reader in Organizational Analysis,* edited by Amitai Etzioni; New York, Henry Holt, 1960.

35. Everett Hughes pointed out that professions require and have to sustain a social license for their operation. See "License and Mandate," pp. 78-87; in Hughes' *Men and Their Work;* Glencoe, Ill., Free Press, 1958. The same points hold for organizations which have professional goals—and for other organizations as well.

36. For interesting studies of community attitudes toward mental illness, see Elaine and John Cumming, *Closed Ranks;* Cambridge, Commonwealth Fund, Harvard Univ. Press, 1957; Marian Radke Yarrow, John A. Clausen, Paul R. Robbins, "The Social Meaning of Mental Illness," *J. Social Issues.*

38. For a review of earlier studies and a report on new data on the function of the family in the recovery of the patient, see Ozzie C. Simmons and Howard E. Freeman, "Familial Expectations and Posthospital Performance of Mental Patients," *Human Relations* (1959) 12:233-242.

39. Many studies have pointed out the therapeutic role of fellow patients. See, for instance, J. Fremont Bateman and H. Warren Dunham, "The State

Mental Hospital as a Specialized Community Experience," *Amer. J. Psychiatry* (1948) 105:445-448.

40. See E. F. Galioni, R. R. Notman, A. H. Stanton, and R. H. Williams, "The Nature and Purpose of Mental Hospital Wards," pp. 327-379; in Greenblatt, footnote 16.

41. Reported by Caudill, footnote 4; p. 330; and Belknap, footnote 14; pp. 171ff.

42. Kurt Lewin, "Group Decision and Social Change," pp. 459-473; in *Readings in Social Psychology* (rev. ed.), edited by Guy E. Swanson, Theodore M. Newcomb, and Eugene L. Hartley; New York, Holt, 1952. Lester Coch and John R. P. French, Jr., "Overcoming Resistance to Change," *Human Relations* (1948) 1:512-532.

43. For statistics on the use of conferences in hospitals, see a report on 316 hospitals by Harry E. Panhorst in "Department Heads Make the Hospital," *Modern Hospital* (1955) 84:No. 1, 81-82.

44. Sydney H. Croog, "Patient Government—Some Aspects of Participation and Social Background on Two Psychiatric Wards," Psychiatry (1956) 19:203-207.

45. See Robert N. Rapoport and Rhona Sofer Rapoport, "'Democratization' and 'Authority' in a Therapeutic Community," *Behavioral Science* (1957) 2:128-133.

46. Caudill, footnote 4; p. 78.

47. See footnote 2; p. 113.

Section II

THE INSTITUTION IN SOCIETY

INTRODUCTION

To take account of extra-institutional variables is to recognize the merit of Etzioni's corrective against overly restrictive interpretation of the "total institution" concept, as employed by Goffman and others. When Parsons and Homans speak of internal and external system problems, they remind us that social system boundaries are seldom if ever completely closed; we only neglect external variables provisionally to see how far we can go in seeking relations among intra-institutional components, just as we set aside internal system relations for the time being to analyze inter-connections between institutions and the social fabric in which they are embedded. From this point of view, then, the either-or theoretical controversy—whether internal or external system variables best explain residential institution—is meaningless; behavior can be explained on many levels, and criteria for selecting the most satisfactory explanations have to do not with the level of explanation, but with ordinary requirements for selecting among explanations, like predictability, parsimony and generality.

Different facets of one general theme—the effect that values of the society outside the institution have on institutional life—are dealt with in the next three articles. Agnew and Hsu, a psychiatrist-anthropologist team, show how awareness of individuals' value orientations can lead to an understanding of their resistance to and acceptance of change. They discuss the Chinese value of dependence on the extended family to highlight, by contrast, the American value of self-reliance. They then go on to show that cultural emphasis on self-reliance led one psychiatric ward's staff and patients to resist an initial attempt at individualizing patients' dress, but that this same value promoted ultimate acceptance of the change. The next paper, by Erikson, focuses on society's specific attitude toward mental illness. The public attitude is marked by ambivalence—whether to view mental patients as passive organisms who happen to be afflicted with a disease over which they have no control, like an infection, or as persons who are responsible and can control their behavior if they wish. The patients, in turn, face the dilemma of which of these roles to adopt for themselves. In this situation, Erikson questions whether psychiatric emphasis on the patient's passive role functions to rehabilitate the patient for his return to society.

The third paper describes prison inmates in terms of the source of their value orientations—whether their reference groups are the law-abiding majority of society's members, the criminal society outside the institution (thieves), or the inmate power structure within the institution (convicts). The latter two deviant sub-groups differ according to Merton's distinction between "cosmopolitan" and "local."[1] Prison conduct for "thieves" is prescribed by the code of loyalty to other criminals, prohibition against "ratting," etc., which obtains in the under-world outside prison, while "convicts" participate in wheeling and dealing to enhance their status and power within the institution.

The last two articles in Section II represent an attempt to relate treatment for the institutional inmate to social systems outside the institution— his family in the first paper, and the community at large, including the family, in the second paper. Fleck and his co-workers are primarily concerned with offsetting deleterious effects of parental interference in their child's hospitalization, while Greenblatt discusses an attempt to provide an intermediary step between total institutionalization and resumption of full participation in the responsibility of family life and work. Erikson would no doubt applaud Greenblatt's efforts to make training for responsibility, with continuing professional support to fall back on, part of the therapeutic task. Indeed each of the papers in this section calls attention to some aspect of the fact that residential institutions function in the service of societal as well as individual needs, and that lack of institutional awareness of their social functions imperils their value both for society and the individuals they seek to return to it.

[1] Robert K. Merton, *Social Theory and Social Structure*, Glencoe, Ill.: Free Press, 1957, Chapter 10.

𝕔𝕖

CHAPTER 10   Introducing Change in

a Mental Hospital*

PAUL C. AGNEW AND FRANCIS L. K. HSU

THE PROBLEM

WITH all their dynamism and emphasis on progress, Americans tend to resist changes like other peoples. There are two reasons for this resistance. On the one hand, any change of any consequence is likely to require some shift in habits to which the individuals involved have been accustomed. On the other hand, since every group is a social system, any change in one of its component parts is likely to require or result in alteration or rearrangement of other parts. Both of these tend to be painful or troublesome.

The purpose of this paper is to indicate one method of dealing with this resistance to change in a mental hospital and an analysis of how this method worked.

THE SETTING

THE setting of the case is the 34-bed psychiatric ward of a 516-bed general medical and surgical Veterans Administration Hospital. This is an open ward used for relatively short term diagnostic work-up and treatment. The staff is psychoanalytically oriented. In addition to individual psychotherapy, the therapeutic armamentarium includes active occupational therapy, recreational therapy, group psychotherapy, drugs and E.S.T. when indicated. Through the team approach, the attempt is made to plan the patient's total hospital experience to supply his individual treatment needs. The patient census includes all diagnostic categories except disturbed psychotics.

On admission to hospital all patients were required to deposit their

* Reprinted from *Human Organization*, 19 (1960–61), 195–198, by permission of the authors and the Society for Applied Anthropology.

civilian clothes at the hospital clothing room and were issued hospital pajamas and robes, or green uniforms. Throughout their stay in the hospital patients were expected to wear this clothing. When leaving the hospital on pass they must turn in the hospital apparel at the clothing room and check out their civilian clothing. On return to the hospital, the reverse must be carried out.

THE PROPOSED CHANGE

THE staff psychiatrists believe that psychiatric patients should wear their own clothing throughout their stay in the hospital. This conviction is based on their experiences and those of others in the planned use of the total milieu to meet dynamically understood therapeutic needs of individual patients. Sivadon, in a recent report on new techniques of sociotherapy employed in a public hospital in the Department of the Seine, France, points out that he has a psychologist to function as a hostess to welcome each new patient, that instead of taking away the patient's personal effects, she gives him whatever he needs—toilet articles, cigarettes, writing paper, and so on.[1] But the therapeutic value of this change is not the issue in this paper and will not be discussed. The Chief of the Psychiatric Service first conveyed to the Director of Professional Services the staff's wish to make the change in October 1958. He presented the reasons in detail. The Director of Professional Services took the attitude that, if the Chief of the Psychiatric Service recommended the change as a "medical" policy, he would support it as policy, but he foresaw many administrative and practical difficulties in the way. He suggested that he call a meeting to include the Director of Professional Services, the Chief of Psychiatry Service, the Registrar, and the Chief of Nursing Service to discuss the matter.

REACTIONS OF THE PERSONNEL

SUCH a meeting was held. The Director of Professional Services presented the proposed change.

The immediate reaction of the Registrar, the Chief of Nursing Service, and others was that the problems involved in making such a change were probably insurmountable:

Where would patients keep their clothing? Who would be responsible for it? How could thievery be prevented? What if a patient did not possess clothing? Who would do the laundry? Would patients elope? Patients would feel "marked" as psychiatric.

These and many more "problems" were brought up as reasons why the change could not be successfully carried out. Had the majority opinion at this meeting prevailed, the whole thing would have been dropped then and there.

The Director of Professional Services decided to hold another similar meeting to discuss the issues further. After the second one, it developed that a series of meetings was held over a four-month period to explore ways in which the change could be worked out.[2] At these meetings a number of ways of solving the anticipated problems were outlined. Some of them were as follows: 1) that the patients should check their clothing out of the hospital clothing room daily and return them at night; 2) a clothing room should be established on the ward, to be operated by the nurses, from which the patients would daily check out their clothes; and 3) individual clothing lockers should be supplied to patients. But each of these suggestions seemed to involve pitfalls making it appear unworkable. Proposals were offered for ways to handle laundry: 1) the hospital laundry could do it; 2) patients and their families could take all laundry responsibility; and 3) laundry could be collected and sent out to local laundries and dry cleaning establishments. Again, each alternative seemed to present new problems which made it appear unworkable.[3]

In this series of six meetings free and open discussion prevailed. Views and ideas of all personnel were expressed with the Director of Professional Services assuming the role of chairman. It would be impractical to present a word-by-word report of these discussions. In essence, over the course of the meetings, there was a shift from seeing the whole proposal as impossible and impractical to reaching workable solutions for all problems involved.

REACTION OF THE PATIENTS

THE patients had frequently complained to the ward personnel about having to wear green hospital uniforms. Professional personnel on the Psychiatric Service all agreed that patients objected to the hospital clothing policy, that they felt it as dehumanizing, as losing individuality and self-respect.[4]

Several weeks before the date set for the changeover to civilian clothes, the matter was presented in detail to the patients' weekly forum.[5] Instead of receiving this news with satisfaction, the patients immediately expressed objections to it:

Where would we keep the clothes? How would the laundry be done? Would we have to pay for dry cleaning? Will we be tagged as "psychos" in the hospital?

Only two patients' forums were held before the clothing change was instituted. The patients' resistance to the proposed change did not diminish until then. But a week or so after the change was brought about, the patients' resistance stopped. It was replaced by an affirmative attitude toward wearing their civilian clothes.

ANALYSIS

THE first reactions of the personnel and the patients are perfectly in line with what we have already pointed out in the introductory section of this paper. Since any and all changes involve rearrangement of thought, habit patterns, and/or human relations and therefore will be painful or trouble-some in some ways to all concerned, the typical first reaction will be blanket resistance to them. However, such pains and troubles may be more tolerated in some milieux than in others. For example, American business and industrial establishments, especially the medium and the big ones, usually aim at bigger volume, better products, and higher profit from month to month and from year to year. The idea of change in the interest of higher efficiency toward these goals, rationalized consciously or unconsciously as progress, is, and must be, accepted by a majority of the employees if they wish to survive. Those who cannot keep up with the pace either voluntarily resign, or are dropped. That is to say, the possible pain or trouble due to the changes are compensated for by the rewards which come with reaching the goals.

However, in a non-profit milieu and especially in a government organi-zation or any highly structured setting such as a hospital where such rewards are not obviously part of the system and where job security is provided for by the bureaucratic structure already, the matter is different. Here any proposed change to the extent that it necessitates alterations of personal habits or organizational routines will tend to be regarded as a nuisance and treated with hostility.[6]

It was obvious that, in their insistence on the status quo, the personnel's resistance took opposite directions. On the one hand, they saw the pro-posed change as entailing more responsibility for themselves with which they did not wish to be burdened. On the other hand, they saw it as leading to more responsibility for the patients which they felt that the patients were not capable of assuming.

These points of resistance were, of course, further disguised under the rationalizing garbs given during the first staff meeting when the question of clothing change was raised. Why did a progressive diminution of the personnel resistance become obvious as the series of meetings progressed? Two factors would seem to be at work. The first is the technique used by the psychiatrists in dealing with the resistances of the personnel; the other concerns the deeper emotional sources of the resistance which can only be understood in terms of the American psychology of self-reliance.

The psychiatrists perceived the resistances of the group and responded as they might to resistances in psychotherapy. They avoided direct frontal attacks on the resistances such as getting angry, pointing them out as unreasonable, branding the personnel's objections as rationalizations, or some other defense. Instead, they encouraged expression of these feelings, but they themselves concentrated on offering, in a calm way, detailed solutions to the real problems involved in implementing the proposed change. On one issue they could be said to have made an interpretation to the personnel. The personnel initially were not aware of their assumption that patients could not assume more responsibility. The psychiatrists gently but effectively conveyed to the group, by detailed descriptions of patients' behavior, that this assumption was not realistic.

How the American psychology of self-reliance was at work in the situation is somewhat more obscure. Elsewhere, one of the authors has dwelt on the subject of individual self-reliance as a basis of American culture and psychology, as contrasted to mutual dependence as a basis of Chinese culture and psychology.[7] Suffice it to say here that self-reliance enjoins the individual, whether as child or adult, to take care of himself, be master of himself, support himself, and to control his own destiny. "Smile and the world smiles with you; cry and you cry alone" is the motto. Self-reliance is practically synonymous in this culture with self-respect. A person who possesses a dependent character is thought to be in need of psychiatric help. The most important expression of this is the tendency on the part of the majority of Americans to insist on making their own decisions and on not following any authority blindly. This is the psychology to which advertisers appeal constantly. Coupled with this insistence on making their own decisions is the American distaste for authority, especially if they are situated at the receiving end of it.

Therefore, as independent members of a great institution, and having been brought up to be self-reliant, the personnel of an American hospital is likely to be much more resistant to change imposed on them by authority from above than is its counterpart in China. To the Chinese, the changes will be infinitely facilitated if they have been suggested or imposed by such persons as father, mother, grandparents, employer, or office superior. The traditional Chinese cultural framework enjoins the individual to submit to authority especially if the authority does not threaten his basic livelihood. The individual in the Chinese culture is, therefore, absolved of any psychological necessity for resisting the change, although he may not like the change for other reasons. Accepting changes imposed by external authority does no violence to his self-respect. To the American, the individual is definitely much more sensitive to imposed authority, and therefore, must resist it much more than would the Chinese. This is why they would give so many rationalizations, some of which are opposed to others. Some of the rationalizations are not necessarily connected with the real motives at all. In fact, the real motives may not be clear to the individuals themselves. When human beings resist change, they often have no particularly coherent or logical reasons in their mind. When pressed, they tend freely to use rationalizations. The true basis of this resistance to the suggested change is that the American individual tends to feel that it is important for him to make his own decisions. Therefore, any kind of blind acceptance of authority means reduction of self-respect.

During the series of conferences, the personnel increasingly reduced its resistance to the proposed change because the individuals involved had gradually internalized, at least in part, the proposed change. As they came to feel they themselves had originated the change, they tended to go along with the change much more easily than before, for if the change came from themselves, it would no longer be seen as threatening to their self-reliance and self-respect.

The substance of this mechanism was utilized, although not described in terms of American self-reliance, in another hospital as reported in Cumming, Clancy, and Cumming. The change attempted there had to do with the reorganization of the lines of authority and communication so that the hospital could operate as one institution instead of a divided one. This involved changes in personnel positions and the introduction of new positions which would inevitably lead to unhappiness on the part of some. What Cumming *et al.* did was to arrange a meeting of all concerned, in which they were given a full description of the new jobs and were, in addition, asked to fill out sociometric ballots indicating which members of the staff they would like to have promoted to these new positions. In this way Cumming *et al.* successfully introduced the change partly because they delegated the decision-making function to a lower echelon which in the past had never . . .

. . . had to assume the responsibility for making decisions about changes, and a feeling of increased status and involvement resulted.[8]

The patients are in a somewhat different situation from the personnel. As Americans, they have also been trained from childhood to be self-reliant and independent; but as patients in a psychiatric ward, they are forced to be utterly dependent and many of them are conscious of this fact. There is thus an inherent contradiction in their very situation of existence and they, like the personnel, also reacted to the proposed change in contradictory directions but for different reasons. The patients' resistance could be conceptualized as follows: patients felt the experience of being in the hospital and of having all clothing and laundry needs supplied by the environment as regressive. When dependent strivings were stimulated, feelings of guilt and loss of self-esteem were also mobilized. The clothing policy was reacted to as a recapitulation of childhood experience with the consequent evocation of dependence and hostility once felt toward parents. When the proposal that patients wear civilian clothes and take care of their own laundry was presented, resistance to giving up dependent gratification was mobilized.[9] After the change had occurred, patients felt the gratification of increased self-esteem at being more independent, and their resistance ceased. The idea of increased individuality tends to reinforce the patients' feeling for self-reliance and tends to override or provide fresh support and new direction for their self-esteem. Hence, their resistance to change subsided and they accepted the change.

Reviewing the reactions of the two groups, the patients' resistance and the personnel's, the common denominator between them is the concept of individual self-reliance. This is a concept which guides American behavior. There are, of course, variations in the degree to which individuals are exposed to this basic American value, but there seems to be little room for dispute that an overwhelming majority of Americans have been, and are continuously being, exposed to this value. Both personnel and patients feared the loss of self-reliance and wished to use the resistance against authority in some fashion as a mechanism of defense. Even though the patients are in a situation of dependence, they will no less feel the conscious need for independence so long as they are not suffering from a major psychosis. They are more likely to be pressed by such a need than patients of another culture in which individual self-reliance as a value is not so important. In fact, the more sensitive they are to this need, the more acutely they will regard their present dependence as a kind of personal disgrace. In order to maintain their feeling of self-reliance or independence, however vague, the one tool at their disposal is to fight against some kind of authority. This is why, when the hospital imposed on them the wearing of the green uniforms as they came in, they complained about it; but when the hospital suggested that they wear their own clothing, even though this is what they had said they wished to do in the first place, they still resisted for the reason that they unconsciously seized it as another opportunity of resisting authority. Their contradictory acts really had nothing to do with wearing the green uniform or wearing their own clothing as such. These acts of opposition merely mitigated for them the disgrace of being dependent, in a cultural environment which promotes self-reliance and independence to the highest degree.

What happened after these initial resistances to change on the part of the patients is open to two different lines of interpretation. On the one hand, we may say that the patients, being in a highly dependent position in the authoritarian framework of a hospital structure, are far less capable of resisting changes imposed on them than the personnel or other freer agents. In this regard they may be compared to children. In the first place, a child may resist his mother by refusing to wear his coat and then resist her later by wearing it; or resist the mother in eating spinach and then resist her by refusing to eat it. The child's object of resistance is neither

the coat nor the spinach, but his mother. But if the mother is really angry
and shows determination by declaring to the child:

Now you are on your own; you can forget about me. Do whatever you please,
but I will not have anything more to do with you,

the child is likely to capitulate and will usually come back to complete
dependence and submission, at least for a short while. Therefore, after the
initial resistance to the green uniforms and then resistance to wearing
their own clothes, the patients really had no alternative when the administration put its foot down. They had in effect been forced to come to terms
with "their parents."[10]

On the other hand, if the Director of Professional Services or the Chief
of Psychiatry Service decided to lay down the law vis-à-vis the personnel,
declaring that, whether you like it or not, we are going to make the
change, it would have been a very different proposition. The Chief of
Psychiatry Service or the Director of Professional Services may be able
administratively to get away with it in this particular issue. They can
order the change and the change will be effected. But the personnel
consists of freer agents than the patient body, who are in a much better
position to sabotage this and other orders when their self-reliance and
self-respect are threatened.[11] In that event the working relationship of the
entire hospital administration will deteriorate.

CONCLUSIONS

THE bearing of this analysis on psychiatric therapy is outside the scope of
the present paper. It does have genuine implications for the administration of large, bureaucratic (including hospital) organizations in which the
profit motive is absent and in which job security does not fluctuate directly
with production.

The following points emerge: A) The experience described in this
paper would indicate that, when an innovation is introduced into an
organization, resistance is to be expected. B) This resistance can be
reduced or eliminated if the American culture pattern of equivalence
between self-reliance and self-respect is taken into consideration. A series
of conferences avoiding any show of authority and emphasizing the independence of all participants seems an effective method. C) A balance
between maximized feeling of independence and the need for enforcing
policy and authority is the most essential part of administrative technique
in American society.

NOTES TO CHAPTER 10

1. Paul Daniel Sivadon, "Techniques of Sociotherapy," *Psychiatry*, XX (Feb-
ruary-November, 1957), 205-210.

2. Cumming and Cumming describe holding meetings as part of their method of bringing about change in a mental hospital. They describe meeting with the staff "for six weeks each morning for an hour, and for the next six months three mornings a week," John and Claire Cumming in M. Greenblatt, D. J. Levinson, and R. H. Williams (eds.), *Social Equilibrium and Social Change in the Large Mental Hospital in the Patient and the Mental Hospital*, The Free Press, Glencoe, Illinois, 1957, p. 61.

3. "A great deal of effort was spent in persuading the staff that things could be done. They found it hard to accept the idea that a routine could be changed wtihout dire consequences." (Cumming and Cumming, *ibid.*, p. 60.)

4. It is not necessarily inferred that psychiatric patients are more sensitive in their reactions to the hospital environment than medical or surgical patients. It probably reflects the greater preoccupation of the psychiatric personnel to the psychiatric patients' sensitivity to such things. This preoccupation is expressed clearly by Alfred H. Stanton and Morris S. Schwartz, e.g., in their study of the mental hospital: "A guiding principle in the improvement of the physical furnishings of the ward was the attempt to deemphasize furnishings that suggested involuntary restraints with precautions which characterized the hospital. Doors were constructed so that the use of keys was an inconspicuous as possible, and all new personnel were instructed to use their keys quietly. To the patients, the key was the most significant symbol of their helplessness . . .," *The Mental Hospital* (A Study of Institutional Participation in Psychiatric Illness and Treatment), Basic Books, Inc., New York, 1954, p. 125.

5. This forum was instituted in November, 1958 in this hospital. It consists of a weekly meeting in which patients meet with ward personnel and are encouraged to express freely and openly their feelings about the hospital, ward rules, etc.

6. John and Claire Cumming observed in another hospital that ". . . a great deal of the daily round is governed by tradition, and in such a situation change is seldom welcomed . . . traditional and static, the mental hospital is hard to change . . . the Administrative officers are vitally concerned with maintaining the status quo. Their natural enemy is the young and enthusiastic doctor with new ideas and a desire to promote change." (*Op. cit.*, pp. 50-51.)

7. Francis L. K. Hsu, *American and Chinese: Two Ways of Life*, Abelard-Schuman, Inc., New York, 1953.

8. Elaine Cumming, I. L. W. Clancey, and John Cumming, "Improving Patient Care Through Organizational Changes in the Mental Hospital," *Psychiatry*, XIX, 249-261. The direct quote is from p. 259. John Cumming and Elaine Cumming made a similar statement in another content: "No staff welcomes programs of general change which they have not themselves initiated." (Cumming and Cumming, *op. cit.*, p. 63.)

9. This observation is based on the consensus of opinion of the psychiatric staff members who had contacts with the patients during the entire episode. After the initial suggestion for the change was made, the Patients' Forum was held several times. This is a regular feature of the Division of Psychiatry in this hospital during which patients can vent their complaints, feel-

ings and views to each other and to the doctors, nurses, and orderlies present. The dependency attitudes on the part of patients in a psychiatric treatment situation is well known. The very process of psychiatric treatment involves first getting the patient to become aware of his helplessness and need for help and then enabling him to mobilize and utilize available resources, from within or without himself, to achieve a socially and culturally acceptable degree of independence. During these forums there was, however, no *direct* evidence showing that patients resisted the proposed change because of their reluctance to giving up dependent gratifications. No patient expressed it overtly in so many words. This is understandable if we take into consideration the American psychology and culture explained before. Being products of a society which equates self-reliance with self-respect Americans, whether they are inside or outside of a hospital, will be loathe to betray their own dependent feelings. In the present instance the inference by the psychiatric staff members is based on the following facts: a) The known relationship between mental patients on the one hand and hospital (especially Government ones) and its staff members on the other; b) the irrelevant and vague nature of the patients' objections to the new clothing policy; c) analysis of the interview material with established interpretive techniques.

10. Some psychiatric thinkers, who emphasize the need for developing the therapeutic community into a "democratic social organization where permissiveness and a spirit of inquiry and helpfulness predominate" (for example, see Maxwell Jones: 'The Treatment of Personality Disorders in a Therapeutic Community,' *Psychiatry,* XX [1957], 217) may view the last part of the analysis with trepidation. They see this analysis as description of an authoritarian approach to mental patients. We can only observe that there is as yet no assurance that the completely democratic approach will prove to be the most therapeutic. The wiser course is probably a compromise between the authoritarian and the democratic, in which direction the trend of general education for our youths is headed today. The present episode is simply part of a total experience in which authoritarian and democratic elements are intertwined.

11. In this connection the reader is referred to the observation of Cumming and Cumming (*op. cit.*, p. 56) that anxiety and hostility among staff may be expressed as continuing non-cooperation, as sabotage of the program.

ॐ

✓CHAPTER 11   Patient Role and Social
Uncertainty—A Dilemma of the Mentally Ill*

KAI T. ERIKSON

T HE concept of role has become widely used in the field of mental
health to relate the behavior of mental patients to the social setting
of their illness. The literature in which this concept has appeared, however, has been largely concerned with the specialized culture of the
mental hospital—the formal and informal structures of ward life—almost
as if the universe to which a patient relates when he enacts a "patient
role" is neatly contained within hospital walls.[1] To the sociologist, who
generally uses the concept of role in a broader social context, this tends to
place a one-sided emphasis on the institution itself as the essential focus of
the patient's social life.

When a person enters a mental hospital for treatment, to be sure, he
abandons many of the social ties which anchored him to a definite place in
society. However, the act of becoming a mental patient effects a fundamental *change* in the person's relationship to the ongoing processes of
society, not a complete withdrawal from them; and while the forms of his
participation are altered, he remains acutely sensitive to outer influences.
Even in the relative isolation of the hospital ward, then, the patient's
behavior to some extent articulates his relationship to the larger society
and reflects the social position which he feels is reserved for him in its
organizational structure. It is this aspect of the role of the patient which
the present paper will consider.

* The research on which this paper is based was supported by a Fellowship from the
Grant Foundation and was conducted under the auspices of the Family Study Center,
University of Chicago. The writer would like to thank Nelson N. Foote, formerly
director of the Family Study Center, for the opportunity to do this study and for many
helpful criticisms.

Reprinted by special permission of The William Alanson White Psychiatric Foundation, Inc., and the author from *Psychiatry*, 20 (1957), 263–274 (copyright by the
Foundation).

DEFINITIONS

ROLE usually is used to designate a set of behaviors or values about behavior which is commonly considered appropriate for persons occupying given statuses or positions in society. For the purposes of this paper, it will be useful to consider that the acquisition of roles by a person involves two basic processes: *role-validation* and *role-commitment*. Role-validation takes place when a community 'gives' a person certain expectations to live up to, providing him with distinct notions as to the conduct it considers appropriate or valid for him in his position.[2] Role-commitment is the complementary process whereby a person adopts certain styles of behavior as his own, committing himself to role themes that best represent the kind of person he assumes himself to be, and best reflect the social position he considers himself to occupy.

Normally, of course, these processes take place simultaneously and are seldom overtly distinguished in the relationship between the person and his community. The person learns to accept the image that the group holds up to him as a more or less accurate reflection of himself, is able to accept as his own the position which the group provides for him, and thus becomes more or less committed to the behavior values which the group poses as valid for him. The merit of making a distinction between these two processes, then, is solely to visualize what happens in marginal situations in which conflict does occur—in which the person develops behavior patterns which the community regards as invalid for him, or the community entertains expectations which the person feels unable to realize. Sociologists, traditional specialists in this aspect of deviance, have generally been more concerned with the process of validation than that of commitment, concentrating on the mechanisms which groups employ to persuade individuals that roles validated for them deserve their personal commitment.

In so doing, sociologists have largely overlooked the extent to which a person can *engineer* a change in the role expectations held in his behalf, rather than passively waiting for others to 'allocate' or 'assign' roles to him. This he does by being so persistent in his commitment to certain modes of behavior, and so convincing in his portrayal of them, that the community is persuaded to accept these modes as the basis for a new set of expectations on its part.

Thus the process by which persons acquire a recognized role may, at times, involve long and delicate negotiations between the individual and his community. The individual presents himself in behavior styles that express his personal sense of identity and continuity;[3] the group validates role models for him that fit its own functional needs.[4] The negotiation is concluded when a mutually satisfactory definition of the individual is reached and a position established for him in the group structure—or when the issue becomes stalemated and suppressive sanctions against deviance are called into play.

The argument to be presented here is that such a negotiation is likely to follow a mental patient's admission to a mental hospital, particularly if he does not qualify as a "certified" patient with a circumscribed disease. In accepting hospitalization, the patient is often caught in the pull of divergent sets of expectations: on the one hand, he is exposed to psychiatry's demand that he make a wholehearted commitment to the process of treatment, and, on the other, he is confronted by a larger society which is often unwilling to validate these commitments. He is left, then, with no consistent and durable social role, with no clear-cut social models upon which to fashion his behavior. The patient is thus often persuaded by the logic of psychiatric institutions to attempt to engineer validation in the role this society provides for the *medical* patient—in which, to be sure, distinctly psychotic patients are presumed to belong. To establish his eligibility for this conventional role, the mental patient must negotiate, using his illness as an instrumentality. He must present his illness to others in a form which they recognize as legitimate, perhaps even exaggerating his portrayal of those behaviors which qualify medical patients for their role. In having to do so, the argument continues, he is often left with little choice but to become sicker or more chronically sick.

THE PATIENT

THIS section is based primarily on data collected in a small, "open" psychiatric hospital which offered analytically oriented psychotherapy for a fairly selective group of patients. Diagnoses in this population ranged, for the most part, from the severe psychoneuroses to borderline psychoses. The institutional setting lacked the scheduled rigidity of closed hospital routines and allowed for an unusual degree of personal initiative. Since the patients received almost daily individual therapy and were, in a certain respect, volunteers for treatment, who recognized the implications of their patienthood, they could hardly be considered representative of the average ward population. But the experienced clinician will be able to determine to what extent generalizations made from observation of this group apply to patients in custodial institutions, whose contacts with the outside world are more limited. No doubt many of the same social forces act upon patients in any hospital situation, even where behavior is more strictly routinized and confined within the limiting boundaries of a closed ward so that it may seem to reflect the common setting in which it took place rather than the common motivations which produced it. Thus it is possible that the uniqueness of the therapeutic setting in which these observations took place simply affords a more spontaneous picture of social forces operating in any psychiatric hospital.

While doing some sociological work in this setting, the writer took a brief inventory of behavior themes which seemed characteristic of the patient group and which appeared to be among the central motifs of the patients' role behavior.

One may begin by noting certain contradictions implicit in the very act of becoming a mental patient. By accepting hospitalization, the patient makes a contractual agreement to cooperate in a therapeutic partnership: he agrees to want and to appreciate treatment, to be realistic about his need for help, to volunteer relevant information, and to act as reliably as possible upon the recommendations of his therapist. Yet it is widely considered a condition of his illness that he is unable to make meaningful contact with any reality, therapeutic or otherwise. In the grip of these discrepant expectations, his behavior is likely to be a curious mixture of the active and the passive, a mosaic of acts which tend to confirm his competence and acts which tend to dramatize his helplessness. He must test the limits of his own uncertain controls and look for consistent expectations to guide him, as the following fragment from a case history illustrates:

One of the outstanding characteristics of this patient is his absolute uncertainty about his illness and what is expected of him in the institution and in therapy. He is uncertain whether he actively produces his hysterical states or whether they come upon him without his being able to do anything about them. He does not know whether he is supposed to show his symptoms or suppress them, to "let go" of his impulses and act out or to exert active self-control and "put the lid on." He is afraid that if he does the former, he is psychotic and will be considered too sick for the open institutional setting here; if he does the latter, he will be a pretending psychopath and considered too well to continue treatment here at all. He does not know what he should expect from himself, from other patients, from his sickness, from other people he knows, or even from his therapist. Perhaps his most crucial problem at the moment is to define for himself what are the conditions of his stay here as a patient.

This fragment sums up the bewildering social situation in which the patient must act, and it is not difficult to understand how the final assumption of a consistent social role might represent to him a clarification and partial adjustment. To demonstrate this, I shall try to isolate a few strands of behavior from this complicated fabric.

All children are taught in this culture that it is impolite to stare at or make reference to the infirmities of cripples. So it is interesting to note that the generous impulse of outsiders to overlook a patient's less visible infirmities is likely to put the patient in an instant state of alarm, and to bring urgent assurances on his part that he is severely sick and in serious need of treatment. Patients often bring this topic into conversation on scant provocation and continue to talk about it even when fairly vigorous attempts are made by visitors to change the subject. The patient is likely to describe this as "accepting the realities of his illness," by which he means that he frankly admits the seriousness of his sickness and refuses to take refuge in some convenient defense that might deny it. Yet to the observer it often appears that this is an attempt to convince *others* of these realities as well as to remind himself, as if he were afraid they would be overlooked entirely. The patient seems to feel it crucial that his illness be accepted as a fundamental fact about himself, the premise on which he enters into relations with others.

Side by side with this severe "honesty," the patient can develop a considerable degree of responsibility in carrying out the therapeutic recommendations of his therapist. And if the hospital tries to foster the patient's social initiative, he may respond with resources that even the therapist did not know were at his disposal. Such initiative is usually in evidence only during certain hospital activities and sometimes appears to belie the very weaknesses which the patient, at other times, displays so insistently. Patients at the hospital in question, for instance, have organized and produced dramatic plays before outside audiences, performing with a skill that surprised professional dramatic observers, and succeeding even when the therapists themselves had severe reservations about the outcome. At a prizewinning performance in a neighboring city, some of the audience were and remained under the impression that the players were members of the medical staff rather than patients of the institution.

Yet as one records this accomplishment, it must be noted that such positive efforts can sometimes be as deceptive as they are surprising, and that, at times, they can produce negative undercurrents that threaten to cancel out the accomplishment altogether. In reporting on the plays performed at the hospital, one journalist noted this. He said that the patients produce and act in plays before paying audiences with a competence which, according to Clifford Odets, who saw one of his plays so performed, is equal to that of any good amateur group. At the same time, the reporter said, one of the doctors had remarked ruefully, "I was very upset when one of my patients, after doing a fine job in the play, went back to the patients' dormitory and tried to set fire to it."

The example is extreme, but it illustrates the conflict a patient encounters in committing himself to positive and constructive activity. Like Penelope, who wove a cloak by day only to unravel it at night, the mental patient often portrays the insecurity of his position by staging, after every advance of this kind, a dramatic retreat into impulsivity and destruction.

Thus at once the patient accepts responsibility for a type of performance rarely asked of the average person, yet is unable to control actions which, in the light of the earlier accomplishment, would seem to be well within his realm of mastery. This seeming paradox is a recurring motif that runs through the whole complex of the patient's role behavior. As has been shown in the case abstract that introduced this section, the patient has potentialities for activity and passivity, for resourcefulness and helplessness, in any given area of action. To organize these into a coherent role pattern, it seems, the patient partitions his hospital world into areas where he considers one or the other of these potential responses specifically appropriate.

In some decisive situations, as has been described, the patient faces his hospital life with remarkable initiative. Yet in others, an overwhelming theme of helplessness seems to dominate his behavior. He is likely to insist, in terms far stronger than the situation would appear to necessitate, that he is unable to control his behavior and must be given a wide license for conduct that is certainly unconventional according to the values prevalent outside the hospital. A patient was asked, "Why did you do that?" His answer, "How should I know? If I knew these things, I wouldn't be here," reflects the values thus emerging in the patient role pattern. Patients have been heard comforting one another by saying, "Of course you can't do it." This process of "giving up defenses" is, of course, presumed to be essential for successful treatment, particularly in intensive analytic therapy, and a certain license for impulsivity and acting out seems to be part of much of psychotherapy in general. But the patient often seems to reserve his right for such license with what appear to be unnecessary claims that he "can't help it."

One might add that whereas clinical evidence indicates that patients often feel a strong guilt at "having let others down," the values of the patient group seldom allow its overt expression—and even supply convenient channels for its projection elsewhere. It is not uncommon for patients to bitterly indict their parents, often for the same weakness they themselves "can't help," sometimes talking as if a kind of deliberate conspiracy was involved in the events that led to their own illness. The weakness of this logic seems evident even to those who use it most persistently, which again indicates that the social usages which allow its expression must have an important social function to the patient group. If a little harsh, it may be one way to deny one's responsibility for being sick, while nevertheless accounting for one's illness in terms that are current outside the hospital walls.

The point is that most of the persons a patient encounters in the hospital, certainly the other patients, are perfectly willing to acknowledge that ego deficiencies are not his "fault" and that he is often compelled to act without the benefit of sufficient controls. To what audience, then, does he address his continual protest that he has the *right* to some license and can't help the fact that he is sick? Largely, one begins to think, these assertions are broadcast not to the audience assembled in the confined orbit of the hospital at all—but to the omnipresent public which, as shall be seen, fails to validate his commitment to therapy. To assume that hospital walls or the implicit ideology of psychiatric institutions protect the patient from this audience would be an unfortunate oversight. The image of the public audience is firmly incorporated within the patient himself, and this image is constantly reinforced by newspapers, movies, radio, and television. The specialized values which psychiatry introduces into the hospital setting cannot entirely overcome the fact that the patient remains sensitive to current public notions about mental illness, and, on certain levels of awareness, even shares them in substance.

What does the outside audience ask of the patient—and its internalized image make him ask of himself? Essentially, he is asked to justify his voluntary retirement to a hospital by demonstrating that he *needs* it, by displaying a distinct illness requiring highly specialized help. The reason for a person's therapy in a residential setting is obviously the wish on everybody's part that he develop adjustive initiative. Yet if large parts of society doubt his claim to illness when he appears to have a certain competence—when, for instance, he rehearses healthy modes of behavior on or off the stage—he is left in the exposed position of one who has to *look* incompetent even while learning to become the exact opposite. A few minutes before going on the stage, a patient-actor announced, "It is a tradition here that the show *never* goes on!" This tradition is of particular interest because it has no basis in fact whatever. The show in question did go on, as had all of its predecessors. Yet even in the act of positive accomplishment the patient feels it important to repeat that failure is the norm among mental patients, for he always anticipates the question, "Look here, if you can do these things so well, why are you here?"

This prominent theme of helplessness which runs through the patient's verbal and behavioral repertoire again reasserts the basic paradox. For while much of the time he may display a passivity that almost suggests disability, he shows a certain ingenuity in organizing his passive behavior strategically; he can put considerable energy into maneuvers which show him to be helpless; in short, he can go to ample expense to give the impression of one who has nothing to expend. This does not imply, of course, that the patient is deliberately staging a deceptive performance. On the contrary, it suggests that the psychological needs which motivate such behavior are as compelling, in a certain way, as those considered to be anchored somewhere in the dynamics and genetics of his illness, and, in fact, tend to reinforce them.

In the absence of clear-cut organic symptoms, a "real" illness which "can't be helped" is the most precious commodity such patients have in their bargaining with society for a stable patient role. It is the most substantial credential available in their application for equal rights with the medical patient, and as such, may come to have an important social value to them. The fatal logic of this may be that the patient will find his social situation better structured for him if he gives in to his illness and helps others to create an unofficial hospital structure which supports the perpetuation of patienthood.

SOCIAL UNCERTAINTY

ALTHOUGH all human groups rely heavily upon the mechanisms they develop to suppress deviant behavior, among the most crucial measures of any society are the provisions it makes for absorbing certain kinds of deviance into its structure. Societies often accomplish this by placing given individuals—usually those whose deviancy is not considered deliberate—in special statuses where their otherwise invalid behavior becomes the expected and legitimate mode of conduct.

In a well-known analysis, Talcott Parsons argues that illness is a form of deviance which the culture shelters in this manner.[5] By setting role expectations for the ill person which both exempt him from his usual social duties and assure that he will return to them as soon as possible, society effectively neutralizes the onus his failure to perform would otherwise imply. The conditions of this special sick role, as Parsons sees them, are four: First, the sick person is exempted from certain of his normal social obligations. Second, the sick person is considered unable to recover by an act of conscious will; that is, he "can't help it." Third, the sick person is considered obligated to *want* to get well, to cooperate with a physician in achieving recovery, and to accept the protection of the sick role only so long as it is therapeutically necessary. Fourth, the sick person is regarded as in need of technically competent help, which implies that accepting the status of "sick person" is conditional upon accepting the status of "patient."

When sociologists speak about societies "doing" something—providing roles, entertaining expectations, and so on—they take for granted that the acts in question are matters of general public agreement, are institutionalized by consensus. One might ask, then, on the basis of what criteria do persons qualify for the sick role? Like the military physician who must determine from day to day which of the many men who report to him are *really* sick, the public at large must have some generally accepted standards for deciding who is eligible for the sick role exemptions. The sick role, of course, is not granted only out of sympathy for a person's discomfort: it is granted as factual recognition that the person is, in fact, *unable* to carry out his normal duties. The first of these criteria, then, to follow Parsons' logic, is that the person must be at least partially disabled either because of the severity of the illness or the requirements for cure. Furthermore, the patient's disability must be considered one that he is unable to erase by a deliberate exercise of will, his willingness and ability to "get well as soon as possible" must remain unquestioned, and his condition must be regarded as within the province of a qualified therapeutic profession. In fact in most medical practice it is the physician, acting in the name of society, who certified his patient as "really" ill.

This brings up an uncomfortable argument. Although the public generally accepts the physician's verbal certificate as indication of legitimate physical sickness, it continues to doubt the medical legitimacy of many forms of mental illness and often fails to accept the mental patient as a qualified candidate for the sick role.

Recent evidence indicates that, despite the public's growing acceptance of psychiatry, current attitudes toward mental illness fall considerably short of the enlightened attitudes promoted in popular publications. The results of these studies have not yet been made available except in scattered summaries, but certain conclusions can be drawn from them that throw the present situation of psychiatry specifically and the field of mental health generally into a fairly harsh focus.[6]

It appears that on the surface the public has developed reasonably tolerant attitudes toward the mentally ill and even a hesitant respect for the practice of psychiatry. People understand the need for increased psychiatric facilities, appreciate the enormity of the mental health problem, and agree that mental illness is a condition requiring specialized treatment and competently trained help. Yet underneath the pleasant surface of these enlightened principles, people have little idea how to recognize the concrete problems that these principles encompass.

The average person, it seems, cannot identify mental illness when he sees it, cannot recognize the symptoms that indicate it, and remains quite uncertain about the very meaning of the term when pressed for a definition. He continues to resist the notion that a person can be mentally ill and not entirely "out of his mind," although willing to accept illness as legitimate if the patient is a potential danger to the community and is securely committed to a custodial institution.[7]

In practice, people make it clear that they do not generally regard behavior as proof of mental illness, unless three interrelated conditions obtain. First of all, they look for a breakdown of intellect, an almost complete loss of cognitive functioning or, in short, a loss of reason. . . . Second, people expect, almost as a necessary consequence of this loss of rationality, that the behavior called mental illness must represent a serious loss of self-control, usually to the point of dangerous violence against others and certainly to the point of *not being responsible for one's acts.* . . . Finally, people feel that, to qualify as mental illness, behavior should be inappropriate—that is, neither reasonable nor expected under the particular circumstances in which the person finds himself.[8]

There seems to be some public agreement that persons not totally psychotic may have "nervous disorders" or other behavioral difficulties. But it is generally felt that these conditions do not amount to "real" sickness—one of the tests being, apparently, that mental illness is not legitimate if one can recover from it—and do not require any specialized help other than consultation or simple encouragement. For this purpose, competent help is available from friends, ministers, and general medical practitioners as well as psychiatrists—perhaps in that order of importance.

Thus the psychiatrist continues to deal with his patient in a context of rather general public uncertainty, if not outright mistrust. He cannot share the physician's license for simply naming his patient to the sick role, confident that the patient's community will substantiate the claim. The psychiatrist can only proceed tentatively: his assurances about a patient's condition or need for special attention, particularly if that patient has not slipped off into a state of colorful sickness visible to the untutored eye, are often contradicted, often ignored, and seldom regarded as the final word of a specialized authority.

Traditional medicine, of course, has had centuries to attract the respect of society and can point to a continued series of new and successful forms of treatment. But it may take more than just time for such authority to be transferred to psychiatry. For it may well be that the very conceptual frameworks which society has acquired through its acceptance of medical and other scientific phenomena do not lend themselves to an understanding of psychiatric subject matter. Injury or disease is conceived as something which has palpable substance, can be located somewhere on the physical organism, can be diagnosed according to an existing body of knowledge, and can be treated with fairly standard instruments in fairly standard ways. In comparison with this set of expectations concerning medical care, the psychiatrist can offer very little. In his role as therapist, he specifically deals with the symbolic, the unique, the personal aspects of human experience, and while his medical arsenal can supply a few standard diagnostic tests, some somatic therapies, and an increasing variety of pills, there is nothing approximating a blueprint after which he can fashion his treatment. When he deals with the dynamics of mental illness, every step he takes is novel and without a precise precedent. As a consequence, many strata of society cannot regard mental therapy as an honest concern of medicine, which, after all, in its traditional objectivity, is supposed to be oriented to substantial and material matters rather than to the intangibles of human experience. If the public makes this distinction too readily, it is using criteria to do so which medicine has advocated for centuries.

The ill person, then, in committing himself to psychiatric treatment and in trying to develop a systematic patient role, is taking on modes of behavior which make little sense to those he adopts them for. It is clear that the public remains skeptical about his claims of sickness, and leaves him in the uncertain position of having to engineer new kinds of access to a legitimate sick role, or, perhaps, turning away altogether into other channels of expression for his deviant motivational needs. How many are shuffled off into marginal areas of society to find a deviant group setting— into criminal gangs, religious sects of one sort or another, into "artists" colonies or hobo camps—one can only guess. However, every physician will agree that an impressive clue to the alternatives of becoming a mental patient is provided by the number of persons who have to translate their discomfort into physical ailments before they are able to recognize it at all.

THE DILEMMA

THIS problem may gain in relevance if one turns from the broader organizational aspect of the patient role and inquires briefly about the social career of the particular patient.

The sick role which Parsons visualizes is a transitory one. It is easy to acquire if eligibility is established, easy to abandon once its functional value is exhausted, so that the experience of being sick poses no necessarily abrupt breaks in the continuity of the medical patient's life. But the mental patient is in double jeopardy. He acquires recognition as a "sick" person only at a considerable emotional price, if at all; later, he is able to withdraw from this recognition only with extreme difficulty, for he then faces the widespread conviction that legitimate mental illness cannot be completely cured anyway.[9] Moreover, the mental patient's treatment is often designed to effect comprehensive ego changes rather than simply to restore him to his former state of health, so that on several counts his experience with sickness may become crucial to his developing sense of direction and identity. The danger is that patienthood may become a model for his image of the future rather than a provisional shelter in which he resets himself for a life already in progress. In some cases of lifelong difficulty, the patient's efforts to be recognized as a patient may be the first definite attempts he has ever made to establish himself in a clear-cut social identity, while his adjustment to the hospital community may be the first successful one he has ever made.

For when the patient has to seek definition as acutely sick and helpless in order to achieve a measure of public validation for his illness—and simultaneously has to use all his remaining strengths to struggle against that illness—a dilemma is posed which he may resolve by simply giving up the struggle altogether and submerging himself in the sick definition permanently. The temptation to embrace such a definition, despite its lack of social approval—perhaps even because of it!—may be quite persuasive, as one of Dostoievski's characters points out:

Oh, if I had done nothing simply from laziness! Heavens, how I should have respected myself then! I should have respected myself because I should at least have been capable of being lazy; there would at least have been one positive quality, as it were, in me, in which I could have believed myself. Question: What is he? Answer: A sluggard. How very pleasant it would have been to hear that of oneself! It would mean that I was positively defined, it would mean that there was something to say about me. "Sluggard"—why, it is a calling and vocation, it is a career. . . . I should have found for myself a form of activity in keeping with it. . . .[10]

This poses a further dilemma for psychiatry. The medical conditions which, it is currently believed, provide the optimal clinical setting for treatment may at the same time be social conditions which put a stamp of permanence on the illness. The danger that the patient will find himself a permanent "form of activity in keeping with" his momentary patient-hood, while trying to engineer access to the medical patient role which psychiatry advocates for him, cannot be overlooked when psychiatrists consider their high readmission rates and their constant struggle with chronicity. It is important to realize that the patient's tendency to see himself as a medical responsibility and make symbolic application for the allowance this implies receives its initial impetus and support from psychiatry, even as psychiatry struggles for its own recognition within medicine. Practically every term in psychiatric usage which identifies patients, treatment, therapeutic settings, and hospital organization is borrowed from medical practice. Certainly a great number of psychiatric procedures are fashioned after medical models, while the physical facilities provided for the treatment of mental patients often duplicate those of the conventional hospital. To the psychiatrist himself, this may be largely a matter of convenience and training, but to the patient it is likely to have an implicit social logic: given the setting, it is only appropriate that he entertain the role expectations of any medical patient.

Perhaps even more important is the manner in which mental mechanisms are likely to be conceptualized by the psychiatrist and his patient alike, providing these mechanisms with an illusion of substance that renders them akin to anatomical organs. In constructing a workable model of psychic processes, psychiatry has tended to visualize the human mind by the use of intricate structural analogies—beginning, perhaps, with Freud's use of topographical terms and continuing throughout a literature in which the ego is likened to a building or machine and disorder is likened to a failure of supports, a weakening or collapse of foundations, and so on. These analogies may well serve the needs of psychiatry to order the dynamic problems it encounters; but they also tend to buttress the patient's already strong tendency to attribute to his illness—in those cases where he cannot actually blame verifiable organic changes—a quasi-organic structure and substance. Substantial disorders, of course, traditionally lie in the province of the surgeon or the practitioner who coaches the organism back to health. Thus, it should be a matter of small surprise if the analogy is taken too seriously and patients enter the therapeutic setting with the passive attitude that they have come to be "fixed," or with the comfortable notion that mental illness is something which has "happened" to them, something in which they are only indirectly implicated, like an "enemy" invasion of germs.

When this disparity between popular attitudes and medical values in psychiatry is pointed out, it is usually proposed that a massive program of public education be initiated in order to create public attitudes receptive to psychiatric realities, thereby creating a consistent patient role for the mentally ill. However, the sociologist may well suggest that these proposals be considered in the light of two crucial issues.

The first of these is the simplest. Would psychiatry be adequately serving its own interests if it *were* able to promote the mental patient's eligibility for the conventional sick role? This role has its roots in a fairly precise line of demarcation between the sick and the well, in that those people who are considered ill enough to need specific exemption are set aside into an identifying social status and expected to perform a fairly well established social role. Medically speaking, there may be some reality to this largely artificial distinction: the physician's practice, at least, is not unduly hampered if the community recognizes different sets of expectations for those whom he regards as his patients. However, to make this clear a social distinction between mental health and mental illness, between the mental patient and the normal citizen, not only puts the psychiatrist in the uncomfortable position of revealing the uncertainty of his knowledge about these groups of phenomena; it puts the patient who does not and should not wish to claim considerable disability into a position of grave jeopardy. Psychiatrists usually prefer to visualize human behavior as falling on a spectrum, in which degrees of illness are recognized as gradations between the polar states of ideal health and total collapse, and thus psychiatrists should be acutely sensitive to the dangers of marking some point on this spectrum as the line between health and illness.[11] Many of them hope to provide preventive and other services to those who remain on the healthier end of the spectrum, for example, and will have every reason to resist the implication that those regarded as in some degree "ill" require special social license. At the present state of knowledge, psychiatrists may find it to their advantage if the state of *being sick enough to need help* and the state of *needing exemptions from normal social duties* are not articulated too clearly within the same role.[12]

The second issue is whether or not psychiatry, especially as it branches out into child guidance and preventive psychiatry, can ever support the contention that it remains an ideological branch of medicine. This is not to question who should carry the *legal* responsibilities for treatment of mental disorders, but to consider how effective scientific analogies are for public education. The public's skepticism about psychiatry as a medical tradition, it must be realized, is not simply a consequence of ignorance or emotional resistance; it has a fairly wide basis in fact and is presented in a framework of fairly sound logic. It cannot be the purpose of this paper to cite the fundamental differences which exist between psychiatric and medical practice on the one hand, and between the mental and medical patient on the other. I am here talking about the *social forms* which the public creates to handle the problem of illness, and considering whether or not a convincing enough logic is available to persuade the public that mental illness belongs to the same social classification as the distinctly organic. Such a logic would have to explain why most medical treatments can become increasingly routinized while psychotherapy must remain individualized and personal. It would have to explain why the objects of physical and mental therapy are basically different, the former restoring the patient to an earlier state of health, the latter changing the very resources with which the patient faces life. Most important, it would have to establish a certain number of predictive criteria, on the basis of which society could estimate the likelihood of recovery in particular cases, the length of treatment required, and the pain or complication the patient could reasonably expect in the meantime. For the sick role is issued by society to help maintain the functional coherence of social processes. It is provisionally assigned, with an implicit expiration date in mind which can be at least vaguely anticipated. To the patient's community, therefore, it is a matter of profound importance whether he asks for a certain period of exemption to recover from an illness or seeks a blank check in order to undergo the uncertainties of psychiatric treatment. The latter instance changes the whole basic relevance of the sick role to the social group which validates its use.

True, psychiatric procedures may, in time, achieve a degree of standardization and a body of knowledge which will make this grouping of medical and mental patients into a single social category reasonable from the public's point of view. Even if one avoids the argument as to whether such a degree of standardization can ever be achieved—or will be good therapeutic practice if it is—it is clear that in the meantime psychiatry's continued attempt to use medical values in the treatment of mental illness may result in continued patient insecurity.

It may then be argued that the time has come for psychiatry to review and perhaps revise its general approach so as to create a more realistic position for the mental patient in society, one which relies less heavily on medical claims and instead takes more firmly into account the social realities that underlie public resistance to the whole ideology of psychiatric practice.

This might call for the sort of re-evaluation which appears to be taking place in certain European treatment centers and is spreading with the growth of the field of social psychiatry. In such centers psychiatrists have joined with social workers, psychologists, and other specialists in the field of social relations to produce a therapeutic atmosphere which relies less on medical analogies than is generally common in the United States. The emphasis seems to be on *re-education and resocialization* rather than on therapy, on *development and training* rather than on reintegration of ego processes, on the *therapeutic community* with its roots in outside society rather than on the hospital with its specialized culture. Certain European institutions, notably the day-hospital which has spread throughout England and the Netherlands, expose patients to a schedule in certain respects far nearer to that of a student than that of a medical patient, while special trade schools and training centers, supervised by clinicians, take over a large bulk of the borderline and even chronically psychotic cases which might be permanently hospitalized or neglected altogether in the United States. It may be that this combination of an educational approach to mental illness and its complementary role of *special student* will provide the richest clue to a clear-cut social position for those now regarded as mentally ill.

It must be admitted in conclusion that the sociologist looks at the patient from a special viewpoint, burdening rather slim threads of evidence with heavy arguments and enjoying a speculative freedom which cannot be shared by those who take the actual and continuing responsibility for treating mental illness. However, the clinician's understanding of the therapeutic environment he creates for his patient may be sharpened by the concepts of the social sciences, particularly where these concepts help to view both patient and psychiatry as participants in the cultural context of social life. The sociologist must point out that whenever a psychiatrist makes the clinical diagnosis of an existing need for treatment, society makes the social diagnosis of a changed status for one of its members. And while the clinician must insist that the treatment which follows and the setting provided for it have to be geared to the inner-dynamic realities of the patient's illness the sociologist proposes that recovery may also depend upon gearing the ongoing treatment to the social realities of the patient's changed status.

NOTES TO CHAPTER 11

1. See, for example, the following: J. F. Bateman and H. W. Dunham, "The State Hospital as a Specialized Community Experience," *Amer. J. Psychology* (1948) 105:445-448; William Caudill, Fredrick C. Redlich, Helen R. Gilmore, and Eugene B. Brody, "Social Structure and Interaction Processes on a Psychiatric Ward," *Amer. J. Orthopsychiatry* (1952) 22:314-334; George Devereux, "The Social Structure of the Hospital as a Factor in Total Therapy," *Amer. J. Orthopsychiatry* (1949) 19:493-500; Howard Rowland, "Interactional Processes in a State Mental Hospital," Psychiatry (1938) 1:323-337; Alfred Stanton and Morris S. Schwartz, "Medical Opinion and the Social Context in the Mental Hospital," Psychiatry (1949) 12:243-249; Stanton and Schwartz, *The Mental Hospital;* New York, Basic Books, 1954.

2. Validation, it might be pointed out, is meant to be more than a community's attempt to impose its moral preferences upon members. The community may validate certain behavior as appropriate for certain individuals even while remaining completely outraged by it. By naming a criminal "habitual" or "confirmed," for instance, people declare their intention of punishing

him, not because his conduct violates their expectations or is "unlike" him, but precisely because it *is* like him and is thus the valid way for him to act.

3. See in this connection, Erik H. Erikson, "The Problem of Ego Identity," *J. Amer. Psychoanal. Assn.* (1956) 4:56-121.

4. See Talcott Parsons, *The Social System;* Glencoe, Ill., The Free Press, 1951.

5. Talcott Parsons, "Illness and the Role of the Physician: A Sociological Perspective," *Amer. J. Orthopsychiatry* (1951) 21:452-460. See also reference footnote 4, Ch. 10.

6. The reference here is to a study conducted by the National Opinion Research Center, University of Chicago. It is based on 3,500 intensive interviews with a representative cross section of the American public. A book describing the results of this study is being prepared by Shirley A. Star, Senior Study Director of the NORC, but in the meantime two short reviews of the general findings are available: Shirley A. Star, "The Public's Ideas about Mental Illness," a paper presented to the Annual Meeting of the National Association for Mental Health, Indianapolis, November 5, 1955; Shirley A. Star, a report on public attitudes in *Psychiatry, the Press and the Public;* Washington, D.C., Amer. Psychiat. Assn., 1956; pp. 1-5.

7. This raises a further problem of interest, which the present paper cannot take time to discuss. In a certain sense it is true that severely psychotic patients may be considered legitimately ill by the general public, but this is at best a special case of the sick role. For it is widely held that mental illness is not legitimate if recovery is possible. Thus, commitment to a custodial institution is regarded far more as leading to a state of permanent constraint than to a provisional role which the patient takes while under treatment which will result in a resumption of normal social obligations.

8. Shirley A. Star, "The Public's Ideas about Mental Illness," reference footnote 6. The italics are mine.

9. An interesting fictional account of this difficulty can be found in Eileen Bassing, *Home Before Dark;* New York, Random House, 1957.

10. F. M. Dostoievski, "Notes from Underground," pp. 442-537; in *A Treasury of Russian Literature,* edited by Bernard Guilbert Guerney; New York, Vanguard, 1943; p. 454.

11. See, in this connection, a report by John Spiegel in *Psychiatry, the Press and the Public,* reference footnote 6, pp. 13-18.

12. This is of outstanding importance in military psychiatry, for instance, where *failure* to offer exemptions to clearly sick persons is often regarded as the best therapeutic measure available. This point was made by Bruce L. Bushard in "The Army's Mental Hygiene Consultation Service," a paper read to the Symposium on Preventive and Social Psychiatry, held under the auspices of the National Research Council and the Walter Reed Army Institute of Research, Washington, D.C., April 15-18, 1957.

ॐ

C H A P T E R 1 2   Thieves, Convicts and

the Inmate Culture*

JOHN IRWIN AND DONALD R. CRESSEY

IN THE rapidly-growing literature on the social organization of correctional institutions, it has become common to discuss "prison culture"
and "inmate culture" in terms suggesting that the behavior systems of
various types of inmates stem from the conditions of imprisonment themselves. Use of a form of structural-functional analysis in research and
observation of institutions has led to emphasis of the notion that internal
conditions stimulate inmate behavior of various kinds, and there has been
a glossing over of the older notion that inmates may bring a culture with
them into the prison. Our aim is to suggest that much of the inmate behavior classified as part of the prison culture is not peculiar to the prison
at all. On the contrary, it is the fine distinction between "prison culture"
and "criminal subculture" which seems to make understandable the fine
distinction between behavior patterns of various categories of inmates.

A number of recent publications have defended the notion that behavior patterns among inmates develop with a minimum of influence from
the outside world. For example, in his general discussion of total institutions, Goffman acknowledges that inmates bring a culture with them to
the institution, but he argues that upon entrance to the institution they
are stripped of this support by processes of mortification and dispossession
aimed at managing the daily activities of a large number of persons in a
small space with a small expenditure of resources.[1] Similarly, Sykes and
Messinger note that a central value system seems to pervade prison populations, and they maintain that "conformity to, or deviation from, the
inmate code is the major basis for classifying and describing the social

* We are indebted to the following persons for suggested modifications of the original draft: Donald L. Garrity, Daniel Glaser, Erving Goffman, and Stanton Wheeler.
    Reprinted from *Social Problems*, 10 (1962), 142–155, by permission of the authors
and the Society for the Study of Social Problems.

relations of prisoners."[2] The emphasis in this code is on directives such as "don't interfere with inmate interests," "don't lose your head," "don't exploit inmates," "don't weaken," and "don't be a sucker." The authors' argument, like the argument in other of Sykes' publications is that the origin of these values is situational; the value system arises out of the conditions of imprisonment.[3] Cloward stresses both the acute sense of status degradation which prisoners experience and the resulting patterns of prison life, which he calls "structural accommodation."[4] Like others, he makes the important point that the principal types of inmates—especially the "politicians" and the "shots"—help the officials by exerting controls over the general prison body in return for special privileges. Similarly, he recognizes the "right guy" role as one built around the value system described by Sykes and Messinger, and points out that it is tolerated by prison officials because it helps maintain the status quo. Cloward hints at the existence in prison of a *criminal* subculture when he says that "the upper echelons of the inmate world come to be occupied by those whose past behavior best symbolizes that which society rejects and who have most fully repudiated institutional norms." Nevertheless, his principal point is that this superior status, like other patterns of behavior among inmates, arises from the *internal* character of the prison situation. McCleery also stresses the unitary character of the culture of prisoners, and he identifies the internal source of this culture in statements such as: "The denial of validity to outside contacts protected the inmate culture from criticism and assured the stability of the social system," "A man's status in the inmate community depended on his role there and his conformity to its norms," "Inmate culture stressed the goals of adjustment within the walls and the rejection of outside contacts," and "Status has been geared to adjustment in the prison."[5]

The idea that the prison produces its own varieties of behavior represents a break with the more traditional notion that men bring patterns of behavior with them when they enter prison, and use them in prison. Despite their emphasis on "prisonization" of newcomers, even Clemmer and Riemer noted that degree of conformity to prison expectations depends in part on prior, outside conditions.[6] Schrag has for some years been studying the social backgrounds and careers of various types of inmates.[7] Unlike any of the authors cited above, he has collected data on both the pre-prison experiences and the prison experiences of prisoners. He relates the actions of inmates to the broader community as well as to the forces that are more indigenous to prisons themselves.[8] Of most relevance here is his finding that anti-social inmates ("right guys") "are reared in an environment consistently oriented toward illegitimate social norms,"[9] and frequently earn a living via contacts with organized crime but do not often rise to positions of power in the field. In contrast, asocial inmates ("outlaws") are frequently reared in institutions: "The careers of asocial offenders are marked by high egocentrism and inability to profit from past mistakes or to plan for the future."[10]

However, despite these research findings, even Schrag has commented as follows: "Juxtaposed with the official organization of the prison is an unofficial social system originating within the institution and regulating inmate conduct with respect to focal issues, such as length of sentence, relations among prisoners, contacts with staff members and other civilians, food, sex, and health, among others."[11] Garrity interprets Schrag's theory in the following terms, which seem to ignore the findings on the pre-prison careers of the various inmate types:

> Schrag has further suggested that all inmates face a number of common problems of adjustment as a consequence of imprisonment and that social organization develops as a consequence. When two or more persons perceive that they share a common motivation or problem of action, a basis for meaningful interaction has been established, and from this interaction can emerge the social positions, roles, and norms which comprise social organization. Schrag suggests that the common problems of adjustment which become the principal axes of prison life are related to time, food, sex, leisure, and health.[12]

Garrity himself uses the "indigenous origin" notion when he says that "the axial values regarding shared problems or deprivations provide the basis for articulation of the broad normative system or 'prison code' which defines positions and roles in a general way but allows enough latitude so that positions and roles take on the character of social worlds themselves."[13] However, he also points out that some prisoners' reference groups are outside the prison, and he characterizes the "right guy" as an "anti-social offender, stable, and oriented to crime, criminals, and inmates."[14] "The 'right guy' is the dominant figure in the prison, and his reference groups are elite prisoners, sophisticated, career-type criminals, and other 'right guys.' "[15] Cressey and Krassowski, similarly, seem confused about any distinction between a criminal subculture and a prison subculture. They mention that many inmates of Soviet labor camps "know prisons and maintain criminalistic values," and that the inmates are bound together by a "criminalistic ideology,"[16] but they fail to deal theoretically with the contradiction between these statements and their observation that the inmate leaders in the labor camps are "roughs" or "gorillas" rather than "right guys" or "politicians." Conceivably, leadership is vested in "toughs" to a greater extent than is the case in American prisons because the orientation is more that of a *prison* subculture than of a criminal subculture in which men are bound together with a "criminalistic ideology."

It is our contention that the "functional" or "indigenous origin" notion has been overemphasized and that observers have overlooked the dramatic effect that external behavior patterns have on the conduct of inmates in any given prison. Moreover, the contradictory statements made in this connection by some authors, including Cressey,[17] seem to stem from acknowledging but then ignoring the deviant subcultures which exist outside any given prison and outside prisons generally. More specifically, it seems rather obvious that the "prison code"—don't inform on or exploit another inmate, don't lose your head, be weak, or be a sucker, etc.—is also part of a *criminal* code, existing outside prisons. Further, many inmates come to any given prison with a record of many terms in correctional institutions. These men, some of whom have institutional records dating back to early childhood, bring with them a ready-made set of patterns which they apply to the new situation, just as is the case with participants in the criminal subculture. In view of these variations, a clear understanding of inmate conduct cannot be obtained simply by viewing "prison culture" or "inmate culture" as an isolated system springing solely from the conditions of imprisonment. Becker and Geer have made our point in more general terms: "The members of a group may derive their understandings from cultures other than that of the group they are at the moment participating in. To the degree that group participants share latent social identities (related to their membership in the same 'outside' social groups) they will share these understandings, so that there will be a culture which can be called *latent,* i.e., the culture has its origin and social support in a group other than the one in which the members are now participating."[18]

We have no doubt that the total set of relationships called "inmate society" is a response to problems of imprisonment. What we question is the emphasis given to the notion that solutions to these problems are found within the prison, and the lack of emphasis on "latent culture"— on external experiences as determinants of the solutions. We have found it both necessary and helpful to divide inmates into three rough categories: those oriented to a criminal subculture, those oriented to a prison subculture, and those oriented to "conventional" or "legitimate" subcultures.

THE TWO DEVIANT SUBCULTURES

WHEN we speak of a criminal subculture we do not mean to imply that there is some national or international organization with its own judges, enforcement agencies, etc. Neither do we imply that every person convicted of a crime is a member of the subculture. Nevertheless, descriptions of the values of professional thieves, "career criminals," "sophisticated criminals," and other good crooks indicate that there is a set of values which extends to criminals across the nation with a good deal of consistency.[19] To avoid possible confusion arising from the fact that not all criminals share these values, we have arbitrarily named the system a "thief" subculture. The core values of this subculture correspond closely to the values which prison observers have ascribed to the "right guy" role. These include the important notion that criminals should not betray each other to the police, should be reliable, wily but trustworthy, cool headed, etc. High status in this subculture is awarded to men who appear to follow these prescriptions without variance. In the thief subculture a man who is known as "right" or "solid" is one who can be trusted and relied upon. High status is also awarded to those who possess skill as thieves, but to be just a successful thief is not enough; there must be solidness as well. A solid guy is respected even if he is unskilled, and no matter how skilled in crime a stool pigeon may be, his status is low.

Despite the fact that adherence to the norms of the thief subculture is an ideal, and the fact that the behavior of the great majority of men arrested or convicted varies sharply from any "criminal code" which might be identified, a proportion of the persons arrested for "real crime" such as burglary, robbery, and larceny have been in close contact with the values of the subculture. Many criminals, while not following the precepts of the subculture religiously, give lip service to its values and evaluate their own behavior and the behavior of their associates in terms relating to adherence to "rightness" and being "solid." It is probable, further, that use of this kind of values is not even peculiarly "criminal," for policemen, prison guards, college professors, students, and almost any other category of persons evaluate behavior in terms of in-group loyalties. Whyte noted the mutual obligations binding corner boys together and concluded that status depends upon the extent to which a boy lives up to his obligations, a form of "solidness."[20] More recently, Miller identified "toughness," "smartness," and "autonomy" among the "focal concerns" of lower class adolescent delinquent boys; these also characterize prisoners who are oriented to the thief subculture.[21] Wheeler found that half of the custody staff and sixty per cent of the treatment staff in one prison approved the conduct of a hypothetical inmate who refused to name an inmate with whom he had been engaged in a knife fight.[22] A recent book has given the name "moral courage" to the behavior of persons who, like thieves, have shown extreme loyalty to their in-groups in the face of real or threatened adversity, including imprisonment.[23]

Imprisonment is one of the recurring problems with which thieves must cope. It is almost certain that a thief will be arrested from time to time, and the subculture provides members with patterns to be used in order to help solve this problem. Norms which apply to the prison situation, and information on how to undergo the prison experience—how to do time "standing on your head"—with the least suffering and in a minimum amount of time are provided. Of course, the subculture itself is both nurtured and diffused in the different jails and prisons of the country.

There also exists in prisons a subculture which is by definition a set of patterns that flourishes in the environment of incarceration. It can be found wherever men are confined, whether it be in city jails, state and federal prisons, army stockades, prisoner of war camps, concentration camps, or even mental hospitals. Such organizations are characterized by deprivations and limitations on freedom, and in them available wealth must be competed for by men supposedly on an equal footing. It is in connection with the *maintenance* (but not necessarily with the *origin*) of this subculture that it is appropriate to stress the notion that a minimum of outside status criteria are carried into the situation. Ideally, all status is to be achieved by the means made available in the prison, through the displayed ability to manipulate the environment, win special privileges in a certain manner, and assert influence over others. To avoid confusion with writings on "prison culture" and "inmate culture," we have arbitrarily named this system of values and behavior patterns a "convict subculture." The central value of the subculture is utilitarianism, and the most manipulative and most utilitarian individuals win the available wealth and such positions of influence as might exist.

It is not correct to conclude, however, that even these behavior patterns are a consequence of the environment of any particular prison. In the first place, such utilitarian and manipulative behavior probably is characteristic of the "hard core" lower class in the United States, and most prisoners come from this class. After discussing the importance of toughness, smartness, excitement and fate in this group, Miller makes the following significant observation:

> In lower class culture a close conceptual connection is made between "authority" and "nurturance." To be restrictively or firmly controlled is to be cared for. Thus the overtly negative evaluation of superordinate authority frequently extends as well to nurturance, care, or protection. The desire for personal independence is often expressed in terms such as "I don't need *nobody* to take care of me. I can take care of myself!" Actual patterns of behavior, however, reveal a marked discrepancy between expressed sentiments and what is covertly valued. Many lower class people appear to seek out highly restrictive social environments wherein stringent external controls are maintained over their behavior. Such institutions as the armed forces, the mental hospital, the disciplinary school, the prison or correctional institution, provide environments which incorporate a strict and detailed set of rules defining and limiting behavior, and enforced by an authority system which controls and applies coercive sanctions for deviance from these rules. While under the jurisdiction of such systems, the lower class person generally expresses to his peers continual resentment of the coercive, unjust, and arbitrary exercise of authority. Having been released, or having escaped from these milieux, however, he will often act in such a way as to insure recommitment, or choose recommitment voluntarily after a temporary period of "freedom."[24]

In the second place, the "hard core" members of this subculture as it exists in American prisons for adults are likely to be inmates who have a long record of confinement in institutions for juveniles. McCleery observed that, in a period of transition, reform-school graduates all but took over inmate society in one prison. These boys called themselves a "syndicate" and engaged in a concentrated campaign of argument and intimidation directed toward capturing the inmate council and the inmate craft shop which had been placed under council management. "The move of the syndicate to take over the craft shop involved elements of simple exploitation, the grasp for a status symbol, and an aspect of economic reform."[25] Persons with long histories of institutionalization, it is important to note, might have had little contact with the thief subculture. The thief subculture does not flourish in institutions for juveniles, and graduates of such institutions have not necessarily had extensive criminal experience on the outside. However, some form of the convict subculture *does* exist in institutions for juveniles, though not to the extent characterizing prisons for felons. Some of the newcomers to a prison for adults are, in short, persons who have been oriented to the convict subculture, who have found the utilitarian nature of this subculture acceptable, and who have had little contact with the thief subculture. This makes a difference in their behavior.

The category of inmates we have characterized as oriented to "legitimate" subcultures includes men who are not members of the thief subculture upon entering prison and who reject both the thief subculture and the convict subculture while in prison. These men present few problems to prison administrators. They make up a large percentage of the population of any prison, but they isolate themselves—or are isolated—from the thief and convict subcultures. Clemmer found that forty per cent of a sample of the men in his prison did not consider themselves a part of any group, and another forty per cent could be considered a member of a "semi-primary group" only.[26] He referred to these men as "ungrouped," and his statistics have often been interpreted as meaning that the prison contains many men not oriented to "inmate culture" or "prison culture"— in our terms, not oriented to either the thief subculture or the convict subculture. This is not necessarily the case. There may be sociometric isolates among the thief-oriented prisoners, the convict-oriented prisoners, and the legitimately oriented prisoners. Consequently, we have used the "legitimate subcultures" terminology rather than Clemmer's term "ungrouped." Whether or not men in this category participate in cliques, athletic teams, or religious study and hobby groups, they are oriented to the problem of achieving goals through means which are legitimate outside prisons.

BEHAVIOR PATTERNS IN PRISON

On an ideal-type level, there are great differences in the prison behavior of men oriented to one or the other of the three types of subculture. The hard core member of the convict subculture finds his reference groups inside the institutions and, as indicated, he seeks status through means available in the prison environment. But it is important for the understanding of inmate conduct to note that the hard core member of the thief subculture seeks status in the broader criminal world of which prison is only a part. His reference groups include people both inside and outside prison, but he is committed to criminal life, not prison life. From his point of view, it is adherence to a widespread criminal code that wins him high status, not adherence to a narrower convict code. Convicts might assign him high status because they admire him as a thief, or because a good thief makes a good convict, but the thief does not play the convicts' game. Similarly, a man oriented to a legitimate subculture is by definition committed to the values of neither thieves nor convicts.

On the other hand, within any given prison, the men oriented to the convict subculture are the inmates that seek positions of power, influence, and sources of information, whether these men are called "shots," "politicians," "merchants," "hoods," "toughs," "gorillas," or something else. A job as secretary to the Captain or Warden, for example, gives an aspiring prisoner information and consequent power, and enables him to influence the assignment or regulation of other inmates. In the same way, a job which allows the incumbent to participate in a racket, such as clerk in the kitchen storeroom where he can steal and sell food, is highly desirable to a man oriented to the convict subculture. With a steady income of cigarettes, ordinarily the prisoners' medium of exchange, he may assert a great deal of influence and purchase those things which are symbols of status among persons oriented to the convict subculture. Even if there is no well-developed medium of exchange, he can barter goods acquired in his position for equally-desirable goods possessed by other convicts. These include information and such things as specially-starched, pressed, and tailored prison clothing, fancy belts, belt buckles or billfolds, special shoes, or any other type of dress which will set him apart and will indicate that he has both the influence to get the goods and the influence necessary to keeping and displaying them despite prison rules which outlaw doing so. In California, special items of clothing, and clothing that is neatly laundered, are called "bonaroos" (a corruption of *bonnet rouge*, by means of which French prison trusties were once distinguished from the common run of prisoners), and to a lesser degree even the persons who wear such clothing are called "bonaroos."

Two inmates we observed in one prison are somewhat representative of high status members of the convict subculture. One was the prison's top gambler, who bet the fights, baseball games, football games, ran pools, etc. His cell was always full of cigarettes, although he did not smoke. He had a job in the cell block taking care of the laundry room, and this job gave him time to conduct his gambling activities. It also allowed him to get commissions for handling the clothing of inmates who paid to have them "bonarooed," or who had friends in the laundry who did this for them free of charge, in return for some service. The "commissions" the inmate received for doing this service were not always direct; the "favors" he did gave him influence with many of the inmates in key jobs, and he reputedly could easily arrange cell changes and job changes. Shortly after he was paroled he was arrested and returned to prison for robbing a liquor store. The other inmate was the prison's most notorious "fag" or "queen." He was feminine in appearance and gestures, and wax had been injected under the skin on his chest to give the appearance of breasts. At first he was kept in a cell block isolated from the rest of the prisoners, but later he was released out into the main population. He soon went to work in a captain's office, and became a key figure in the convict subculture. He was considered a stool pigeon by the thieves, but he held high status among participants in the convict subculture. In the first place, he was the most desired fag in the prison. In the second place, he was presumed to have considerable influence with the officers who frequented the captain's office. He "married" another prisoner, who also was oriented to the convict subculture.

Since prisoners oriented either to a legitimate subculture or to a thief subculture are not seeking high status within any given prison, they do not look for the kinds of positions considered so desirable by the members of the convict subculture. Those oriented to legitimate subcultures take prison as it comes and seek status through channels provided for that purpose by prison administrators—running for election to the inmate council, to the editorship of the institutional newspaper, etc.—and by, generally, conforming to what they think administrators expect of "good prisoners." Long before the thief has come to prison, his subculture has defined proper prison conduct as behavior rationally calculated to "do time" in the easiest possible way. This means that he wants a prison life containing the best possible combination of a maximum amount of leisure time and a maximum number of privileges. Accordingly, the privileges sought by the thief are different from the privileges sought by the man oriented to prison itself. The thief wants things that will make prison life a little easier—extra food, a maximum amount of recreation time, a good radio, a little peace. One thief serving his third sentence for armed robbery was a dish washer in the officers' dining room. He liked the eating privileges, but he never sold food. Despite his "low status" job, he was highly respected by other thieves, who described him as "right," and "solid." Members of the convict subculture, like the thieves, seek privileges. There is a difference, however, for the convict seeks privileges which he believes will enhance his position in the inmate hierarchy. He also wants to do easy time but, as compared with the thief, desirable privileges are more likely to involve freedom to amplify one's store, such as stealing rights in the kitchen, and freedom of movement around the prison. Obtaining an easy job is managed because it is easy and therefore desirable, but it also is managed for the purpose of displaying the fact that it can be obtained.

In one prison, a man serving his second sentence for selling narcotics (he was not an addict) worked in the bakery during the entire term of his sentence. To him, a thief, this was a "good job," for the hours were short and the bakers ate very well. There were some rackets conducted from the bakery, such as selling cocoa, but the man never participated in these activities. He was concerned a little with learning a trade, but not very seriously. Most of all, he wanted the eating privileges which the bakery offered. A great deal of his time was spent reading psychology, philosophy, and mysticism. Before his arrest he had been a reader of tea leaves and he now was working up some plans for an illegal business involving mysticism. Other than this, his main activity was sitting with other inmates and debating.

Just as both thieves and convicts seek privileges, both seek the many kinds of contraband in a prison. But again the things the thief seeks are those that contribute to an easier life, such as mechanical gadgets for heating water for coffee and cocoa, phonographs and radios if they are contraband or not, contraband books, food, writing materials, socks, etc. He may "score" for food occasionally (unplanned theft in which advantage is taken of a momentary opportunity), but he does not have a "route" (highly organized theft of food). One who "scores" for food eats it, shares it with his friends, sometimes in return for a past or expected favor, but he does not sell it. One who has a "route" is in the illicit food selling business.[27] The inmate oriented to the convict subculture, with its emphasis on displaying ability to manipulate the environment, rather than on pleasure, is the inmate with the "route." The difference is observable in the case of an inmate assigned to the job of clerk in the dental office of one prison. This man was known to both inmates and staff long before he arrived at the institution, for his crime and arrest were highly publicized in the newspapers. It also became known that he had done time in another penitentiary for "real crime," and that his criminal exploits had frequently taken him from one side of the United States to the other. His assignment to the dental office occurred soon after he entered the prison, and some of the inmates believed that such a highly-desirable job could not be achieved without "influence" and "rep." It was an ideal spot for conducting a profitable business, and a profitable business was in fact being conducted there. In order to get on the list to see the dentist, an inmate had to pay a price in cigarettes to two members of the convict subculture who were running the dental office. This practice soon changed, at least in reference to inmates who could show some contact with our man's criminal friends, in or out of prison. If a friend vouched for a man by saying he was "right" or "solid" the man would be sitting in the dental chair the next day, free of charge.

Generally speaking, an inmate oriented to the thief subculture simply is not interested in gaining high status in the prison. He wants to get out. Moreover, he is likely to be quietly amused by the concern some prisoners have for symbols of status, but he publicly exhibits neither disdain nor enthusiasm for this concern. One exception to this occurred in an institution where a thief had become a fairly close friend of an inmate oriented to the prison. One day the latter showed up in a fresh set of bonaroos, and he made some remark that called attention to them. The thief looked at him, laughed, and said, "For Christ's sake, Bill, they're *Levi's* (standard prison blue denims) and they are always going to be Levi's." The thief may be accorded high status in the prison, because "rightness" is revered there as well as on the outside, but to him this is incidental to his being a "man," not to his being a prisoner.

Members of both subcultures are conservative—they want to maintain the status quo. Motivation is quite different, however. The man oriented to the convict subculture is conservative because he has great stock in the existing order of things, while the man who is thief oriented leans toward conservatism because he knows how to do time and likes things to run along smoothly with a minimum of friction. It is because of this conservatism that so many inmates are directly or indirectly in accommodation with prison officials who, generally speaking, also wish to maintain the status quo. A half dozen prison observers have recently pointed out that some prison leaders—those oriented to what we call the convict subculture—assist the officials by applying pressures that keep other inmates from causing trouble, while other prison leaders—those oriented to what we call the thief subculture—indirectly keep order by propagating the *criminal* code, including admonitions to "do your own time," "don't interfere with others' activities," "don't 'rank' another criminal." The issue is not whether the thief subculture and convict subculture are useful to, and used by, administrators; it is whether the observed behavior patterns originate in prison as a response to official administrative practices.

There are other similarities, noted by many observers of "prison culture" or "inmate culture." In the appropriate circumstances, members of both subcultures will participate in fomenting and carrying out riots. The man oriented to the convict subculture does this when a change has closed some of the paths for achieving positions of influence, but the thief does it when privileges of the kind that make life easier are taken away from him. Thus, when a "prison reform" group takes over an institution, it may inadvertently make changes which lead to alliances between the members of two subcultures who ordinarily are quite indifferent to each other. In more routine circumstances, the thief adheres to a tight system of mutual aid for other thieves—persons who are "right" and "solid"—a direct application in prison of the norms which ask that a thief prove himself reliable and trustworthy to other thieves. If a man is "right," then even if he is a stranger one must help him if there is no risk to himself. If he is a friend, then one must, in addition, be willing to take *some* risk in order to help him. But in the convict subculture, "help" has a price; one helps in order to gain, whether the gain be "pay" in the form of cigarettes, or a guarantee of a return favor which will enlarge one's area of power.

RELATIONSHIPS BETWEEN THE TWO SUBCULTURES

IN THE routine prison setting, the two deviant subcultures exist in a balanced relationship. It is this total setting which has been observed as "inmate culture." There is some conflict because of the great disparity in some of the values of thieves and convicts, but the two subcultures share other values. The thief is committed to keeping his hands off other people's activities, and the convict, being utilitarian, is likely to know that it is better in the long run to avoid conflict with thieves and confine one's exploitations to the "do rights" and to the members of his own subculture. Of course, the thief must deal with the convict from time to time, and when he does so he adjusts to the reality of the fact that he is imprisoned. Choosing to follow prison definitions usually means paying for some service in cigarettes or in a returned service; this is the cost of doing easy time. Some thieves adapt in a more general way to the ways of convicts and assimilate the prisonized person's concern for making out in the institution. On an ideal-type level, however, thieves do not sanction exploitation of other inmates, and they simply ignore the "do rights," who are oriented to legitimate subcultures. Nevertheless, their subculture as it operates in prison has exploitative effects.[28]

Numerous persons have documented the fact that "right guys," many of whom can be identified as leaders of the thieves, not of the convicts, exercise the greatest influence over the total prison population. The influence is the long run kind stemming from the ability to influence notions of what is right and proper, what McCleery calls the formulation and communication of definitions.[29] The thief, after all, has the respect of many inmates who are not themselves thieves. The right guy carries a set of attitudes, values and norms that have a great deal of consistency and clarity. He acts, forms opinions, and evaluates events in the prison according to them, and over a long period of time he in this way determines basic behavior patterns in the institution. In what the thief thinks of as "small matters," however—getting job transfers, enforcing payment of gambling debts, making cell assignments—members of the convict subculture run things.

It is difficult to assess the direct lines of influence the two deviant subcultures have over those inmates who are not members of either subculture when they enter a prison. It is true that if a new inmate does not have definitions to apply to the new prison situation, one or the other of the deviant subcultures is likely to supply them. On the one hand, the convict subculture is much more apparent than the thief subculture; its roles are readily visible to any new arrival, and its definitions are readily available to one who wants to "get along" and "make it" in a prison. Moreover, the inmate leaders oriented to the convict subculture are anxious to get new followers who will recognize the existing status hierarchy in the prison. Thieves, on the other hand, tend to be snobs. Their status in prison is determined in part by outside criteria, as well as by prison conduct, and it is therefore difficult for a prisoner, acting as a prisoner, to achieve these criteria. At a minimum, the newcomer can fall under the influence of the thief subculture only if he has intimate association over a period of time with some of its members who are able and willing to impart some of its subtle behavior patterns to him.

Our classification of some inmates as oriented to legitimate subcultures implies that many inmates entering a prison do not find either set of definitions acceptable to them. Like thieves, these men are not necessarily "stripped" of outside statuses, and they do not play the prison game. They bring a set of values with them when they come to prison, and they do not leave these values at the gate. They are people such as a man who, on a drunken Saturday night, ran over a pedestrian and was sent to the prison for manslaughter, a middle class clerk who was caught embezzling his firm's money, and a young soldier who stole a car in order to get back from a leave. Unlike thieves, these inmates bring to the prison both anti-criminal and anti-prisoner attitudes. Although it is known that most of them participate at a minimum in primary group relations with either thieves or convicts, their relationships with each other have not been studied. Further, criminologists have ignored the possible effects the "do rights" have on the total system of "inmate culture." It seems a worthy hypothesis that thieves, convicts and do rights all bring certain values and behavior patterns to prison with them, and that total "inmate culture" represents an adjustment or accommodation of these three systems within the official administrative system of deprivation and control.[30] It is significant in this connection that Wheeler has not found in Norwegian prisons the normative order and cohesive bonds among inmates that characterize many American prisons. He observes that his data suggest "that the current functional interpretations of the inmate system in American institutions are not adequate," and that "general features of Norwegian society are imported into the prison and operate largely to offset any tendencies toward the formation of a solidary inmate group. . . ."[31]

BEHAVIOR AFTER RELEASE

IF OUR crude typology is valid, it should be of some use for predicting the behavior of prisoners when they are released. However, it is important to note that in any given prison the two deviant subcultures are not necessarily as sharply separated as our previous discussion has implied. Most inmates are under the influence of *both* subcultures. Without realizing it, inmates who have served long prison terms are likely to move toward the middle, toward a compromise or balance between the directives coming from the two sources. A member of the convict subculture may come to see that thieves are the real men with the prestige; a member of the thief subculture or even a do right may lose his ability to sustain his status needs by outside criteria. Criminologists seem to have had difficulty in keeping the two kinds of influence separate, and we cannot expect all inmates to be more astute than the criminologists. The fact that time has a blending effect on the participants in the two deviant subcultures suggests that the subcultures themselves tend to blend together in some prisons. We have already noted that the thief subculture scarcely exists in some institutions for juveniles. It is probable also that in army stockades and in concentration camps this subculture is almost nonexistent. In places of short-term confinement, such as city and county jails, the convict subculture is dominant, for the thief subculture involves status distinctions that are not readily observable in a short period of confinement. At the other extreme, in prisons where only prisoners with long sentences are confined, the distinctions between the two subcultures are likely to be blurred. Probably the two subcultures exist in their purest forms in institutions holding inmates in their twenties, with varying sentences for a variety of criminal offenses. Such institutions, of course, are the "typical" prisons of the United States.

Despite these differences, in any prison the men oriented to legitimate subcultures should have a low recidivism rate, while the highest recidivism rate should be found among participants in the convict subculture. The hard core members of this subculture are being trained in manipulation, duplicity and exploitation, they are not sure they can make it on the outside, and even when they are on the outside they continue to use convicts as a reference group. This sometimes means that there will be a wild spree of crime and dissipation which takes the members of the convict subculture directly back to the prison. Members of the thief subculture, to whom prison life represented a pitfall in outside life, also should have a high recidivism rate. However, the thief sometimes "reforms" and tries to succeed in some life within the law. Such behavior, contrary to popular notions, is quite acceptable to other members of the thief subculture, so long as the new job and position are not "anti-criminal" and do not involve regular, routine, "slave labor." Suckers work, but a man who, like a thief, "skims it off the top" is not a sucker. At any rate, the fact that convicts, to a greater extent than thieves, tend to evaluate things from the perspective of the prison and to look upon discharge as a short vacation from prison life suggests that their recidivism rate should be higher than that of thieves.

Although the data collected by Garrity provide only a crude test of these predictions, they do support them. Garrity determined the recidivism rates and the tendencies for these rates to increase or decrease with increasing length of prison terms, for each of Schrag's inmate types. Unfortunately, this typology does not clearly make the distinction between the two subcultures, probably because of the blending process noted above. Schrag's "right guys" or "antisocial offenders," thus, might include both men who perceive role requirements in terms of the norms of the convict subculture, and men who perceive those requirements in terms of the norms of the thief subculture. Similarly, neither his "con politician" ("pseudosocial offender") nor his "outlaw" ("asocial offender") seem to be what we would characterize as the ideal-type member of the convict subculture. For example, it is said that relatively few of the former have juvenile records, that onset of criminality often occurs after a position of respectability has already been attained in the civilian community, and that educational and occupational records are far superior to those of "right guys." Further, outlaws are characterized as men who have been frequently reared in institutions or shifted around in foster homes; but they also are characterized as "undisciplined troublemakers," and this does not seem to characterize the men who seek high status in prisons by rather peaceful means of manipulation and exploitation. In short, our ideal-type "thief" appears to include only some of Schrag's "right guys"; the ideal-type "convict" seems to include some of his "right guys," some of his "con politicians," and all of his "outlaws." Schrag's "square Johns" correspond to our "legitimate subcultures" category.

Garrity found that a group of "square Johns" had a low parole violation rate and that this rate remained low no matter how much time was served. The "right guys" had a high violation rate that decreased markedly as time in prison increased. In Garrity's words, this was because "continued incarceration [served] to sever his connections with the criminal subculture and thus to increase the probability of successful parole."[32] The rates for the "outlaw" were very high and remained high as time in prison increased. Only the rates of the "con politician" did not meet our expectations—the rates were low if the sentences were rather short but increased systematically with time served.

Noting that the origins of the thief subculture and the convict subculture are both external to a prison should change our expectations regarding the possible reformative effect of that prison. The recidivism rates of neither thieves, convicts, nor do rights are likely to be significantly affected by incarceration in any traditional prison. This is not to say that the program of a prison with a "therapeutic milieu" like the one the Wisconsin State Reformatory is seeking, or of a prison like some of those in California, in which group counseling is being used in an attempt to change organizational structure, will not eventually affect the recidivism rates of the members of one or another, or all three, of the categories.

However, in reference to the ordinary custodially-oriented prison the thief says he can do his time "standing on his head," and it appears that he *is* able to do the time "standing on his head"—except for long-termers, imprisonment has little effect on the thief one way or the other. Similarly, the routine of any particular custodial prison is not likely to have significant reformative effects on members of the convict subculture—they will return to prison because, in effect, they have found a home there. And the men oriented to legitimate subcultures will maintain low recidivism rates even if they never experience imprisonment. Garrity has shown that it is not correct to conclude, as reformers have so often done, that prisons are the breeding ground of crime. It probably is not true either that any particular prison is the breeding ground of an inmate culture that significantly increases recidivism rates.

NOTES TO CHAPTER 12

1. Erving Goffman, "On the Characteristics of Total Institutions," Chapters 1 and 2 in Donald R. Cressey, Editor, *The Prison: Studies in Institutional Organization and Change,* New York: Holt, Rinehart and Winston, 1961, pp. 22-47.
2. Richard A. Cloward, Donald R. Cressey, George H. Grosser, Richard Mc-Cleery, Lloyd E. Ohlin, and Gresham M. Sykes and Sheldon L. Messinger, *Theoretical Studies in Social Organization of the Prison,* New York: Social Science Research Council, 1960, p. 9.
3. *Ibid.,* pp. 15, 19. See also Gresham M. Sykes, "Men, Merchants, and Toughs: A Study of Reactions to Imprisonment," *Social Problems,* 4 (October, 1957), pp. 130-138; and Gresham M. Sykes, *The Society of Captives,* Princeton: Princeton University Press, 1958, pp. 79-82.
4. Cloward, *et al., op. cit.,* pp. 21, 35-41.
5. *Ibid.,* pp. 58, 60, 73.
6. Donald Clemmer, *The Prison Community,* Re-issued Edition, New York: Rinehart, 1958, pp. 229-302; Hans Riemer, "Socialization in the Prison Community," *Proceedings of the American Prison Association,* 1937, pp. 151-155.
7. See Clarence Schrag, *Social Types in a Prison Community,* Unpublished M.S. Thesis, University of Washington, 1944.
8. Clarence Schrag, "Some Foundations for a Theory of Correction," Chapter 8 in Cressey, *op. cit.,* p. 329.
9. *Ibid.,* p. 350.
10. *Ibid.,* p. 349.
11. *Ibid.,* p. 342.
12. Donald R. Garrity, "The Prison as a Rehabilitation Agency," Chapter 9 in Cressey, *op. cit.,* pp. 372-373.
13. *Ibid.,* p. 373.
14. *Ibid.,* p. 376.
15. *Ibid.,* p. 377.

16. Donald R. Cressey and Witold Krassowski, "Inmate Organization and Anomie in American Prisons and Soviet Labor Camps," *Social Problems*, 5 (Winter, 1957-58), pp. 217-230.
17. Edwin H. Sutherland and Donald R. Cressey, *Principles of Criminology*, Sixth Edition, New York: Lippincott, 1960, pp. 504-505.
18. Howard S. Becker and Blanche Geer, "Latent Culture: A Note on the Theory of Latent Social Roles," *Administrative Science Quarterly*, 5 (September, 1960), pp. 305-306. See also Alvan W. Gouldner, "Cosmopolitans and Locals: Toward an Analysis of Latent Social Roles," *Administrative Science Quarterly*, 2 (1957), pp. 281-306 and 2 (1958), pp. 444-480.
19. Walter C. Reckless, *The Crime Problem*, Second Edition, New York: Appleton-Century-Crofts, 1945, pp. 144-145; 148-150; Edwin H. Sutherland, *The Professional Thief*, Chicago: University of Chicago Press, 1937.
20. William Foote Whyte, "Corner Boys: A Study of Clique Behavior," *American Journal of Sociology*, 46 (March, 1941), pp. 647-663.
21. Walter B. Miller, "Lower Class Culture as a Generating Milieu of Gang Delinquency," *Journal of Social Issues*, 14 (1958), pp. 5-19.
22. Stanton Wheeler, "Role Conflict in Correctional Communities," Chapter 6 in Cressey, *op. cit.*, p. 235.
23. Compton Mackenzie, *Moral Courage*, London: Collins, 1962.
24. *Op. cit.*, pp. 12-13.
25. Richard H. McCleery, "The Governmental Process and Informal Social Control," Chapter 4 in Cressey, *op. cit.*, p. 179.
26. *Op. cit.*, pp. 116-133.
27. See Schrag, "Some Foundations for a Theory of Correction," *op. cit.*, p. 343.
28. See Donald R. Cressey, "Foreword," to Clemmer, *op. cit.*, pp. vii-x.
29. "The Governmental Process and Informal Social Control," *op. cit.*, p. 154.
30. "But if latent culture can restrict the possibilities for the proliferation of the manifest culture, the opposite is also true. Manifest culture can restrict the operation of latent culture. The problems facing group members may be so pressing that, given the social context in which the group operates, the range of solutions that will be effective may be so limited as not to allow for influence of variations resulting from cultures associated with other identities." Becker and Geer, *op. cit.*, pp. 308-309.
31. Stanton Wheeler, "Inmate Culture in Prisons," Mimeographed report of the Laboratory of Social Relations, Harvard University, 1962, pp. 18, 20, 21.
32. *Op. cit.*, p. 377.

ॐ

CHAPTER 13 Interaction between
Hospital Staff and Families*

STEPHEN FLECK, ALICE R. CORNELISON,
NEA NORTON, AND THEODORE LIDZ

IN THE COURSE of our study of the family environment of schizophrenic patients, we have become increasingly aware of the need for constant examination of the interrelationship between the hospital staff and the families of patients. Without attention to this relationship, family attitudes toward the hospital or staff attitudes toward the family may affect the patient deleteriously or even catastrophically. Here we wish simply to provide an initial report on a few of the many significant problems that can arise between staff and family.[1]

The hospital as a social system has been scrutinized repeatedly during recent years, with particular emphasis on the effects of staff attitudes and staff disharmony upon patients. While Simmons and Wolff have studied the social hierarchy in the general hospital,[2] Caudill and Stainbrook,[3] Jones,[4] Stanton and Schwartz,[5] and others have reported in detail on the interaction between the mental hospital team and their patients. Some attention has also been given to the relationship between the patient and his family during the period of hospitalization,[6] but few systematic studies have been carried out. On the practical side, therapy has been provided for the mothers of hospitalized children by Szurek,[7] for mothers of schizophrenic patients by Abrahams and Varon,[8] and for the marital partners of patients.[9]

In many hospitals, social service case work with the families of psychiatric and other patients is carried out routinely, with varying degrees of intensity.[10] However, the interaction between hospital personnel and the families of psychiatric patients has been almost completely neglected,

* Reprinted by special permission of The William Alanson White Psychiatric Foundation, Inc., and the authors from *Psychiatry*, 20 (1957), 343–350 (copyright by the Foundation).

even though it has commonly been recognized that families can disrupt the therapeutic relationship between the patient and the hospital, and that what transpires at home can influence the hospitalized patient profoundly. Richardson's pioneering book, *Patients Have Families*,[11] which focused attention upon some of the problems involved, has not been followed by studies of the families of patients in mental hospitals. However, Inwood has described his experiences with complaining families of psychotic soldiers;[12] Fetterman has considered assigning participant roles to family members in the treatment of psychotic patients, whether hospitalized or not;[13] and Tennant,[14] Brody,[15] and Faris[16] have studied the effects of careful case work service for families of patients in private psychiatric hospitals.

The Yale Psychiatric Institute long ago established the policy of providing social case work for family members of every patient, in order to obtain essential data from families, to provide adequate liaison between the family and staff, and to clarify and seek to modify family problems that affect the patient. In the research reported here the same worker interviews all families to provide a more uniform screen against which family reactions can be observed and evaluated. Her interaction with each family member is discussed regularly with the entire research team, and the information is shared with the staff. Knowledge and understanding of the families are enhanced by the use of projective tests for all members. Only upper- and middle-class families have been studied, who are usually well educated and sophisticated, and less likely to be awed by the authority of the hospital personnel than those of lower socioeconomic levels.

GENERAL OBSERVATIONS

ADMISSION to a psychiatric hospital differs from admission to a general hospital. The former often occurs under duress; the patient may be committed despite his expressed opposition to hospitalization, and responsible family members may also act under pressure from neighbors, friends, or even the authorities. Family members may disagree as to the necessity or wisdom of commitment, or may experience the same conflict within themselves. Other more tangible differences concern the usual curtailment of visiting, the indefiniteness of diagnosis and prognosis, the greater difficulty in understanding psychiatric treatment methods as compared to medical or surgical procedures, and the comparatively personal information requested, often by social workers rather than a physician.

Furthermore, the families of schizophrenic patients may in themselves present many problems, which may or may not have something to do with why the patient is schizophrenic, but nevertheless must be taken into account. Among these are the following:

(1) Frequently one parent—usually the mother—is overambitious and obsessively anxious, believing that no one can understand or properly care for her child except herself. Such a mother suffers severe anxiety when separated from the child. She may have to withdraw the patient from the hospital to allay this anxiety, just as earlier she had to fasten her child to her to be secure. While she may withdraw the patient early in the hospitalization, she is more likely to do so later, when the patient shows signs of independence which the therapist considers improvement.[17] This rather classic occurrence of a parent's sabotaging treatment just as it begins to work can be avoided by appropriate attention to the parent's needs. Recognition and amelioration of the parent's plight are in order, rather than rebuffing an "intolerable schizophrenogenic mother" or an "intractable domineering father."

(2) Divisions or schisms between family members which have existed openly or covertly long before the hospitalization of the patient are apt to become disagreements about what needs to be done for the patient. The more dominant spouse may insist upon hospitalization, while the other may consider loving care at home essential. The one who does not have his way can still sabotage treatment. Or, because one parent likes one hospital, the other prefers treatment elsewhere. The hospital staff can be caught up in such struggles just as the patient has been, and must guard against antagonizing one parent by seeming to side with the other.

(3) Intense guilt reactions may occur in parents who feel that they are to blame for the patient's illness. Such parents feel impelled to do everything for the patient, even to the detriment of their other children. The guilt is often so extreme that it must be projected on to the doctors or the hospital, expressed in incessant fault-finding with the therapy. Other projections may lead to shifting blame to the other parent, to outsiders such as teachers, or to some happenstance. There may ensue an extensive search for etiologic factors, in which the parent scrutinizes every detail of the patient's history and solicits opinions from every conceivable source.

(4) A serious product of the parental disharmony and the parental guilt is the recrimination by one parent against the other. The manifest or latent hostilities gathered through the years break forth when a parent, guilty concerning his or her own deficiencies as a parent, condemns the other for shortcomings that he thinks made the child ill. The battle is noted by the patient, who is often an artist in splitting the parents, and affects his hospital course even though the family discord remains unnoted by his psychiatrist. Often, however, the hospital is involved in the struggle, as each parent seeks to gain the solace of having hospital personnel side with him against the other.

The task of the hospital is to treat the patient and prevent the family's problems from interfering with the therapeutic program. Even though understanding of the parental problems is not a primary interest, the parents' disharmony may be a prime source of the patient's dilemma, and modification of the family environment can be useful or even essential to promoting improvement in the patient. From among the numerous problems that can arise to disturb the family-staff relationship, we shall select two of significance to serve as illustrations, which we shall call the problem of *family decompensation* and problems which arise through *staff exclusiveness*.

FAMILY DECOMPENSATION

THE schizophrenic illness of a family member can change the tenuous equilibrium of the family and precipitate disorganization that deprives its members of emotional support from each other just when they need it most. The patient, who already feels overwhelmed, may be caught in the midst of the family disorganization. The disruption of the object relationship can precipitate illness in other members of the family, further increasing the stresses on all of the members.

The critical situation of the Neuberg family following the admission of Arthur, their fifteen-year-old son, in a state of catatonic excitement will illustrate some of the problems involved.

The Neuberg family equilibrium had been precarious for many years. Mrs. Neuberg had married her strange but ardent suitor after becoming pregnant with the patient. Both parents were strongly attached to their parental families; this had fostered jealousy and strife, and had resulted in the Neubergs' failing to establish a nuclear family of their own. For instance, the mother refused to move from the apartment house in which her married sisters lived, although this meant that Mr. Neuberg had to travel over two hours each day to work. Mr. Neuberg felt that he was excluded from the family and that his wife was more attached to her family than to him; on the other hand, he spent much of his free time with his mother, whom his wife would not visit. During the year before Arthur's admission Mr. Neuberg had planned to move the family to the west coast when his mother and brother moved there, but Mrs. Neuberg had threatened to separate from him rather than go along.

Mr. Neuberg had unusual aptitudes, but the plans he evolved for utilizing them were often impractical, if not paranoidally grandiose. He worked hard at his hobbies and schemes, to the exclusion of socialization with his family. Mrs. Neuberg became increasingly resentful that the entire burden of raising the three children rested upon her. She resented her husband's absences from home, but could not tolerate his incessant talk when he was at home, and disapproved of the bizarre ideas he expressed to the children.

When Arthur was admitted to the hospital, Mr. Neuberg was in a highly excited state, showing signs of paranoid distortion. He sought to blame Arthur's illness upon any one of a number of events in Arthur's recent or distant past: his guilt over an injury to his sister, masturbation, overwork in high school, disappointment in his first crush, and so on. Mr. Neuberg circumstantially repeated one such story after another to the staff, elaborating the details in his effort to convince them.

It was soon apparent that the long-standing conflict between the parents had now flared into mutual recrimination. The father felt guilty because he had often been reprimanded for his neglect of his family; the mother felt guilty because she had raised a schizophrenic son and because she had not left the father, whom she privately believed was an ambulatory psychotic. The father was openly blamed for the son's psychosis by the wife and her family, particularly by one sister who attacked him viciously, with complete disregard for his despair over his son's illness. Mrs. Neuberg, whom the social worker found to be feeling depressed and lost, confided that she would leave her husband now that she saw that maintaining a home with this bizarre man had damaged the family.

The first crisis arose because of Mr. Neuberg's energetic and excited efforts to treat his son, which were disturbing and could not be controlled, and made it necessary to stop his visits. Separation from his son heightened his anxiety, and led him to feel that the hospital also blamed him for his son's illness. He wished to remove his son from the hospital and devote all his time to caring for him. Mrs. Neuberg was terrified lest he be permitted to carry out this plan. The social worker recognized Mr. Neuberg's incessant talk as paranoid and possibly psychotic and arranged that a senior psychiatrist see him regularly. It proved possible to allay his guilt, by permitting expression of the hostility toward his wife's family. This helped to diminish the projection of blame against his wife and against the hospital. Through regular discussions of his problems and of the difficult family situation, he gained the support he needed during this critical period and quieted down so that he could resume visiting the patient.

At the same time, with the help of the social worker, Mrs. Neuberg began to recognize that her husband was not solely responsible for the family problems, and that the difficulties had been heightened by her attachment to her family and the meddling sabotage of her sister. She realized that she was fond of her husband, who was childishly dependent upon her, who deeply admired her, and who had sought to be a good husband and faithful provider. Through further discussion, she recognized that her son probably had been frightened by the threats of separation, and needed his father despite the difficulties in the father's relationship with all members of the family.

It was possible to re-establish and maintain some degree of family unity, so that each parent could give the other some support and so that both could strive to attain a new equilibrium. Mr. Neuberg began to spend more time with his other children, and sought to help his wife. Mrs. Neuberg came to recognize, at least in part, that she did not have to rely on her sister but was herself able to guide her children.

A later crisis arose when Mr. Neuberg impetuously decided to remove his son, in response to the boy's pathetic pleading. This was headed off by the social worker, who understood his need to prove that he would sacrifice anything for his son, by suggesting that leaving the boy in the hospital and waiting patiently for his recovery required a great deal of self-sacrifice and self-restraint.

The differences between the parents again threatened to become acute during preparations for the patient's discharge, and once again it seemed that the patient would become the focal point of their controversies. The staff had suggested that they send the boy to a boarding school for a year. Mr. Neuberg agreed, despite the severe financial burden, expecting his wife to object. She did object, taking our recommendation as an implied condemnation of her and the home. Moreover, the prospect of further prolonged separation from Arthur virtually precluded re-establishment of the close relationship between herself and her son, just as it deprived the father of the much desired opportunity to demonstrate that he was a good father for Arthur. However, when she saw the patient's enthusiasm for the school plan, she agreed. Then her husband, who had very easily agreed at first, changed his mind and had to be persuaded again.

We felt that unless the parents had been permitted to voice their objections and work through their resistances, they might have agreed to the plan without expressing their opposition, but they probably would have eventually undermined the patient's adjustment at school. Actually the parents have been pleased, because the patient has been doing very well since discharge. Had he returned home, the family would have had to readjust again after having barely achieved a tenuous equilibrium.

STAFF EXCLUSIVENESS

STAFF exclusiveness is manifested by prohibition of family visits and by ineffectual communication by the therapist and staff with the family. Sometimes all communication between family and hospital ceases. Families may find this isolation intolerable, and it is rarely helpful to their efforts to adjust to the hospitalization. Moreover, the therapist may deprive himself of useful information or may even be misled by the patient's statements or behavior, and both can impede or even stop therapeutic progress. For instance, Arthur's fear that the family might break up was quite realistic, but this could be established only from the family's communications and not from his psychotic productions, which avoided the topic.

Since the tendency is to concentrate all efforts upon the patient who is admitted to the hospital for treatment, the psychiatrist is apt to resist and resent forces that interfere with his relationship with the patient. Yet the very complex relationship between the patient, the family, and the hospital can, unless given very careful consideration, impede or even founder the therapeutic effort. This is particularly true of young schizophrenic patients who are still deeply involved with their parents, and are often in a close relationship with a parent who is seriously disturbed. The family disequilibrium or schism may have much to do with the patient's illness and can continue to affect him in the hospital. Isolation from the family is sometimes necessary, but in itself it is not an effective means of coping with the problems, for they cannot be dodged indefinitely. The hospital must endeavor to modify the parents' attitudes toward the patient and toward each other, particularly when the patient remains dependent upon the parents.

The Lamb family may be used as an illustration of some of the ways in which excluding relatives may affect therapy. This family, whose son,

Daryl, was a schizophrenic patient, appeared less bizarre and pathological as individuals than did the Neuberg family, in part because we had little contact with them for many months after Daryl's admission.

The Lambs had had serious difficulties for many years, chiefly because of Mr. Lamb's infidelity and drinking and his jealousy of Daryl, the oldest child. Daryl had not been wanted by the father, and was never permitted to interfere with their social life or with Mr. Lamb's interests. Mrs. Lamb, however, was happy with her mother role, although beset by many difficulties caused by her husband's jealousy of the child. As Daryl grew up, Mr. Lamb always belittled him and mocked at his effeminate traits and artistic inclinations. The father had much less difficulty, however, in accepting Daryl's only sibling, a sister seven years younger. Mrs. Lamb's submissiveness and indecisiveness were pronounced in her dealings with the entire family. In particular, she could not impose realistic restrictions upon Daryl; she attempted to compensate for her husband's contemptuous treatment of him, and she feared to undermine or block his artistic inclinations.

Daryl was a very sensitive child whose social awkwardness had been noted as early as kindergarten. Although above average intelligence, he did poorly in the early grades. Later he received superior marks but encountered many difficulties in school because of his bizarre and effeminate behavior and his mendacity. This behavior led to psychiatric treatment during his senior year at a boarding school and, when it continued despite therapy, to hospitalization. He was eighteen when admitted, a shy, sensitive boy whose appearance and awkwardness suggested very early adolescence. In the hospital, he at first isolated himself almost completely, hardly communicating with anyone and then only in a haughty, contemptuous manner. After several frustrating months of extremely patient and persistent effort on the part of the therapist, Daryl began to communicate meaningfully with him, although not with other staff members and patients; and when the therapist left the hospital, about six months after Daryl's admission, he refused for some time to communicate with his new doctor.

From the time of his admission Daryl insisted that his parents did not love him and demanded that they not be permitted to visit him. Moreover, we knew that Daryl's father was openly jealous of his son, which placed both Daryl and his mother in a particularly difficult position when the patient visited at home. Both therapists feared that opposing Daryl's demands to exclude his family would destroy their relationship with him.

Lacking adequate contact with the family, we had no evidence that the isolation from the patient bothered them. The mother, passive and fearful, abided by our decision, made soon after admission. When she was seen again, she appeared quite depressed, and Daryl's sister, his only sibling, had also become disturbed and was worried about the absence of contact with her brother. Mrs. Lamb began to discuss her own indecisiveness and indulgence of Daryl's demands with the social worker, and we came to realize that the hospital was behaving as the mother had in the past, by permitting Daryl to decide if and when she could visit. The staff finally persuaded the therapist to insist that Daryl see his family.

Later it came to light that, as Daryl had perceived it, we had not only behaved like the undemanding mother by giving in to him, but also had unwittingly imitated the father, who explicitly expected nothing from Daryl, and
who also sought to separate his wife and son. At the same time, the fact that the
parents abided by our decision meant to Daryl that they were less interested in
him than ever. The mother, on the other hand, needed the social worker's help
to be more assertive with both her children. Her guilt feelings had been aggravated by our stand, because she took it as confirmation of her fear that she
was an unfit mother, making her more uncertain than ever in her relationships
with her children.

Although the social worker helped Mrs. Lamb considerably, enabling her to
deal more effectively with both her children, we were unable to influence the
basic family difficulty. Amelioration of Mr. Lamb's severe alcoholism and rejection of his son, which were rooted in similar experiences in his own background,
would have required intensive individual psychotherapy, which he was unwilling to undertake. He rarely came to the hospital even after we permitted it, and
continued to maintain the pretense of being a highly competent and self-
sufficient person.

Therapeutic benefits for the patient ensued from the mother's visits, not from
the separation. Some months later home visits became possible, and Daryl's interest in life outside an institution was thereby stimulated considerably. He finished his high school work successfully while still a patient in the Institute, and
this achievement, together with his regular trips home, facilitated therapeutic
consideration of his ambivalences in all his personal relationships. The ultimate
prognosis for him and the family, however, remained guarded.

In this case, as in others, staff exclusiveness had undermined an already
precarious family equilibrium, had deprived the staff of important information, and had interfered with therapy instead of facilitating it.

We have presented only a few of the very complex interactions among
young schizophrenic patients, their families, and the hospital staff, from
the wealth of material made available through the study. While it is true
that the hospital team's tasks can often be eased temporarily in many respects by exclusion of the family from the hospital experience, such simplification of a complex problem ignores reality, necessity, and opportunity.

We believe that maximal inclusion of certain family members, if not
the entire family, into the hospital experience opens important new
therapeutic potentialities. The aim should be to reconcile therapeutic
indications for both patient and family. Young schizophrenics are still
closely attached to their parents, and it is unrealistic to try to sever such
bonds abruptly upon hospital admission, no matter how unwholesome
the attachment may seem at the moment. The patient's effort to withdraw
from his family is often motivated by fear of his hostile or libidinal aggression, or by disillusionment, but it is usually highly ambivalent, for

there are also deep needs for attachments to one or both parents. Many patients, however, are excited by contact with a parent who is also upset, and in occasional extreme cases this disturbing interaction must be prohibited.[18]

It is quite common for inexperienced therapists to encourage the expression of hostility and even rebellious behavior against parents, because it is sometimes wrongly believed that such behavior indicates developing independence and maturity.[19] We have found the reverse usually to be true. In such situations, the patient uses the staff as a shield from behind which he can safely attack his relatives without assuming responsibility for his behavior, instead of examining his impulses and feelings in treatment.

No matter how desirable prohibition of family visits appears to be on therapeutic grounds, it becomes a wise decision only if there is evidence that the family can tolerate it. Otherwise, family disorganization may be transformed into interference with treatment. Even if the patient is not removed from the institution altogether, disagreement between staff and family may affect the patient adversely, just as does disagreement among staff members, so aptly described by Stanton and Schwartz.[20] Moreover, we have evidence that chronic controversy and disunity have characterized many of these families throughout the patient's life, and that, not infrequently, the patient has been caught and torn by this schism.[21] It is incumbent upon hospital staffs to make certain that the patient does not simply move from a position of being the focus of family disunity to one of being the center of a struggle between staff and family.

It has been stated that if a recovered young schizophrenic patient returns to live with his family, the likelihood of recurrence is increased.[22] We can neither confirm nor deny this principle at present. We have found that preparation for disposition of the patient must begin at admission, because the success of any plan, whether the patient returns home or not, depends upon the family's readiness and ability not only to accept it but also to feel comfortable with it. Active cooperation cannot be expected unless the family is helped to recover, first of all, from the disorganizing and possibly overwhelming experience of the hospitalization of the patient. The expectation that relatives of patients will differ from other human beings in the possession of some miraculous ability to change unconsciously determined behavior, simply because they are told they must, disregards all psychodynamic knowledge. A tacit hope prevails, however, that families will quickly give all the necessary information and then disappear to leave the staff alone with the patient. Such assumptions may prepare the way for therapeutic failure for which staff and family will blame each other. If the relatives are to participate in the management of the patient, as we believe they should, continued contact with them is necessary, because the family situation is not static.

Here we would like to make a few observations and speculations concerning the patient committed to a state hospital—a more common situation than those discussed in this paper. Whereas in the upper-middle-class families we have studied it is often difficult to persuade the family to accept a plan which entails having the patient live apart from them following recovery, a reverse situation often exists in families of lower social class. They frequently break off contact with the hospital altogether if hospitalization goes on for any length of time and are quite unprepared to receive the patient back following his discharge. This happens even in families considered "cohesive" on cultural grounds. It has also been observed that, to some extent, the state hospital patient's fate and recovery actually depend on the family's activity and the interest which they maintain in him, as well as on their prodding hospital staffs into renewed therapeutic efforts with chronic patients.[23]

The details and dynamics of family equilibrium cannot be discussed here, but our findings suggest that two things may happen following the commitment of a family member: First, the family may remain in a precarious state of equilibrium but make recurrent efforts to reunite the family, including the patient, and this results in such active behavior with hospital staffs as just mentioned. Second, the family may re-establish equilibrium by excluding the patient and then be hard put to it to shift toward an older equilibrium which may have been less stable, or to a totally new state of balance required by the readmission of the patient into their midst. This second group may well contain the families who discontinue contact with patient and hospital, or who make no effective demands for treatment or discharge. Probably there are many gradations between these alternatives, and further research will be required to establish the validity of these hypotheses.

Hospitalization of psychiatric patients occurs at various stages of illness, and also at different stages of family disorganization. It is not known at this time whether class differences are a significant factor in determining how early or late hospitalization occurs, in terms of either illness or family disorganization. However, it is obvious that the upper-middle-class families we have studied have recourse to many more facilities short of hospitalization than do families from lower socioeconomic groups—for instance, special schools, long vacations, and private psychiatric care. Occasionally, the moment of hospitalization may be determined by agencies outside the family, such as school authorities, employers, or neighbors, but in most instances the family's capacity to tolerate the disturbed member in their midst and their attitude toward mental hospitals appear to be the decisive factors.

We have also found that the reactions of relatives to hospitalization offer an important opportunity for research into the interaction in families under stress and provide data which transcend our immediate goal of studying the families of schizophrenic patients.[24] Opportunities for research aside, we conclude with Fetterman that "he who neglects the family neglects the patient."[25]

NOTES TO CHAPTER 13

1. Data on the influence of family attitudes upon patients prior to hospitalization have been collected by Nea Norton, Alice R. Cornelison, and Stephen Fleck, and will be reported elsewhere.
2. L. W. Simmons and H. G. Wolff, *Social Science in Medicine;* New York, Russell Sage Foundation, 1954.
3. William Caudill and Edward Stainbrook, "Some Covert Effects of Communication Difficulties in a Psychiatric Hospital," Psychiatry (1954) 17: 27-40.
4. Maxwell Jones, *The Therapeutic Community;* New York, Basic Books, 1953.
5. Alfred H. Stanton and Morris S. Schwartz, *The Mental Hospital;* New York, Basic Books, 1954.
6. George Devereux, "The Social Structure of the Hospital as a Factor in Total Therapy," *Amer. J. Orthopsychiatry* (1949) 19:492-500. J. A. Rose, "Relation of Family to Hospital," in "Symposium on Pediatrics," *Medical Clinics of North America* (1952) 36:1551-1554. S. A. Szurek, "Some Lessons from Efforts at Psychotherapy with Parents," *Amer. J. Psychiatry* (1952) 109: 296-302.
7. Szurek, reference footnote 6.
8. Joseph Abrahams and Edith Varon, *Maternal Dependency and Schizophrenia;* New York, International Univ. Press, 1953.
9. Eugene Brody, "Modification of Family Interaction Patterns by a Group Interview Technique," *Internat. J. Group Psychotherapy* (1956) 6:38-47. E. R. Inwood, "Therapeutic Interviewing of Hostile Relatives," *Amer. J. Psychiatry* (1952) 109:455-458.
10. Mildred T. Faris, "Casework with Mentally Ill Patients and their Relatives," *J. Psychiat. Soc. Work* (1955) 24:108-112. Norton, Cornelison, and Fleck, reference footnote 1. M. A. Tennant, "Psychiatric Social Work in a Private Mental Hospital," *J. Psychiat. Soc. Work* (1954) 23:234-241.
11. H. B. Richardson, *Patients Have Families;* New York, Commonwealth Fund, 1945.
12. E. R. Inwood, reference footnote 9; see also "The Problem of the Hostile Relative," *U.S. Armed Forces Med. J.* (1953) 4:1734-1747.
13. J. L. Fetterman, "Better Doctor-Family Cooperation as an Aid to the Mentally Ill Patient," *Medical Clinics of North America* (1948) 32:631-640.
14. Tennant, reference footnote 10.
15. Brody, reference footnote 9.
16. Faris, reference footnote 10.
17. Ruth W. Lidz and Theodore Lidz, "The Family Environment of Schizophrenic Patients," *Amer. J. Psychiatry* (1949) 106:332-345. Theodore Lidz, Beulah Parker, and Alice R. Cornelison, "The Role of the Father in the Family Environment of the Schizophrenic Patient," *Amer. J. Psychiatry* (1956) 113:126-132.

18. Gwen E. Tudor, "A Sociopsychiatric Nursing Approach to Intervention in a Problem of Mutual Withdrawal on a Mental Hospital Ward," Psychiatry (1952) 15:193-217.
19. Elvin V. Semrad, Doris Menzer, James Mann, and Christopher T. Standish, "A Study of the Doctor-Patient Relationship in Psychotherapy of Psychotic Patients," Psychiatry (1952) 15:377-384.
20. Reference footnote 5.
21. Abrahams and Varon, reference footnote 8; Lidz, Parker, and Cornelison, reference footnote 17; C. W. Wahl, "Some Antecedent Factors in the Family Histories of 392 Schizophrenics," *Amer. J. Psychiatry* (1954) 110:668-676.
22. Paul Federn, *Ego Psychology and the Psychoses;* New York, Basic Books, 1953; J. R. Paul, "Preventive Medicine, Yale University School of Medicine 1940-1949," *Yale J. Biol. Med.* (1950) 22:199-211.
23. B. Roberts and J. Meyers, unpublished data.
24. Reference footnote 1.
25. Reference footnote 13.

ꙮ

CHAPTER 14   The Transitional Hospital:

A Clinical and Administrative Viewpoint*

MILTON GREENBLATT

THE hospital administrator is vitally interested in "social psychiatry," not only for the insights he gains as to how the hospital community functions, and the assistance given him in producing favorable institutional change, but also because social psychiatry promises both the clinician and administrator new dignity and scientific status in their functions of patient care and treatment. From this perspective we view clinical administrative problems as related to two broad goals. The first is to create a "therapeutic community" within the hospital (beginning in most instances from an essentially custodial level). The second is to develop a "community mental hospital" by stimulating joint responsibility and collaboration of both hospital and community in many aspects of mental illness and health.

In this discussion we have purposely omitted references to specific modalities or facilities for patient care (such as day hospital, halfway house, clubs, or even drugs, psychotherapy, etc.) which are adequately discussed elsewhere. We also appreciate the preliminary nature of these formulations which in a short text can be developed only in a simple general outline.

CREATION OF THE THERAPEUTIC COMMUNITY

THE concept of the therapeutic community has already received explicit attention in many articles and books (Belknap 1956, Caudill 1958, Cumming and Cumming 1957, Denber 1960, Greenblatt *et al.* 1957, Greenblatt *et al.* 1955, Jones 1953, Stanton and Schwartz 1954, von Mering and King 1957), and some institutions have achieved a social

* Reprinted from the *Journal of Social Issues*, 16 (1960), 62–69, by permission of the author and the *Journal*.

program with impressive advantages suggesting a successful movement towards the ideal. Where this has been accomplished, the steps taken have been somewhat as follows:

1. *Development of the Therapeutic Potential of Staff.* This involves recognition of role problems of each occupational group, encouragement of individual expression, enhancement of selfesteem, improvement of social life, greater participation in the therapeutic program, removal of barriers between upper- and lower-level staff, reduction of hierarchical status differences, and facilitation of upward as well as downward flow of communication, especially between administrative personnel and ward staff. More democratic relations between management or senior personnel and ward personnel are thus encouraged.

The attendant, for instance, is now seen in his social context as "low man on the totem pole"—least trained, least paid, least rewarded, given the most difficult assignments, and permitted to work with least support and at greatest distance from administrative staff. He often suffers social discrimination at the hands of superiors. The privilege of communicating what he knows about patients, and his education and growth as a person are often neglected (Brown 1948, Greenblatt *et al.* 1957, Hall 1952, Hyde 1955, Hyde *et al.* 1956, Wells *et al.* 1956).

Now it is recognized that the attendant often holds the key to the patient's well-being, and that his morale is the crucial factor in patient care. If not respected as a person, he tends to displace his dissatisfaction onto his relations with patients. Staff's anger, resistances, feuds are all recognized as vital elements in therapy. And with the emergence of such recognition have come the collaboration of psychiatrists with social scientists, and the flowering of a modern "social psychiatry."

2. *Removal of Punitive, Restrictive Barriers Between Staff and Patient.* Enhancement of the value of staff members appears to result in a reduction of routinization of roles and development of closer personal relationships between staff and patients, reflecting in a sense the closed gap between the various levels of staff. Ward "emotional climate" in general is markedly improved, and fear of punishment and coercion diminished. Specific practices, such as seclusion, tubs, packs, forced feedings, physical restraints, over-medication, removal of clothes and possessions, and denial of civil rights are reconsidered as to their true contribution to patient care, and in many instances long-standing routines of management are scrapped as negative or maltherapeutic.

3. *Development of the Social Environment as a Therapeutic Force.* The nature of psychiatric illness demands that there be available a rich social environment to help the patient emerge from his withdrawn state when he is psychologically ready to do so. The concept is different from the "total push" philosophy of the past (Myerson 1939, Semrad and Corwin 1940, Tillotson 1939), which tried to *force* the patient into inter-

action. The modern approach is to *remotivate* the patient (von Mering and King 1957) by various means to make beneficial use of an enriched social program. Practically, when patients come out of their withdrawn state, they need occupational therapy, together with recreation, work, and social opportunities such as are available to citizens in the community. As he continues to improve, he seeks more interaction with the environment and requires satisfaction of now outwardly-directed energies. At this time, staff, if properly motivated, becomes increasingly helpful in developing new ways of reaching the patient. In fact, both patients and staff enter into a complementary ward and hospital life.

4. *Participation of Patients in the Therapeutic Process.* Dispersion of responsibility and authority, and broader participation of staff, now lead to patients' participation in their own therapeutic program. Self help and patient organization towards that end become additional modalities. The patients turn to self-government, become a board of inspectors, manage many aspects of ward life, including feeding, recreation, etc., and may even, after appropriate training, participate in some managerial decisions concerning their welfare.

DEVELOPMENT OF THE COMMUNITY MENTAL HOSPITAL

Now we are confronted with the new challenge—the attainment of a "community mental hospital," one closely in touch with the community, guiding the community in its mental health developments and benefiting thereby. It is the necessary outcome of social advances heretofore achieved within the hospital. It is increasingly clear that a mental hospital's progress toward a therapeutic community can be sharply limited by a prevailing low level of enlightenment in the outer community. The hospital is not only dependent on the community for basic sustenance and support but needs the enlightened cooperation of its citizens in order to guarantee the social and emotional acceptance of the patients it discharges. Any clinician of experience knows how quickly the work of the hospital can be vitiated if the patient meets an intolerant, rejecting environment when he is released.

As the development of the therapeutic community within a hospital implies breaking down barriers between staff and patients, so the development of a *community mental hospital* implies breaking down of barriers between hospital and community—the merging of inner and outer communities to desirable goals of successful resettlement of the discharged patients and mutual support of the health of community and hospital (Greenblatt and Simon 1959, Milbank Memorial Fund 1957, World Health Organization 1953).

The community mental hospital implies bilateral responsibility, collaborative effort and coordinated programming. Such a program can only be regarded as an exploratory effort, for although some successful collaborative models have been described, many new problems and complexities are to be expected of each new endeavor, based on local conditions and potentials.

Techniques, instrumentalities and modalities in the achievement of the ideal *community mental hospital* can be discussed best in relation to the following desiderata:

1. *Patient Contact with the Community.* Staff is trained to prepare the patient for discharge beginning at admission. Expectation of long hospitalization and dependence on the hospital are discouraged. It is now recognized that much therapeutic or rehabilitation work can be done in aftercare or transitional facilities. We assume that reality problems of adaptation to the community are generally best dealt with *in vivo*, and the patient should not therefore be encouraged to surrender to dependency on the hospital for passive gratification of sick needs.

At the point of discharge, resistances develop in both staff and patients. In patients, there is an aggravation of symptoms or acting out. Staff is often threatened by exacerbation of the patient's psychopathology, and in itself has often developed dependence upon the patients such that, in some instances, the staff need the patient more than vice versa. But firm emphasis by management on early discharge planning and looking to the outside for therapeutic aid will encourage staff to resolve its ties to sickness and actively seek early mobilization of family, job and community to the patients' benefit.

Altogether we are speaking here of greater flexibility in patient management as regards use of both hospital and community resources, a less serious view of risks in discharging a patient, and a greater value put on the community as a therapeutic ally. Thus the patient is permitted earlier visiting privileges, weekends and evenings out; he continues to utilize the social-recreational advantages of the outside, such as baseball, theater, gyms, parks, picnics, beaches; and wherever the situation warrants he is permitted to work in the community while resident in the hospital, or paid contract work can be brought into the hospital to provide tangible and realistic incentives to combat apathy and retreat.

2. *Relatives' Contact with Patient and Hospital.* Relatives are the proximal group representing the community with whom the hospital has contact. Potentially they constitute a body of individuals, most likely greater in size than the patient population. Consider this fact: in the state of Massachusetts some 30,000 patients are hospitalized, presumably representing at least 30,000 relatives who were at some time in contact with the hospital and challenged by the problems of mental disease. If during their lifetime approximately 10 per cent of the citizens in the Commonwealth may be expected to be hospitalized, then presumably at least this number of relatives will have had an opportunity to experience the mental hospital

and the problems of mental illness. For this very large group, no well-thought-out plan exists to cultivate favorable attitudes to mental illness. Mere contact alone with the hospital does not necessarily change attitudes favorably; it is, rather, the nature of contact that matters—its educational and growth-enhancing values. If the contact is carefully planned and full advantage taken of learning opportunities provided by this experience, relatives may become more enlightened and accepting of mental hospital and mental illness and thereafter become effective ambassadors and catalysts of goodwill and community understanding. If the contact is negative, threatening or anxiety-provoking, where the threat and anxiety have no opportunity to be "worked through," relatives may become more resistant to mental illness and driven further away from hospital and patient.

How can the relatives' contribution to the hospital be enhanced; how can the relative get more out of the role as relative? The first problem, which has received scrutiny in some advanced hospitals, is the problem of visiting (Hotchkiss, 1956). Some have asked, What is the nature of the visiting experience; how do patient, relatives and staff meet; is the visit conducive to a relaxed, meaningful exchange, or is it a formal, duty-bound affair? Does the relative have an opportunity to come into contact with staff and to have his questions properly answered?

Several hospitals have successfully extended their visiting time. In one center, visiting time has been increased from one hour daily to nearly eight. This has been accomplished without increased stress upon staff; instead of visitors coming in one large rush or traffic jam during the designated hour, they now come throughout the longer period in smaller numbers, and are easier to handle. The visitor is now free to stay for a "natural" period instead of for the prescribed hour. His visit may be in any part of the hospital where he can see activities, observe patients, and at times join with them in their daily life. The next step is for the visitor to become a social and recreational partner; in participating thus he may acquire a more positive feeling for the hospital and help the patient to feel more "at home." A freer relative who has an opportunity to *do* something rather than sit and force conversation may be a happier relative and a healthier link between patient and outside.

Relatives are being encouraged increasingly to enter into individual or group discussions with staff (Greenblatt *et al.* 1957, Kahn and Prestwood 1954, Steele 1948). In some instances these are primarily informational, in others the relative becomes a "client" himself. This recognizes the role of family members in mental illness. As staff deals more with family members, new light is cast on the meaning of illness and of hospitalization. Family members meeting in group sessions are usually eager to share problems with each other and often gain considerably from mutual exchange and expression of emotionally charged concerns. These kinds of group activities help greatly, we believe, to prepare the family to receive the patient on discharge and to weather crises that so frequently arise in the adjustment period.

Family's participation with the patient in the hospital is a preparatory step to incorporation of family members in the hospital organization, especially its auxiliary or volunteer groups. They can be invited to contribute as welfare-minded citizens to help the hospital and, thus, to add a new role to that of patient's relative.

Staff contact with family is a preliminary step to staff visits in the patient's home setting and staff appreciation of family dynamics. Such visits are very useful in aiding the transition from hospital to home, and in aftercare as well as in prevention of relapse. They should also be explored for their possible utility in prehospitalization orientation of patient and family, and even in prevention of hospitalization. The latter has been systematically attempted by two clinics in Boston recently and with notable success (Freedman *et al.* 1960, Moore *et al.* 1960).

3. *Staff Contact with Community.* The movement of patients into the community can best be accomplished if staff, too, is interested in the community and properly adapted there. Too often in the past the mental hospital has been a place of retreat or haven of refuge for staff members, many of whom themselves found life in the community too anxiety-provoking. They sought security in living within the confines of the hospital with room provided free or at low rent, meals served, and financial stresses minimized by steady income. However, only when staff appreciates problems of living in the community and experiences ways of solving them can they help patients face reality with courage and confidence. Based in the community and working in the hospital, staff members live more like the average citizen. Since they are more *en courant* with community facilities, they may more readily participate with patients in their contacts outside of hospital grounds.

As we have said regarding relatives, staff may become better community ambassadors of goodwill, interpreting the hospital's program to friends and associates, and participating in community organizations. Furthermore, staff is encouraged to take an active part in public lectures, panels, and other media of communication. Thus, if patients in transition are in a sense becoming alumni of the hospital, the staff should not be a narrow cloistered group but a "community faculty."

4. *Community Contact with the Hospital.* The community mental hospital will not only encourage visiting of relatives but will hold open house and conduct tours for interested organizations or groups. Volunteers and auxiliary personnel have already proved their worth (Evans 1955, Frank 1949, Hyde and Hurley 1950, Malamud 1955, Spingarn 1959). Volunteer hospital organizations now include not only citizens but also students from universities who may become a source of enthusiastic and creative manpower. This has been amply demonstrated

in the activities, for example, of the Harvard-Radcliffe student group (and others from surrounding Boston universities) (Greenblatt *et al.* 1957, Jurkowitz 1956, Spencer 1957, Umbarger *et al.* 1960) as part of the mental health volunteer effort of the Phillips Brooks House, a Harvard student center. This student resource, if expanded and developed throughout the nation, would, we predict, greatly benefit students and patients alike.

Churches and community organizations have an unusual opportunity to apply themselves to the cause of the needy. Some churches have adopted wards, and some communities have shown special interest in citizens hospitalized from their area. Some citizens' groups have played a prominent role in helping discharged patients, setting up expatient clubs, halfway houses, etc. Those citizens in strategic positions in industries that are willing to hire expatients can be an exceptional source of strength, for work is vital to rehabilitation and self-respect.

IMPLICATIONS FOR STAFF

THE new developments in hospital-community transition suggest that staff needs instruction on the importance of discharge, rehabilitation, community psychiatry, home visits, continuity of patient care from prehospital to posthospital period, and the more flexible and creative use of hospital and other facilities such as day and night units and halfway houses. In the future, staff will be trained to see the hospital as a temporary care facility, to be used not longer than the patient's vital needs require. This will hopefully lead to a new concept of the mental health center of the future with less emphasis on new construction, more on personalized care during part of the day or brief total periods with the expectation that patients move on selectively to settings or environments most appropriate to their prevailing needs and current growth potentialities.

Thus, a new orientation to training of psychiatrists, ancillary and ward personnel, rehabilitation workers, volunteers and community participants is emerging as a necessary ingredient in the development of the community mental hospital of the future.

REFERENCES

Belknap, Ivan: *Human Problems Of A State Mental Hospital.* McGraw-Hill Book Co., New York, 1956.
Brown, Esther Lucile: *Nursing For The Future.* Russell Sage Foundation, New York, 1948.
Caudill, William: *The Psychiatric Hospital As A Small Society.* Harvard University Press, Cambridge, 1958.
Cumming, Elaine and John Cumming: *Closed Ranks.* Harvard University Press, Cambridge, 1957.

Denber, Herman C. B. (ed.): *Research Conference On Therapeutic Community.* Charles C. Thomas, Springfield, Illinois, 1960.

Evans, Ruth L.: Volunteers in a Mental Hospital. *Mental Hygiene, 39,* 111-117, January 1955.

Frank, Marjorie H.: Volunteer Work with Psychiatric Patients. *Mental Hygiene, 33,* 353-365, July 1949.

Freedman, T. T., P. Rolfe and S. E. Perry: Home Treatment of Psychiatric Patients. *American Journal of Psychiatry, 116,* 807, March 1960.

Greenblatt, Milton, Daniel J. Levinson and Richard H. Williams (eds.): *The Patient And The Mental Hospital.* The Free Press, Glencoe, Illinois, 1957.

Greenblatt, Milton and Benjamin Simon (eds.): *Rehabilitation Of The Mentally Ill: Social And Economic Aspects.* Publication No. 58 of American Association for the Advancement of Science, Washington, D.C., 1959.

Greenblatt, Milton, Richard H. York and Esther Lucile Brown: *From Custodial To Therapeutic Patient Care In Mental Hospitals.* Russell Sage Foundation, New York, 1955.

Hall, Bernard H.: *Psychiatric Aide Education.* Grune & Stratton, Inc., New York, 1952.

Hotchkiss, Georgina: The Psychiatric Patient's Visitors. *Nursing Outlook, 4,* June 1956.

Hyde, Robert W.: *Experiencing The Patient's Day.* G. P. Putnam's Sons, New York, 1955.

Hyde, Robert W., Milton Greenblatt and Frederic L. Wells: The Role of the Attendant in Authority and Compliance: Notes on Ten Cases. *Journal of Genetic Psychology, 54,* 107-126, 1956.

Hyde, Robert W. and Catherine F. Hurley: Volunteers in Mental Hospitals. *Psychiatric Quarterly Supplement, 24,* Part 2, 233-249, 1950.

Jones, Maxwell: *The Therapeutic Community.* Basic Books, Inc., New York, 1953.

Jurkowitz, Maeda: College Volunteers in a State Mental Hospital. Honors thesis submitted to Social Relations Department, Radcliffe College, April 1956.

Kahn, Shirley W. and A. Rodney Prestwood: Group Therapy of Parents as an Adjunct to the Treatment of Schizophrenic Patients. *Psychiatry, 17,* 177-185, May 1954.

Malamud, Irene T.: Volunteers in Community Mental Health Work: The Respective Roles of Laymen and Professionally-Trained Persons. *Mental Hygiene, 39,* 300-309, April 1955.

Milbank Memorial Fund, 34th Annual Conference, Part I: *An Approach To The Prevention Of Disability From Chronic Psychoses: The Open Mental Hospital Within The Community.* Milbank Memorial Fund, New York, 1957.

Moore, Robert F., Robert S. Albert, Mary J. Manning and Betty A. Glasser: Explorations in Alternatives to Hospitalization. Presented at American Psychiatric Association Annual Meeting, May 1960.

Myerson, Abraham: Theory and Principles of the "Total Push" Method in the Treatment of Chronic Schizophrenia. *American Journal of Psychiatry, 95,* 1197-1204, 1939.

Semrad, Elvin V. and William Corwin: Total Push Treatment of Chronic Schizophrenia at the Metropolitan State Hospital: Preliminary Report. Archives of Neurology & Psychiatry, *44*, 232-233, July 1940.

Spencer, Steven M.: They Befriend the Mentally Ill. *The Saturday Evening Post*, October 5, 1957.

Spingarn, Natalie Davis: *The Volunteer And The Psychiatric Patient.* American Psychiatric Association, Washington, D.C., 1959.

Stanton, A. H. and M. S. Schwartz: *The Mental Hospital.* Basic Books, Inc., New York, 1954.

Steele, Muriel H.: Group Meetings for Relatives of Mental Hospital Patients. Thesis submitted to Smith College, 1948.

Tillotson, Kenneth J.: The Practice of the "Total Push" Method in the Treatment of Chronic Schizophrenia. *American Journal of Psychiatry, 95,* 1205-1213, March 1939.

Umbarger, Carter C., Andrew P. Morrison, Peter R. Breggin and James S. Dalsimer: *The College Student And The Mental Patient.* Unpublished book, 1960.

Von Mering, Otto and Stanley H. King: *Remotivating The Mental Patient.* Russell Sage Foundation, New York, 1957.

Wells, Frederic L., Milton Greenblatt and Robert W. Hyde: As the Psychiatric Aide Sees His Work and Problems. *Genetic Psychology Monographs, 53,* 3-73, 1956.

World Health Organization, Technical Report Series No. 73: *Third Report Of The Expert Committee On Mental Health.* Geneva, September 1953.

Section III

INTERNAL STRUCTURE AND
PROCESSES OF INSTITUTIONS

INTRODUCTION

THE story is told, at one residential treatment center for children, of an adolescent girl patient who was taking a group of professional visitors on a tour of the grounds. As the group passed various staff members on the way, the patient-guide would indicate to her group, "That's Mr. White, the Assistant Director," or "That's Mrs. Smith; she's a social worker." Finally one of the visitors asked, "And what is your title?" "Child," was the reply.

This anecdote illustrates one difference between the sociological approach to studying business organizations and the study of institutions for residential treatment. The client of a business firm is not ordinarily included in describing positions within the organization, but in treatment institutions the inmate is always with us, occupying a definable position, and a description of the institutional structure is not complete unless all three kinds of internal relationships—those among staff, among clients, and between clients and staff—are included.

Yet in spite of the differences, students of the internal structure of treatment institutions can take an important cue from studies of industrial organizations. In mental hospitals and prisons, as in factories and business offices, patterns of informal relationships are frequently more important, for understanding behavior within the organization, than formally prescribed chains of command and segments of responsibility.

Articles included in this section represent analyses of relationships, formal and informal, between positions *within* the institution; that is, they focus on *internal* structure. The positions themselves may be formally prescribed, for example, by professional title, or they may be informal, arising from convergence of informal group expectations and individuals' behavior in relation to these expectations.

We shall use the major role distinction between institutional staff and clients (patients, inmates) to arrange the articles in this section. Those dealing with intra-staff relations are presented first. Following them are studies of client interaction, and analyses of staff-client relations conclude the section.

"The Formal Structure of a Psychiatric Hospital," by Jules Henry, describes official supervisory responsibility with a conceptual scheme applicable to all task-performing organizations. The special circumstances of the psychiatric hospital give rise to situations of "multiple subordination," in which one worker is subordinate to many chiefs. Henry presents an analysis of stresses resulting from this organizational structure and suggests that administrators' problems often derive from basic structural defects rather than from individuals' shortcomings in carrying out job requirements.

In contrast, Scheff's paper highlights the informal side of staff structure. He shows the techniques through which attendants in a mental hospital, formally subordinate to physician-administrators, are able to exercise considerable control over their superiors by means of an informal system of sanctions and rationalizations.

Whereas Henry uses the theory of formal organizations and Scheff relies on a description of informal mechanisms to explain problems in a hospital administration, Martin employs role-set theory to analyze strains in carrying out the duties of incumbents of one position on which he focuses—the psychiatric resident. Five social mechanisms—differential role involvement, differential power distribution, insulation from observability, observability of conflicting expectations, and role-set abridgement—are used to discuss the resident's status and role relations.

The fourth article on intra-staff relations deals with conflicts between incumbents of two different staff positions. It is based on interviews conducted with cottage parents and caseworkers in two correctional institutions for boys. Piliavin found lack of respect for each other's profession among caseworkers and cottage parents, both at the custodially oriented institution he studied, and at the more therapeutically oriented one. Such conflict is inevitable as these institutions are presently structured, in his opinion, and he suggests structural changes to alleviate the problem.

Interrelations among clients are described in the paper by Bloom, Boyd and Kaplan. They identified two cliques on an open psychiatric ward, a leadership clique and a dissident clique, each of which performed different social functions for the total group ward. Dentler and Erikson, in the next paper, report investigations to support the hypothesis that deviancy need not have disruptive consequences for a group, but indeed may strengthen its cohesiveness.

In "The Triple Bind," client interaction processes are intensively revealed among a clique of four boys. In addition to describing the informal role relationships in this sub-group of a cottage of delinquents, the authors relate each member's position in the subgroup to his personality structure and dynamics, and then proceed to indicate how the group system functions to maintain itself in opposition to institutional values.

The paper by Stanton and Schwartz has achieved the status of a classic in describing patient-staff relationships. Employing participant observation, they observed a connection between disagreement among staff members and excited behavior on the part of the patients. As the authors point out, the process is a triangular one; dissension in staff relations is somehow communicated to the patients, and this affects them adversely. Unfortunately, efforts to substantiate Stanton and Schwartz's finding with quantitative data have yielded negative results. An example is the next paper by Dinitz and his co-workers. These investigators caution that their study is an attempt to establish whether intra-ward disagreement among staff personnel is related to patients' overt functioning; it does not inquire into effects on therapeutic goals for patients. Another study by Wallace and Rashkis,[1] which is reprinted in another reader, also failed to confirm the Stanton-Schwartz hypothesis.

The last article in this section reports research on staff-inmate relations in correctional institutions, based on questionnaires administered to inmates and staff. Street studied four institutions which differed in structure because each had a different goal. One aimed at discipline. Another combined treatment and custody, but not in a well-integrated way. The other two institutions were primarily treatment-oriented, one stressing milieu therapy, and the other, individual psychotherapy. These structural differences, it was found, resulted in institutional differences in staff attitudes and in inmate attitudes. In the treatment-oriented institution, attitudes of staff toward inmates and inmates toward staff were more positive than in the more custodial settings. Further, the difference in administrative goals has an impact on inmate structure: leadership and integration in the inmate group are more strongly associated with positive feelings toward staff and institution in the treatment settings, especially so in the institution emphasizing milieu therapy.

Studies of residential institutions, even more than analysis of other kinds of organizations, call attention to strains, or disfunctions, in system operations. The papers in this section focus primarily on identifying structural sources of disfunction. In Section IV, when disfunctions are discussed, they will be related to the four universal functions of social systems.

[1] Anthony F. C. Wallace and Harold A. Rashkis. "The Relation of Staff Consensus to Patient Disturbance on Mental Hospital Wards," in Neil J. Smelser and William T. Smelser (eds.) *Personality and Social Systems,* New York: Wylie, 1963, pp. 630-36.

CHAPTER 15   The Formal Social Structure
of a Psychiatric Hospital*

JULES HENRY

THIS paper is an attempt to communicate some of the conceptualizations and hypotheses regarding formal organizational structure which
the author arrived at as the result of intensive study of a psychiatric unit of
a general hospital. I present these in the hope that some of the conceptualizations of the way that stress is created by organizational structure, which
I have formalized in two equations, can be further tested by other workers. On the basis of my observations, I feel that when people fail to
function adequately in an organization, the areas of stress in the formal
organization itself must be examined. In other words, before one identifies
certain people as operating inappropriately within the organization, some
attention should be focused on the difficulties inherent in the organization
itself. On the basis of my data, I have constructed certain typical situations that arise in hospital administration, involving, for example, the
charge nurse, or the administrators of different wings of a hospital. Some
of these situations will be recognized by people working in other hospitals
as typical of their own organizations, too.

The emotional relations among the workers in any task-performing
organization are important; but in a psychiatric hospital they are especially so because of the direct effect of workers on patients. It has long
been one of the guiding principles of sociology and anthropology that the
specific quality of emotional relations between people is in large part a
function of the over-all *formal* social matrix in which they live, and this
paper will be devoted to the development of hypotheses regarding the
relationship between the formal structure of a psychiatric hospital as a
task-performing organization and the attitudes of the workers toward

* Reprinted by special permission of The William Alanson White Psychiatric Foundation, Inc., and the author from *Psychiatry*, 17 (1954), 139–151 (copyright by the
Foundation).

each other.[1] I feel that it is legitimate at this time to stress formal organization, for the reason that so many of the important pioneering sociological studies[2] of psychiatric hospitals have analyzed patient-personnel relationships in terms of *informal* social structure. The point of view presented in the following pages stresses the importance of understanding the underlying formal matrix of such an organization as a precondition for understanding the nature of informal relationships that develop within it.[3]

THE IMAGE OF SOCIAL STRUCTURE

IN this discussion I mean by formal structure *the image a member of a task-performing group has in his mind* of (1) the pattern of rules according to which the regular tasks of the organization are to be carried out and (2) the pattern of rules according to which the people in the organization ideally relate to each other in task-performance.[4] In our culture such structures are frequently represented on organizational charts.

It is characteristic of people in our culture to imagine many aspects of the world, both tangible and intangible, to have shape.[5] The universe has been imagined as a globe with our world 'inside,' and the atom as a planetary system; and in the same way, social systems are endowed with shape. Organizational perfection in industry, government, and the Army is exemplified in the so-called line organization. In the last twenty-five years, this way of organizing work has, without exception, been advocated by writers on public administration.[6] Diagrams of 'good' institutional organization often look like trees—sometimes like pine trees—with a central trunk and branches radiating horizontally.[7] Figure 1 illustrates the point.

Military organization typifies this kind of arrangement: the trunk is the line of command descending vertically to the subordinate officers, who bring to execution the orders issued by the general; the branches, radiating *horizontally* from the trunk, represent the regiment, battalion, platoon, and company, in descending order. The line organization is the stereotype of good organization in our culture.

FIG. 1

LINE ORGANIZATION

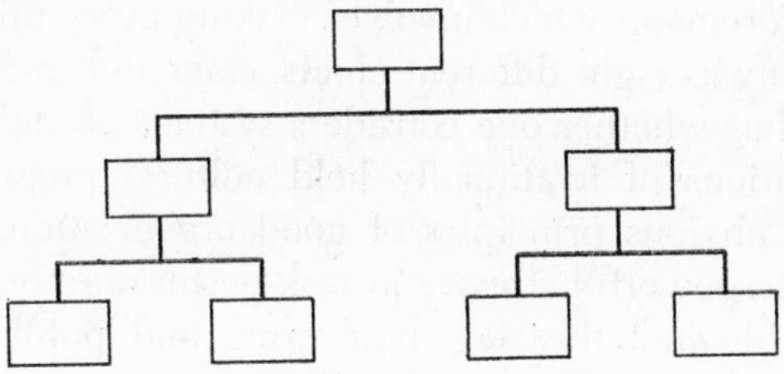

Obviously a social organization really has no "shape": there is no central "trunk," no "line," no "branches," and authority does not "descend." Rather, the image that a culture has of an organization represents, in part, the way in which people in that culture expect things to get done—that is, a set of values. In our culture these values include responsibility, authority, command, obedience, dominance, and submission.

The fact that an organization is conceptualized as a shape means many things to the people who must work in it. A shape has boundaries, long and short lines between points,[8] and, under propitious circumstances, definiteness and dependability. It is important to a worker in an organization not only (1) that the shape of the organization is that which he has learned to expect as a member of a particular culture, but also (2) that he can expect the shape to remain the same day after day.

The image of the pine has been so firmly impressed upon our imaginations that the image of the oak, with branches extending *diagonally* upward and outward from the trunk, is horrifying to specialists in industrial organization. *Whereas the image of the pine postulates a single direct line of command from the chief of an organization to his subordinate, the image of the oak suggests several lines of authority from more than one chief to a single subordinate.* This is the so-called functional type of organization. Figure 2 illustrates the image of the oak.

FIG. 2

IMAGE OF THE OAK

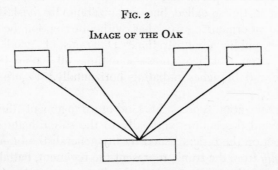

The subordination of one worker to several chiefs, which I shall call *multiple subordination,* is unworkable in our culture.[9] Without exception outstanding writers on industrial management in the twentieth century have criticized Taylor, the father of scientific management, for his idea of the "functional foreman," which involves making every production worker subject to as many as eight different chiefs, each an expert in a particular kind of work. Thus whether one considers systems of multiple subordination to be violations of irrationally held cultural prejudices or simply deviations from obvious principles of good organization, it is clear that today they create powerful stresses in task-performing organizations, and are not acceptable in industrial engineering and public administration theory. I have, by means of the hypotheses and analysis that follow, endeavored to conceptualize the processes involved.

THE ORGANIZATIONAL STRUCTURE OF A
PSYCHIATRIC UNIT OF A GENERAL HOSPITAL

THE hypotheses presented in this paper are based on my study of the formal organizational structure of the psychiatric unit of a private general hospital. The hospital had between 700 and 800 beds; one floor, containing 29 of the 54 beds in the psychiatric unit, was studied intensively. The methods of study were interviewing and direct observation, supplemented by attendance at staff conferences and rounds, and by many informal conversations with all varieties of personnel at lunch, coffee, and casual meetings. Intensive observation and interviewing were carried out from September 1951 to February 1952; this was followed by less intensive interviewing as needed, while the analysis of the data was in progress. The approximately 70 hours devoted to direct observation were scattered throughout the days and nights, and the days of the week, in a random way. Observation periods of interaction between patients and personnel ranged from ten minutes to nine hours and fifteen minutes, with a mean of two hours and thirty-five minutes.

The formal structure of the hospital studied has both pine-tree and oak-tree characteristics (see Figure 3). From the director to the several departments, the authority is of the line type; from the departments to the supervisor of psychiatric nursing, authority is of the functional or oak-tree type. From the supervisor to her head nurses and below, authority is again of the line variety; but from the staff nurses to the attendants, authority is of the oak-tree type—almost any supervisor can tell an attendant what to do.

One can see how readily a system of multiple subordination comes into being in a psychiatric hospital, for a large number of tasks must be performed for each patient. The patient must be prevented from killing himself or injuring others, he must be fed properly, given psychotherapy, kept clean, and kept from falling out of bed, and he must be supervised in O.T., recreation, and other activities such as bathing. He must be given medications, and have his temperature taken; and he must not lose his money or false teeth, break his glasses, or steal the property of other patients. Of course, which of these tasks will be performed depends also on the character of the hospital. At any rate it is readily understood that a psychiatric hospital is a place *par excellence* where not only the personnel, but especially the patients have to be controlled in order that nothing unforeseen happens. Thus in a psychiatric hospital tasks are numerous, frequently unrelated to each other, and characterized at times in addition by the quality of *emergency*. The tasks are said to be unrelated because, for

FIG. 3

ORGANIZATIONAL CHART OF A GENERAL HOSPITAL WITH REFERENCE TO THE
PSYCHIATRIC UNIT (HIGHLY SIMPLIFIED)

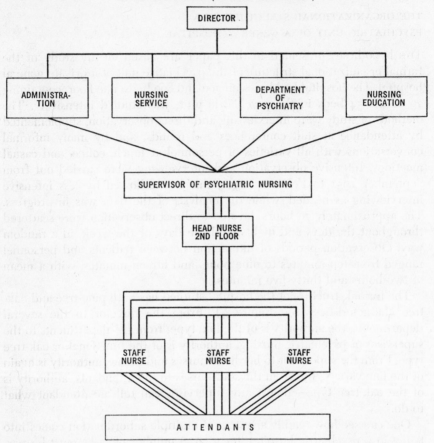

example, there is no relationship between seeing that a patient does not lose his false teeth and giving him psychotherapy. Yet the same nurse is sometimes supposed to do just that: be custodian of false teeth and give patients the kind of thoughtful attention expected of psychiatric nurses in some hospitals.

Thus it is easy to see, in view of the functions of the psychiatric hospital, how a system of multiple subordination comes into being. Yet interviews showed that the organizational structure was not considered satisfactory by the personnel; the data showed much agreement that it was difficult to work in the system, that there was a problem of definition of function, and that information did not 'behave' as it should. I should now like to examine in more detail the operations of the system, and offer some hypotheses as to the ways in which stress is related to the formal structure.

From the study of this institution, and from examination of the literature in industrial engineering and public administration, it seems possible
to set up general hypotheses about the development of *stress* in systems
of multiple subordination. I shall present these in terms of the *administrative units* (such as departments) of which the systems are composed, the
power of the units, the extent to which the units *overlap* in their functions,
and the degree to which the administrative units are in *agreement* on
policies and methods. It was clear in the hospital studied—and the
theoretical and empirical analyses of task-performing organizations in the
literature provide overwhelming supporting evidence—that much of the
tension experienced by workers in carrying out their day-to-day tasks
within systems of multiple subordination is a direct result of the stresses
inherent in such systems by virtue of their very structure. As I studied the
hospital and reviewed the literature, it became clear to me that administrative units, their relative power with respect to one another, and the
degree of consensus among the units about goals and methods, were
indeed the central variables that determined the character of the stresses.
In formulating the hypotheses, therefore, I have used only those variables
which seem to me crucial and central.

In order to make the matter clearer, let us imagine a general hospital
with three building units. While the entire hospital has a director, each of
the three buildings has an assistant director, X, Y, and Z. The hospital has
four basic departments, dealing with medical services, nursing, administration, and nursing education, and the operations of these departments
extend throughout the three buildings. Now if X, Y, and Z have purely
coordinating functions—that is, functions that are concerned only with
ensuring that operations decided on by the departments are carried out
properly—then the functions of X, Y, and Z do not overlap with those of
the departments, and problems of power do not arise. If, however, X, Y,
and Z have executive powers so that they can temporarily delay or stop
action on decisions made by the departments, then the powers of X, Y, and
Z tend to approach those of the departments, and overlap them. Thus, for
example, if the department of psychiatry decides that all patients shall be
permitted to carry their own cigarettes, but Z prevents its being done on
the grounds that cigarettes should be carried only by convalescing patients
in order that disturbed patients may have an incentive to get well, then
Z's functions overlap those of the department of psychiatry and, in this
instance, Z is also more powerful than the department. Let us assume on
the other hand that a patient's relatives come to take him home, but find
that the ward will not release him because no order to that effect has been
left by his physician. They may then get Z to ask the ward to release the
patient anyway. If the ward does not release the patient, the department
of psychiatry is said to have greater power in that instance than Z, who
represents the administration. If a number of such situations arise, in
which now a given department overrules the administration, now the

administration overrules the department, and if in addition the two frequently confer about many details of day-to-day operation, it may be said that the administration and the department have approximately equal power and much overlap. An example of nonoverlap would be a situation in which the department of psychiatry decides to give a patient electrotherapy, but the administration does not concern itself with the basic therapeutic plan at all.

Thus the relative power of units can be measured in terms of the number of situations in which a unit (such as a department) has authority to issue an incontrovertible command, has veto power over the commands of other units, or has power to hire and fire. Functional overlap is measurable in terms of the number of operations performed by one unit that are also performed by other units. Consensus measures may be obtained by counting the number of times the departments are in agreement in actual operations. The difficult problem of stress may be approached by measuring the frequency of cases in which people quit or the frequency of statements about quitting and by counting the frequency of hostile statements and statements about loss of interest in the job which can be attributed to administrative operations. Other measures of stress are statements about confusion and fatigue in task performance.

On the basis of these considerations, I have formulated the following hypotheses about systems of multiple subordination:

(1) In an organization composed of units of approximately equal power the firmness of any decision is a function of consensus, provided, always, that in any matter under consideration, all the chiefs are interested.

(2) The more of such equipotential units (that is, units of approximately equal power) there are involved in any decision, the less likely it is to be firm.

(3) The multiplication of such units produces a system stress (T) that is directly proportional to the power of the units (P) and to the functional overlap or degree of similarity of their functions (Sf), and inversely proportional to the extent of consensus (C). This relationship may be expressed in the following quasi-mathematical form:[10]

$$T \to f\left(\frac{P \times Sf}{C}\right)$$

Equation 1

This enables one to deduce the following subsidiary hypotheses:

(a) Where units are powerful and have greatly similar functions (high degree of functional overlap), stress will be high in an organization if consensus is low.

(b) Low stress level is possible in an organization of powerful units even in the presence of much functional overlap provided consensus is high.[11]

(c) Even where the units have little power or functional overlap stress will be high if consensus is low (that is, the goals and/or the methods of the units are different).

(d) Regardless of the value of the numerator, stress will always be high as consensus approaches zero. This would mean that even when things seem to be going smoothly, such a system is prone to periodic spasms because of sudden disagreements. This underscores the great vulnerability of such systems, and their *dependence on identity of basic goals in the different units.*

So far I have considered the organization as a whole and the question of stress as it arises from the total organizational structure. I will now, in the succeeding sections, turn to more specific situations which arise within such a structure, and the ways in which they affect individual workers.

COMMUNICATIONS AND CONTROL

IN Figure 3, representing the formal structure of a general hospital containing psychiatric wards, the supervisor of psychiatric nursing is a key figure, for the policies and directives emanating from the four basic departments channel through her. In figurative terms she is a transmitter of messages to all employees from the department heads. She can decode, transmit, block, interpret, scramble, or unscramble messages that come to her from above and below. At every moment of operating time on her shift she must make decisions with respect to descending messages coming from four different departments as to whether messages are consistent with each other and whether present messages are consistent with past ones. She must also decide whether messages either ascending or descending should be transmitted or blocked. In terms of action on a message coming from above, she must decide whether she will act or whether she will ask someone else to act (that is, whether the message pertains to her reserved or delegated authority). If she asks someone else to act, she must select the actor with precision and dispatch. All of this would be difficult enough to do if she transmitted only one kind of information. When she must transmit four different kinds of information, the difficulties are great, and these multiply if the messages from the different departments are incompatible with each other. It thus becomes evident that *the efficiency of a communications network is closely related to the formal structure of the social system it is intended to bind together.* In other words, a communications network can be no more efficient than the organization of which it is part. This statement is no tautology if one starts, as I do here, from the assumption that in setting up an organization one sets up the formal structure first and then plans the communications system.

In view of the number of persons to whom she is responsible and whose directives she must transmit, the supervisor is already in a rather complicated situation. However, it is not unusual for some systems to be complicated even further by persons in relatively high echelons bypassing the supervisor and giving orders directly to persons in the lower or even in the lowest echelons, thus extending their own control. I have called this process *blanketing,* for its end result is that the persons in the lower echelons become blanketed by directives. In fact, in a system that permits members in the highest echelons to give orders directly to those in the lowest, the lower one is in the hierarchy the more persons one will receive directives from. It is thus true also that the lower one is in the hierarchy the greater is the intensity of the process of multiple subordination.

Blanketing takes place, however, not just because "people don't have any sense" or because they "don't know how to administer." The causes of this process, it seems to me, are inherent in the system dynamics themselves. But before giving my reasons for thinking so, it is necessary to analyze an important aspect of the functioning of a psychiatric hospital —the task of the psychiatric nurse.

TASK PERFORMANCE

In all task-performing organizations the "rationality" of the operations is important:[12] such things as number of commands (Nc), the number of persons a worker must respond to (Np), the consistency of the commands he receives (Cs), and the interrelatedness of his operations (Ir), all affect the individual worker's stress-in-task-performance (S).[13] The relationship among all these factors may be condensed in the following quasi-mathematical model.

$$S \rightarrow f \left(\frac{Nc \times Np}{Cs \times Ir} \right)$$

Equation 2

From what has been said, it can be understood that Equation 2 has a special relevance to a psychiatric ward, because of the peculiarities of the organization of work. The equation, however, has a special relevance also to the analysis of a system of multiple subordination, for it is when a worker has multiple superiors that the number of persons giving orders, the number of orders given and their consistency, and the interrelatedness of the tasks may become acute issues.

From Equation 2 one may now derive, among others,[14] the following subsidiary hypotheses:

(1) Though stress-in-task-performance may tend to increase as a worker has to respond to more and more commands from more and more people, his stress will increase sharply when the commands lack consistency and the tasks he is to perform are not clearly related to each other.

(2) Where multiplicity of chiefs cannot be avoided, an antidote to the worker's stress is increased coordination of chiefs, resulting in increased consistency in commands and interrelatedness of tasks.

(3) Workers may show relatively great tolerance for multiplicity of commands as long as consistency and interrelatedness remain high. The view of Gulick, therefore, that "a workman subject to orders from several superiors will be confused, inefficient, and irresponsible"[15] would not appear to be necessarily correct without considering these other factors.

RANDOMNESS

I would now like to suggest one more hypothesis about task-performing organizations in our culture:

The greater the number of tasks to be performed, the greater the chances of the occurrence of random—that is, unpredicted—events in the event sequences involved in task performance. Since human society has a horror of random—unpredictable—behavior, this assumption may be used to derive a *law of diminishing randomness: In all human societies efforts are made to reduce the chances of the occurrence of random events.*[16]

I shall call this horror of randomness in social systems *system anxiety*. Efforts to prevent the occurrence of random events—whether these be incorrect performances of tasks or simply failures to perform tasks—express themselves in the multiplication of controls—supervisors, foremen, systems of cost accounting, and so on—in task-performing organizations.[17] But since each control added to a system is *itself a new task*, the question is raised as to *how this new task is to be controlled.* Thus in the very act of attempting to diminish the chances of random events occurring, the chances are increased. In this way very large enterprises may become 'overanxious,' inefficient systems because of the proliferation of control devices. On the other hand such organizations may diminish supervision through granting more autonomy to individual subunits. This apparently tends to diminish system anxiety while increasing efficiency of operations.[18]

It is now, I think, somewhat clearer why blanketing may take place on a large scale in a task-performing organization. The causes seem to be: (a) the multiplicity of tasks that have to be performed, and the ensuing problems of the control of randomness; and (b) the difficulties of operating a system of multiple subordination, with its inherent difficulties in coordination. Taken together these factors cause considerable stress, or, as I have called it, system anxiety, which leads to blanketing—that is, to greater and greater efforts at control all down the line. However, since blanketing increases the number of persons to whom a worker must respond, and hence increases the chances for the development of inconsistencies in orders, it may actually increase stress throughout the system. In this way, in the very act of attempting to decrease stress, through introducing greater control, stress may be increased.

I think it is now possible to understand certain aspects of the natural history of supervisors who attempt to operate in hospitals characterized by the features outlined in the preceding paragraphs. If a supervisor has the potentialities for the development of authoritarian behavior, she may tell everybody to "go hang," and that she will run things as she sees fit. In this way she shuts out many of the conflicting stimuli that impinge upon her from the various levels of the hierarchy, and gets some consistency and order into her operations. On the other hand, if she lacks this potentiality and is a permissive, yielding sort of person, she may want to obey everyone. This can lead only to wide swings in behavior, and, possibly, to ultimate total failure to function. The permissive supervisor in such a system may communicate her own confusion to her subordinates, while the authoritarian supervisor on the other hand, seems to give her subordinates a straight line of policy to follow, and the wards seem to function in an orderly way. Thus a system of the kind described here may be able to function only by *generating rebels against itself.*

Obviously the foregoing implies no judgment by the writer as to what the 'best' type of supervisor is. In American culture the occupation of a key position by an authoritarian figure may have serious and undesirable implications for maximal personality functioning both of the patients and of the personnel. The tendency of authoritarian figures to rigidify the social processes of an institution, with all that that implies in terms of resistance to innovation, must also be taken into account. One needs to take account of the institutional goals as well. If orderliness and smoothness of operations are major goals, and take primacy, for example, over flexibility, permissiveness, and the giving of a strong sense of personal autonomy to both personnel and patients, then a supervisor who is strict with everybody may be just what the central administration of the hospital needs. Meanwhile the administration sacrifices the values of flexibility, autonomy, and willingness to experiment, which may, but need not necessarily, come with the so-called permissive supervisor.

FUNCTIONAL DEFINITION

BEFORE leaving the subject of formal structure and its consequences for supervisors, it seems necessary to give some attention to the problems of functional definition. Not infrequently in American task-performing organizations a new functionary is introduced into the structure because some need is vaguely felt. For example, a hospital may introduce a person between the chief of nursing service and the floor supervisor. While the need is vaguely felt, however, the new functionary's functions are equally vague. It is believed—and this is not an unusual situation—that by exercising his vaguely defined functions the new functionary may "make a place for himself." Thus much of the burden of defining his functions may be placed on a new person. It can readily be seen, I think, that where functions are not clearly defined, improvisation must occur and may reach considerable dimensions. Not only does the new functionary improvise about his job (outward improvisation) but also everybody else does (inward improvisation). The new functionary must try to figure out what he is to do; and those with whom he works and those subordinate to him also try to figure out what he is supposed to do. This produces a spiralling effect, for once uncertainty enters the system at any point, improvisation may enter at all points.

In a competitive, status-conscious society, vague definition of function sometimes eventuates in feelings of reference, hostility, secrecy, and betrayal. This operates as follows: If A's function is defined in such a way as to appear to overlap the functions of B, then the members of the system tend to become divided, some belonging to A's camp and others to B's camp. X, a fellow worker of Y's, may belong to A's camp, while Y belongs to B's camp. Hence X and Y become involved in questions of loyalty to one another, and become suspicious and hostile toward each other. There develops a tendency toward secrecy because people do not wish to state that A "really" does not have the right to the functions he performs or to the position he occupies; hence they become fearful that their opinion of A's "rightful" position might become known. Meanwhile things begin to happen to both A and B: they appear to be undercut or by-passed in terms of their own definitions and interpretations of their functions, and their attitudes toward day-to-day happenings may become permeated by the feeling that "there is more to this than meets the eye"; or "A [or B] is out to get me." Thus the net stress effects of multiple subordination for the organization as a whole, the stress in task performance (as defined in Equation 2), the blanketing, and the lack of clarity in the definition of functions may ultimately seriously lower the efficiency of the personnel or even cause them to leave the organization.

SOME OVERT AND COVERT CONSEQUENCES OF STRESS

THE occurrence of vaguely defined functions in a system, accompanied by the difficulties in obtaining consensus and time synchronization which are usually present in systems of multiple subordination, tends to increase stress. Under these conditions workers are observed to behave in one or more of the following ways:
(1) They tend to become more and more dependent on the supervisor for direction (which might be called centripetal or focussed drift). (2) They tend to avoid the supervisor because of her observed indecision (centrifugal drift). (3) They tend to seek or to create an all-powerful being, such as a moderator, who will be outside or above the system (another aspect of centripetal drift). (4) They tend to become apathetic about their work, feeling there is no solution to their problems. (5) They tend to seek now one person, now another, to whom to tell their troubles, and of whom to ask advice. (6) They tend to develop covert social structures more suited to their needs than the overt one.

Put another way, in a system of this kind *uncertainty becomes a drive,* and hence much behavior is directed toward the reduction of uncertainty. The six modes of behavior named above are ways of reducing the uncertainty drive. In this section only items 3, 5, and 6 will be discussed.

The moderator.—When, for reasons already given, the operation of a system of multiple subordination becomes difficult, a moderator may be introduced. Thus a moderator, or rather his work, is an instrument for maintaining the system in a steady state. The usefulness of a moderator is, however, in a certain sense, illusory: *he can bring no more balance into the system than is provided by the basic underlying structure.* For if consensus cannot be obtained because of disagreements in values and/or objectives, or if there is no reduction in the number of equipotential units while functional overlap persists at a high level, the moderator simply works hard without increasing efficiency. Under such circumstances the moderator may become the central focus of the system: it tends to rely on him. Since the more severe the basic problems, the harder the moderator has to work, the magnitude of his work (Mw)[19] becomes an expression of the underlying tension (T). Hence:

$$T \to f\,(Mw)$$

Equation 3

Thus it is seen that *the harder the moderator works, the greater the stress in the system.* This paradox can be understood when it is realized that the office of moderator permits underlying problems of the organization to go unsolved, and even to multiply.[20]

The covert social structure.—In the presence of stress within the formal organization, workers attempt to develop informal social structures more in conformity with their needs; and thus the formal organization is thwarted as people take their troubles where they think they will get the most satisfaction. From this it follows that in an organization, conceived as a system of communications circuits, there is a circular relationship between interpersonal tensions and circuit-jumping (Cj) (that is, not "going through channels") such that the greater the tension in the system the greater the Cj and the greater the Cj the greater the tension. It is also true that Cj tends to increase functional overlap and is likely to increase the difficulty of arriving at consensus. (See Equation 1.)

Telegraphic signals can be said to have destination only if there is a receiver somewhere along the line, and someone to decode and interpret the signals. Analogically speaking, in a social system information will travel from person to person only if there are active receivers—that is, listeners. The magnitude of Cj therefore is a function also of the presence in the system of people who are willing to listen to the information that comes to them. In a system under stress almost everyone becomes a receiver because of his own need to send. Hence information about trouble (stress) often gets to places where it should not, and the resulting stress is fed back into the system, with consequent increase in stress. In this way the entire organization may begin to buzz with suspicion, gossip, rumor, and some truth.

The communications universe.—Every human being has an ideal communications universe, defined as the persons or groups whom he considers have the right to knowledge of his thoughts and behavior; and the persons or groups about whose thoughts and behavior he feels he should have knowledge. The communications universe varies depending on the kind of thoughts and behavior that are concerned: a nurse may feel that almost anybody has a right to know what her routine of work is; but that only certain people have the right to know how much time she spends on each of her tasks; and that still different persons—possibly only her best friend—have the right to know whom she dates. Similar considerations apply to incoming information—that is, information about others. A supervisor may feel that she has the right to know all about a nurse's difficulties in task performance, but she may be completely uninterested in the nurse's dating behavior, and thus feel that the nurse is justified in keeping such information from her.

The stresses operating on a person or within an organization are in part a function of the extent to which the ideal communications universe is violated. This stress, however, is related also to the *status* of the people who, in relation to a particular person, have information about him he would rather they did not have, and to the *number* of such people. It makes a big difference whether the superintendent of the hospital sees an orderly put his arm around a nurse while on duty, or whether just a friendly nurse sees it. It also makes a big difference whether only a few people know about it or the whole hospital knows about it.

I am dealing here, perhaps, with another one of those often illusory human needs: *the need to have some control over information that has to do with oneself,* whether that information is supposed to come to one, or whether that information is about one. When people feel that they have lost control over information they begin to get upset. On the other hand, when people become upset they change their behavior toward information: they may scatter information about themselves, attempt overcontrol of it, run about trying to get more and more information, or cut themselves off from it. How human beings treat information and how they feel about its behavior therefore become indexes of their feelings of security. Thus when information behaves in such a way as to violate the communications universes of many people and to jump circuits; when people "clam up" or actively try to worm things out of other people, it is a sign that administrative steps are necessary.

To summarize what I have said about the overt and covert conse-

quences of stress: Difficulty in achieving consensus, unsatisfactory definition and overlap of functions, and the presence of units of approximately
equal power in a task-performing organization may result in circuit-
jumping, with much consequent stress, which in turn leads to further
circuit-jumping. For example, the nurse who cannot get satisfaction by
communicating with her immediate superior seeks out a distant superior
in another part of the system from whom she does get the kind of advice
and counsel she needs. Meanwhile her immediate superior, offended that
the nurse has gone to the distant superior, becomes hostile, thus intensify-
ing the nurse's avoidance of her and the nurse's dependence on the distant
superior. In this way these stresses become self-reinforcing.

A staff confronted with inconsistencies, urgent multiple choices, and a
feeling of uncertainty will try to reduce stress by seeking all-powerful
figures and by developing informal social structures that seem more
satisfying to their needs than the formal one. In the long run, however,
the efforts by the staff at *immediate* reduction of stress may actually increase the stress.

If stress increases in the system, the number of people who receive
information about trouble increases also, because people who themselves
have stressful information to communicate are likely to become active
listeners to the troubles of others. The entire system may begin to buzz,
and the communications universes of many may be violated. But at the
same time that information about trouble seems to get around to almost
everybody, a contrary tendency—to keep quiet about everything—also
manifests itself. Thus scattering information about trouble and holding on
to it so it will not roam may come to exist side by side.

SUMMARY AND CONCLUSIONS

IN recent years much attention has been given by students of human
relations to problems of informal social systems in task-performing organizations in our society. These informal systems have their being within a
matrix of formal organizational structure, which, in very considerable
part, may come to be determinative of the quality of the informal relations. Because the emotional character of these relations is so important in
psychiatric hospitals, the formal structure of the psychiatric hospital becomes a crucial issue. One might even be tempted to say that the kind of
care the patient ultimately gets, and even the course of his illness, is in no
small part a function of the informal relations among the personnel as
determined by the formal matrix in which they operate.

It is in connection with these relations that the problems inherent in a
system of multiple subordination—or "functional organization" as it is
called in the literature—arise. One can see, of course, how readily a
system of multiple subordination comes into being in a hospital, for since

each patient has to have so many different things done for him, un-simplified functional operation seems to be the natural way to do things. However, such operations, as Gulick[21] and many others have pointed out, lead to overlap and multiplication of contradictory orders, with all that implies for the efficiency of the organization.

In these circumstances the problem of reduction of randomness be-comes a critical one, for everyone in the upper echelons may become concerned that tasks will not be performed according to organizational hopes. This leads to the projection of persons from the upper levels of the organizational hierarchy deep into the lower levels as they exercise anxious surveillance.

In any system of multiple subordination the problems of spheres of activity of different departments raises issues of the definition of func-tions. This leads to inward and outward improvisation: a worker impro-vises his own theories as to his functions, and other people improvise theories about his functions. Thus when the functions of a worker are not clearly defined, a guessing game develops and is eagerly pursued by both the functionary and those on whom he impinges. Often the two guess at cross purposes. Out of vagueness of definition of function and multiplicity of signals there grow hostility, secrecy, conflicts over personal loyalties, and feelings of betrayal.

Under these conditions nurses and orderlies may be observed to be-have in one or more of the following ways: They may become more and more dependent on a supervisor, may avoid the supervisor, may seek out all-powerful figures, may become apathetic in their work, may seek out now one person, now another to whom to tell their troubles, or may foster the development of informal covert social structures. One of the results of these behaviors is that information about trouble starts to wander in an almost random way throughout the system; and since this eventuates in the violation of the communications universes of many people, stress is again added to the system.

It would appear that a psychiatric hospital organized as a system of multiple subordination may not be able to provide that "therapeutic fitness" of which Devereux speaks in discussing the social structure of a schizophrenic ward.[22] By *dividing* the personnel and thus facilitating the development of all those emotional problems consequent on a divided world, such an *external* system simply reproduces the *internal* system of the schizophrenic and, in no small part, the internal systems of many others suffering from mental illness.

Clearly any organization in our culture starts its operations with in-dividuals having certain personalities. An organization based on the most perfect engineering principles, therefore, could readily be wrecked were the positions in it filled by people who were stupid, inflexible, hostile, and so on. The message of this paper, however, has not been that a good organizational blueprint is magic that will bring about excellent interpersonal relations in task performance. What I have attempted to suggest, rather, is that an organization having specific characteristics can, through repetitively creating particular situations for the personnel working within it, bring about stresses in interpersonal relations, so that many persons, regardless of their personalities, will experience similar tensions. Obviously these tensions will have different ultimate effects on different people. A person subject to mood swings, for example, may experience wider and wider swings as stress mounts throughout the organization; while on the other hand a relatively phlegmatic person may experience only mild malaise.

Yet failure of a member to function adequately in an organization ought not to be too readily diagnosed as a symptom of some deep-going psychopathology—a point which may be particularly important to remember in an organization containing many persons skilled in psychiatric diagnosis. Rather, so it seems to me, in the presence of poorly functioning personnel, an administrator might ask himself *first* whether the poor functioning might not be due to some underlying defect in the organizational structure. It is not possible to put a group of even basically well-integrated persons into a poorly conceived organization and expect them to function without much stress. "Good Joes" are not enough. The structure must be "good" too.

NOTES TO CHAPTER 15

1. Perhaps Dr. Kirkbride should be given credit for having first stressed the importance of the formal structure of a mental hospital to the welfare of patients. See Earl D. Bond, *Dr. Kirkbride and His Mental Hospital;* New York, Lippincott, 1947; pp. 153-154. William C. Menninger, in speaking of a psychiatric hospital, has said that "above all, it must be a highly organized, efficient institution." See his "Therapeutic Methods in a Psychiatric Hospital," *J. Amer. Med. Assn.* (1932) 99:538-542. See also: Chester I. Barnard, *The Functions of the Executive;* Cambridge, Harvard Univ. Press, 1938. Burleigh B. Gardner, "The Factory as a Social System"; in *Industry and Society,* edited by William Foote Whyte; New York, McGraw-Hill, 1946.

    There is no reason why the hypotheses developed here need be thought of as applying to psychiatric hospitals only, even though they were developed in the course of the study of one.

2. J. Fremont Bateman and H. Warren Dunham, "The State Mental Hospital as a Specialized Community," *Amer. J. Psychiatry* (1948) 105:445-448. William Caudill, Fredrick C. Redlich, Helen R. Gilmore, and Eugene B. Brody, "Social Structure and Interaction Processes on a Psychiatric Ward," *Amer. J. Orthopsychiatry* (1952) 22:314-333. Howard Rowland, "Interaction Processes in the State Mental Hospital," *Psychiatry* (1938) 1:323-337. Rowland, "Friendship Patterns in the State Mental Hospital," *Psychiatry*

(1939) 2:363-373. Charlotte Green Schwartz, Morris S. Schwartz, and Alfred H. Stanton, "A Study of Need-Fulfillment on a Mental Hospital Ward," Psychiatry (1951) 14:223-242. A. H. Stanton and M. S. Schwartz: "The Management of a Type of Institutional Participation in Mental Illness," Psychiatry (1949) 12:13-26. "Medical Opinion and the Social Context in the Mental Hospital," Psychiatry (1949) 12:243-249. "Observations on Dissociation as Social Participation," Psychiatry (1949) 12:339-354. "A Social Psychological Study of Incontinence," Psychiatry (1950) 13:399-416.

3. See Gardner, reference footnote 1. It is my understanding that in forthcoming publications Caudill and Stainbrook, and Stanton and Schwartz also stress formal structure.

4. Obviously this definition takes care of such behavior complexes as role, status, technique, authority, and so on.

5. The tendency among us to impose shape on the outer world is so strong that such conceptions as Brahman or *mana*—according to which the supernatural is essentially formless—are intolerable to most religious persons. This is true also for the common man in India: for while the *yoga* knows that true Being is formless, the simple Hindu must have his anthropomorphic gods. Karl Deutsch has done a service in bringing together descriptions of shapes that have dominated Western thought in the past 500 years. See his "Mechanism, Organism, and Society: Some Models in Natural and Social Science," *Philosophy of Science* (1951) 18:230-252.

6. See, for example: Alvin Brown, *Organization of Industry;* New York, Prentice-Hall, 1947. H. Gulick and L. Urwick (eds.), *Papers on the Science of Administration;* New York, Inst. of Public Admin., 1937. Delbert C. Miller and William H. Form, *Industrial Sociology;* New York, Harper, 1951. James D. Mooney, *The Principles of Organization;* New York, Harper, 1947. Paul D. O'Donnell, *Production Control;* New York, Prentice-Hall, 1952.

7. One is reminded in this connection of the Mundugumor conception of their social organization as made up of what they call *ropes.* See Margaret Mead, *From the South Seas;* New York, William Morrow, 1939; p. 176.

The conception of organizations (particularly of states) as organisms, with a ruling head and with obedient limbs and internal organs responding to impulses emanating from it, is a variant of the tree theme. The idea apparently has a very ancient history in European culture. See F. J. C. Hearnshaw, *The Social and Political Ideas of Some Great Medieval Thinkers;* New York, Holt, 1923.

8. Alexander Bavelas, "A Mathematical Model for Group Structures," *Applied Anthropology* (1948) vol. 7, no. 3, 16-30.

9. ". . . the evolution of the British Army is instructive. Today it is coordinated in a single department, the War Office. Everyone regards this piece of organization as a matter of course. Naturally an army must have one head, must be coordinated. In the year of Waterloo a British commander in the field had to deal with more than a dozen independent and separate ministers or departments in Whitehall on the affairs of his army. It required a hundred years of struggle, of incessant royal committees and commissions, of recurrent scandals due to maladministration, before the last vestige of conflicting authorities had disappeared. . . ." L. Urwick, "Organization as a

Technical Problem"; in Gulick and Urwick, reference footnote 6. No wonder Taylor's view was unacceptable: theories of multiple subordination
might lead to the military collapse of modern nations! See Frederick Taylor,
The Principles of Scientific Management; Norwood, Mass., Plimpton Press,
1911; pp. 123-128.

The Soviet experience has paralleled ours and that of the British. Before
the Sixteenth Party Congress, Soviet industry was organized according to
the principle of *funktsionalka,* which made each enterprise directly subordinate to a group of central commissariats. This caused so much confusion
and inefficiency that it was denounced by Stalin at that Congress. In place
of the old system they now have the relatively autonomous factory manager,
responsible to his regional *glavk* or Central Board of Industrial Management. While this reduces very considerably the confusion implicit in the old
funktsionalka system, however, the factory Party committees, the labor
unions, and other agencies still limit considerably the autonomy of the
factory director, and thus make him still subject to a *de facto* system of
multiple subordination. See A. Vucinich, *Soviet Economic Institutions;*
Stanford, Calif., Stanford Univ. Press, 1952 (Hoover Inst. Studies, series E,
no. 1).

10. Sometimes misunderstandings have arisen about the way I intend these
symbolic statements to be taken, and they have been criticized in terms of
mathematical logic. It seems to me that to do this is to lose sight of the fact
that while these images, like many others used in our culture, are not 'exact'
descriptions of the outer world, they have the utility of enabling one to
quickly see a variety of possibilities inherent in a situation—a variety that
might not, perhaps, become so quickly evident, were a statement not made
in this concise form. I have attempted to underscore the heuristic function
of these equations by using an arrow rather than an equals sign to indicate
the relationship between the left and right sides.

11. The objection to this hypothesis on the grounds that competition for power
between units that functionally duplicate each other would cause stress is
not valid, because in such a case it could be argued that the goals of the
units are not the same. A more valid objection might come in terms of the
apathy that might develop from repetitions of the same job by different
units, and frustration from seeing the job one intended to do already performed by others.

12. See L. Gulick, "Notes on the Theory of Organization"; in *Papers on the
Science of Administration,* reference footnote 6.

13. In Equation 1, P is a measure of the power of the various units in an administrative structure; Sf measures the extent to which such units may overlap each other's functions, and C is the measure of agreement among the
units. T is a measure of the stress *throughout the entire system.* In Equation 2, on the other hand, the rationality of the task is looked at from the
standpoint of the *individual worker* performing the task, so that S is a measure of the individual's stress as he carries out a *particular* function or set of
functions.

14. Not all the possible hypotheses are stated but only some of the less obvious
ones.

15. Gulick, reference footnote 12. Such is the horror of multiple direction in our culture that John Lee sees in the principle of unitary direction the expression of a "human need." He says, "The error which Taylor made in his eight functional foremen was to overlook the human need on the part of the workers for such definite direction as is incarnated in one person." Thus the list of items in the encyclopedia of human needs is determined not only by culture but by the specific job the encyclopedist holds in a particular culture. See John Lee, "The Pros and Cons of Functionalization"; in Gulick and Urwick, reference footnote 6.

16. Obviously this derives from the concept of negative entropy.

17. The often complex and rigid kinship structures of some primitive societies, which strictly control marriage, economic, and ceremonial relations, are excellent examples from a different area of social science of this human horror of unpredicted events.

18. See James C. Worthy, "Organizational Structures and Employees' Morale"; in *Readings in Industrial and Business Psychology*, edited by Harry W. Karn and B. von Haller Gilmer; New York, McGraw-Hill, 1952. It is interesting to observe, in this connection, what has happened in the Soviet factory system. It became evident to the Russians in the 1930's and early 1940's that absolute centralization would not work. The result was a movement in the direction of giving individual factories, and even single shops within factories, considerable apparent autonomy. However, this was accompanied by multiplication of local supervisory agencies and voluntary groups. The present result is that a large number of supervisory operations, often overlapping, are constantly being performed, so that everybody's business is everybody else's. See Vucinich, reference footnote 9; p. 41.

19. Measurable in terms of hours spent in conferences on organizational matters.

20. An important reason why this state of affairs may continue is that the moderater often has no real power to enforce even the agreements he can bring about. See Alvin Brown, reference footnote 6; pp. 71-73.

21. Reference footnote 12; pp. 15, 22, 23.

22. George Devereux, "The Social Structure of a Schizophrenic Ward and Its Therapeutic Fitness," *J. Clin. Psychopathol.* (1944) 6:231-265.

ઝ

Chapter 16   Control Over Policy by
Attendants in a Mental Hospital*

THOMAS J. SCHEFF

A CENTRAL problem in the study of organizations is the extent of participation in policy decisions by organization members. On one extreme are autocracies, in which policy is formed almost completely within the superior group; on the other, examples of dominance or control by subordinate groups: "bureaucratic sabotage" in government, and restriction of production by work groups in industry are two examples. Whether the situation is that of autocracy, control by subordinate groups, or "codetermination," these different modes of policy formation may be used to illustrate the social bases which underlie decision processes in complex organizations.

PROBLEM AND METHOD

THE question raised is: How is it possible for subordinate groups in an organization to exert control over organization policy? This question is particularly relevant in the United States to custodial organizations such as prisons and mental hospitals, since there are concerted efforts underway to find an effective method of changing the traditional policies of these organizations. The data of this study are based on participant observation in a large state mental hospital. The administration of this hospital had launched a vigorous and ambitious program of reform in the hospital in 1957. Despite the administration's energetic efforts, the program was largely frustrated by the lower staff, particularly by the attendants.[1] How did this come about?

The explanation given here is in terms of the system of social control operative in the hospital. In order for a subordinate group to exert control

* Reprinted from the *Journal of Health and Human Behavior*, 2 (1961), 93–105, by permission of the author and the American Sociological Association.

over organization policy, it must, first, exact compliance from the superior group and, then, maintain discipline and a united front among its own members. These two requirements imply a system of social control which is effective between and within groups in the organization.

Any system of social control has two components: one, overt actions (sanctions), the other, verbal statements (rationalizations). Considering one special type of sanction in their discussion of the stability of governments, political scientists have noted that force by itself is usually incapable of maintaining a stable system of control. Power must be converted into authority through legitimation by the persons ruled. Like force, social sanctions used by a group are usually accompanied by rationalizations which legitimate its own practices and "neutralize" (deny the legitimacy) of those of its opponents.[2] Social control, then, arises out of the interplay of sanctions and rationalizations.[3]

CONTROLS BY A SUBORDINATE GROUP: HOSPITAL ATTENDANTS

IN the hospital observed, a subordinate group was influential in shaping hospital policy (1) through the vulnerability of the administration to control by its physicians, (2) the techniques used by the attendants to control the physicians, and (3) the techniques employed to maintain a united front within the attendant group. These techniques can be understood better in the light of the situation in the hospital at the time of this study.

"Western State," as it will be called, is a 4,000-bed state mental hospital located in a middle-sized Western city. It is relatively old, dating back over a hundred years. Early in 1957, the administration of this hospital initiated a program which was intended to change radically the character of the hospital.

The central feature of the new program, as seen by the staff, was the ward meeting, which was called "the T.C." (Therapeutic Community) by the staff and patients.[4] The administration hoped that this meeting would: (1) function as a treatment procedure for individual patients, like an enlarged group therapy session and, more importantly, (2) serve to break down traditional staff practices by providing channels of communication between patients and ward staff, supervisors, and physicians. It was thought that custodial practices could be eliminated and replaced by "social treatment."

Meetings were not begun on all wards in the hospital; the adoption of the meeting was left up to each ward staff. Three wards volunteered initially. After a one year trial, by the end of 1957, there were some nine wards out of a total of 44 holding meetings. The administration had hopes that meetings would be adopted on all wards throughout the hospital. To further these hopes, it had conducted a series of intensive lectures and demonstrations for the entire hospital staff, to convince the staff of the benefits of the program.

The reaction of the staff to the new program was largely negative, however. The attendants, particularly, who were by far the largest staff group (about six hundred persons), reacted strongly against the program, deeming it impractical, fraudulent, and immoral. At the time the present study began, in the early part of 1958, the furor of discussion and condemnation of the new program had reached a peak. At times, the reactions of the staff were visible even in public meetings. One incident at a hospital-wide meeting provides an example.

The meeting was part of the series of demonstrations of the "Therapeutic Community." A period had been left for questions, with the superintendent in charge. Initially, staff members were slow to raise questions, but after the early minutes had passed, questions came rapidly. The rejection of the program soon became evident from the character of the questions. Toward the end of the hour, the meeting nearly broke up when one staff member asked if it were true that the administration condoned intimate contacts between male and female patients. The superintendent answered that the administration did not condone improper behavior, but the phrasing of his answer was not direct enough to satisfy the audience. In what was virtually a demonstration, the audience jeered and hooted the superintendent.

By the last part of 1958, it was clear that the new program was not going to be adopted by the entire hospital in the near future, if at all. Although the administration's program was carefully conceived and implemented, the resistance of the staff was so determined as to force the abandonment of sections of the program. The staff's victory was manifested at a later meeting, when in response to staff questions, the superintendent announced that "Therapeutic Community" was not necessary for every ward; it was just one more technique added to the hospital's battery of treatment procedures. This was the announcement that the conservative staff had waited to hear: like all earlier innovations, the ward meetings could also be absorbed into the traditional hospital structure. What had begun as a revolutionary new program ended as only one more treatment procedure.

One factor in this result was the vulnerability of the administration to control by the staff.

VULNERABILITY OF THE WARD PHYSICIAN

THE focal point of staff control over the administration was the ward physician. The ward physician was the sole representative of the administration in most wards in the hospital. In this capacity, the physician was responsible for the treatment of the ward patients, and for insuring staff obedience to hospital regulations. The ward physician found it difficult to carry out his duties as the representative of the administration, however. Typically, the doctor facing the ward staff was in a weak position, relative to the staff, because of his short tenure on the ward and his lack of training and interest in administration. The problem of the length of tenure of ward physicians will be considered first.

During this study, the modal length of stay of a physician on a ward was approximately two and one-half months. Complaints about the turnover of physicians were raised in several ward meetings. One "charge" (supervisory attendant) stated: "Just about the time we have them broken in to our ward, off they go to somewhere else." The high turnover rate of ward physicians was due to the large number of separations from the hospital and to the administrative practice of periodic changes in assignments.

Separations from the hospital were frequent among the physicians. Five out of the hospital's total of thirty left during the study period of six months. According to informants, this high rate of separation (33 per cent per year) was not unusual for the physician group.

Had turnover been due solely to separation, only one ward in three would have been affected during any given year. In actuality, the turnover due to separation was magnified by the administrative policy of reassignment. During the year, a physician was likely to be transferred within the hospital from two to five times. At times, transfers were made for training purposes; the administration tried to expose a doctor in training to a variety of wards.

More frequently, the administration appeared to be juggling the particular skills and interests of the physicians against the special demands of the various wards. On one occasion, in a hospital policy meeting, a replacement was being discussed for a receiving ward physician who was leaving the hospital. One administrator suggested the name of a staff physician. Another said, "Oh, no, not him. We need a 'live one' for this ward." The final outcome of this discussion was that five physicians were transferred: one to replace the physician who was leaving, one to replace the replacement, and so on. This practice magnified the effect of separation many times.

As a result of these conditions, the typical ward physician was a newcomer. The ward staff, in contrast, was all but rooted to the ward. The supervisory staff of many wards had been as long as five years in the same assignment. Although the rank-and-file attendants were moved more frequently, even the most mobile of them usually had more seniority on the ward than the physician.

The typical ward physician was not only a newcomer, but also, as far as most ward problems were concerned, an amateur. By training, the physician is prepared to give medical treatment to individual patients. Yet the demands of the ward physician's role are for a ward administrator and leader. The making of ward policy and the command of the ward staff and patients were duties which pressed for immediate attention. None of the physicians was prepared for these duties by their training.

The physicians were not only unprepared for administrative duties, they were also apt to look upon them with distaste. Oriented toward the individual patient, many considered time spent outside of psychotherapy or medical treatment as an irritating distraction from their "real" job.[5] One psychiatrist, a respected young resident, said:

I've spent three years in medical school, and two years as a psychiatric resident, yet I could have done as well in this job (ward physician) after the first six months of medical school. There is practically no time for psychotherapy here. The best we can offer is a social cure.

Another ward physician made a similar comment. "I seldom use anything I learned in medical school. Practically all I do is go to meetings."

By its emphasis on individual treatment, the physician's training had focused his attention and interest elsewhere, making it difficult for him to learn from experience on the ward. In a mental hospital ward, preparation for private practice comes very close to being a "trained incapacity" for ward leadership.

Without training or interest in administration, the new physician was confronted by a ward staff which was relatively permanent and well-organized. Given this situation, the doctor was in the position described by Weber, that of the "political amateur" leading a bureaucracy.[6] Lipset notes this condition in his discussion of a governmental succession:

The new ministers, like most politicians, were amateurs in their respective departments. None of them had ever had administrative experience in a large organization.[7]

This condition, Lipset believes, is the typical setting for "bureaucratic sabotage." In it the reform aims of the succeeding government easily become enmeshed in the traditional pattern of bureaucratic operation, and are transformed or replaced.

According to Weber, the amateur successor quickly becomes dependent on his staff, to the point that he is partially or completely captured. In many cases capture took place in the mental hospital ward. If the doctor too readily took the side of the patients in the ward meetings, or sought to advance the administrative position, the staff had procedures available to control the doctor. Often these procedures were successful because of the physician's impossible span of control.

The ward physician, even if assigned to only one ward, had many other duties besides those in his ward. Admission and physical examination, conferences on various administrative levels, and in-service training and workshops made demands on his time. In the back wards, a physician might be assigned as many as four wards. Most physicians, therefore, were present on their wards a maximum of three or four hours a day.

TECHNIQUES USED TO CONTROL THE ADMINISTRATION: SANCTIONING OF THE PHYSICIAN

ONE type of sanction was withholding information. During the physician's absence of twenty or more hours during the day, and on weekends, he was dependent on the staff for reports of the behavior of the patients who were in his care. If the doctor was too demanding of the ward staff, he found that the information he needed to evaluate his patients was not forthcoming, or given only in part. One physician, for example, complained bitterly that his ward staff told him only half-truths.

A second type of sanction used by the staff involved the manipulation of patients. One of the traditional duties of the ward staff was to allow only patients with appointments to see the doctor. The writer has witnessed occasions on both a back ward and on a front ward which were very nearly mob scenes. Patients who would have ordinarily been shunted away from the doctor were encouraged by staff members to accost him with their requests. This tactic apparently had developed out of dissatisfaction with the doctor's performances in ward meetings earlier in the same week. In such a situation, the physician, whose time on the ward was limited, found it difficult to get off the ward gracefully.

A third type of sanction was outright disobedience. This tactic was used with some physicians, but more usually, against psychologists and social workers. On one front ward, a psychologist had begun daily group psychotherapy sessions with a small group of patients. He found, however, that he could not get the cooperation of the nursing staff:

Every day at the specified time I went to start the session. The attendants would say, 'Oh, is it two o'clock already!' I would have to round up the patients myself. Patients would then leave or be taken from the group while I was getting the others. I finally gave up the session for patients. We'll have to work on the staff first.

The fourth, and probably the most important, sanction was available chiefly to the supervisory personnel: the withholding of cooperation. The ward physician is legally responsible for the care and treatment of each ward patient. This responsibility requires attention to a host of details. Medicine, seclusion, sedation and transfer orders, for example, require the doctor's signature. Tranquilizers are particularly troublesome in this regard since they require frequent adjustment of dosage in order to get the desired effects. The physician's order is required to each change in dosage. With 150 patients under his care on tranquilizers, and several changes of dosages a week desirable, the physician could spend the major portion of his ward time in dealing with this single detail.

Given the time-consuming formal chores of the physician, and his many other duties, he usually worked out an arrangement with the ward personnel, particularly the charge (supervisory attendant), to handle these duties. On several wards, the charge called specific problems to the doctor's attention, and the two of them, in effect, would have a consultation. The charge actually made most of the decisions concerning dosage change in the back wards. Since the doctor delegated portions of his formal responsibilities to the charge, he was dependent on her good will toward him. If she withheld her cooperation, the physician had absolutely no recourse but to do all the work himself.

Of course, the ward doctor could buck the ward staff and seek to rely upon his own devices. In this situation, he must stay on the ward virtually all of his waking hours in order to keep up with his responsibilities. This happened only once at Western State, to the writer's knowledge. In this case the doctor flouted the traditional routine of the staff and sought to impose reform on the ward under his personal direction. He found his position on the ward untenable, however, and was transferred at his own request.

The physician was caught, then, between administrative and ethical imperatives, on the one hand, and the demands of the staff, on the other. There appeared to be two common resolutions to this dilemma. The first resolution occurred often among the psychiatrists and younger physicians. The encroachments of the ward staff on the doctor's prerogatives, and the atmosphere of resistance strengthened their resolve to be quit of the hospital as soon as possible. Their feeling was that they could easily find a job involving higher pay, use their medical skills, and find a more appreciative and co-operative staff. Thus, the role dilemma of the physician, which arose in part from the high separation rate of the physicians, became a cause of further separations, creating a vicious circle.

The second solution to the physician's role conflict was to reach a tacit understanding with the staff. To the extent that the physician sided with the staff, he found his relations with the staff improving, and that he was able to leave the ward after a reasonable expenditure of time. The physician new to the ward soon got the point, and arrived at a working arrangement which involved the continuation of much of the old ward system in return for cooperation from the staff.

Although the working arrangement between staff and physician brought relief to the physician from some of the strains in his role, this resolution was not completely free of tension. In yielding to the demands of the ward staff, he was in some danger of reprimand by the administration. The administration did not go too far, however, in its censure of physicians. For the past several years, the hospital has been unable to fill its vacant posts for physicians. The administration treated its physicians, therefore, with deference. This is not to say that the administration was improperly lenient with physicians. It simply did not seek trouble with the physicians, in order to keep the staff it had.

A second source of embarrassment for the physicians who compromised with the staff was in the ward meeting itself. Patients with grievances against staff members told all to the new ward doctor in the staff meeting. For example, on one back ward, a patient stated heatedly in ward meeting that she had been held and choked by three staff members. Even though the staff members named resolutely denied everything, and made counter-charges against the complaining patient, the situation was somewhat embarrassing to the doctor. As a representative of the administration, and as a professional, he should take action to find the truth of the matter. But since he had arrived at an understanding with the staff, such action would jeopardize his relationship with the staff. The way in which this impasse was handled by the doctor and the staff was characteristic of the hospital, and will be treated now in detail.

RATIONALIZATIONS USED AGAINST THE ADMINISTRATION

THERE was a strong feeling of solidarity among the staff in the hospital in the face of attack from the administration. "Whitecoats stick together" was a motto of the attendants. The feeling of solidarity was so strong that it was difficult, even in a staff meeting in which no outsiders were present, for any criticism of a staff member to be voiced. Even the reform-oriented staff members felt this imperative. As a result, ward problems were virtually never discussed directly and forthrightly. They were trans-formed, rather, into problems of patients.[8]

Because of this convention, the misbehavior of single patients was discussed for days running. Often the breach of the rules seemed rather trivial in comparison with the extended and heated argument that re-sulted from it. The outsider, who is unaware of the conflicts within the staff, is apt to be puzzled by the seemingly endless discussion of a negligible offense by a patient.

On one occasion in a back ward, the question of demoting a patient, Jenny White (pseudonyms are used for all patients and staff) from her position as clothesroom helper, lasted four days, and crowded what seemed to be pressing problems from discussion. The argument centered about the question of whether this patient was faking seizures in order to avoid the heavy work connected with the clothesroom. The final result of this extended discussion was that the patient was transferred to another ward.

Curious about the heated argument, the writer questioned several of the staff members in private about the patient. It was stated that this patient was the center of a dispute between two ward factions. Her supporters, a group of older attendants, had made her a favorite among the patients, and treated her with small indulgences. For instance, they allowed her to keep her clothes and cosmetics in the clothesroom in excess of the space allotted to the other patients. A group of younger attendants, on the other hand, felt that Jenny was the "pet" of the older group and that the indulgences were unfair.

The writer asked one informant if arguments between these two staff groups had occurred over other "pets." The answer was in the affirmative; there had been many similar frustrating discussions about other "pets." The writer asked if the problem was actually the conflict between the staff groups, and not the patients. The informant seemed surprised, but said that might be the case. The writer then asked why the difference in the points of view of the staff groups were not discussed. The informant appeared embarrassed. She said:

"You can't talk about things like that around here."
"Why not?"
"It's not right." (said with conviction)
"Why not?"
"Oh, you can't talk about that in front of the doctor and everybody."
"What about when there's no one there but the attendants?"
"Oh, I don't know. We don't do it then either. Nobody wants to start."

By transforming the ward's problems into problems of patients, the staff protected the legitimacy of traditional practices.[9] With this technique, the ward doctor and the staff, in collaboration, dealt with the impasse in ward meetings mentioned earlier, when the patient complained of mistreatment by a staff member. This staff member resolutely denied the charge, and made counter-charges against the patient. Other staff members joined in, making the patient's charges an occasion for recalling the history of the patient's past misdeeds. In the general confusion, the doctor and still other staff members found it easy to obscure the issue further by asking misleading and obfuscating questions of the complaining patient. The patient saw the futility of his complaints in this situation and sat down.

After several weeks of such behavior by a doctor, the patients no longer turned to him in staff meetings. An outsider, if one was present, or other staff members, was addressed instead. On several occasions the writer has seen patients stating a complaint, turning from staff member to staff member, as he spoke, as if seeking a sympathetic listener.

The other important type of rationalization was neutralizing the claims to legitimacy of an opponent. This technique was used effectively against the reforms urged by the administration. One technique was to characterize all reforms as coming from "outside," and not really part of the hospital. Gouldner noticed the same device in the factory, as an aspect of "mock" bureaucracy.[10] Thus, with no justification, many of the staff identified in 1957 reforms solely with the acting-superintendent, rather than with the superintendent himself, who was on a short leave. One staff member stated: "All this nonsense will stop when our superintendent gets back." This feeling persisted in spite of the fact that the superintendent had been present when the reforms were initiated, and had expressed himself as strongly in favor of the changes.

The theme of outsiders arose continually in ward discussion. The psychologists and social workers were favorite targets for ridicule as outsiders. One typical comment was their lack of acquaintance with ward problems. On one occasion an attendant complained about the social worker attached to the ward:

> Always criticizing our doctor. She doesn't understand what it's really like here. You can't handle these patients as if they were ordinary people.

At times the maneuver to neutralize opposing policies was subtle. One of the back wards had a series of techniques of defense against an outsider, differentiated according to the length of time he was on the ward. The one-day visitor was given the "tour," arranged so that the more creditable aspects of the ward were shown. If an observer was to be on the ward for any length of time, emphasis shifted from misleading to discrediting him. On one occasion a social worker was asked his opinion of a matter being discussed in staff meeting. Since the worker had been on the ward only a week at the time, he was flattered to be brought into the discussion. He proceeded to give his opinion. He later learned that he had been taken in by a ruse. He was purposely asked a question about a problem which the staff knew to be an intricate one, in the hope that he would make a fool of himself.

TECHNIQUES OF CONTROL WITHIN THE STAFF: SANCTIONS

PERHAPS the most pressing problem faced by the staff in its maneuvers was keeping discipline among its own members. A sizable minority of the staff was in sympathy with the administration's program. Particularly with the advent of the ward meeting, coalitions between dissidents and reforming physicians were possible. Other workers were tempted to break ranks in their sympathetic treatment of particular patients. Yet in spite of these possibilities, most of the staff were kept in their place. How was this accomplished?

The system of social control which operated within the staff had both direct and subtle aspects. One potent set of practices stemmed from the ward supervisors, the attendant charges. These leaders had control over work assignments and influence in promotions. The control exercised by the leadership has been described by Belknap, and will not be discussed here.[11]

Other practices were more subtle. One procedure was to control the staff through sanctioning of patients. The system of patient control operated in the back wards with a clarity and force that was somewhat puzzling. The vigor with which patients were controlled seemed excessive relative to the patient behavior which supposedly called it forth. By

far the greatest number of the patients were quite abject in their relations
to the staff. From time to time, one of a small group, consisting of not
more than six or seven patients, behaved insolently, or was insubordinate
toward a staff member. Such behavior was unusual, even in this group.
Moreover, the control activities were not centered on this "insubordinate"
group, but extended to most of the patient population.

Also puzzling was the relationship of the most outspoken of the conservative members of the staff toward the patients. Although these staff
members raised their voices against the patients at almost every opportunity, in their personal relations with patients, they were often cordial;
their behavior often seemed to belie the contempt for patients they expressed publicly. The longer the author stayed in back wards, the more
obvious the paradoxical nature of the control measures became. How can
these discrepancies be accounted for?

The explanation of the intensity of the sanctions in the back wards lay
in the fact that the control of the patients was only one aspect of a larger
system of control. The sanctions which kept the patients in their place also
operated indirectly upon the staff members. The intensity and incon-
sistency of the staff behavior mentioned above arose because the patients
were not their main target. The target was those staff members who would
allow the patients to forget their place. By disparaging the patients in
forceful terms, these staff members were warning the reform-oriented
members of the staff and, indirectly, attacking them.

Of the sanctions which controlled staff behavior, the coercive measures
used by the leaders figured largely. Control through formal leaders was
only an aspect of the system of control, however. The operation of informal measures such as gossip and ridicule, which found all staff members
participants, was also important. One example was the use of ridicule in
staff meetings. The bitter invective which was aimed at patients also
implied the unworthiness of a staff member who would fraternize too
closely with the patients. On several occasions, several members were
accused of being "soft" with the patients. This pattern of reproach is
similar to the use of stinging epithets by Southern whites against those
who would break the "color lines." "Nigger-lover" is one such term. These
terms pose a scarcely veiled threat to the person's reputation and self-
esteem, and are therefore potent measures of control.

Often the control measures were more covert. Reformist staff members
occasionally ventured to suggest trials of various aspects of the administration's program. On several of these occasions, conservative staff members,
rather than attacking the program or its advocates directly, brought the
discussion around to descriptions of the current behavior of some of the
ward patients. By their accurate descriptions of the behavior of these
patients, they undercut the suggestions of the reformers on the staff. The
assumption of the reform program was that patients as a group are
worthy of the time and effort required to transform the hospital. By im-

plying the unworthiness, repulsiveness and contemptible nature of the patients as a group, the conservative staff members effectively attacked this assumption, and easily won the argument, since the reformers were unable to answer these hidden attacks.

A final example of the operation of sanctions within the staff is provided by a situation which occurred frequently in one of the back wards. It was the custom of the afternoon shift attendants to sit together before the entrance to the ward office during a quiet period of the day. With the exception of two of the attendants who manned an outer office, and the afternoon "charge," who often was inside the office, the entire afternoon shift sat in a semicircle, guarding the office. Sitting in this position, they talked among themselves and watched the patients. If the doctor was in the office, they kept the patients from seeing him. Very few patients approached this barrier. A patient who did come to this group, with a request for a dental appointment, for example, was usually teased or taunted until she gave up. Under these conditions a civil conversation between patient and staff members was impossible.

All of the shift participated in this activity, including the most reform-oriented staff members. In order to honor a patient's request in a situation like this, a staff member would have had to oppose, however gently, another staff member in the presence of a patient. Since this was counter to one of the unspoken rules of the staff, it seldom occurred. Similar kinds of control are exercised in groups of adolescent boys. All of the boys, not only the leader, use the epithet "chicken" for the person who does not conform. Staff members on the afternoon shift, similarly, kept each other from consorting with patients, even when the shift leader was absent.

RATIONALIZATIONS USED WITHIN THE STAFF

STAFF members were controlled through the operation of sanctions such as those used by the leadership, and through informal measures such as gossip and censure in face-to-face interaction. Of greater importance than sanctions in the control of the staff, however, were rationalizations that were shared by the staff members. Unlike the patients, the staff members were not overwhelmed by the operation of sanctions; staff members could themselves strike back against the shift leadership if provoked. That they seldom did so was the result not only of the power of the leadership, but also of the fact that the bulk of the staff was caught up in the system of rationalizations which prevented organized opposition. Even in wards where a stable reform group existed, the actions of the group were highly variable and inconsistent. The rationalizations which kept this group and similar groups on other wards captive are discussed below. Three types of rationalization will be considered: patient labels, ridicule of patients, and fictions concerning patients.

The Use of Labels. The use of convenient labels for the patients operated to justify and maintain traditional hospital practices. Terms such as "vegetable," (a withdrawn patient) which were at once an attack on the patient's moral worth, and a justification of inactivity of the staff, were used by most of the staff in referring to a patient, rather than the more neutral psychiatric term.[12] This particular term, "vegetable," was no longer used openly, since its use had been forbidden by the administration. In the informal discussions in which most ward business was conducted, however, it was still used.

There were two main reasons for its continued use. The nursing staff had little training in the use of psychiatric terminology. Mainly, however, they felt that the diagnostic terms were pretentious and irrelevant to hospital problems, with some justification. Although an official diagnosis was attached to each patient, little use was made of it in the entire course of treatment.[13] The nursing staff thought of diagnosis as one more of the hospital formalities which had little relation to actual hospital practices.

Rather than using psychiatric terminology, the nursing staff described patients either in terms of organic conditions, or in terms of their ward behavior. Examples of the former usage were "ep" (epileptic), and "lobotomy" (as in the statement by one of the reform group: "You will never get anywhere with her, she's a lobotomy." That is, the patient was brain-damaged and therefore permanently unresponsive). Further examples were: "feebie" (feeble minded), "luie" (luetic: a patient with syphilis), "drug addict," and "alcoholic." Examples of labels based on behavior were: "pest," "nuisance," "manic," "suicide," "untidy" (incontinent), "promiscuous," "runaway," "hebie" (hebephrenic-silly), "queen bee" (referring to patients who tried to keep themselves attractive through the use of cosmetics, dress and so on. Usually this term had the connotation of persons who thought themselves superior to the other patients), "withdrawn," and "combative."

All of these terms carried disparagement, both for the individual patients, and for the patients as a group. Often, however, these terms were used not to disparage, but simply for convenience. The ward culture possessed no other generally accepted terms which did not disparage. In these cases, the patient's low status was reaffirmed even when there was no intention to do so.

Ridicule of Patients. There is a great deal of nervous laughter in the mental hospital ward. Staff members faced with a constant array of immediate, yet recurring, problems frequently tell jokes at the patients' expense. The types of humor considered here are: "identity" jokes, ridicule of patients, and other humor.[14]

Identity jokes refer to real or pretended mistaken identities, mistaking a patient for a staff member, or vice versa. In the staff dining room an attendant who was first in line with a group of attendants said to the staff food-handlers: "I get so tired of taking these people (i.e., patients) to eat."

Jokes about letting staff members and others on and off a locked ward with a key are frequent. These sometimes have a hostile edge. On the author's first visit to a men's ward, when he asked to be let off the ward, one attendant said: "These people come in and then they want to get out right away." The other attendant said: "You have to go through the (disposition) clinic if you want to get out, just like the others."

Staff members often complained that the dress of some of the physicians make it impossible to distinguish them from the patients. This declaration was usually met by a smile or laughter from other staff members present, as if it were malicious to admit such a mistake for someone with so high a status as a doctor. The humor in this situation was based on the unstated assumption of the lowly, undesirable status of the patient. The fact that staff members laughed at jokes like these was an inadvertent affirmation of these underlying assumptions.

Ridicule occurred, even on front wards, when a patient's record was read to the staff for the first time in ward "intake" conferences. Some typical situations which occurred in a front ward "intake," where the physician in charge was an extremely conscientious psychiatrist:

1.

Doctor: "We have a liberal dose of psychosis this morning. This patient has always thought she was Honeybear Warren. Better write to Warren and tell him he is a bigamist." (Laughter.)

Attendant: "Married to a woman 35 years and then . . ." (she laughs) The patient was brought in. She told her story and was taken out. Turning to the social worker after the patient left, the physician said: "Would you check on this?" (Laughter.)

2.

Another patient, an American Indian. The physician read from her record: "She was doing a war dance on Highway 99. (Laughter.) She was heading West on the wrong side of the road."

Attendant: "All good Indians go West." (She laughed.)

3.

Another patient: the doctor read from her record: "She sets off fire alarms." (Laughter.) "She thought her hotel was full of rubber snakes and some of them weren't rubber." (Laughter.)

4.

This patient was a middle-aged woman with her hair in ring curls. The patient had finished her story of plots on television to "get her," men watching her doing her wash, and planning earthquakes when she dried her clothes. At this point in her story, she interjected: "Things like that would make most people mentally ill. Thank God I'm not crazy." At this point, staff members coughed, covered their mouths, and took other steps to avoid laughing out.

5.

After the "intake" was over, during which one patient had said that she was Greg Sherwood, an attendant said to another: Do you think Pat Boone looks you in the eye when he's on TV?" (They both laughed.)[15]

The Power of Fiction. In the back wards there was a large body of beliefs about patients which was based partly on experience, but depended mostly on being transmitted from employee to employee. Some of these beliefs were stated frequently and openly: (1) Epileptics have a very bad disposition—there is an "epileptic" personality consisting of being willful, stubborn, changeable and deceptive, and so on. (2) A series of beliefs were related to the notion that patients are like children; and that patients are happy. (3) Female patients are wilder and stronger than male patients. (4) Persons lose all sense of morality when they become mentally ill. This conviction was related to staff beliefs about patient sexuality. Other convictions were held firmly, but seldom discussed openly. Two examples will illustrate the tenor of a large body of similar beliefs.

One attendant stated that the reason there was so much incontinence was that when a person becomes mentally ill, he loses control of the sphincter. She said that the doctor would agree to that. Author: "Why is it then, that there is so much incontinence here and so little on some of the other wards?" Attendant: "Because our patients are so much sicker."

A front ward attendant, a person who was an unusually competent nurse and was sympathetic with the patients when in actual contact with them (although she "talked tough" with the other attendants) stated, as an aside from the main topic of conversation, that all mental patients have a distinctive odor: "You get in the showers with them sometimes. It just pours off them."

On back wards such beliefs were firmly held by most of the staff. Since practically all of the staff shared these beliefs, they were validated by consensus. On front wards, however, these beliefs were much more of an individual matter, so that the staff member was much less certain of their validity.

Of all the aspects of patient behavior discussed by the staff, the most prominent was the patients' sex life. The nursing staff had the strong belief that patients' sex life was abnormal and should be strictly regulated. In one staff conference, the misbehavior of a patient on the grounds was the topic of discussion. A number of rumors of misbehavior by this patient had been discussed. The argument appeared to be resolved, however, when a student nurse indicated that she was an eye-witness to the incident.

Student nurse: "Lola was carrying on with a male patient near the tennis court." (Said with rolling of eyes and gestures indicating a serious offense.)

Social worker: "What was she doing?"

Attendant: "That's just like Lola. I wouldn't put it past her." At this point there was a great deal of tsk-tsking, nodding of heads, and giggling. Staff members began to whisper to each other about other aspects of the "patient sex problem."

Social worker: "Just exactly what was she doing? Were they having intercourse?"

Student nurse: "No." (This came as a surprise, since everyone had assumed that had been what she meant.) "They were just kissing, but Lola was the aggressor; he was trying to bring her back to the ward, and she kept dragging him back."

Social worker: "Maybe she was out of line, but there was nothing terribly wrong about what you saw, which is the idea you gave us at first."

Student nurse: "I guess what she was doing was all right, *but not for a patient in a State Mental Hospital.*"

The student nurse felt, and the other staff strongly concurred, that such behavior was inappropriate for a person with the status of a patient. Although patients occasionally were promiscuous, there was no factual basis for most of the stories that circulated through the staff.

The cumulative result of the stream of rationalizations, the labels, ridicule, and fictions was that an image of the patient was created and maintained in the ward, an image that was congruent with traditional practices. The administration sought to break up this image in its training of the attendants, and in its formal presentations. But the image offered by the administration was vague in outline, and heard infrequently on the back wards.

The circumstance which sealed off the possibility of escape from the ward frame of reference was the condition of the patients. The administration program rested on the assumption that patients were worthy human beings, yet the evidence afforded by the staff's own eyes seemed to belie the assumption. Most of the patients on back wards were pitiful in appearance, at best, living under crowded and harrowing conditions. Without adequate clothing and washing conveniences, cut off from support from the outside community, abandoned by their relatives, they were a sorry picture to the staff. Under the impact of the ward rationalizations, the staff was selectively sensitized to only the worst features of the patients, and often overlooked the courage and decency that accompanied these features. In these circumstances, the rationalizations presented in staff discussions seemed to be confirmed daily, and the administration's program seemed Utopian and fanciful.

With the combined impact of sanctions and rationalizations, the members of the neutral and conservative groups were kept firmly in their place as traditional staff members. Even the members of the reform group, who had their own defenses against these controls, were not able to act consistently to further hospital reform. These staff members had no "place to stand" psychologically, because of their isolation. Because of the continual, but disguised verbal assaults on the patients, in which they occasionally participated, they were unable to maintain their ideological bearings, and drifted back and forth in their opposition to traditional ward practices.

SUMMARY

This analysis of the reaction of the staff of a large mental hospital to an administrative program of change has revolved around the question: How was the staff able to resist the program introduced by the administration? It suggests that the answer lay in the differing structures of the administrative and staff groups.

The staff of the hospital was a stable and highly organized community. Within this community, over the years, an informal system of sanctions and rationalizations had evolved. These techniques were described. They enabled the staff to exert control over the administration and to keep discipline within its own ranks. The system of social control was sufficiently effective to stalemate a vigorous program of reform introduced by the administration. The system was also so pervasive that even the sizable group within the staff who wished to participate in hospital reform were confused or neutralized.

The administrative and medical personnel, by contrast, were highly mobile and lacking in the training and interest necessary to provide leadership in the staff community. Due to the shortages of personnel and resources, and the nature of the physicians' training, the administration relied largely on formal controls, without the informal system of controls which usually supports changes in organizations.[16] In this situation, the defensive tactics of the staff were effective to the point that the program did not reach completion.

Assuming that the shortages of personnel and resources that the administration faced will not be greatly changed in the near future, the problem of planning change in existing mental hospitals and similar custodial organizations becomes a problem of understanding the informal techniques of control used by the staff, and of counter-techniques to be used in instituting new programs.

NOTES TO CHAPTER 16

1. For a case study of staff reaction to a similar program in a prison, cf. Richard McCleery, *Policy Change in Prison Management* (East Lansing: Governmental Research Bureau, Michigan State University, 1957).
2. Rationalization is not used here in the disparaging sense of fictional excuses, but in the neutral, social psychological sense of "definition of the situation." The use of the term "neutralize" follows Gresham M. Sykes and David

Matza, "Techniques of Neutralization: A Theory of Delinquency," *American Sociological Review*, 22 (1957) 774-840.

3. The pervasive influence of social control, when control occurs through both sanctions and rationalizations, was first noted by Emile Durkheim. In *The Elementary Forms of the Religious Life*, he suggested that religious practices and religious beliefs were mutually sustaining elements in the survival of religious institutions. For a critical exposition, see Talcott Parsons, *The Structure of Social Action* (New York: McGraw Hill, 1937), Chapter X.

4. Another aspect of the new program was the encouragement of outside research in the hospital. This report was made possible through the cooperation and financial support of the hospital administration. The author was attached to the hospital staff as a research sociologist, and permitted to follow his own research interests. Free from formal duties, he was able to spend from four to six hours a day in the wards in informal discussions with staff and patients, and in attending staff and ward meetings, for a period of six months. The report on the larger study of which this paper is a part is *Staff Resistance to Change in a Mental Hospital* (unpublished doctoral dissertation, University of California, Berkeley, 1960). The observations reported here were made largely on four wards: two receiving wards and two "chronic" wards.

5. The Cummings noted the same phenomena in the hospital they studied. Cf. Elaine Cumming and John Cumming, "The Locus of Power in a Large Mental Hospital," *Psychiatry*, 19 (1956), 371-383. See particularly the first paragraph on page 364.

6. Max Weber, *The Theory of Social and Economic Organization* (New York: Oxford University Press, 1947), p. 128.

7. Seymour M. Lipset, *Agrarian Socialism* (Berkeley and Los Angeles: University of California Press, 1950), p. 262.

8. Caudill called attention to what may have been the same techniques: "The tendency to focus on a particular patient as the source of a problem, rather than also utilizing knowledge about the wider context in which the problem occurs, seems to be a very general phenomenon in a psychiatric hospital." William A. Caudill, *The Psychiatric Hospital as a Small Society* (Cambridge: Harvard University Press, 1958), pp. 322-323.

9. The transformation of the problems of the staff into problems of patients was a process which pervaded staff discussion to the point where most staff meetings would have been incomprehensible to the listener unless he understood this technique. The process of transformation may be germane to a proposition suggested by Stanton and Schwartz. Alfred H. Stanton and Morris S. Schwartz, *The Mental Hospital* (New York: Basic Books, 1954), pp. 342-366. They propose that the "disturbed behavior" of a patient might be caused by covert conflict among members of the staff over that patient. In a subsequent study, this proposition was not supported. See Anthony F. C. Wallace and Harold A. Rashkis, "The Relation of Staff Consensus to Patient Disturbance in Mental Hospital Wards," *American Sociological Review*, 24 (1959) 829-836. If the same kind of transformation described here occurred in the small hospital they studied, it is possible that it is not "disturbed behavior" that arises from covert conflict, but *staff discussion* of the

patient's "disturbed behavior." Since disturbances are relatively frequent in mental hospital wards, it is possible that Stanton and Schwartz inadvertently selected only those disturbances which were called to their attention by protracted staff discussion.

10. Alvin W. Gouldner, *Patterns of Industrial Bureaucracy* (Glencoe: The Free Press, 1954), pp. 182-183.

11. Ivan Belknap, *Human Problems of a State Mental Hospital* (New York: McGraw-Hill, 1956), pp. 180-190.

12. Even the supposedly neutral psychiatric terms often carry disparagement. Caudill noted what appears to be a similar technique in the hospital he studied (op. cit., p. 62):

"... Some thought was given to the meaning of diagnosis as a security operation. Within a hospital, diagnosis may be thought to serve two functions: on the one hand, it is a useful way of classifying a patient in terms of the etiology and symptoms of his illness; but, on the other hand it is also a way of disposing of a patient by labeling him. For example, if a patient's behavior comes to be continually explained by the 'fact' that he 'has' schizophrenia, then the chance of the patient being relegated to a chronic hospital career are increased. In this latter case, diagnosis may be thought of as a security operation meaning that uncertainty about a patient is removed by labeling him and that many communications from him may now be safely ignored."

For a speculative but more general discussion of the moral condemnation implicit in psychiatric terminology, see Sebastian de Gratzia, *Errors of Psychotherapy* (Garden City: Doubleday, 1952).

13. The relative unimportance of the official classifications of patients was noted by Belknap in "Southern State Hospital," see Belknap, *op. cit.*, p. 128.

14. For a bibliography of studies of humor as an instrument of social control, see Russell Middleton and John Moland, "Humor in Negro and White Subcultures: A Study of Jokes Among University Students," *American Sociological Review*, 24 (1959), 61-69.

15. Goffman reports instances of the "discrediting" of patients which involve subtle ridicule, in his study of St. Elizabeth's Hospital. Cf. Erving Goffman, "The Moral Career of the Mental Patient," *Psychiatry*, 22 (1959), 136-137.

16. Cf. Chester Barnard, *The Functions of the Executive* (Cambridge: Harvard University Press, 1938). According to Samuel A. Stouffer, *et al.*, *The American Soldier: Combat and Its Aftermath* (Princeton: Princeton University Press, 1949), Vol. 2, p. 114:

"One important function of the existence of formal sanctions was that when imposed they called into *automatic* (italics mine) operation informal sanctions, both social and internalized. The existence of these informal sanctions gave the formal sanctions much of their force."

This quotation illustrates the importance of the informal system of control. However, it is questionable whether the informal sanctions are *automatically* called into operation to support the rule. They may, as has been pointed out here, subvert it. The conditions under which the informal system supports or subverts the formal system can only be answered through empirical investigation.

CHAPTER 17 Structural Sources of Strain in a Small Psychiatric Hospital*

HARRY W. MARTIN

A characteristic of hospital environments is a more or less chronic state of strain in the interpersonal relations of staff members. This paper examines the social structure of a small psychiatric hospital in an attempt to locate the stress points which pattern and contribute to such intrastaff tensions. The focus is on the psychiatric resident status and role-set—that is, those with whom the resident has role-relations—and it is "organizational" in the sense that attention is confined to the structure and processes within the hospital.[1] More precisely, the focus is on that part of the structure designated by Parsons as the operative system,[2] and on only a part of that.

Organizational research in mental hospitals suggests that the stress-producing factors stem less from the nature of the work done than from the social definitions under which it is done, which involve a complex division of labor, of statuses, and of authority. Henry has examined what he calls systems of multiple subordination, which, he maintains, still enjoy exuberant development in hospitals.[3] Other organizational sources of stress are described in the work of Stanton and Schwartz,[4] Belknap,[5] and Caudill.[6] Loeb has pointed out problems which arise from the interaction of occupational label, skills, and individuality of personnel.[7] Strains also arise, according to Smith, from blocked mobility; the necessity to standardize care, which often conflicts with the individuation of treatment; and the charismatic authority of physicians.[8] Other conditions conducive to a tension-ridden environment derive from the patterning of communication flow along the status hierarchy[9] and the interprofessional competition as representatives of different disciplines converge in the hospital context.

* Reprinted by special permission of The William Alanson White Psychiatric Foundation, Inc., and the author from *Psychiatry*, 25 (1962), 347–353 (copyright by the Foundation).

The observations providing a base for this paper were made in a 40-bed hospital operated by the department of psychiatry of a medical school. The hospital is psychodynamically oriented; psychotherapy is the treatment of choice, with drugs and electroshock following in that order. Emphasis is placed upon the hospital milieu as a part of patient care. The administration and staff are oriented toward equalitarianism and the team concept. Treatment, research, and teaching are carried on in the hospital; the psychiatric staff views teaching as its primary activity, while other personnel tend to be service-oriented. Psychiatric residents and interns in psychology, occupational therapy, and social work train in the hospital, and, in addition, medical and nursing students rotate through the hospital for instruction in psychiatry. Usually the staff consists of three senior psychiatrists, four first-year psychiatric residents, seven psychiatric nurses, two social workers, two occupational therapists, a senior psychologist, aides and orderlies, and Red Cross volunteers. These statuses, along with those of patients and their families, comprise the role-set of the psychiatric resident.

As observation accumulated, it became clear that residents, more often than any other status group, were central targets of criticism. The most frequently and openly critical persons were, in order, nurses, social workers, and occupational therapists. Actual and alleged incidents and situations provoking criticisms of residents were numerous: Refusing or failing to communicate information about patients and their families; unilaterally removing patients from ward meetings and occupational therapy; ignoring hospital policies; refusing or forgetting to see members of patients' families; encouraging patients to act out without due regard for the effects on other patients and nursing staff; obtaining information on patients from student nurses rather than from nurses; and, generally, being defensive about their status and authority. As one social worker put it, "They act as if we were going to take something away from them."

The consequences of such conditions were most clearly seen in the attitudes and behavior of nurses. One prevalent attitude was expressed in such statements as, "This hospital does not want professional nurses; they want us to do aides' work," "There is no opportunity to use your professional skills," and "Residents think that nurses are not people." Failure of nurses and residents to comply with each other's expectations and communication breaks between them were perennial sources of tension— although the latter were often more symptomatic of tensions than a cause of them. Their disagreements caused nurses and residents to withdraw from one another. One nurse reported in speaking of her problem with a resident, "Somehow, we just seem to forget to carry out Doctor A's orders." Sometimes nurses would come to tears in conferences or angrily walk out, slamming doors behind them, and occasionally some nurses would boycott scheduled staff meetings. Beyond such measures, the nurses' chief weapons were to complain to the Clinical Director, to threaten resignation, or actually to resign.

In an attempt to deal with some of these problems, the Clinical Director instituted an hourly conference each week, attended by the nursing supervisor, the two head nurses, the senior social worker, and the senior occupational therapist. The Clinical Director acted as discussion leader, and the sociologist sat in as an observer. After a few meetings, the nurses, the social worker, and the occupational therapist began to side together against the residents—who were not present, but whose side of the problems discussed was presented by the Director. The sociologist suggested that the residents should attend the meetings, but the Clinical Director was opposed to this on the grounds that their schedules would not permit it. Had the group pressed for their attendance, the Director would probably have agreed; however, the group felt that this would be too threatening and would stifle discussion.

As the meetings proceeded, the Director incurred considerable resentment, not only because he was presenting the residents' point of view, but also because he conducted the meetings in the fashion of nondirective therapy and resisted taking direct administrative action to control the residents' behavior. He was accused of defending the residents, of doing therapy in the discussions, of assuming that complainants were distorting reality, and of being a poor administrator.

Purely sociological or purely individual-psychological explanations may be invoked to explain such intraorganizational tensions. As one might expect, the latter are more often resorted to in a psychodynamically oriented setting—but, it may be added, not without some deleterious results. Both orders of explanation must be employed to fully understand particular incidents.[10] The aim here, however, is not to examine particular instances but to call attention to general structural features and latent definitions of the interactional setting in which the psychological dynamics of actions are influenced and displayed. I proceed from the assumption that certain characteristics of the psychiatric-resident status make it one of the most unstable points in the hospital's organizational structure.[11]

Since the focus is on the status and role-set of the psychiatric resident, I shall present a brief review of the concepts of Merton which I shall be using.[12] A *status* is a position located in a social structure. Each status has several roles associated with it. The status of resident, for example, entails role relationships with patients, nurses, social workers, and so on. These are the resident's role-partners, and together they comprise his role-set.

Merton posits six social mechanisms which articulate the roles in role-sets. These are: (1) *Differential role-involvement.* Not all role-partners are concerned with equal intensity about the performance of persons in a given status. The expectations of and demands upon a given position are differentially distributed among role-partners. This allows latitude for action and eases the problem of dealing with the conflicting demands which may arise from different quarters of the role-set. (2) *Differential power distribution.* Power refers to the conditions permitting an imposition of one's will upon others even against their resistance. Usually this capacity is unequally distributed within role-sets. Varying degrees of freedom to act result from power coalitions in role-sets, from being unobserved or unattended during power struggles among role-partners, and, in some instances, from one's own status power. (3) *Insulation from observability.* Interaction among role-partners is structurally segmented and intermittent; one does not engage with all role-partners simultaneously and continuously. Under this condition, performance takes place under varying degrees of insulation from observability. Generally, such insularity tends to diminish pressures from competing expectations. (4) *Observability of conflicting expectations.* Conditions or events may lead to a recognition by role-partners of their contradictory demands upon a status-occupant. However, this recognition occurs only when role-partners, by whatever means, attempt to resolve their incompatibilities. (5) *Role-set abridgment.* Sometimes status occupants attempt to deal with conflicting demands by severing or reducing interaction with role-partners. (6) *Social support.* This comes into play when occupants of like statuses band together, however loosely, to share their common misery or to combine their forces for attack.

I shall, in analyzing the resident's status and role-relations, discuss these in terms of the first five of Merton's six mechanisms.

In the teaching and treatment functions in the hospital, the status of resident is the key structural unit. Although the residents are under the tutelage and supervision of senior psychiatrists, they assume first-level responsibility for diagnosis, treatment, and management of patients. They and the nurses are, as it were, the upper and lower stones of the therapeutic mill. Thus, residents are simultaneously the chief workers in the hospital and the chief object of its training program. While these two divisions of the resident-status tend to merge, the resident is subject to charges of neglecting one for the other, or, conversely, of excusing or being excused for defaults in one area because of pressures in the other. As a worker, he is under constant pressure to make himself available to patients and other professional persons working with patients. As a trainee, he must find time to study. He pressures himself and is pressured by others to prove himself as a healer of illnesses whose diagnosis and treatment can be elusively intangible. His performance is under the surveillance of his tutors and the eyes of staff members at all levels, some of whom may find advantage or satisfaction in depreciating his performance.

Of the statuses comprising the resident role-set which I have enumerated, I shall now consider those with which the resident is most centrally involved:[13] psychiatric supervisor, nurse, social worker, occupational therapist, patient, and patient's family member or members. The role-relationships between the resident and each of these statuses rarely remain simple dual systems of interaction. Decisions and actions in each role-relationship often have important implications for other role-relationships. Generally, the relationships have a tendency to coalesce into a series of interlocking triadic forms—for example, resident, nurse, and patient; resident, social worker, and family; and so on. Coalitions frequently develop within these triads.[14] As long as the coalitions are between the resident and the other professional person, things go relatively well. But not infrequently, the professionals in the triad are wittingly or unwittingly aligned against each other. When senior staff members are brought in to arbitrate matters in, say, a resident-patient versus nurse situation, a new triangle of supervisor, resident, and nurse develops. Only rarely can a supervisor find a solution which avoids the implication of siding with either resident or nurse. In short, the role-set of the resident tends to be segregated into several triangular clusters in which the resident status is the primary interlocking unit.

Differential role-involvement. Many of the status occupants in the resident's role-set have relatively little power to exert direct demands upon the resident or little reason to do so. Role-involvement in any particular role-relationship, although bilateral, is not necessarily or always symmetrical; that is, role-partners may or may not be equally interested in the meaning or outcome of the relationship.[15] Only two of the resident's relationships—resident-patient and resident-supervisor—approach symmetry; the others are more asymmetric. The attitudes and behavior of the resident are of primary significance to nurses and other ancillary professionals, since their work and the satisfactions they derive from it are strongly affected by his actions and attitudes. Although the resident may be evaluated in terms of how he works with ancillary professionals, his situation is much less affected by them. Thus, it is not unusual for residents to display real or seeming indifference in these role-relationships. Such asymmetry tends to deny the equalitarian ideology and to place the burden of maintaining relational equilibrium upon the less powerful members of the role-set. This, in turn, contravenes associative, tolerative, and accommodative processes, opening the way to conflict.[16] Differential role-involvement, then, occurs and has a high stress-producing potential.[17]

Differential power distribution. The power structure of the hospital is composed of four levels: the senior psychiatric staff, the resident staff, the ancillary professional staff, and the so-called nonprofessional staff. Here I shall discuss differential power only as it is reflected in the exercise of authority in patient care.[18] Except for the senior staff, no status group in the hospital is as powerful as the resident, and those at lower levels have few formal sanctioning devices for shaping his behavior. Nurses tend to rely mainly on policies and procedures stipulated by hospital administration. But these can be abrogated by the uncodified rule that when a doctor's orders are in conflict with hospital policy, they take precedence. There is scarcely an opportunity for any coalition within the role-set which has greater force than the resident alone. Who does what, when, and where with his patients is of concern to the resident, and his veto power as a physician over any such matters can be negated only by his superiors. While the resident would thus seem to be virtually impregnable, his role-partners are not helpless, for they can attempt by informal sanctions to bring him in line when he deviates from expectations.[19] They may give him the silent treatment or otherwise snub him, withhold information from him, forget to carry out his orders, or employ other pressure techniques. Thus, the differential distribution of legitimate power among the key members of the resident role-set gives rise to disruptive mechanisms and processes. In any concrete instance, it should be observed, the extent to which these conditions obtain depends upon how a given resident chooses to exercise his authority.

Although the authority of the resident is almost unassailable, several factors tend to keep him insecure. In the final analysis, his authority is based on his having achieved the status of physician and presumably being armed with conventional medical knowledge and skills. He could have entered almost any other medical specialty with some degree of expertness; but when he begins psychiatric training, his expertise is of little value. He must now learn to think and act like a psychiatrist, which often requires some divestment of attitudes and behavior patterned after role models who may have been nonpsychiatric physicians. Unlike his conventional medical knowledge, which in great part is being surrendered, the knowledge and expertise he now aspires to gain are not exclusively his own. Not only the new knowledge, but often also its application, have already been shared with others—a source of some irritation. In the learning and work context, the resident proceeds under the observation of nonphysicians who may know more about psychiatry and mental patients than he, and, under the equalitarian doctrine, they can question and pass judgment on his performance. All of this adds up to a situation with much potential for status anxiety. While some residents deal with this fairly readily and comfortably, the general pattern is for residents to fall back defensively onto the fact that they are physicians. During the early stage of training, excessive use of the "After all, I am the Doctor" defense arouses hostility.

Insulation from observability. Merton maintains that to the extent to which the role-structure insulates status occupants from direct observation, they are not uniformly subjected to competing pressures from members of the role-set.[20] However, observability also functions as one means of social control. The mechanism of insulation from observability allows the status occupant to meet disparate expectations without offending the various role-partners. My observations indicate that a small teaching hospital affords the resident relatively little insulation, for much of his role-activity is directly or indirectly under the observation of role-set members. Although he is maximally insulated from observation in his supervisory hours and in doing psychotherapy, in the former he may have to reveal the interactions occurring in the latter,[21] and leaks can and do occur in the psychotherapy relationship with patients. Patients at times compare notes on their relationships with the same or different therapists and on their doctors' behavior during psychotherapy. And, generally, the resident's performance in diagnosis and management of patients is subject to observation by the staff at all levels. It is impossible to say how effective this observability is as a means of social control over the resident. It undoubtedly has some effect in this regard, but it may be more effective in generating anxiety and defensiveness.

Observability of conflicting expectations. As I have just discussed, a certain amount of veiling, or insulation from observability, serves to articulate roles. Observability, however, may also serve an articulative function when it derives from conditions which lead role-partners to an awareness of their incompatible expectations of other status-occupants. Given the interaction among the resident's role-partners and the degree of observability which he is subjected to by them, it would seem probable that they would come to recognize the contradictory demands upon him. This, indeed, seems to be the case; nevertheless, there are sectors in which this visibility seems to be ineffective as a reductive mechanism. For example, procedures which maximize the resident's training may be viewed by nurses and others as thwarting or delaying the therapeutic process. The resident, then, is not infrequently caught in the diverse expectations from these dual sources.

A similar situation arises in the resident-nurse-patient relationship. Patients may pressure therapists for individual privileges and greater freedom from ward routine, while nurses tend to pressure residents for greater control over patients. Other things being equal, such demands by patients fit with the residents' desire to individuate treatment, but this tends to conflict with the necessity imposed upon the nursing staff to maintain a modicum of order and routine in hospital ward life. Some patients play the nurse and resident off against each other in such situations. Although the pathology of the patient cannot be discounted, the unstable structural features remain. When conflicts are taken to supervisors for settlement, the patient is only indirectly involved in negotiations among supervisor, resident, and nurse. The opportunity for mutual awareness of the conflicting norms and behavior leading to such incidents is relatively high among these three statuses and frequently leads to measures for resolution. However, such actions tend to occur only after tensions have mounted to considerable proportions. Several factors reduce the probability of reaching continuing effective solutions. First, there is a tendency to overlook the individuation-standardization gap and the different norms and expectations governing each side of this dichotomy. Second, the role-structure in which such conflicts arise, and in which solutions are often sought, are triads which tend toward an unbalanced power distribution of two against one. Finally, there is a predilection for seeking explanations at the personality level, which tends to ignore the influence of structural factors.

Abridgment of the role-set.   This is, as Merton says, the limiting mode of dealing with contradictory demands upon status-occupants. It involves breaking off certain relationships in the role-set; and in order for the measure to be effective, the person resorting to it must be able to continue to function within the now truncated role-set. Obviously, it is usually possible to discontinue only peripheral relationships, and it is therefore unlikely, except in unusual circumstances, that these role-partners have been able to exert stringent contradictory demands. This mode of adapting to pressure is virtually unavailable to the central members of the resident role-set. The role-structure is tightly morticed, and their performance is greatly dependent upon their interaction with the resident. Abridgment of the role-set—with the exception of patients—as a mode of adapting to pressure is, however, accessible to the resident. By narrowing his focus to psychotherapy and discounting the importance of the patient's interaction with others in the hospital, the resident can severely limit his contact with role-partners. However, ignoring role-partners and their expectations creates disturbance in the system. By such abridgment the resident does not remove himself from the system, and he now becomes a target of increased criticism and sanctions intended to bring him back into line with the norms which govern him as learner-worker. My observations show that numerous abortive attempts at abridgment are made through bilateral and unilateral withdrawal, with role-partners shutting off communication and refusing to work together. These measures exacerbate the tensions generated by conflicting demands and unfulfilled expectations. Generally, the notion of role-set abridgment appears to be most useful in aiding understanding of disarticulative processes within role-sets; it functions as an articulative mechanism in relatively rare situations.

NOTES TO CHAPTER 17

1. For a review and evaluation of research in this area, see Amitai Etzioni, "Interpersonal and Structural Factors in the Study of Mental Hospitals," *Psychiatry* (1960) 23:13-22.

2. Talcott Parsons, "The Mental Hospital as a Type of Organization," pp. 108-129, in Milton Greenblatt, Daniel J. Levinson, and Richard H. Williams, *The Patient and the Mental Hospital;* Glencoe, Ill., Free Press, 1957; see pp. 125*ff.*

3. Jules Henry, "The Formal Social Structure of a Psychiatric Hospital," *Psychiatry* (1954) 17:139-151; and "Types of Institutional Structure," pp. 73-90, in *The Patient and the Mental Hospital,* footnote 2.

4. Alfred H. Stanton and Morris S. Schwartz, *The Mental Hospital;* New York, Basic Books, 1954.

5. Ivan Belknap, *Human Problems of a State Mental Hospital;* New York, McGraw-Hill, 1956.

6. William Caudill, *The Psychiatric Hospital as a Small Society;* Cambridge, Harvard Univ. Press, 1958.

7. Martin B. Loeb, "Role Definition in the Social World of a Psychiatric Hospital," pp. 14-19, in *The Patient and the Mental Hospital,* footnote 2.

8. Harvey L. Smith, "Professional Strains and the Hospital Context," pp. 9-13, in *The Patient and the Mental Hospital,* footnote 2; and "Two Lines of Authority Are One Too Many," *Modern Hospitals* (1955) 84:59-64.

9. See footnote 6; pp. 231-265.

10. Compare Chris Argyris, *Personality and Organization;* New York, Harpers, 1957; p. 7.

11. To fully sustain this argument, all other statuses within the hospital would have to be compared with that of the resident. This is not now possible.

12. Robert K. Merton, *Social Theory and Social Structure* (rev. ed.); Glencoe, Ill., Free Press, 1957; pp. 368-369.

13. The interaction system is the core of the social matrix in which work is done. Hughes points out that one of the common failures of research is to overlook part of this system. See Everett C. Hughes, "Social Role and the Division of Labor," *Midwest Sociologist* (Spring, 1956), p. 37.

14. Coalitions are an inherent and pervasive part of social life. Their appearance in, and consequences for, organizational life need systematic study. Sociological interest in triadic relations and coalitions stems back to Georg Simmel. For a bibliography of prior research and theory and a recent theoretical formulation on this phenomenon, see William A. Garrison, "An Experimental Test of a Theory of Coalition Formation," *Amer. Sociological Rev.* (1961) 26:565-573.

15. These structurally defined patterns of interest may be modified by other modes of identity such as age, sex, race, and so on.

16. See John L. Gillin and John P. Gillin, *Cultural Sociology;* New York, Macmillan, 1948, for a general discussion of these social processes.

17. The functional relationship among status differentials, role-involvement, and ideology has important implications for intrastaff discontent. One study shows that acceptance of status differentials and a desire for greater differences is a function of high objective status, while the opposite is a function of low status. However, on psychotherapeutically oriented wards all status occupants were found to minimize status distinctions, but expressed high discontent with the existing status situation. On medico-organically oriented wards less discrepancy between real and ideal status differences was ob-

served. See Simon Dinitz, Mark Lefton, and Benjamin J. Pasamanick, "Status Perceptions in a Mental Hospital," *Social Forces* (1959) 38:124-128.

18. This is an oversimplification; however, distinctions between power, influence, and the various forms of authority cannot be dealt with here. See Robert Bierstedt, "An Analysis of Social Power," *Amer. Sociological Rev.* (1950) 15:730-738.

19. For a discussion of conformity with respect to observability and authority, see Rose Laub Coser, "Insulation from Observability and Types of Social Conformity," *Amer. Sociological Rev.* (1961) 26:28-39.

20. See footnote 12; p. 374.

21. This, of course, depends upon the nature of the supervision. Apparently it would occur most often in "process-centered" supervision. See Group for the Advancement of Psychiatry, "Trends and Issues in Psychiatric Residency Programs," Report No. 31, March, 1955; p. 9.

CHAPTER 18   Conflict between Cottage
Parents and Caseworkers*

IRVING PILIAVIN

IT has been frequently observed that the achievement of therapeutic goals by institutional-care programs is greatly dependent upon the degree to which the efforts of personnel within these settings are integrated. The need for integrated effort has been particularly stressed in relation to the work of personnel providing individualized treatment and those responsible for the day-to-day care of people in institutions.[1] Yet, analyses of institutional programs have indicated only a minimum of co-operation and co-ordination among workers providing these services. Specifically, within institutions for delinquent and/or emotionally disturbed children, in which these roles are generally performed by caseworkers and cottage parents respectively, reports reveal that working relationships of these employees are often characterized by resentment, differences of opinion, and lack of mutual respect.[2] Most writers concerned with institutional care agree on the gravity of the cottage-parent–caseworker conflict problem but do not agree in their beliefs about its causes. Perhaps the dominant view is that these disputes stem from cottage parents' resentment of the accurate perception of the professional workers that resident staff members fail to perform in a manner consistent with therapeutic dictates. Writers have attributed this failure in turn to a variety of factors, including cottage parents' lack of allegiance to program aims,[3] their lack of training for therapeutic endeavor with disturbed children, as well as their emotional inadequacies and problems.[4] An alternative formulation, however, sees conflict between cottage parents and caseworkers as a product of competition among these workers for the affection and loyalty of children under care,[5] while a third explanation is that the conflict results from caseworkers' unrealistic expectations of cottage staff.[6]

The above views have served as bases for a wide variety of proposals for mitigating relationship problems that occur between cottage parents and caseworkers. Examples of such remedies include attracting more mature and emotionally secure cottage personnel through provision of higher salaries and promotional opportunities, insuring better resident staff performance by means of training programs and professional supervision, and increasing the flow of communication between professional and non-professional staff members to develop better understanding. While many of these recommendations have been put to use within institutional settings, systematic assessment of their effect has yet to be reported. This is the intent of the present paper. Specifically, the research on which it is based sought to furnish data on three questions: (1) How do the treatment ideologies of cottage parents in institutions employing procedures to reduce cottage-parent–caseworker conflict differ from those of cottage parents in settings not utilizing such procedures? (2) How do cottage parents and caseworkers evaluate one another in these two types of settings? (3) What are the implications of these evaluations for cottage-parent–caseworker relations and programs in these facilities?

DESCRIPTION OF SETTINGS

BECAUSE of limitation of funds, it was necessary to restrict the study to two institutions, one voluntary and one state-supported.[7] The settings were roughly similar in that they were large, cottage-based correctional institutions for boys.[8] However, as suggested by the staffing patterns presented in Table 1, the agencies differed widely in their provision of services.

The model within which Institution A most readily fit was that of a residential treatment center. All clinic personnel were professionally trained social workers, and all had small caseloads. Each cottage, manned by a husband-wife team, housed at most twenty boys. Psychiatric consultation to program staff was liberally provided. Finally, the agency took a number of steps to insure the adequacy of performance of cottage parents and the integration of the efforts of these workers with those of caseworkers. These steps included the following: (1) providing comparatively high remuneration to cottage parents in order to attract better applicants; (2) financing cottage parents' attendance at training institutes given by nearby social work schools;[9] (3) furnishing professional supervision for cottage staff;[10] (4) instituting formal, weekly case conferences for clinic and cottage personnel; and (5) narrowing the range of "communication partners" among caseworkers and cottage parents by organizing the cottages into four autonomous units, each with its own complement of clinic and resident staff workers.

The institutional model most resembled by Institution B was that of a so-called custodial institution. Its caseworkers, three of whom had no social work training, had little time to provide direct service. Its cottage parents,[11] although better paid than those at Institution A, had no access to staff-training programs, were supervised only in administrative matters, and had to care for cottage populations half again as large as those at Institution A. Finally, formally arranged contacts between cottage parents and caseworkers were virtually non-existent. They occurred only when some crisis event, such as a runaway took place.

STUDY METHOD

THE data on which the study was based were obtained in "focused interviews" with cottage parents and clinic workers.[12] Preliminary interviews

TABLE 1.

Selected Staffing Characteristics of Institutions A and B

| | INSTITUTION | |
CHARACTERISTIC	A	B
Approximate average population	320	500
Clinic program:		
Total budgeted casework positions	19	7
Budgeted administrative and supervisor positions	5	1
Budgeted practitioner positions	14	6
Mean caseload per practitioner position	23	83
Mean caseworker-youth contacts per month	3.3	0.8
Cottage program:		
Total cottages	16	16
Mean number of children per cottage	20	31.2

revealed that many of the resident staff workers were reluctant to be interviewed individually.[13] Consequently, rather than risk high refusal rates, couple members were interviewed together.

Job vacancies, the desire to limit respondents to those workers with at least six months' experience in their present agency, and the refusal of one couple at Institution A to be interviewed made it necessary to limit the number of respondents to fourteen caseworkers and fourteen cottage couples at Institution A and seven caseworkers and fifteen cottage couples at Institution B.

While no systematic assessment of response reliability was made, replies to several "trap" questions suggested that, with the exception of one Institution A couple, workers' replies were valid. The responses of this couple were omitted from the analysis.

Responses were coded by the writer. Twenty-five per cent of the interviews were subsequently recoded by another worker, whose codings were in agreement on 86 per cent of the replies.

FINDINGS

Workers' treatment ideologies. All respondents were asked two questions designed to ascertain treatment orientation. The first query was intended to tap their beliefs about the primary purpose of the agency, while the second sought to determine, in a general sense, their opinions about the means necessary to fulfill this purpose. Responses to the first question revealed no differences among workers. All stated that helping boys to become law-abiding was the primary concern of the program.[14] This unanimity did not carry over, however, in relation to workers' conceptions regarding the proper means to achieve this aim. While all case-workers agreed that meeting individual needs was the appropriate approach for effecting their agency's aims, cottage couples' opinions showed strong agency-related differences. Eleven of the fourteen cottage couples in Institution A and only three of the fifteen couples in Institution B believed that an individualized treatment approach was the preferred pathway to rehabilitation of delinquent boys. The remaining couples in the two agencies believed this goal could be achieved only by training and exercise of discipline. These differences are in accord with the previously cited commentaries on institutional staff relations and make plausible the inference that the efforts put forth at Institution A to improve cottage parents' operations did tend to develop among these workers a treatment ideology congruent with that of professional social workers.

Mutual evaluations of cottage parents and caseworkers. Unexpectedly, however, the degree of similarity among the treatment ideologies of cottage parents and caseworkers apparently had little bearing on the evaluations these workers made of one another. At both Institution A and Institution B these mutual assessments were essentially negative.

Thirteen of the fourteen caseworkers at Institution A found fault with the operations of their cottage-parent colleagues. Their criticisms covered one or more of the following areas: the cottage parents' emphasis on control, their intrusion into caseworkers' responsibilities by counseling youth, and their failure to carry out treatment plans developed by clinic workers and agreed upon in case conferences. Significantly, 71 per cent of the professional staff members regarded these presumed inadequacies in the performance of cottage parents as the result of psychological or training limitations. Portions of assessments of cottage parents made by two caseworkers suggest the flavor of the dominant professional point of view:

The cottage parents do what they please and what they need to do out of their own particular personality situations. . . . Further, most of them are not even high-school trained. Supposedly they are equal to us administratively, but everyone knows they are not. And this is why they cannot take direction—because they are so threatened. I think direction should be given to cottage parents, but around here you are constantly barking up an impossible tree.

Sometimes cottage parents recognize what I am trying to explain to them. They see the therapeutic value of it, but they find themselves emotionally blocked from implementing my plan.

The above assessments found some parallel at Institution B, in which five of the seven caseworkers noted specific shortcomings in the cottage parents' operations, and three regarded these shortcomings as the consequences of the individual inadequacies of the cottage parents. Significantly, these complaints were confined to the presumed overemphasis of cottage parents on control. The lack of concern about cottage parents' possible treatment ventures[15] apparently stemmed from the marginal position of the professional workers in the agency's rehabilitation program. One caseworker described the situation as follows:

The cottage parent gives the boys something they receive from no one else on the grounds. The rest of us deal with the boy cursorily. The cottage parent deals with him directly and knows more about him than anyone else.

The attitude of Institution B cottage parents toward caseworkers was essentially one of indifference. Thirteen couples professed ignorance about caseworkers' activities and expressed, further, the belief that clinic workers had insufficient contact with youth and resident staff to affect the actions of either. But, if the stance of these workers toward clinicians was one of insouciance, that of the Institution A cottage parents was one of anger and resentment. Ten of the thirteen couples interviewed held that caseworkers were either unrealistic in their treatment of youth or in their appraisal of the possibilities of program implementation within cottages. In addition, eight of these ten couples, and one other, voiced resentment about the depreciating appraisal of them by clinic personnel. Also, while cottage parents did not deny that they at times departed from established treatment plans or counseled members of their cottages, their rationale for these actions was at variance with that of the clinicians. First, all the cottage parents stated that maintaining order within their cottages was one of their primary responsibilities and that when implementation of treatment plans interfered with control this implementation had to be postponed. Furthermore, eleven of the thirteen couples believed that counseling or advising the boys was an appropriate cottage-parent function. They defended this practice on the ground that caseworkers were not always available to youngsters who desired help and/or on the assumption that they, and not the caseworkers, were the most important treatment personnel within the institution.[16]

Consequences of staff conflict for institution programs. Although two major lines of inquiry were followed in an attempt to analyze the impact of cottage-parent–caseworker relationships on institutional operation, only one of these, the analysis of informal-communication[17] patterns among cottage and clinic personnel, can be discussed here.

The significance of informal-communication networks among organization personnel has been discussed in numerous studies.[18]Perhaps the major function of such networks lies in the fact that they do not involve either formal outlets or "going through channels." Consequently, they offer workers opportunity to exchange essential information much more quickly than do formal-communication networks.[19] Obviously, the importance of informal networks depends on the tasks assigned to workers. When only one individual is responsible for turning out a product, or when activities of personnel are routine, the need for communication with co-workers becomes minimal. At the opposite pole, however, when workers' actions are highly varied and require collaboration, the use of informal communication becomes essential.[20] It is at this latter pole that correctional settings, mental hospitals, and children's institutions are most appropriately located. To the extent that these settings are concerned with rehabilitation, the activities of staff must be sufficiently flexible to respond to the changing needs presented by inmates. Without the communication links between workers such as are provided by informal-communication networks, staff performance becomes less responsive to the various manifestations of inmate needs, and program achievements are reduced.

Given, then, the importance of informal communication in institutional settings, the findings of this research are striking, for they reveal that such communication was rare between cottage parents and caseworkers at both of the institutions studied. At Institution B, cottage couples, by their own estimates, averaged one informal contact with a casework practitioner every eight weeks, while the average of casework practitioners' estimates of their informal contacts with cottage parents was once in five weeks.[21] At Institution A, these contacts, as reported by resident and clinic personnel, averaged once in six weeks and once in four weeks, respectively.[22]

This mutual isolation was explained by most workers at Institution B on the ground that clinic staff, because of their lack of contact with inmates, could provide little assistance to the efforts of cottage workers. This, however, did not furnish the basis for the estrangement found at Institution A. As shown in Table 2, cottage-parent "isolates" placed the responsibility on the intractability of the caseworkers. The assumed disinterest of the professional workers in cottage programs and their mistrust of cottage parents were seen by most couples as the reasons why caseworkers did not visit cottages and why they, the resident staff, had little inclination to talk to clinic personnel.

Institution A caseworkers, on the other hand, saw their failure to have more informal contact with cottage personnel as due either to the pressure of other clinic duties or to the intractability of non-professional staff members. It must be noted, furthermore, that four caseworkers who attributed their meager contact with cottage parents to the higher priority of other tasks had also described the resident workers as inadequately prepared for their jobs. The neutrality of the responses of these clinicians may have been more apparent than real.

In any case, at both agencies studied, the co-ordination of clinic and cottage services relied mainly on formal-communication channels. The negative effects of this reliance may have been limited at Institution B, in view of the marginal position of clinic workers in the agency's treatment program.[23] Such was not the case, however, at Institution A. Both clinic and cottage personnel of this agency had frequent contacts with inmates. Presumably, these contacts supplied insights having important implications for treatment. Yet, because of antagonisms and mistrust, communication regarding these insights was so infrequent as to put into question the efficacy of this agency's program.[24]

DISCUSSION

IN brief, then, the major finding of this study is that staff conflict as well as its dysfunctional consequences can endure in treatment-oriented insti-

---

TABLE 2.

*Primary Reason Reported by Staff for Limited Informal Contacts between Caseworkers and Cottage Parents by Institution**

| | INSTITUTION | | | |
| | A | | B | |
REPORTED REASONS	CASE-WORKERS	COTTAGE PARENTS	CASE-WORKERS	COTTAGE PARENTS
Total	9	11	5	15
Intractability of cottage parents	4	—	2	—
Pressure of other duties	5	2	—	2
Intractability of caseworkers	—	8	—	—
Marginal position of caseworkers	—	1	3	13

* Asked only of non-administrative personnel who reported that informal contacts took place less often than once in two weeks.

tutional-care settings despite the use of measures generally advocated for its reduction. In the present section, an attempt will be made to identify some reasons for this persistence.

It is possible that, as most caseworkers in this research argued, cottage parents were simply not capable of carrying out their assigned responsibilities. This explanation, however, ignores a potent source of conflict among organizational personnel, namely, specialization itself. Two means by which specialization can lead to interdepartmental conflict are of particular relevance to the findings of this research.

First, because workers with different specializations have responsibilities and problems unique to their respective positions, they typically differ in the degree to which they emphasize various organizational goals and tasks.[25] Second, in seeking to attain their assigned goals, workers are led on occasion to expand the scope of their activities into realms regarded by others as reserved only for them.[26] It is only a brief step from these structurally induced practices to staff conflict itself. Disputes about these concerns are generally controlled in organizations largely through use of such conflict-neutralizing mechanisms as communication, supervision, value infusion, and selective recruitment. However—and this is the crucial point of this discussion—it is likely that these mechanisms are of limited utility in organizations of the type examined in the present study. This point is dramatically demonstrated by comparing institutional-care settings to commercial organizations.

In commercial enterprises, as a rule, organizational goals are well articulated;[27] the tasks of workers, particularly those of lower-echelon staff, are standardized,[28] and the appropriateness of workers' operations for achievement of organizational goals has been demonstrated.[29] Thus, to the extent that workers share organization goals, their expectations of one another are likely to have considerable congruence. Second, because of relative clarity in the means-goal chain, obstacles to efficient performance resulting from organizational defects, workers' failure to share goals, or interdepartmental disputes can be either controlled or accounted for, thus helping to stabilize workers' activities and expectations.[30]

In institutional-care settings, however, these conditions do not apply. Although service goals may be shared among workers, their implications for performance have not been empirically established or even clearly implied. Moreover, workers' roles have yet to be satisfactorily articulated.[31] Thus, in the absence of a demonstrable link between workers' activities and long-range treatment goals, no criteria are available to determine the validity of either professional or non-professional workers' conceptions of the scope of the cottage worker's treatment role. Similarly, no empirical justification is available for the applicability of the caseworker's treatment norms in a group-living situation, in which not only control problems exist, but in which therapeutic actions are carried out in a group rather than dyadic situation. Finally, the lack of programing involved in the cottage parents' organization roles suggests that, regardless of their appropriateness, treatment-plan prescriptions given to these workers will lack operational clarity. That is, their specific application in concrete situations will not be well defined.

These conditions permit institution workers to have objectives, role conceptions, and operating procedures frequently in conflict with and yet unaffected by one another's expectations. In fact, the possibility cannot be discounted that not only may communication between personnel fail to resolve their disputes, it may serve also to increase the visibility of their discordant views and further amplify their conflict.

The above considerations, in brief, lead to the inference that conflict between caseworkers and cottage parents may be an inescapable feature of residential treatment centers as well as of custodial institutions, as these facilities are currently organized. Assuming this inference to be valid, what steps might be taken to resolve the dilemma that follows? While the current state of organization theory does not permit definitive answers to this query, two possible approaches deserve brief mention.

The first approach involves the relocation of caseworkers from their relatively isolated clinic offices to cottages. This move would increase informal communication opportunities among professional and non-professional staff members, would provide a common exposure to the daily activities of the institution, and presumably would enable professional staff members to develop clearer understanding of the responsibilities and problems faced by cottage workers in carrying out their assigned roles. A second, more radical, innovation calls for the assignment of both cottage-parent and caseworker responsibilities to one professional worker. Such action obviously removes the opportunity for conflict between cottage parents and caseworkers. It also offers increased assurance that cottage staff performance will be based on the needs of those being served.[32]

The above courses of action certainly do not exhaust the possible means by which conflict among institutional personnel can be reduced. Furthermore, the feasibility of these, as well as of alternative approaches, still needs to be assessed. However, to the extent that the findings of this research are applicable to institutions generally, introduction and appraisal of such measures must be regarded as among the major needs of the institutional-care field.

NOTES TO CHAPTER 18

1. Norman Lourie and Rena Shulman, "The Role of the Residential Staff in Residential Treatment," *American Journal of Orthopsychiatry*, XXII (October, 1952), 801-4. Similar views have been expressed by a number of

writers. See, for example, Hershel Alt and Hyman Grossbard, "Professional Issues in the Institutional Treatment of Delinquent Children," *American Journal of Orthopsychiatry*, XIX (April, 1949), 279-94; Maurice Harmon, "The Importance of Staff Teamwork in a Training School," in *Selected Papers in Group Work and Community Organization Presented at the National Conference of Social Work, 1952*, pp. 109-17; Swithun Bowers, "The Social Worker in a Children's Residential Treatment Program," *Social Casework*, XXXVIII (June, 1957), 283-88.

2. George H. Weber, "Conflicts between Professional and Non-professional Persons in Institutional Delinquency Treatment," *Journal of Criminal Law, Criminology, and Police Science*, XLVIII (June, 1950), 26-43; Eva Burmeister, "Training for Houseparents," *Child Welfare*, XXXVI (January, 1957), 27-31; Robert A. Cohen, "Some Relations between Staff Tensions and the Psychotherapeutic Process," in *The Patient and the Mental Hospital*, ed. Milton Greenblatt, Daniel J. Levinson, and Richard H. Williams (Glencoe, Ill.: Free Press, 1957), pp. 301-8.

3. This inability to secure allegiance has been accounted for by the failure of institutions to provide cottage staff adequate status, compensation, and promotional opportunities. See, for example, Mayer Zald, "The Correctional Institution for Juvenile Offenders: An Analysis of Organizational Character," *Social Problems*, VII (Summer, 1960), 63.

4. References to either or both of these possible sources of cottage-parent malfunctioning may be found in Burmeister, "Training for Houseparents," *op. cit.*, pp. 27-31; R. L. Jenkins, M.D., "Treatment in an Institution," *American Journal of Orthopsychiatry*, XI (January, 1941), 85-91; Jerome Goldsmith, "The Communication of Clinical Information in a Residential Treatment Setting," in *Casework Papers, 1955* (New York: Family Service Association of America, 1955), pp. 43-52; Howard Polsky, "Changing Delinquent Subcultures: A Social-Psychological Approach," *Social Work*, IV (October, 1959), 3-15; Ella Reese, "The Professional Child Welfare Worker: Institutional Child Welfare Worker," *Child Welfare*, XXXV (December, 1956), 8-10; Elliot Studt, "Therapeutic Factors in Group Living," *Child Welfare*, XXXV (January, 1956), 1-6; Child Welfare League of America, "Report of the Committee on Standards for Group Care" (undated, mimeographed).

5. Goldsmith, "The Communication of Clinical Information . . . ," *op. cit.*, p. 48.

6. These unrealistic expectations, it is asserted, derive from the failure of caseworkers to appreciate the range of tasks and problems faced by cottage parents in performing their roles. See Lloyd Ohlin, "The Reduction of Role Conflict in Institutional Staff," *Children*, V (March-April, 1958), 65-66; Robert Vinter and Morris Janowitz, "Effective Institutions for Juvenile Delinquents: A Research Statement," *Social Service Review*, XXXIII (June, 1959), 118-30.

7. Hereinafter referred to as "Institution A" and "Institution B."

8. Although the organization of services for the care of delinquents may differ in some respects from that for non-delinquents, sufficient similarities exist in the two forms of care to suggest that the findings of this study may be relevant to settings serving non-delinquent youth.

9. About one-third of the cottage parents had attended at least one such institute.

10. Of the four supervisors of cottage parents at this institution, two were graduate social workers, one held a Master's degree in psychology, and the fourth had obtained a bachelor's degree in education.

11. As at Institution A, cottages were under the supervision of married couples.

12. Robert K. Merton and Patricia Kendall, *The Focused Interview* (Glencoe, Ill.: Free Press, 1956).

13. These objections were largely based on workers' resistance to give time to the study, as well as some anxiety about being interviewed without partners.

14. While this question may seem superfluous, it was asked because of the possibility that staff members believed other goals, such as punishment or community protection, directed their day-to-day activities.

15. While five Institution B caseworkers stated that counseling inmates was an appropriate cottage-parent function, none of the Institution A caseworkers voiced this belief.

16. Twelve Institution A cottage couples believed resident staff to be more important than clinic workers for purposes of treatment; eleven of the caseworkers held the diametrically opposite view.

17. The term "informal communication" refers to that communication taking place among workers as a result of voluntarily "getting together."

18. Herbert A. Simon, *Administrative Behavior* (New York: Macmillan Co., 1958), pp. 160-64; Peter M. Blau, *The Dynamics of Bureaucracy* (Chicago: University of Chicago Press, 1955), p. 142; Philip Selznick, *TVA and the Grass Roots* (Berkeley and Los Angeles: University of California Press, 1949), pp. 251-52; Alfred H. Stanton and Morris S. Schwartz, *The Mental Hospital* (New York: Basic Books, 1954), pp. 234-43.

19. The concern here for the merits of informal-communication channels is not to denigrate those of formal communication, which are necessary in the development and communication of official agency decisions and policy.

20. Simon, *op. cit.*, p. 156.

21. The contact rates of the two groups are in fairly close agreement since there were approximately twice as many cottage parents as clinicians in the institution.

22. Since there are approximately as many caseworkers as cottage couples at the private agency, these rates as given by the two groups show considerable disparity. Nevertheless, at best, the informal contact rate was low.

23. This is not intended to imply that the program of Institution B was adequate. Rather it is to recognize that, whatever the level of adequacy of the program, clinic personnel were not in a position to influence it significantly.

24. Because of the mistrust between several caseworkers and cottage parents, some of this information was not exchanged even in formal conferences. One clinic worker said: "I just feel that basically they do not have 'it,' the minimum amount necessary to give those kids a healthy living situation. All my fancy explanations usually fall on dead ears. . . . I have to be very guarded in what I discuss, for I am not sure how these cottage parents would use it."

25. Alvin Gouldner, *Patterns of Industrial Bureaucracy* (Glencoe, Ill.: Free

Press, 1954), pp. 233-36; Neal Gross, Ward S. Mason, and Alexander W. McEachern, *Explorations in Role Analysis* (New York: John Wiley & Sons, 1958), pp. 183-92; Peter Blau and W. Richard Scott, *Formal Organizations* (San Francisco: Chandler Publishing Co., 1962), pp. 173-74.

26. Gross, *et al.*, *op. cit.*, pp. 123-26; Marshall E. Dimock, "Expanding Jurisdictions: A Case Study in Bureaucratic Conflict," in *Reader in Bureaucracy,* ed. Robert K. Merton *et al.* (Glencoe, Ill.: Free Press, 1952), pp. 282-91.

27. Thus, according to Simon, commercial organizations are concerned with obtaining the greatest net money return. "This goal is relatively easily measured and thus can serve as a criterion for assessing the adequacy of workers' operations" (Simon, *op. cit.*, pp. 172-73).

28. Peter Blau, *Bureaucracy in Modern Society* (New York: Random House, 1956), p. 18.

29. *Ibid.*, p. 32.

30. James G. March and Herbert A. Simon, *Organizations* (New York: John Wiley & Sons, 1958), p. 145.

31. These problems as they exist in social work practice are discussed in Joseph W. Eaton, "A Scientific Basis for Helping," in *Issues in American Social Work,* ed. Alfred J. Kahn (New York: University Press, 1959), pp. 270-92; see also Alt and Grossbard, "Professional Issues in the Institutional Treatment of Delinquent Children," *op. cit.*

32. Advocacy of this dual responsibility of professional staff members can be found in other writings. See, for example, Lloyd Ohlin and William C. Lawrence, "Social Intervention among Clients as a Treatment Problem," *Social Work,* IV (April, 1959), 3-13; and Howard W. Polsky, "Changing Delinquent Subcultures: A Social Psychological Approach," *Social Work,* IV (October, 1959), 3-15.

ॐ

C H A P T E R 1 9   Emotional Illness and Interaction
Process: A Study of Patient Groups*

SAMUEL W. BLOOM, INA BOYD, AND HOWARD B. KAPLAN

S TUDIES of the mental hospital as a social institution have tended to
emphasize the special purposes of the hospital rather than its generic
similarity with other social institutions. However, beginning with the
pioneering studies of Rowland[1] the informal life of the mental hospital
has been the subject of virtually constant and ever increasing descriptive
study. One result has been to establish a view of the hospital as a social
system and to direct attention to the cultural patterns which fundamentally determine and control behavior within such a system. Goffman has
described patterns of "inmate culture" in a mental hospital which he
argues are generic to all "total institutions." Studies of prisons are his
most frequent source of analogy.[2] In common with most other hospital
studies, however, Goffman shares a preoccupation with conflict and
breakdown in the social system. The interests and values of patients, he
argues, are basically at conflict with those of the hospital staff. The "staff-
inmate split" which results is controlled by an autocratic authority structure in which the patient is subordinate. It is for this basic reason,
Goffman argues, that a *sub rosa* patient culture develops in the mental
hospital very similar to the undercover inmate cultures observed in
prison.[3]

In this tradition, we have attempted to study a mental hospital as an
institution of socialization, both in its formal and informal aspects. The
major purpose of this paper is to identify and describe informal patient
groups, and to discuss the reciprocal effects of the socialization process

* Revision of a paper presented at the twenty-fourth annual meeting of the Southern Sociological Society, Miami Beach, Florida, April 1961. This research was supported in part by Grant number 511.888 from the Hogg Foundation for Mental Health
and by the Veterans Administration Hospital, Houston, Texas.
Reprinted from *Social Forces*, 41 (1962), 135–141, by permission of the authors
and The University of North Carolina Press.

in such groups upon the more formal structures and functions of the psychiatric ward.

We have selected for study two types of psychiatric patient groups. One type, the friendship clique, is informal, the product of spontaneous processes of social interaction which are assumed to be common to all social institutions. The second is a formal social unit, selected and continuously under the control of the staff; it is organized for purposes of group psychotherapy, a function specific to this type of institution.

THE SETTING OF THE STUDY

WE have been studying a psychiatric ward in a general Veterans Administration Hospital in the southwestern part of the United States. At the outset of the study, this ward, consisting of 46 beds, and usually operated at near capacity, was one of six psychiatric wards in the hospital. Ward 612, as it is known in the hospital, has been an open ward since 1954, dedicated to the principles of "the therapeutic community" as originally outlined by Maxwell Jones.[4] It has since that time been distinctive from other wards in the hospital. Ward 612 is, in effect, an experimental ward, a place where new methods of patient care are tried. When these ideas seem to be effective, they are adapted in other parts of the hospital psychiatric service. One example is group therapy; another is patient government. Both were first tried at this particular hospital on Ward 612, and later introduced on other psychiatric wards.[5]

The nickname among hospital patients for Ward 612 is "The Penthouse." Quite obviously, this is not simply because it is on the top floor of the psychiatric wing. The ward is known as a "good place to be." This is to be expected by the nature of the therapeutic community orientation with its emphasis upon the humane and the democratic.[6] More than that, however, Ward 612 has become known as a "last stop" in hospitalization. Patients have been selected for the ward on the assumption that they will benefit sufficiently to become candidates for discharge within a limited period of time, usually within three to six months. Anxiety reaction, depressive reaction, and personality and character disorder are the major diagnoses. The more severe psychotics can hope to get to Ward 612 only after they become "responsible," and show evidence of being able to benefit from a therapeutic program which requires patients to monitor their own behavior to a large extent. Transfer to Ward 612, therefore, has come to be thought of as an "honor" among patients; it is a step up, figuratively as well as literally.[7]

The staff of the ward consisted of a psychiatrist, psychologist, social worker, nurse, and three aides. In addition to these full-time staff personnel, two psychologists and a psychiatric resident participate as regular leaders of group psychotherapy. The hospital maintains departments of occupational, correctional, industrial, and educational therapy. All are utilized by the ward, thus making their personnel contributors to the total ward staff. Although the life of the ward is autonomous to a large extent, there are strong links between the ward and the total hospital social system. There is a fundamental dualism in the identity of each staff member on this ward. He is on the one hand, part of Ward 612 and subject therefore to its special structure of authority and values. He is also a member of a hospital department, such as nursing or psychology, and subject therefore to a second structuring of authority and a value-system which is quite independent of Ward 612.

INFORMAL SOCIAL STRUCTURE IN THE PATIENT WORLD

THE informal patient life of Ward 612 was studied over a fifteen month period by participant-observation and sociometric techniques. The observation was intermittent, except for a six week period when a medical student engaged in full-time observation of the ward. A sociometric questionnaire was administered to the entire ward patient population of five different times during the fifteen months.

Our analysis of these data suggested that the ward characteristically appears to possess two distinct types of cliques[8] which have immediate and significant consequences for the maintenance and change of the formal ward structure.

One type of clique is a leadership group, and the second is a group of dissenters.

The leadership clique functions as a means of socialization and social control for the prevailing values of the staff. The second clique expresses sentiments of dissent from the staff values by testing the limits of the ward and hospital codes of behavior.

The leadership clique assumes several responsibilities. For example it runs the patient government. The actual dominant leader of the patients is not always the ward's elected president, but he is generally very influential in deciding who will be the president. For example, just prior to the recent patient government election, the leadership clique gathered in conversation and decided that a certain patient should be elected ward president. The reason given to the observer for his choice was, "It will be good for him" meaning that it was an act designed to help the patient in his illness. The patient in question did "have ability," but they (the leadership clique) were not thinking of the office or the specifications for leadership as much as they were, in this instance, of the individual patient. Later at the ward meeting, this chosen patient was indeed elected.

A second responsibility of the leadership clique is the education of new patients in their patient roles, and in the details of ward culture. This may be illustrated by a small group of patients which was transferred together from another ward in the hospital to 612. This group stayed close together, avoiding association with other men on the ward. It became known that they were outcasts on the ward, that the other men were not willing to accept them.

Quick action was taken by the leader of the clique when he became aware of the "outcasts." He, together with others at the nucleus of the leadership clique, sought out the new patients, assuring them that they were not being rejected on the ward. Similar examples may be found frequently among our field notes, indicating that the leadership clique watches closely the behavior of all the patients, taking action to help, to correct, and to punish.

A third responsibility of the leadership clique is the training of "heirs to the throne." We have followed closely the careers of several patient leaders. Each one was found to participate, first, as a second-ranking figure in the leadership clique prior to becoming himself the top man.

The second type of clique we call the dissident clique, intending the name to express deviation from the majority in attitudes toward the prevailing codes of behavior. This type of clique, in general, seems to be a less permanent part of the ward culture than the leadership clique. It appears to emerge, much as a social movement, as a symptom of rebellion against the prevailing mores, waxing or waning according to the climate of the ward. Nevertheless, it is a typical, if only periodically recurring, aspect of the social structure of the ward.

A particularly interesting example of the dissident clique was a group referred to by the patients as "the playboys." The playboys were observed regularly to test the limits. They smuggled liquor into the ward, gambled, stayed up late, noisily engaged in prankish behavior, and otherwise took liberties with various ward rules, thus expressing their rejection of the current patient and staff leadership. To a large extent, however, this clique did not show its deviation directly to the staff. There was a duplicity in their behavior, not unlike the "playing it cool" reported by Goffman.[9]

The leader of the playboys was a former important figure on the ward who had been in the leadership clique. While he was in the leadership clique, he behaved according to the appropriate role prescription; he was a guardian of the prevailing norms. His defection appears to be connected with his discharge from the hospital. As he became aware that discharge was to come soon, he split with the leadership clique, taking with him a few close associates. This group became the nucleus for the dissident clique. This attenuation from the leadership clique and the ward as a whole did not occur suddenly; it was a gradual process over several weeks. It persisted for a short time following the discharge of the playboy leader, then dissipated, to be replaced later by another dissident clique.

The patient typically goes through four stages in his patient career. He is initiated, socialized, integrated, and, finally, separated from the ward culture. While the leadership clique is the guardian of the ward values, the dissident clique provides a mechanism of deviation which apparently arises in response to the heightened anxiety and sense of loss which characterizes the final stage of patienthood.

As a result of expectations of discharge, any such patient represents a threat to the maintenance of the legitimate ward structure. However, this threat is intensified when the patient about to be separated formerly occupied a nuclear position in a leadership clique. As evidenced by the leader of the playboys, the impact of impending separation defies even the strength of a leadership position. The leader, like other patients, goes through a separation experience usually accompanied by feelings of disenchantment and criticism of the ward, the staff, and the hospital. In the process, the ward culture loses an erstwhile *supporter* of the legitimate norms and at the same time gains a *dissident* who is all the more threatening by dint of his continuing (at least for a while) popularity since he swells the ranks of the deviant not only with himself but also with some of his close followers.

This general experience was found in each of the three cases of patient leaders who were selected for special case study.[10]

The equilibrium of clique structure as we have described it is unstable. That is, over short-run periods of time, relationships among the cliques change according to a number of elements in the total ward situation. Each major clique possesses as its nucleus a small core around which rotates a number of individuals or pairs. When the spirit on the ward is strongly united in purpose and mood, these subgroups are held together by bridging relationships among representatives from the different cliques. In times of upheaval, however, the links weaken and the subgroups become more separate and more competing. When, for example, a change in the ward program was decided but not yet started, a feeling of some uneasiness became apparent among the staff and patients. The current leader of the patients effectively used his personal prestige to keep the patients loyal to the staff. However, a dissident group formed which became known as the "hell-raisers." Also, a clique of "strangers" who had been transferred from another ward resisted the leader's overtures, isolating themselves from the rest of the patients. Before long, the leader himself entered a characteristic separation phase in his own patient career. It was not long before his leadership power was spent. An heir whom he had trained for leadership took over, but the general climate of the ward was so disturbed that for more than a month the leadership clique was not effective.

THE THERAPY GROUP

In contradistinction to the informal patient groups discussed above, the therapy group represents a formal, institutionalized aspect of the social structure of this psychiatric ward.

TABLE 1.

*Tendency of Patients to Make Friendship Choices Within One's Own Therapy Group According to Chi-Square Analysis of In-Group to Out-Group Sociometric Choices**

THERAPY GROUP	QUESTIONNAIRE NO. 1 2ND MONTH OF STUDY	NO. 2 5TH MONTH	NO. 3 12TH MONTH	NO. 4 14TH MONTH	NO. 5 15TH MONTH
1	(N = 4) P < .001	(N = 5) N.S.	(N = 8) P < .01	(N = 6) P < .001	(N = 11) N.S.
2	(N = 6) N.S.	(N = 8) P < .05	(N = 4) N.S.	(N = 8) P < .05	(N = 7) P < .001
3	(N = 7) N.S.	(N = 9) N.S.	(N = 10) P < .001	(N = 4) P < .001	(N = 10) N.S.
4	(N = 6) P < .001	(N = 6) P < .02	(N = 9) P < .001	(N = 5) P < .001	(N = 5) P < .001
5	(N = 10) P < .001	(N = 8) P < .001			(N = 8) P < .001
6				(N = 7) P < .001	(N = 7) P < .001
7				(N = 4) P < .001	(N = 9) P < .001
8			(N = 6) P < .001		
9			(N = 5) P < .001		
10	(N = 5) P < .001				
11	(N = 4) N.S.				
12	(N = 2) P < .001				
13	(N = 2) N.S.				
14		(N = 8) P < .001			
Total N	46	44	42	34	57
	5/9				

* When P<.05, tendency is asserted to be significant for choosing within own therapy group. Blank spaces indicate that no group is active for corresponding therapist at the time.

[286]

In keeping with the therapeutic community philosophy, group psycho-therapy is well established as the single most important organized activity on Ward 612. Every patient assigned to the ward participates in a therapy group. The groups themselves, during the period of this study, ranged in size from 2 to 11 persons.

The procedure of these groups is not uniform, some meeting daily, others meeting two or three times a week.

In general our purpose is to describe and discuss the reciprocal effects of formal and informal patient groups. The preceding discussion suggested some of the mechanisms by which informal patient life affects the formal aspects of ward structure. However, in like manner, the formal patterns of patient interaction were found to influence the patients' mode of relationship in informal groups.

Both the general impression of the staff and the analysis of sociometric data suggested that therapy group membership did influence other parts of the patients' experience on the ward.

The latter data, for example, indicated that the therapy group tends to be the focus of friendship choices.

As Table 1 demonstrates, at each administration of the sociometric questionnaire, there was a significant tendency on the part of the majority of therapy groups to focus friendship choices within their respective groups.

Anywhere from 56 percent to 100 percent of the therapy groups may demonstrate this tendency, depending upon the time of the administration. Such variation, occurring as it did concurrently with certain changes on the ward, suggested that there was a negative relationship between ward stability and the tendency for friendship and therapy groups to be congruent. That is, in times of social disorganization, there was a tendency for informal group relationships to be articulated with the more formal, institutionalized structure. Early in the study, the ward was a stable community. The therapeutic community philosophy with modifications based upon local experience was well established. The prestige of the ward in the hospital was high. In this situation of stable predictable norms, the clique structure appeared to be at its highest level of significance in the informal life of the ward. When, however, the ward's therapeutic program was changed,[11] the ward community reacted by becoming very unstable, at least during the period of transition while the day hospital was being added. At this time, the therapy group became increasingly important to the patients and the cliques became relatively weak and ineffectual. It was observed, for example, that the election of leaders in the patient government lacked purpose and significance to the men. "They just don't seem to care," a staff member observed, as a patient was elected chairman who had long aspired to the office but who previously had been steadfastly opposed by the leadership clique.

In Table 1, the fourth column shows data collected just at this point of change in the ward program. In this column, every therapy group tended to focus friendship choices upon their respective therapy groups. Thus, we find some support for the hypothesis that in periods of unstable community norms, the formal, more goal-directed type of patient group assumes increased importance in the informal social behavior of patients.

According to the evidence, this relationship between a formal special-purpose activity group (the therapy group) and an informal group (the friendship group) is to a degree constant. That is, the therapy group is always a significant determinant of friendship. Only in the degree of influence does the stability-instability of the ward's social organization result in more or less significance in the relationship between these two structures.

DISCUSSION

FRIENDSHIP cliques in a psychiatric ward such as have been described above represent a form of social behavior which is characteristic of all formal organizations including the prison, school, and factory. There are variations, however, in both the structure and function of these types of groups.

In the present context, two types of informal patient groups tended to arise, and apparently had both functional and dysfunctional consequences for their members *and* for the formal organization of the ward. In a similar way, the existence of a formal patient organization (the therapy group) had important effects on the more informal life of the patient population.

Two types of informal patient groups were isolated: the leadership clique and the dissident clique.

The former served the functions of supporting the formal aspects of ward life as represented by the values of the staff, by providing a patient government which would, in turn, replace itself with others who would judge themselves by these same values, and by acting as a quasi-formal socializing agency for new patients.

The dissident group served an important function for the individual by providing a means of withdrawing from this dependence on institutional values thus permitting him to adapt to societal standards with which the institution's values were not always in congruence. However, at the same time there were apparently dysfunctional consequences for the formal ward structure. The existence of this "withdrawal mechanism" helped to deplete the membership of needed leadership and helped to increase the ranks of the deviant group with followers of these leaders. The followers were not themselves ready to utilize this withdrawal agency and merely served to undermine the broader associational values.

A third type of informal patient group may be distinguished which did not have direct or apparent consequences for the formal structure of the ward, but appeared to have beneficent consequences for the individual. This is the friendship clique which cannot be identified with either the leadership or dissident clique. What, more precisely, are the major function(s) which appear to be served by these groups?

In the prison, a major function of inmate cliques is *defense*. That is, the clique serves to defend the individual inmate psychologically from the onslaught against his self-esteem which he perceives both in society at large and in the staff.[12] The clique also serves as a defense of criminal culture against the prevailing social culture.[13]

If one analyzes the status of the prisoner in society, a hypothetical explanation of the characteristic functions of his cliques is suggested. The prisoner's role is defined by the prevailing culture to include "responsibility for one's own state." The prisoner, by definition, has violated social norms, for which he is being "punished" by incarceration, and "rehabilitated" for a return to normal society. As a result of this definition of his role, the prisoner is informed and constantly reminded that he has been fundamentally a "bad" human being. His reinstatement in society is made dependent upon a fundamental change in "self." Even in highly enlightened, progressive prisons and reformatories, prisoners have testified to the feeling of "psychological onslaught" which results from these implicit assumptions in the definition of the role. Only from fellow inmates, linked culturally with the criminal sub-world outside the prison, does the individual prisoner find social acceptance which does not degrade and "strip" him of his basic sense of identity. Thus, the defensive function of the clique fits into the inmate social system which, by its very nature, requires mechanisms of defense against a hostile prevailing community.

A second possible function for the individual patient is *development*. In the high school for example, the clique's function has been interpreted to be mainly *developmental*. It is a "mechanism" which fits the special needs of the adolescent in finding his "identity," in enabling him to develop from childhood to adulthood.[14] The adolescent in our culture finds himself between two well defined statuses; he is under pressure to assume the obligations of one (adulthood) while at the same time he is denied certain basic privileges of that status. He is in a phase of growth and of discovery concerning himself. Therefore, it may be speculated that the clique finds a logical fit in the adolescent culture as a protective social structure which facilitates this developmental process.

In a similar manner, for the mental patient, the therapeutic process implies the development of a self-concept that is favorable from the point of view of the patient and reality-oriented within the context of the broader social milieu. On the assumption that no change in self-image

can be effected outside of the context of social interaction, it is suggested
that the informal friendship group provides an optimum opportunity for
the patient to perceive and react to the image which he presents to
others. Ideally, such a group could function as a mechanism which facilitates the continuous reevaluation and testing of the patient's self-image.

Above, we suggested various functions and dysfunctions of informal
patient groups, both for the individual and for the formal structure of the
ward. In a reciprocal manner, as we have previously mentioned, the
existence of a formal structure such as the therapy group has important
effects upon the informal group life of the patients. A good deal more
research must be directed toward the discovery of the manifest and latent
functions of both types of groups in the therapeutic process.

NOTES TO CHAPTER 19

1. Howard Rowland, "Interaction Processes in the State Mental Hospital,"
   Psychiatry, 1 (1938), pp. 323-337; "Friendship Patterns in the State Mental
   Hospital," *Psychiatry*, 2 (1939), pp. 363-373.
2. Erving Goffman, "Characteristics of Total Institutions," in *Symposium on
   Preventive and Social Psychiatry* (Washington, D.C.: Walter Reed Army
   Institute of Research, 1957), pp. 43-84; "The Moral Career of Mental Patients," *Psychiatry*, 22 (May 1959), pp. 123-142; *Asylums* (New York:
   Anchor Books, 1961).
3. Goffman, *op. cit.*, 1957.
4. Maxwell Jones, *The Therapeutic Community* (New York: Basic Books, Inc.,
   1953).
5. More recently (since January 1961), Ward 612 has been the testing ground
   of a program of day hospital care. This change was introduced by the Chief
   of Psychiatric Services in the hospital, following a policy change in the
   national organization of Veterans Hospitals. The in-patient group continues
   to be the same size, varying from about 43 to 46 patients. In addition, there
   were at last count 14 patients on day care. Patients who are on day care
   only are added to the normal routine of ward activity, participating with
   the in-patients in group therapy, patient government, and various forms of
   occupational, recreational, educational, and other therapies. Since this
   change is so recent, however, most of our general comments about the
   ward's image in the hospital refer to its former program when it was a
   completely in-patient service.

   The policy change at the national level is still tentative. This hospital and
   several others in the country are participating in a pilot study of new methods of admission and care aimed at a more effective use of in-patient facilities and the reduction of the length of hospitalization.

   Not all day patients participate in the full program. On an individual
   basis the decision is made what the degree of participation will be. As this
   is written, for example, only five day patients out of 14 remain at the
   hospital for a full day. The remainder come to the hospital only for group
   therapy.

6. The therapeutic community program was recently characterized in the following terms:
   1. It is oriented to productive work and quick return to society.
   2. Educational techniques play an important role in reorienting the patients and there is liberal use at the same time of group dynamics and group pressures for constructive purposes. The attitude seems to be that for some purposes groups can be treated more effectively than individuals.
   3. A marked diffusion of authority to personnel and to patients is a peak characteristic of the system. The operation is strongly democratic and represents a flight from authoritarianism. See Herman C. B. Denber (Editor), *Research Conference on Therapeutic Community* (Springfield, Ill.: Charles C. Thomas, 1960), p. 6.
7. The psychiatric service does *not*, however, use a "step-ladder" system, whereby a patient may expect to graduate from the "poor" wards to the "better" wards, as his disturbed behavior improves. There are other open wards for responsible patients, but Ward 612 has acquired a special reputation in the hospital.
8. There are, of course, other friendship cliques of variable size on the ward at any given time. However, we have been able to discuss at this point only two types which are of apparent significance for the formal structure of the ward.
9. Goffman, *op. cit.*, 1957.
10. This is discussed more fully by the authors elsewhere. See S. W. Bloom, I. Boyd, H. B. Kaplan, "The Problems of Institutional Care: A Case Study" (mimeographed, 1961).
11. See Table 1, No. 8.
12. R. A. Cloward, "Illegitimate Means, Anomie, and Deviant Behavior," *American Sociological Review*, 24 (April 1959), pp. 164-176; see also by the same author, "Social Control in the Prison," *Theoretical Studies of the Social Organization of the Prison*, Bulletin No. 15 (New York: Social Service Research Council, 1960), pp. 20-48.
13. *Ibid.*; see also Goffman, *op. cit.*, 1957.
14. Erik H. Erikson, *Childhood and Society* (New York: W. W. Norton and Co., 1950).

CHAPTER 20   The Functions of
Deviance in Groups[*]

ROBERT A. DENTLER AND KAI T. ERIKSON

A LTHOUGH sociologists have repeatedly noted that close similarities exist between various forms of social marginality, research directed at these forms has only begun to mark the path toward a social theory of deviance. This slow pace may in part result from the fact that deviant behavior is too frequently visualized as a product of organizational failure rather than as a facet of organization itself.

Albert Cohen has recently attempted to specify some of the assumptions and definitions necessary for a sociology of deviant behavior (3). He has urged the importance of erecting clearly defined concepts, devising a homogeneous class of phenomena explainable by a unified system of theory, and developing a sociological rather than a psychological framework—as would be the case, for example, in a central problem which was stated: "What is it about the structure of social systems that determines the kinds of criminal acts that occur in these systems and the way in which such acts are distributed within the systems?" (3, p. 462). Cohen has also suggested that a theory of deviant behavior should account simultaneously for deviance and conformity; that is, the explanation of one should serve as the explanation of the other.

In this paper we hope to contribute to these objectives by presenting some propositions about the sources and functions of deviant behavior in small groups. Although we suspect that the same general processes may well characterize larger social systems,* this paper will be limited to small groups, and more particularly to enduring task and primary groups. Any set of propositions about the functions of deviance would have to be shaped to fit the scope of the social unit chosen for analysis, and we have elected to use the small group unit in this exploratory paper primarily

* Reprinted from Social Problems, 7 (1959), 98–107, by permission of the authors and the Society for the Study of Social Problems.

because a large body of empirical material dealing with deviance in groups has accumulated which offers important leads into the study of deviance in general.

With Cohen, we define deviance as "behavior which violates institutionalized expectations, that is, expectations which are shared and recognized as legitimate within a social system" (3, p. 462). Our guiding assumption is that deviant behavior is a reflection not only of the personality of the actor, but the structure of the group in which the behavior was enacted. The violations of expectation which the group experiences, as well as the norms which it observes, express both cultural and structural aspects of the group. While we shall attend to cultural elements in later illustrations, our propositions are addressed primarily to the structure of groups and the functions that deviant behavior serves in maintaining this structure.

PROPOSITION ONE

Our first proposition is that *groups tend to induce, sustain, and permit deviant behavior*. To say that a group *induces* deviant behavior, here, is to say that as it goes through the early stages of development and structures the range of behavior among its members, a group will tend to define the behavior of certain members as deviant. A group *sustains* or *permits* this newly defined deviance in the sense that it tends to institutionalize and absorb this behavior into its structure rather than eliminating it. As group structure emerges and role specialization takes place, one or more role categories will be differentiated to accommodate individuals whose behavior is occasionally or regularly expected to be deviant. It is essential to the argument that this process be viewed not only as a simple group adjustment to individual differences, but also as a requirement of group formation, analogous to the requirement of leadership.

The process of role differentiation and specialization which takes place in groups has been illuminated by studies which use concepts of sociometric rank. Riecken and Homans conclude from this evidence: "The higher the rank of a member the closer his activities come to realizing the norms of the group . . . and there is a tendency toward 'equilibration of rank'" (11, p. 794). Thus the rankings that take place on a scale of social preference serve to identify the activities that members are expected to carry out: each general rank represents or contains an equivalent role which defines that member's special relationship to the group and its norms. To the extent that a group ranks its members preferentially, it distributes functions differentially. The proposition, then, simply notes that group members who violate norms will be given low sociometric rank; that this designation carries with it an appropriate differentiation of the functions that such members are expected to perform in respect to the group; and that the roles contained in these low-rank positions become institutionalized and are retained in the structure of the group.

The most difficult aspect of this proposition is the concept of *induction* of deviance. We do not mean to suggest that the group creates the motives for an individual's deviant behavior or compels it from persons not otherwise disposed toward this form of expression. When a person encounters a new group, two different historical continuities meet. The individual brings to the group a background of private experience which disposes him to certain patterns of conduct; the group, on the other hand, is organized around a network of role priorities to which each member is required to conform. While the individual brings new resources into the group and alters its potential for change and innovation, the group certainly operates to rephrase each member's private experience into a new self-formula, a new sense of his own needs.

Thus any encounter between a group and a new member is an event which is novel to the experience of both. In the trial-and-error behavior which issues, both the functional requirements of the group and the individual needs of the person will undergo certain revisions, and in the process the group plays an important part in determining whether those already disposed toward deviant behavior will actually express it overtly, or whether those who are lightly disposed toward deviating styles will be encouraged to develop that potential. *Inducing* deviance, then, is meant to be a process by which the group channels and organizes the deviant possibilities contained in its membership.

The proposition argues that groups induce deviant behavior in the same sense that they induce other group qualities like leadership, fellowship, and so on. These qualities emerge early and clearly in the formation of new groups, even in traditionless laboratory groups, and while they may be diffusely distributed among the membership initially they tend toward specificity and equilibrium over time. In giving definition to the end points in the range of behavior which is brought to a group by its membership, the group establishes its boundaries and gives dimension to its structure. In this process, the designation of low-ranking deviants emerges as surely as the designation of high-ranking task leaders.

PROPOSITION TWO

BALES has written:

The displacement of hostilities on a scapegoat at the bottom of the status structure is one mechanism, apparently, by which the ambivalent attitudes toward the . . . 'top man' . . . can be diverted and drained off. These patterns, culturally elaborated and various in form, can be viewed as particular cases of mechanisms relevant to the much more general problem of equilibrium (2, p. 454).

This comment provides a bridge between our first and second propositions by suggesting that deviant behavior may serve important functions for groups—thereby contributing to, rather than disrupting, equilibrium in the group. Our second proposition, accordingly, is that *deviant behavior functions in enduring groups to help maintain group equilibrium.* In the following discussion we would like to consider some of the ways this function operates.

Group performance. The proposition implies that deviant behavior contributes to the maintenance of optimum levels of performance, and we add at this point that this will particularly obtain where a group's achievement depends upon the contributions of all its members.

McCurdy and Lambert devised a laboratory task which required full group participation in finding a solution to a given problem (7). They found that the performance of their groups compared unfavorably with that of individual problem-solvers, and explained this by noting the high likelihood that a group would contain at least one member who failed to attend to instructions. The group, they observed, may prove no stronger than its weakest member. The implication here, as in the old adage, seems to be that the group would have become correspondingly stronger if its weakest link were removed. Yet this implication requires some consideration: to what extent can we say that the inattentive member was acting in the name of the group, performing a function which is valuable to the group over time? To what extent can we call this behavior a product of group structure rather than a product of individual eccentricity?

As roles and their equivalent ranks become differentiated in a group, some members will be expected to perform more capably than others; and in turn the structure of the group will certainly be organized to take advantage of the relative capabilities of its members—as it demonstrably does in leadership choice. These differentials require testing and experimentation: the norms about performance in a group cannot emerge until clues appear as to how much the present membership can accomplish, how wide the range of variation in performance is likely to be, and so on. To the extent that group structure becomes an elaboration and organization of these differentials, certainly the "weak link" becomes as essential to this process as the high-producer. Both are outside links in the communication system which feeds back information about the range of group performance and the limits of the differentiated structure.

As this basis for differentiation becomes established, then, the group moves from a state in which pressure is exerted equally on all members to conform to performance norms, and moves toward a state in which these norms become a kind of anchor which locates the center of wide variations in behavior. The performance 'mean' of a group is of course expected to be set at a level dictated by 'norms'; and this mean is not only achieved by the most conforming members but by a balance of high and low producers as well. It is a simple calculation that the loss of a weak-link, the low producer, would raise the mean output of the group to a point where it no longer corresponded to original norms unless the entire structure of the group shifted as compensation. In this sense we can argue that neither role differentiation nor norm formation could occur and be maintained without the "aid" of regular deviations.

Rewards. Stated briefly, we would argue that the process of distributing incentives to members of the group is similarly dependent upon the recurrence of deviant behavior. This is an instance where, as Cohen has urged, an explanation of conformity may lead to an explanation of deviance. Customarily, conformance is rewarded while deviance is either unrewarded or actively punished. The rewards of conformity, however, are seen as "rewarding" in comparison to other possible outcomes, and obviously the presence of a deviant in the group would provide the continual contrast without which the reward structure would have little meaning. The problem, then, becomes complex: the reward structure is set up as an incentive for conformity, but depends upon the outcome that differentials in conformity will occur. As shall be pointed out later, the deviant is rewarded in another sense for his role in the group, which makes it "profitable" for him to serve as a contrast in the conventional reward structure. Generally speaking, comparison is as essential in the maintenance of norms as is conformity: a norm becomes most evident in its occasional violation, and in this sense a group maintains "equilibrium" by a controlled balance of the relations which provide comparison and those which assure conformity.

Boundaries. Implicit in the foregoing is the argument that the presence of deviance in a group is a boundary maintaining function. The comparisons which deviance makes possible help establish the range in which the group operates, the extent of its jurisdiction over behavior, the variety of styles it contains, and these are among the essential dimensions which give a group identity and distinctiveness. In Quaker work camps, Riecken found that members prided themselves on their acceptance of deviations, and rejected such controls as ridicule and rejection (10, pp. 57-67). Homans has noted that men in the Bank Wiring Group employed certain sanctions against deviant behavior which were felt to be peculiar to the structure of the group (5). A group is distinguished in part by the norms it creates for handling deviance and by the forms of deviance it is able to absorb and contain. In helping, then, to give members a sense of their group's distinctiveness, deviant behavior on the group's margins provides an important boundary-maintaining function.

PROPOSITION THREE

KELLEY and Thibault have asserted:

It is common knowledge that when a member deviates markedly from a group standard, the remaining members of the group bring pressures to bear on the deviate to return to conformity. If pressure is of no avail, the deviate is rejected and cast out of the group. The research on this point is consistent with common sense (6, p. 768).

Apparently a deviating member who was *not* rejected after repeated violations would be defined as one who did not deviate markedly enough. While there is considerable justification to support this common-sense notion, we suggest that it overattends to rejection and neglects the range of alternatives short of rejection. The same focus is evident in the following statement by Rossi and Merton:

What the individual experiences as estrangement from a group tends to be experienced by his associates as repudiation of the group, and this ordinarily evokes a hostile response. As social relations between the individual and the rest of the group deteriorate, the norms of the group become less binding for him. For since he is progressively seceding from the group and being penalized by it, he is the less likely to experience rewards for adherence to . . . norms. Once initiated, this process seems to move toward a cumulative detachment from the group (8, p. 270).

While both of the above quotations reflect current research concerns in their attention to the group's rejection of the individual and his alienation from the group, our third proposition focuses on the common situation in which the group works to prevent elimination of a deviant member. *Groups will resist any trend toward alienation of a member whose behavior is deviant.* From the point of view of the group majority, deviants will be retained in the group up to a point where the deviant expression becomes critically dangerous to group solidarity. This accords with Kelley and Thibault's general statement, if not with its implication; but we would add that the point at which deviation becomes "markedly" extreme—and dangerous to the group—cannot be well defined in advance. This point is located by the group as a result of recurrent interaction between conforming members who respect the central norms of the group and deviating members who test its boundaries. This is the context from which the group derives a conception of what constitutes "danger," or what variations from the norm shall be viewed as "marked."

From the point of view of the deviant, then, the testing of limits is an exercise of his role in the group; from the point of view of the group, pressures are set into motion which secure the deviant in his "testing" role, yet try to assure that his deviation will not become pronounced enough to make rejection necessary. Obviously this is a delicate balance to maintain, and failures are continually visible. Yet there are a great many conditions under which it is worth while for the group to retain its deviant members and resist any trend which might lead the majority membership and other deviant members to progressive estrangement.

ILLUSTRATIONS OF PROPOSITIONS

EACH of the authors of this paper has recently completed field research which illuminates the propositions set forth here. Dentler studied the relative effectiveness of ten Quaker work projects in influencing conformity with norms of tolerance, pacifism, democratic group relations, and related social attitudes (4). One interesting sidelight in this study was the finding that while all ten groups were highly solidary, those with relatively higher numbers of sociometric isolates exhibited higher degrees of favorable increased conformity.

Case study of five of the ten groups, using interviews and participant observation, revealed that the two groups achieving the greatest favorable changes in tolerance, democratism, pacifism, and associated attitudes not only had the highest proportions of social isolates, but some of the isolates were low-ranking deviants. Of course none of the groups was without at least one isolate and one deviant, and these roles were not always occupied by the same member. But in the two high-change groups low-rank deviants were present.

In one group, one of these members came from a background that differed radically from those of other members. Although these were cooperative living and work projects, this member insisted upon separately prepared special food and complained loudly about its quality. Where three-fourths of the group members came from professional and managerial families, and dressed and acted in conformity with upper-middle-class standards, this deviant refused to wear a shirt to Sunday dinner and often came to meals without his shoes. He could not hold a job and lost two provided by the group leader during the first two weeks of the program.

His social and political attitudes also differed radically from group norms, and he was often belligerently assertive of his minority perspectives. He had no allies for his views. In an interview one of the group leaders described the group's response to this deviant:

At first we didn't know how to cope with him though we were determined to do just that. After he came to Sunday dinner in his undershirt, and after he smashed a bowl of food that had been fixed specially for him—as usual—we figured out a way to set down certain firm manners for him. There were some rules, we decided, that no one was going to violate. We knew he was very new to this kind of life and so we sought to understand him. We never rejected him. Finally, he began to come to terms; he adapted, at least enough so that we can live with him. He has begun to conform on the surface to some of our ways. It's been very hard to take that he is really proud of having lost his first two jobs and is not quiet about it. Things have gone better since we made a birthday cake for him, and I feel proud of the way our group has managed to handle this internal problem.

The same group sustained another deviant and even worked hard to retain him when he decided to leave the group. Here a group leader discusses group relations with this member:

X left our group after the first four weeks of the eight-week program. He had never been away from home before although he was about 21 years old. He couldn't seem to adjust to his job at the day camp, and he just couldn't stand doing his share of the housework and cooking. This lack of doing his share was especially hard on us, and we often discussed privately whether it would be good for him to relieve him of any household chores. We decided that wouldn't be right, but we still couldn't get him to work. Funny, but this sort of made housework the center of our group life. We are proud that no one else has shirked his chores; there is no quibbling now. . . . Anyway, X kept being pressured by his mother and brother to come home, but we gave him tremendous support. We talked it all out with him. We let him know we really wanted him to stay. This seemed to unify our group. It was working out the problem of X that seemed to unify our group. It was working out the problem of X that seemed to help us build some group standards. He began to follow some of our standards but he also stayed free to dissent. His mother finally forced him to come home.

In the second high-change group, there were also two extreme deviants. Here a group leader comments on one of them:

I've never got over feeling strongly antagonistic toward K. K has been a real troublemaker and we never really came to terms with him or controlled him significantly. He is simply a highly neurotic, conflicted person as far as life in our group goes. Personally, I've resented the fact that he has monopolized Z, who without him would have been a real contributor but who has become nothing more than a sort of poor imitation of K. After we had been here about half the summer, incidentally, a professional came out from staff headquarters and after observing our meetings he asked why K hadn't been dismissed or asked to leave the group early in the summer. But K didn't leave, of course, and most of us wouldn't want him to leave.

Finally a group leader described the reaction to the departure of its second deviant, who was repeatedly described in interviews as "kind of obnoxious:"

On the night N was upstairs talking with your interviewer, the group got together downstairs suddenly to talk about getting up a quick party, a farewell party for him. In 15 minutes, like a whirlwind, we decorated the house and some of the fellows wrote a special song of farewell for N. We also wrote a last-minute appeal asking him to stay with the group and people ran about asking, "What are you doing for N?" There seemed to be a lot of guilt among us about his leaving. We felt that maybe we hadn't done enough to get him more involved in the life of our group. I think there was some hidden envy too. After he had left, a joke began to spread around that went like this: If you leave now maybe we'll have a party for you.

The group with the lowest amount of change during the summer contained two low-ranking members, one of whom deviated from the group's norms occasionally, but no evidence came to light to indicate that this group achieved the same intensity in social relationships or the same degree of role differentiation as did groups with more extremely deviant members. Members of this low-change group reflected almost without exception the views expressed in this typical quotation:

Objectively, this is a good, congenial group of individuals. Personally they leave me a little cold. I've been in other project groups, and this is the most congenial one I've been in; yet, I don't think there will be any lasting friendships.

All these quotations reflect strong impressions embodied in our observational reports. Taken as a whole they illustrate aspects of our three postulates. While this material does not reveal the sense in which a group may induce deviance—and this is perhaps the most critical proposition of all—it does show how groups will make great efforts to keep deviant members attached to the group, to prevent full alienation. By referring to our findings about attitude change we have hoped to suggest the relevance of deviance to increasing conformity, a functional relationship of action and reaction.

In 1955-6, Erikson participated in a study of schizophrenia among basic trainees in the U.S. Army, portions of which have been published elsewhere (1). Through various interview and questionnaire techniques, a large body of data was collected which enabled the investigators to reconstruct short histories of the group life shared by the future schizophrenic and his squad prior to the former's hospitalization. There were eleven subjects in the data under consideration. The bulk of the evidence used for this short report comes from loosely structured interviews which were conducted with the entire squad in attendance, shortly after it had lost one of its members to the psychiatric hospital.

The eleven young men whose breakdown was the subject of the interviews all came from the north-eastern corner of the United States, most of them from rural or small-town communities. Typically, these men had accumulated long records of deviation in civilian life: while few of them had attracted psychiatric attention, they had left behind them fairly consistent records of job failure, school truancy, and other minor difficulties in the community. Persons in the community took notice of this behavior, of course, but they tended to be gently puzzled by it rather than attributing distinct deviant motives to it.

When such a person enters the service, vaguely aware that his past performance did not entirely live up to expectations current in his community, he is likely to start negotiating with his squad mates about the conditions of his membership in the group. He sees himself as warranting special group consideration, as a consequence of a deviant style which he himself is unable to define; yet the group has clear-cut obligations which require a high degree of responsibility and coordination from everyone. The negotiation seems to go through several successive stages, during which a reversal of original positions takes place and the individual is fitted for a role which is clearly deviant.

The first stage is characteristic of the recruit's first days in camp. His initial reaction is likely to be an abrupt attempt to discard his entire "civilian" repertoire to free himself for adoption of new styles and new ways. His new uniform for daily wear seems to become for him a symbolic uniform for his sense of identity: he is, in short, overconforming. He is likely to interpret any gesture of command as a literal moral mandate, sometimes suffering injury when told to scrub the floor until his fingers bleed, or trying to consciously repress thoughts of home when told to get everything out of his head but the military exercise of the moment.

The second stage begins shortly thereafter as he fails to recognize that "regulation" reality is different from the reality of group life, and that the circuits which carry useful information are contained within the more informal source. The pre-psychotic is, to begin with, a person for whom contacts with peers are not easy to establish, and as he tries to find his way into these circuits, looking for cues to the rhythm of group life, he sees that a fairly standard set of interaction techniques is in use. There are ways to initiate conversation, ways to impose demands, and so on. Out of this cultural lore, then, he chooses different gambits to test. He may learn to ask for matches to start discussion, be ready with a supply of cigarettes for others to "bum," or he may pick up a local joke or expression and repeat it continually. Too often, however, he misses the context in which these interaction cues are appropriate, so that his behavior, in its over-literal simplicity, becomes almost a caricature of the sociability rule he is trying to follow. We may cite the "specialist" in giving away cigarettes:

I was out of cigarettes and he had a whole pack. I said, "Joe, you got a smoke?" He says "yes," and Jesus, he gave me about twelve of them. At other times he used to offer me two or three packs of cigarettes at a time when I was out.

Or the "specialist" in greetings:

He'd go by you in the barracks and say, "What do you say, Jake?" I'd say, "Hi, George, how are you?" and he'd walk into the latrine. And he'd come by not a minute later, and it's the same thing all over again, "What do you say, Jake?" It seemed to me he was always saying "hi" to someone. You could be sitting right beside him for ten minutes and he would keep on saying it.

These clumsy overtures lead the individual and the group into the third stage. Here the recruit, almost hidden from group view in his earlier overconformity, has become a highly visible group object: his behavior is clearly "off beat," anomalous; he has made a presentation of himself to the squad, and the squad has had either to make provisions for him in the group structure or begin the process of eliminating him. The pre-psychotic is clearly a low producer, and in this sense he is potentially a handicap. Yet the group neither exerts strong pressures on him to con-form nor attempts to expel him from the squad. Instead, he is typically given a wide license to deviate from both the performance and behavior norms of the group, and the group in turn forms a hard protective shell around him which hides him from exposure to outside authorities.

His duties are performed by others, and in response the squad only seems to ask of him that he be at least consistent in his deviation—that he be consistently helpless and consistently anomalous. In a sense, he be-comes the ward of the group, hidden from outside view but the object of friendly ridicule within. He is referred to as "our teddy bear," "our pet," "mascot," "little brother," "toy," and so on. In a setting where having buddies is highly valued, he is unlikely to receive any sociometric choices at all. But it would be quite unfortunate to assume that he is therefore isolated from the group or repudiated by it: an accurate sociogram would have the deviant individual encircled by the interlocking sociometric preferences, sheltered by the group structure, and an important point of reference for it.

The examples just presented are weak in that they include only failures of the process described. The shell which protected the deviant from visibility leaked, outside medical authorities were notified, and he was eventually hospitalized. But as a final note it is interesting to observe that the shell remained even after the person for whom it was erected had withdrawn. Large portions of every squad interview were devoted to arguments, directed at a psychiatrist, that the departed member was not ill and should never have been hospitalized.

DISCUSSION

THE most widely cited social theories of deviant behavior which have appeared in recent years—notably those of Merton and Parsons (8; 9)—have helped turn sociologists' attention from earlier models of social pathology in which deviance was seen as direct evidence of disorganiza-tion. These newer models have attended to the problem of how social structures exert pressure on certain individuals rather than others toward the expression of deviance. Yet the break with the older social disorgani-zation tradition is only partial, since these theories still regard deviance from the point of view of its value as a "symptom" of dysfunctional struc-tures. One aim of this paper is to encourage a functional approach to deviance, to consider the contributions deviant behavior may make toward the development of organizational structures, rather than focusing on the implicit assumption that structures must be somehow in a state of disrepair if they produce deviant behavior.

Any group attempts to locate its position in social space by defining its symbolic boundaries, and this process of self-location takes place not only in reference to the central norms which the group develops but in reference to the *range* of possibilities which the culture makes available. Specialized statuses which are located on the margins of the group, chiefly high-rank leaders and low-rank deviants, become critical referents for establishing the end points of this range, the group boundaries.

As both the Quaker and Army illustrations suggest, deviant members are important targets toward which group concerns become focused. Not only do they symbolize the group's activities, but they help give other members a sense of group size, its range and extent, by marking where the group begins and ends in space. In general, the deviant seems to help give the group structure a visible "shape." The deviant is someone about whom something should be done, and the group, in expressing this concern, is able to reaffirm its essential cohesion and indicate what the group is and what it can do. Of course the character of the deviant behavior in each group would vary with the group's general objectives, its relationship to the larger culture, and so on. In both the Quaker groups and Army squads, nurturance was a strong element of the other members' reaction to their deviant fellow. More specifically in the Army material it is fairly sure that the degree of helplessness and softness supplied by the pre-psychotic introduced emotional qualities which the population—lacking women and younger persons—could not otherwise afford.

These have been short and necessarily limited illustrations of the propositions advanced. In a brief final note we would like to point out how this crude theory could articulate with the small group research tradition by suggesting one relatively ideal laboratory procedure that might be used. Groups composed of extremely homogeneous members should be assigned tasks which require group solution but which impose a high similarity of activity upon all members. If role differentiation occurs, then, it would be less a product of individual differences or the specific requirements of the task than a product of group formation. We would hypothesize that such differentiation would take place, and that one or more roles thus differentiated would be reserved for deviants. The occupants of these deviant roles should be removed from the group. If the propositions have substance, the group—and this is the critical hypothesis—would realign its members so that these roles would become occupied by other members. While no single experiment could address all the implications of our paradigm, this one would confront its main point.

This paper, of course, has deliberately neglected those group conditions in which deviant behavior becomes dysfunctional: it is a frequent group experience that deviant behavior fails to provide a valued function for the structure and helps reduce performance standards or lower levels of interaction. We have attempted here to present a side of the coin which we felt was often neglected, and in our turn we are equally—if intentionally—guilty of neglect.

SUMMARY

This paper has proposed the following interpretations of deviant behavior in enduring primary and task groups:

1. Deviant behavior tends to be induced, permitted, and sustained by a given group.

2. Deviant behavior functions to help maintain group equilibrium.

3. Groups will resist any trend toward alienation of a member whose behavior is deviant.

The substance of each proposition was discussed heuristically and illustrated by reference to field studies of deviant behavior in Quaker work projects and Army basic training squads. A laboratory test was suggested as one kind of critical test of the paradigm. The aim of the presentation was to direct attention to the functional interdependence of deviance and organization.

REFERENCES

1. Artiss, Kenneth L., ed., *The Symptom as Communication in Schizophrenia* (New York: Grune and Stratton, 1959).
2. Bales, Robert F., "The Equilibrium Problem in Small Groups," in *Small Groups*, A. Paul Hare, et al., eds. New York: Knopf, 1955), 424-456.
3. Cohen, Albert K., "The Study of Social Disorganization and Deviant Behavior," in *Sociology Today*, Robert K. Merton, et al., eds. (New York: Basic Books, 1959), 461-484.
4. Dentler, Robert, *The Young Volunteers* (Chicago: National Opinion Research Center Report, 1959).
5. Homans, George W., *The Human Group* (New York: Harcourt, Brace, 1950).
6. Kelley, Harold H., and John W. Thibault, "Experimental Studies of Group Problem Solving and Process," in *Handbook of Social Psychology*, Vol. II, Gardner Lindzey, ed. (Cambridge: Addison-Wesley, 1954), 759-768.
7. McCurdy, Harold G., and Wallace E. Lambert, "The Efficiency of Small Human Groups in the Solution of Problems Requiring Genuine Cooperation," *Journal of Personality*, 20 (June, 1952), 478-494.
8. Merton, Robert K., *Social Theory and Social Structure*, rev. ed. (Glencoe: Free Press, 1957).
9. Parsons, Talcott, *The Social System* (Glencoe: Free Press, 1951), 256-267,

321-325; and Talcott Parsons, Robert F. Bales and Edward A. Shils, *Working Papers in the Theory of Action* (Glencoe: Free Press, 1953), 67-78.

10. Riecken, Henry, *Volunteer Work Camp* (Cambridge: Addison-Wesley, 1952), 57-67.
11. Riecken, Henry, and George W. Homans, "Psychological Aspects of Social Structure," in *Handbook of Social Psychology*, Vol. II, Gardner Lindzey, ed. (Cambridge: Addison-Wesley, 1954), 786-832.

ॐ

C H A P T E R 2 1   The Triple Bind: Toward a
Unified Theory of Individual and Social Deviancy*

HOWARD W. POLSKY, IRVING KARP, AND IRWIN BERMAN

HAWTHORNE Cedar Knolls School has pioneered for over sixty years
in the study and treatment of emotionally disturbed delinquent children. Its clinic established thirty years ago, has made important contributions in the treatment of delinquent psychopathology.[1][2][3] A major focus in
recent years has been the conceptualization of its semi-autonomous subcultural resident units.[4][5][6] It has experimented continuously with the
fashioning of the environment into a therapeutic instrument.[7] Over the
last year the Peer Culture Project[8] has been engaged in formulating a
unified theory of individual and social deviancy. Its purpose is to enlarge
the effective unit of treatment from the caseworker-individual relationship
to the residents' primary groups. We want to remove the institutionalization of theoretical orientations and social structures which focus either on
the disturbed individual or the pathological social environment. We do
not see pathology as an either/or proposition, but as a spectrum of behavior, individual and social, which social scientists and clinicians can
better understand and treat by working together.

The sociological insistence that society shapes deviant subcultures is a
critical corrective to psychological explanations. The explanation of subcultural delinquency as an exclusive product of social conditions, however, fails to take into account psychopathology—which, to be sure, arises
from a social base—but once risen, is more or less autonomous. How
pathological defenses are interwoven and supported by the social structure is of supreme importance in residential treatment, and, indeed, in
other settings as well.

Subcultural delinquencies are unacceptable ways to society of achieving
instinctual, status, and material gratification. Deception, manipulation,

* Reprinted from the *Journal of Human Relations*, 11 (1962), 68–87, by permission
of the authors and the *Journal*.

and physical coercion are the delinquents' modalities. The "ideal" delinquent gets what he wants regardless of what society or his conscience demands of him. He has poor capacity to tolerate internal stress. Interpersonal conflict is substituted for grappling internally with fears ranging from homosexuality to loss in social esteem.[9] In contrast to the schizoid adolescent, who avoids external stimulation by retirement into a fantasy world, the mobile delinquent is in antagonistic conflict with society.[10]

The emotionally disturbed delinquent has gone awry early in the socialization process in his struggle with adult authority.[11] He has internalized a defective psychic representative (superego) of parents and neighborhood, which disables him from participating normally in society as he grows older.[12] By "defective" we do not mean that the delinquent has necessarily projected a distorted image of early adult models upon reality; not infrequently he is nurtured in a coercive and manipulative milieu. His present situation, however benign, is distortedly perceived in accordance with past projections and experiences, as if it were hostile. The delinquent feels rejected and exploited and is disposed to distrust and outmaneuver the enemy. The focus of the conflict is *between* him and the external world, not within himself.

As he grows older, the delinquent becomes increasingly vulnerable to society's sanctions. More discipline is expected of him as he matures. To withstand these pressures he draws increasingly upon peer support. He becomes more wary and versatile in his attack against adult authority. Since the superego is derived from identification with parental figures from whom the delinquent is now alienated, affiliation with peers provides substitute emotional attachments for his parents. The peer group is a substitute for what he has lost with increased distance from his own family. When he combines with boys with similar problems, a new social phenomenon emerges.

In their interaction, the aggressive delinquents reinforce each other's hostility and evolve a common perceptual outlook toward adults, their common enemy, who are to be subverted by any means.[13] For delinquents, interpersonal tension is more manageable than intrapsychic conflict, so that the gang in seeking, encouraging, and challenging community rejection is in forward momentum. The delinquent group's hostility to outsiders is enhanced by severe punishment, accommodation, and/or inadequacy of adults in contact with them. The more hostile society is to them, the more the boys' distorted perceptual system is confirmed.

The delinquent leader's function in the group is crucial. He protects the group's social system against outsiders. An authoritarian group morality evolves in an intensified struggle with society. Each boy cannot always mobilize himself, however, to fit the group's standards, so that an internal threat to its solidarity is omnipresent. Internal group discipline moreover, recreates for each member transference problems related to prior familial adaptations.

In order to conceptualize how pathological defenses interlock within the peer subculture, we have to analyze the group social structure. At Hawthorne each boy lives in a web of social relations in the cottage. The roles that the boys evolve in the peer culture bring into play transference phenomena that tie their past with their current social practice. Instead of group solidarity among delinquents, we have witnessed a coercive peer social system. How does the intensively exploitative situation within the peer culture square with the boys' need to maintain an efficient common attack against society?

The solution to this problem entails conceptualization of three systems —individual, peer subculture, and community—as they feed back into each other and trap the delinquent in a *triple bind*. Since early childhood these boys have been in extreme conflict with authority. Would this not characterize their internal relations as well? But how? Against society, they transfer attitudes and behavioral patterns typified by their struggles with their own parents; but in the peer pecking order, depending upon their status, they assume either the same or the reciprocal of the aggressor-aggressed role set vis-a-vis adults. This is why the "queer," "rat," or "mutation" (the scapegoat at the bottom of the pyramid) must be "invented" if someone with predisposing talents cannot be found. In the gang, the leader imposes his will in relative isolation from disapproving adults. Even the lowly bushboy, however manacled he may be by "his" gang, will have moments of solidarity in the fight against other gangs or adults.

Our work is a logical extension of current subculture theory. Albert Cohen, for example, carried his investigations to the point of the rejected (the delinquents) rejecting the rejectors.[14] He did not, however, develop the implications for the impact of these external relations upon the internal organization of the peer culture; and, the impact of peer roles upon the members' psychic structures. The study of these interchanges and mechanisms which feed back upon one another is the focus of our orientation. For in the process of mobilizing against the "aggressive" adult world, delinquents identify with that aggressor and create an authoritarian structure in which the leadership exploits its followers by imposing the "same" suppressive controls which adults impose upon them. It is in the peer social organization, the reconstituted "family" that the boys' pathology is reinforced in a fantasy system through mutually supportive transferences. Society's suppression of the peer group reinforces the entire circular process.

Thus, the delinquent is pinned in a peer culture which is evolving a value system opposed to society; he is enmeshed in a system of exploitative internal peer relations; and both processes reinforce defective super-ego functioning. In effect, the delinquent is caught in a "triple bind." By "bind" we mean the pathological articulation of two systems—between individual and group or between groups—whereby a pathological balance is maintained through the pressure of each system upon the other. It may be likened to two fencers momentarily transfixed by the pressures emanating from the continuous equal force of their foils upon each other.

In our subculture studies at Hawthorne, Bind I is the pathological articulation of the peer group (or the individual in the role of a group member) and the community.[15] Bind II refers to the systems of peer group roles awaiting the newcomer.[16] The relationship of the individual's intrapsychic structure and his role in the peer group constitutes Bind III.[17] In the remainder of this paper we illustrate each bind and their interconnections.

A CASE STUDY

FOR the last year an interdisciplinary team consisting of a sociologist, clinician, group worker, and psychologist have been studying cottage subgroups. The team observed a high conflict subgroup of four boys in a senior cottage for several months.

The boys' relationship was felt by the staff to be so destructive that the dominant member of the subgroup, Joel Mechanic, was transferred to another cottage. Six weeks after the boys were separated, however, we brought them together in Dr. Nathan Ackerman's studio at the Jewish Family Service and experimented with reproducing on film the boys' social field in the cottage. The boys were simply asked by the clinical group worker who was with them in the cottage to describe their life at Hawthorne. In the studio they instantly reconstructed their natural subgroup as it had been observed by the two researchers in the cottage for several months.

A CONFLICT SUBGROUP: BIND II

THE key concept for studying social relations is *role*—a pattern of behavior an individual enacts in the group which is oriented by and to other members. The concept of role induction refers to behavior as it is molded by the expectations of "significant others" in the individual's milieu. The first task is to locate the subgroup in the cottage and institution in a historical perspective. Art Noble, Steve Leopard, and a third boy constituted a high status group in Cottage 17. Noble, the leader, urged his roommates to "stay out of trouble." They were, "close and equal." Subsequently, Joel Mechanic from 19, a tougher cottage, was moved into Cottage 17, into Noble and Leopard's room in the place of the third boy. The aura of comradeship was shattered. The new arrival, Joel Mechanic, made it clear that he was to be the dominant person in the room and cottage. Leopard shifted his allegiance from Noble to Mechanic, and the two ridiculed and denigrated Noble. Mechanic and Leopard began to steal together and support each other in ignoring and defying adult authority. Whenever the new, inexperienced cottage parents ventured to control Mechanic, he belligerently responded, "Are you threatening me?" making them withdraw. Noble confronted the cottage parents: "If you let Mechanic con you, I'm going to do these things too." A fourth boy, Kritic, who came into cottage 17 with Mechanic, sought to join up with Mechanic. The subgroup organization is epitomized in the boys' epithets of each other: Mechanic, the "big man," was Kritic's "ace" and "guardian angel"; Kritic was the "chickie" (lookout); Leopard was regarded as Mechanic's "handyman" and "pushover"; and Noble was the "progressive" —who was playing "cool to get out of Hawthorne." In summary, Joel Mechanic, the aggressive con leader inducted Leopard into delinquency, ranked (denigrated) Noble and flaunted cottage parental authority. Kritic ingratiated himself into Mechanic's orbit.

The group's aggressive value system is reproduced on the film in the opening scenes and pervades the entire proceedings. Note how Kritic elaborates Joel Mechanic's aggressive role, as the latter recalls his entrance into Cottage 17 from 19. (Mr. Karp is the clinical group worker and interviewer).

Karp: All right . . . how was 19 different from 17?
Mechanic: (*Bragging*) Well, we had guys with guts . . . 17 had nobody.
Noble: I wouldn't say that. (*Leopard Laughs*)
Mechanic: They still do . . . they can stomp out 17 like nothin'.
Karp: Well, what did 19 have, specifically . . . as a cottage . . .
Mechanic: Everyone stuck together . . . (*Pause*)
Karp: Do you remember your reaction, Joel, when you heard there was going to be seniority in 17?
Kritic: (*Glances at Karp*) I'll tell you what his reaction was . . . (*Mimicking Mechanic's Voice and Posture*) . . . When I'm there, there's not going to be *no seniority!*
Karp: What would happen if there were seniority?
Kritic: . . . 19 had no seniority, 17 is no better . . . so we figured if somebody comes over and starts bothering you, he'll land on his ass or something . . .

In the film Leopard's shift from Noble to Mechanic is re-enacted. In the extract below Leopard remarks that all three were friends at first and reverses himself in less than a minute in reacting to Mechanic's continuous pressure upon Noble.

Karp: Now what happened to you? Joel is in the room now.
Leopard: Well, we started to get to be good friends all three of us . . . (*During this speech Noble faces Leopard and Listens attentively*) . . . but uh, I don't know what happened or when it happened (*Smiling*) but Joel and I started doing things together, you know, we would see something we liked, we wouldn't say a word, we

would just pick it up and take it into the room. (*Noble flicks ash, then turns to Leopard again. Mechanic just stares ahead, no expression*) Whatever it was we did, it was together . . . whether it was wrong or right, it was together. Arty Noble seemed to be left out . . .

Noble: (*To Karp*) I saw conflict where me and Steve (Leopard) used to talk Jewish at night (*Leopard turns to Mechanic and smiles at him knowingly*) and me and Steve were talking a little bit and Joel said he didn't like it and . . . uh . . . we got into an argument about that and (*Earnestly*) that's where the break started to occur . . .

Mechanic: (*To Noble Haughtily*) There never was nothin' to break, it was always broken. (*Looks away disdainfully*)

Leopard: Yeah, that was true . . . ever since the first day. (*Looks down*)

The film catches three systems in transaction: the individual youngster, the peer group, and society, represented by the clinical group worker and the camera. Within the rigid aggressive framework that Mechanic imposes upon the group, Noble launches a skillful, diversified attack against Mechanic, banking upon the superego support of the group worker and the "camera." He discourses at length on another aggressive leader, Barry, who preceded Joel Mechanic. Barry had "personality," and didn't have to use force all the time. Noble is implying that something is wrong with Joel Mechanic because the latter uses threatening "power" all of the time.

Noble: . . . and when Barry left and Joel came in, I didn't look up to Joel. Joel was one of the bigger guys. Joel wasn't as big as Barry (*Looks over at Mechanic*) and Joel didn't have the personality of Barry. Because me and Barry, when we fought, we were friends. We could always talk about something.

Mechanic: (*Firmly*) I'm *glad* I don't have the personality of Barry . . . (*Leopard smiles self-knowingly*)

Noble: I liked Barry a lot, but that's not the point. And Barry . . . (*Mechanic Laughs*)

Mechanic: You cleaned his pipe.

Noble: I never cleaned his pipe . . . (*Mechanic laughs, ridicules*) We used to get together. We all felt important, you know. It wasn't a continuous battle (*Mechanic laughs with body*) for power. Barry didn't have to use force, it was there. But with Joel was a different setup. (*Mechanic and Leopard Whisper and Laugh*) Joel was always more or less a threatening power . . .

Mechanic: (*Looking away from them, fingers arm of chair, sighs*) I never enforced nothin'.

Noble: True, but whenever you spoke, you spoke in a tone, "Well, (*To Mechanic*) come on and do something about it if you don't like it." Or something like that.

In this manner Noble reproaches Mechanic for three-fourths of the first half hour of the film; then in a dramatic obligatory scene, Joel Mechanic, Leopard, and Kritic join forces in a devastating counterattack which strips Noble of his pretensions. Kritic plays the pivotal role in turning the group upon Noble:

Kritic:	(*Rocks chair*) When Joel did leave, something split inside. You ... practically ran the cottage.
Mechanic:	That's right, and you're trying to run it *now*.
Noble:	(*To Mechanic, shaking head and dragging on Cigarette*) No sir! No sir! I *never* tried to run the cottage!
Kritic:	At the time that Joel left you did try to run the cottage.
Mechanic:	(*Talks, Overlaps Kritic*) The day I left (*Points finger at Noble*) you changed all the furniture around the room . . . You were taking advantage of him. (*Indicating Leopard with thumb*)
Noble:	I wasn't taking advantage of him.
Mechanic:	(*Rapidly, Malice evident*) Because you know, it would have went against you. You wanted to get back at him!
Noble:	Maybe!
Mechanic:	And (*points finger for emphasis at Leopard*) you wanted revenge.
Noble:	I didn't want revenge against *you* (*Emphasis*) (*Leopard Laughs*)
Mechanic:	. . . Now that I was out of the cottage you had known that you were top man (*Using finger for emphasis*) and that wasn't saying much . . .
Kritic:	Without asking anybody, you walk right over to the television set and said, (*Mimicking Noble*) This is weak and turned the channel . . .

BIND I. SUBGROUP AND COMMUNITY

WHAT is the relationship between the internal processes in this subgroup and the institution? Mechanic "selected" two key adult figures as models. His closest adult friend was the toughest child care counselor on the campus who wakened Mechanic in the morning by tossing him out of bed. The other major figure was the unit supervisor, with whom Mechanic was in a constant power struggle, but could not defy openly. Mechanic infrequently saw his social worker. The cottage parents were viewed as powerless figures who could not prevent Mechanic and Leopard's acting out:

Karp:	I understand when you fellows had the TV, other fellows had the idea, but you told them they'd better not . . .
Leopard:	No one had the guts enough to walk down and take it. We just decided we needed a television for the day and we forgot to bring it back down . . .
Karp:	And if you saw something you wanted . . .
Leopard:	We would take it without any question. (*Mechanic nodding in agreement*)

Mechanic:	And we always slimed our way out of it . . . if they asked us where we got it from.
Karp:	So you managed to get away with a lot, quite a bit more than the other boys in the cottage.
Leopard &	(*Leopard starts to bite nails quickly*)
Mechanic:	Yeah.
Karp:	How did you manager to get away with so much?
Leopard:	(*Pauses*) (*To Mechanic for Confirmation*) That's a secret. That's a secret. (*Laughs*)
Mechanic:	(*Rubbing Leg*) We had a technique that was good. When we did borrow something, we did it only on occasion, not every other day. (*Noble Yawns*) . . .

Thus Mechanic was manipulative in his dealings with the two power figures who impinged upon him and disdainful of weak adult figures like the cottage parents who could not "catch" him. How did these attitudes feed back into the peer group? In the excerpt below, Joel Mechanic reveals his contemptuous attitude not only towards Noble, his sworn adversary, but also Leopard, his ally:

Karp:	How did you size up the group? Now here were these two fellows . . .
Mechanic:	(*With Grin to Karp*) Two *schmucks!* (*Noble momentarily stops shaking cigarette out of pack and smiles weakly at Mechanic*)
Karp:	All right.
Leopard:	(*Protesting*) Hup! Hup! (*Noble is facing away from Mechanic, putting Cigarette into mouth*)
Mechanic:	That's right, when I first moved in, that's what you were!
Karp:	All right . . . so what . . .
	(*Kritic coolly looks at Mechanic*)
Mechanic:	Compared to the guys in our cottage you were two *schmucks.*
Karp:	So how do you figure it, now what are you going to do about it: Here you were in the room with two *schmucks* . . . as you say . . . how, how did you get close with one? (*Noble has finished lighting cigarette and looks at Mechanic*)
Mechanic:	(*Struggling*) Dunno. We just drifted together, that's all. He liked the things I liked. He liked to rob (*Smiles*) and everything . . . (*He stretches out legs. Leopard Laughs*)
Karp:	You mean you both had ideas on how to work angles?
Mechanic & Leopard:	Yeah.

Why do we refer to the institution-subgroup complex as a bind? Here the film is nonpareil in capturing tensions and conflicts that less sensitive instruments blur. Mechanic is in a tight position during the filming: on one side, Noble has been attacking him as a bully, on the other the camera threatens to expose him as such. He must be careful not to reveal too much to the authorities who have power over him; yet he must be sure to put the *schmucks* in their place. All of this is sharply etched in a sequence which takes less than ten seconds to enact:

Karp: So you were trying to settle . . . so what were you trying to settle with him, (*Noble*) Joel?
Mechanic: I was going to put it to him. I wasn't going to take it from no one. And I was going to be on top. (*Puts candy in mouth*)
Karp: All right. So this was a way of proving it. You feel that . . .
Mechanic: Proving what?
Karp: That you were on top.
Mechanic: I didn't want to prove nothing.
Karp: Well, what is it that . . .
Mechanic: I just wanted to whip him, that's all.
Karp: For what reason?
Mechanic: (*To Karp*) I don't know. Maybe I didn't like him. I don't know, I can't remember back that far.

In his flagrantly insincere relations with staff, Mechanic has the added burden of masking his aggression in the peer group.

BIND III. INDIVIDUAL—PEER GROUP RELATIONSHIP

So FAR we have outlined the relationship between this miniature peer group system and the institution, and the feedback into the boys' internal relations. The next crucial issue is this: How do the boys' defenses reinforce these two systems of interaction—within the peer group and between it and the institution? We shall briefly summarize the boys' psychodynamic pictures and draw upon the film for behavioral validation. Then we shall illustrate how the boys' unconscious distortions complement each other in the peer group social system.

Since the behavior in the group is the product of personality predispositions and the social situation, how can the two be separated for analysis? We have to estimate each boy's patterned distortion in the context of his intrapsychic structure and history. Sappenfield refers to this process as *perceptual identification:* . . . "interpreting two or more objects or events as if they were identical." Perceptual identification, in other words, involves imputing to different stimuli, which are in fact not identical, an equivalent (identical or nearly identical) meaning. Whenever two processes, two objects, two symbols, a symbol and an object, etc., are interpreted as having identical value for the satisfaction or frustration of an active motivational pattern, perceptual identification may be said to occur.[18]

THE SUBGROUP MEMBERS

MECHANIC

A LARGE, muscular, 16 year-old oral character disorder, Mechanic was in institutional placement since the age of six. He has a history of bullying weaker boys and leading them into delinquency. The world is hostile, full of depriving adults and competing peers. Mechanic has repressed his superego and projected it on to watchful adults who must be subverted in order for him to achieve insatiable material and status gratification. Peers who express adult values are perceptually identified as hostile superego representatives who must be punched out of existence. Noble, for example, has "the kind of look that you like to punch in."

According to Noble, Mechanic "wasn't afraid to punch a guy in the face, and he wouldn't feel bad about it . . . he'd suffer no qualms." This is what Leopard meant when he referred to Mechanic as "cold-blooded." Whereas Noble, initially recalled that all three were together at first, and in this he is supported by Leopard, Mechanic insists that "it (relationship) was always broken," and hence "there was never nothin' to break." During Leopard's and Mechanic's acting out, Noble (according to Mechanic) "was never around when we did things like that." One of Mechanic's favorite words is "stomp out" which he uses in the film several times.

Finally, he brags in the film about his prowess for outmaneuvering the staff: "we always slimed out of it [when caught with stolen articles] . . . if they asked us where we got it from . . . we had a technique that was good. When we *did* borrow something, we did it only on occasion, not every other day . . . we never did get caught. . . ."

LEOPARD

A soft, light complexioned 16 year-old, neurotic, accident-prone youngster, Leopard stems from a Jewish orthodox home; at puberty he became unmanageable and truant from school. His inner state is chaotic. His fragile ego cannot integrate libidinal wishes, his harsh superego and external reality demands. He outflanks this conflict by "letting" others use him. Referring to his stealing and acting out with Mechanic, Leopard says: ". . . but then Joel came in. I dunno what happened, I just went. I dunno where I went, but I went."

The libidinal picture is confused, because he has investments apparently on all levels: a constant floating up and down the psychosexual scale with no real object cathexis taking place. Leopard enjoys having two boys fight over him and tells Kritic: ". . . you were enjoying it too!"

Instead of making compromises as do many adolescents when they are in conflict, Leopard vacillates between enacting the impulse and enacting the defense. He does not enact the original impulse, but a watered-down symbolic version and derives alleviation of guilt through punishment. Leopard is the most neurotic of the boys and derives sexual satisfaction by being overpowered.

Leopard does not see a connection between the injury he sustains and his guilt which was present as a result of enacting an impulse which violated his superego. His outstanding trait, his ambivalence, pervades all of his activity and indeed his very speech pattern throughout the film:

"Well before Joel came in, our room, you might say, was the honor room, though we all got into trouble" (Bursts into an embarrassed chuckle and looks down). And in another place, "We stayed out of riots, though we always got blamed for it" (laughs self-consciously).

Leopard cautions Mechanic not to say anything into the microphone, and avoid trouble: ". . . they can hear it." A few moments later he laughs appreciatively at Mechanic's raspberry and later on stimulates him to make disruptive noises into the microphone.

NOBLE

A 16 YEAR-OLD, borderline paranoid, schizophrenic boy, Noble was referred to Hawthorne for shooting a rifle in a school yard, and incorrigible behavior at home. He had threatened to kill his older brother and mother. Shortly after the film was made his father did shoot at the mother, wounded her, and killed himself. Noble speaks of gang fights and slashing a boy's face with a belt buckle. He had a series of fights with boys when he first arrived at Hawthorne, but later took on the role of reformed convert.

Noble is threatened by strong homosexual and destructive urges. He attempts to repress and deny these urges by projecting them onto the environment. He disavows personal responsibilities for the "jungle" which he sees as originating in others rather than within himself. In the film he repeatedly views the sources of trouble as *external* and above himself: "*Things were happening* in the cottage and it more or less started *coming down to us . . .*"

Although Noble tries to dissociate himself from evil acting out he reveals his own emotional investment in it: "We stayed out of riots . . . none of this crap was for us . . . we don't wanna get blamed for what the other guys are doing, so we stayed out and we just watched and we were having *just as much fun.*"

He can criticize his own past, but always as a counterpart to his present reformed behavior. "I was really gone, I didn't give a damn about anybody, about anybody's feelings. All I cared for was myself . . ."

Noble is a moralist who elicits the sympathy of adults by talking to them about this "jungle." He tries to convince staff and peers that he is a good boy: "I always talked nicely . . . I told him if he didn't like it he could change it . . . " When he becomes overly dependent, he becomes anxious and paranoid.

Structurally, Noble has a severe ego weakness, which induces him to rely heavily on projections. He converts people to his point of view in order to have a congenial environment; he projects his unacceptable wishes on to some adults and peers and converts others into an alliance against them; thus he transforms his internal aggression into interpersonal and intergroup battles.

KRITIC

A SMALL 15 year-old, "pre-oedipal, oral biting" youngster, Kritic was referred to Hawthorne because he was unmanageable at home and school. He stayed out late, had temper tantrums and fought his siblings. He stole at school and did poor school work. He associated with older boys whom he felt he had to impress with his aggressiveness. Kritic feels that he is small in a world of big, capricious adults and tough aggressive peers. He has a need to prove he is as big as they.

Teasing in a biting fashion as an interpersonal defence dominates his psychic picture. He wants to be accepted by the big boys and, like a jackal, share in the feast. If he's allowed to hang around, he'll share the spoils; where there is action, some of it is going to rub off on him. He has a need to prove that he's really as big as the other guys, so that he can be admitted into the fold. His reality testing is quite seriously defective on this score. He provokes people beyond their point of tolerance. There is a naive optimism about what he can do and this is suggestive of some ego defect in an otherwise shrewd capacity to size up situations. He has an extreme tendency to find other's weak spots, and provoke them by cutting them down to his size.

Kritic not only volunteers to speak for Mechanic, but in doing so *mimics* Mechanic's tough voice and posture: ". . . I'll tell you what his reaction was: "When I'm there, there's not going to be *no* seniority!"

Kritic ridicules Noble's attempt to mask aggression. ". . . you walked right over to the television set and said, *"this is weak,"* and turned the channel . . ." ". . . and I came over to you and you said, 'get the hell outta here.'"

Kritic graphically summarizes the conflict between Mechanic and Noble: it was to see ". . . *who was the bigger man.*" Kritic dares to contradict Mechanic who responds, "Oh we knew that," and Kritic quickly rejoins, ". . . no, we didn't know that."

Kritic convinces himself that he is the equal of the bigger men, but they don't share his image of him. Mechanic and Leopard ridicule him as ". . . bringing in crackers and pretzels," which makes Kritic uncomfortable, and which he tries to shrug off.

THE FANTASY SOCIAL SYSTEM

How do the boy's distortions interlock in the peer subgroup? Noble and Mechanic project different parts of the psychic establishment. Noble projects unacceptable aggressive wishes on to others; Mechanic represses the superego and projects it on to adults and peers, like Noble, whom he suspects of supporting staff. Mechanic and Leopard regarded the new cottage parents as weak representatives of authority. In this vacuum, Noble becomes the substitute target. He inherits hostility that is primarily directed at the staff, but he offers the advantage to Mechanic and Leopard of being around to be abused as they feel the need, without impunity. They sense Noble's hypocrisy and enjoy undermining his judgmental posture of their delinquency. Their counterattack to Noble's pretenses is direct as if to say: "You are not strong, we can make a *schmuck* out of you, You are a *schmuck*, and we shall treat you accordingly." Mechanic's rigid hostility towards Noble is intensified by Noble's extreme identification with the staff:

Noble: And when I heard Joel was coming in, I didn't like the idea but
            I says, well, if he's coming in there's nothing we can do about it
            . . . (*Cautiously, Looking Uncertainly at Joel*) . . . that's the way
            the staff wants it. (*Leopard Flaps his Arms a Bit*) We accepted
            him right away, into the thing.
Mechanic: (*Facing Noble*) you didn't have no choice. (*Noble Turns to
            Mechanic*)

Mechanic and the others sense that Noble wants to commit antisocial acts too. At the same time, Noble represents superego inhibitions.

This formulation is related to the boys' diametrically opposed relations to the staff. Noble ingratiates himself with adults and seeks their support to help him repress his instinctual drives. He is eager to share his inner world with adults because he wants them to understand and join him in his fight against the jungle and to buttress his fragile defenses. Mechanic distrusts adults, with whom he is flagrantly insincere. He is suspicious that adults are watching him all the time and he will not divulge any information which exposes himself. Staff ideals threaten to contaminate him and curb aggressive impulses which are gratified through manipulation, bullying, and the buildup of an elaborate precautionary network. Noble, on his side, shifts his allegiance from the peer group to the staff; as the two opposing value systems become polarized he throws himself on the side of the staff and alienates himself further from his peers. By projecting his unacceptable impulses on to peers and aligning himself with the cottage parents, he fictitiously controls his own aggressive impulses.

But by playing along with the cottage parents, Noble becomes game for the boy's hostility and contributes to that jungle that is smothering him. To have external justification that the world is a jungle right in his own room, relieves him of the burden of projecting his aggressive impulses further out into the environment. His intrapsychic struggle is transformed into an interpersonal battle between himself and Mechanic. Moreover, his expectations for adults to be strong authority figures is unrealistically heightened, and when they disappoint him he threatens to abandon them. The role which Mechanic and Leopard carved out for Noble as the rejected "superego" is reinforced by the latter's pathology. Noble derives gratification in the role of the group superego because it fulfills his defense of projecting unacceptable aggressive wishes on to others. The more vigorously he plays the role of the staff superego in the subgroup, the more he is denigrated by Mechanic and the more his paranoia is supported by actual persecution.

When a person is cast in a role supported by the unconscious distortions of his associates, the social structure coheres because of, and not in spite of, severe overt conflict. Noble's decision not to leave the bedroom is related to his unconscious compliance with the abusers and opposition to them, rather than coming to grips with his own aggression. Mechanic has transferred the projected superego from the staff to Noble, whom he rigidly and mechanically puts in his place. Leopard, in turn, derives vicarious gratification out of the suppression of Noble, and indirectly, his own superego, and is brought into a closer symbiotic bind with Mechanic. In the film, Leopard's provocation of Mechanic to act out is vividly and continuously dramatized.

Leopard emerges most clearly in our analysis for the exemplification of the splitoff of intrapsychic processes in the group structure and their interlocking into a fantasy social system. Mechanic and Noble are the two external representatives of Leopard's internal conflict between id impulses and superego prohibitions. Leopard became attracted to Mechanic because he represented guilt free libidinal acting out. Mechanic's defense is not to appear guilty. Guilt accompanies Leopard everywhere, and his ambivalence makes him raw with it. In this turmoil, Leopard selects not any bad boy, but someone well defended against guilt. Mechanic fits this role perfectly.

Kritic is the outsider. He senses that Mechanic and Leopard are forming an alliance to get what they want and he wants in also. He is rejected by them for two reasons: (1) they saw a "little *schmuck*" weak and puny. He was only excess baggage, and (2) his biting and sarcastic criticism frequently punctured their bloated self-image. Kritic tried to join in by projecting an image of a powerful figure and convince them that they could be stronger with him in, but they could not see it that way. Mechanic recoiled from the small, pretentious boy who potentially could prick his omnipotent bubble. Kritic contributes to Mechanic's and Leopard's manipulation and aggression by his admiration and repeated attempts to be identified with him.

Mechanic constantly reproduces a social field populated by inferior, hated rivals and dependent symbiotic allies. One is either for or against Mechanic. Both Noble, his opponent, and Leopard, his ally, consciously and unconsciously reinforce his aggressive and manipulative outlook.

Interwoven with the power struggles is the boys' latent homosexuality. The aggressor is masculine and his target is in effect castrated. When the target submits, he is in danger of being cast in the feminine role. Mechanic refers to Noble as the "pipe-cleaner" of Barry, the former tough leader.

What we have in effect are two power pyramids: (1) the subordinate position of the peer group to the staff; and, (2) the internal pecking order of the peer subgroup. Both structures are interwoven with the boys' psychopathology. The boys are caught in a triple bind. They oppose staff authority by varying forms of subversion. In their own group, through identification with the "aggressor," they create stereotyped, coercive relationships. These two systems reinforce the boys' pathological defenses.

We have tried to demonstrate that the gang code evolves from the struggle of the residents against the staff, in the authoritarian management of peers of one another, and that both processes are rooted in each boy's pathological defenses and developmental history. Their interrelationships can be summarized as follows: The boys' conflict with society is qualitatively strengthened by their combinations in the peer culture. They transform individual opposition into collective antagonism to societal norms.

In their peer social structure the delinquent leadership imposes severe controls upon compeers. The boys' social system is reinforced through mutually supportive transferences in what we call a fantasy social system. Society's suppression of the peer group reinforces the entire circular process.

CONCLUSION

WE BELIEVE that the theoretical model developed above has important implications for psychosocial treatment. To be maximally effective, residential treatment must be integrated at three levels in order to "unbind" psychopathology and its social reinforcements: the caseworker must become more clearly aware of the social systems in which his charges function; the clinical group worker and the residential administrator must understand more clearly how the boys become locked in deviant peer subcultures and the accommodation of the staff to them. Together we must devise an intervention program which can trace the reverberations of treatment at community, peer culture and individual levels so that the interweaving of psychotherapy and planned social living can be transformed from a vague ideal into a specific strategy for tracing the transactional effects of individual and social systems upon each other.

NOTES TO CHAPTER 21

1. Goldsmith, Jerome M., Schulman, Rena, Grossbard, Hyman, "Integrating Clinical Processes with Planned Living Experiences," *American Journal of Orthopsychiatry*, Vol. 24, April 1954.

2. Lander, Joseph M., "The Role of Residential Treatment for Children," *American Journal of Orthopsychiatry*, Vol. XXV, October, 1955, 675-678.
3. Magnus, R., Kohn, Martin, "Countertransference in a Clinical Group," mimeographed, July, 1956, Hawthorne.
4. Polsky, Howard W. and Kohn, Martin, "Participant-Observation in a Delinquent Subculture," *American Journal of Orthopsychiatry*, Vol. XXIX, No. 4, October 1959, pp. 737-751.
5. Polsky, Howard W., "Changing Delinquent Subcultures: A Social Psychological Approach," *Social Work*, Vol. 4, No. 4, October 1959, pp. 3-15.
6. Polsky, Howard W., *Cottage Six: "The Social System of Delinquent Boys in Residential Treatment,"* Russell Sage, N.Y., 1962.
7. Grossbard, Hyman, *Cottage Parents, What They Have To Be, Know and Do,* Child Welfare League of America, N.Y., 1960.
   Alt, Herschel, *Residential Treatment for the Disturbed Child,* International Universities Press, N.Y., 1960.
8. The Peer Culture Project was supported jointly by Russell Sage and Hawthorne Cedar Knolls School.
9. Adler, Jack, Berman, Irwin, "Ego-Superego Dynamics in Residential Treatment of Disturbed Adolescents," Paper presented at American Orthopsychiatric Association Meeting, Feb., 1960, Chicago, Ill.
10. Mower, Orval, "Learning Theory and the New Neurotic Paradox," in *Learning Theory and Personality Dynamics*, Ronald Press Co., New York, 1950.
11. Johnson, Adelaide M., "Superego Lacunae of Adolescence," in Eissler, K. R., Ed. *Searchlights in Delinquency: New Psychiatric Studies,* pp. 225-245, International University Press, New York, 1949, p. 227.
12. Glueck, Sheldon and Glueck, Eleanor, *Unravelling Juvenile Delinquency,* Harvard University Press, Cambridge, 1950. See especially Chapter XVIII, "Character and Personality Structure" and Chapter XVIX, "Dynamics of Temperament."
13. Miller, Walter B., Geertz, Hildred, Cutter, Henry S. G., "Aggression in a Boys' Street-Corner Group," Psychiatry: *Journal for the Study of Interpersonal Processes*, Vol. 24, No. 4, November, 1961.
14. Cohen, Albert, *"Delinquent Boys, The Culture of the Gang."* The Free Press Glencoe, Ill., 1955, pp. 132-133 and 136-137.
15. The group-community relationship is based upon opposing norms, for example, the injunction against ratting upon all gang members. The key process between staff and peer group is *accommodation,* the implicit or explicit reinforcement of negative peer values by the staff. See Chapter 9, "Double Standard Complementarity" in *Cottage Six, The Social System of Delinquent Boys in Residential Treatment,* to be published by Russell Sage, June 1962.
16. The peer group system is maintained by the juxtaposition of complementary role positions: big man-punk; con man-bushboy, etc. The chief process in the peer system is *role induction:* Chapter 51 "The Cottage Social Structure," *op. cit.*
17. Extreme projection of past models into current social relations is *transference.*

18. For an enlightening discussion of perceptual identification as it relates to identification of (1) two external objects, (2) self with another person or object, and (3) self with a group, see Chapter 10, "Perceptual Identification," in *Personality Dynamics,* Bert R. Sappenfield, Alfred A. Knopf, 1954, N.Y., pp. 278-288.

৪৯

CHAPTER 22   The Management of a Type of Institutional Participation in Mental Illness*

ALFRED H. STANTON AND MORRIS S. SCHWARTZ

THE HOSPITAL WARD AS A SOCIAL ORGANIZATION

THE project, from which this is the first report, has as a broad purpose the improvement in the day-to-day decisions of administrative psychiatrists in a mental hospital. We have turned to the social sciences in the hope that students of groups and institutions have succeeded in providing concepts and methods adequate to provide very practical guidance in the management of patients who live an institutional life for a longer or shorter period. From this social science standpoint, the so-called medical opinion of the psychiatrist is regarded as serving a function in the social organization as a whole. The psychiatrist and the nurse function not only as physician and nurse, but also as the government of the patients—executive, legislative, and judicial. They disburse economic favors, educate, chaperone and discipline, advise and protect. The psychiatrist's so-called medical opinion—which is not based on data he learned in medical school—may fulfill all of these functions and many others.

The conception of the ward as a social organization can be illustrated by a figure of speech. It is analogous to a group of interlacing whirlpools where, if *one* whirlpool is altered by a person's sticking a finger in it, the whole pattern, and each part of it, will be altered to a greater or lesser extent. The analogy fails primarily in that no one, including the medical staff, can be regarded as putting a finger in from above, but all are themselves parts of the pattern of whirlpools.

* This investigation was supported (in part) by a research grant made to the Washington School of Psychiatry by the Division of Mental Hygiene, U.S. Public Health Service. The remainder of the project was supported directly by the Washington School of Psychiatry.

Reprinted by special permission of The William Alanson White Psychiatric Foundation, Inc., and the authors from *Psychiatry*, 12 (1949), 13–26 (copyright by the Foundation).

METHOD

THE method used to provide the material for the present paper has been the keeping of detailed daily records of contacts we have had with staff, relatives, and patients in the course of the ordinary daily work.

One author, the sociologist, has spent long periods upon the ward with no duties other than observation. The other author, the psychiatrist, is responsible for the care of all patients on the ward and for dealing with the patients' relatives, occupational therapists, nurses, and the psychotherapist. Consequently, his duties require relatively frequent contact with every important person in the patients' immediate social environment.

Certain phenomena within the social organization have been found to fall within definite patterns. In many cases the recognition of these patterns has been preceded by a somewhat intuitive sense that various occurrences somehow belong together; but the very act of recording and reviewing them has resulted in clarifying, revising, and often amplifying the picture of occurrences which generally come together. It has usually been a considerable period before a consensus of all trained observers has been reached upon the existence of a particular syndrome.

The gathering and clarifying of data have always proceeded in a clinical setting: we have tried to keep the therapeutic goal paramount, and research which might hamper the clinical program of the hospital has been rigorously excluded. Thus some observations have probably been missed, but, on the other hand, the demand for therapeutic action has led to an additional validation for the work. The psychiatrist, because he is a part of the social organization, is continuously taking action on the ward as difficulties arise. As he finds that a difficulty is part of a particular pattern, new and better ways of intervening may be suggested by this finding and must be tried for ethical reasons. If the intervention does in fact prove beneficial, there is both an assurance that the pattern is not a figment of the investigator's imagination and an opportunity to assess how important the pattern is in the lives of those participating in it. Each recurrence of the pattern provides a new opportunity for prediction and validation. This operational test is an approach to experimental method in the social science field. The great advantage a mental hospital has as an area for social science research lies in the fact that to some extent decisions are made by scientifically trained and interested persons.

THE PROBLEM

ONE of these social patterns is the subject of the present discussion. It forms almost as clear a syndrome of difficulty in the group as the clinical symptoms and signs of acute appendicitis do in the individual. Variations occur and some instances have escaped notice except in retrospect; but to one familiarized with the technique of looking at nurses, patients, and doctors, including oneself, within the same field of vision, the problem is often clear as it occurs.

THE RECOGNIZED PROBLEM

CERTAIN aspects were well known before the present study was undertaken. The following sequence of events had been generally recognized:

One nurse is noticed to be taking a so-called "special interest" in a particular patient, and her care of this patient tends to become conspicuous. The patient seems to become peculiarly dependent upon her care, improving when she is on duty and worse than usual when she is not. The patient begins to complain of the other nurses, comparing them unfavorably to the nurse who is, according to the cliché, "involved" with the patient. If the patient is a man, he is likely to express erotic fantasies and to consider marriage with the nurse. Often the care of the particular patient is left to this nurse by the others; and if this does not occur, she and the patient may themselves attempt to arrange for her to be assigned to him. In general, at these times, staff members, particularly the nurse's immediate superiors, become quietly concerned and discuss the situation in somewhat hushed voices, as if facing a very "delicate" problem. These supervising nurses will then often seek out a psychiatrist for advice on how to intervene. Frequently the psychiatrist's advice is vague or uncertain, and is often couched in such general terms as an "erotic countertransference," mixed with, or replacing "hostility." In general the problem has been handled in the past in one of the following ways: the nurse is transferred to another ward; the supervisor is advised to consult with the patient's doctor over the proper handling of the delicate situation; or the nurse is advised to seek personal psychotherapy.

These techniques of intervention leave much to be desired. The nurse has generally become defensive by this time and justifies her actions on the grounds that the patient's need requires special attention. His specious improvement supports her belief. She is generally particularly alert to refute in advance all attempts to intervene, especially denying any suggestion of an erotic involvement.

If psychotherapeutic discussions with the nurse occur, the nurse is likely to recognize that she likes the patient, but soon her attention turns to another nurse or to her superiors in the hospital organization; this together with general dissatisfaction with the management of the patients and broad complaints about the hospital are likely to be the earliest preoccupations.

FURTHER OBSERVATIONS ON THE PROBLEM

THE further course of events, previously unsuspected, was uncovered in the present study.

Occasionally the so-called attachment seems to wither away without incident, but more frequently the nurse finally and suddenly becomes aware of anger at the patient. If this is expressed to the patient, the nurse is profoundly chagrined at her offense to nursing ethical principles, almost always dutifully reports it to the physician in charge, and ordinarily either resigns or takes the first step toward resignation. Within a few hours the patient's clinical condition is reported markedly improved. There may or may not be an outburst of anger on the part of the patient directed toward the nurse.

A woman patient had not eaten enough voluntarily for some years. The symptom remained remarkably constant, but it was generally known that by considerable effort and time, it was possible to induce the patient to take adequate food without being tube-fed. However, several experiments in the past had demonstrated that the attempt to feed the patient this way apparently always led to increasing demands upon the nurse's time until the nurse would give up. Miss Jannison, the charge nurse, may be described as quiet, canny, politically-minded, and ambitious; she apparently generally believed herself above showing any feelings. She had relied upon the tube-feeding in a quite routine fashion until she heard that the patient was to see a psychotherapist of whom she was remotely fond. Shortly after this she mentioned to the administrative psychiatrist casually one day that she would like to try to see if the patient would not eat if sufficiently encouraged. As it became clear that she wanted to do this herself, rather than delegate it to another nurse, a faint blush appeared. She undertook the program with initial success, at least in the sense that the patient took more and more food. About a week later, Mr. Robertson, a nurse who is ordinarily thought of as almost too indulgent, approached the psychiatrist and remarked, with a knowing smile, that Miss Jannison just had to try to do things that other people failed at. He went on to state that she should be permitted to find out that it would not work.[1] A few days later, after two hours with the patient, Miss Jannison volunteered to the psychiatrist, quite quietly and coldly, and contrary to hospital tradition, "Oh, I don't know. Sometimes I don't think she's worth the effort. After all, what will she be if she recovers." Relatively routine tube-feeding was reinstated. Miss Jannison was never again present at the tube-feeding and apparently dismissed the patient as completely as her position would permit. Two days later she began ruminating out loud about the desirability of another hospital some distance away and about two weeks later resigned and went to this hospital.

Miss G, a schizophrenic, was ordinarily a quiet, tense, depressed patient, and had a rather pronounced and continuously irritated or sulky expression on her face; she was inactive, but able to live upon the convalescent floor. Occasionally she became wildly excited and was brought to the disturbed floor where she would struggle in a frenzied fashion to get to the door, stating only, "I have got to get home, I have got to get home, I have got to get home." At times, though she was a small person, three people were required to hold her away from the door. She improved somewhat under the administrations of Miss Jonathan, a thoroughly experienced, open and friendly nurse, who was in charge of the ward, but she remained confused, very over-active and sleepless. Miss G expressed many times her appreciation of Miss Jonathan's care, and Miss Jonathan in her turn went out of her way to state that she liked Miss G and hoped she would get well. Miss Jonathan was worried about Miss G's psychotherapist.[2] After a few days on the ward, Miss G was struggling toward the door and Miss Jonathan suddenly lost her temper and, to her own utter horror, slapped the patient in the face. She sought out the psychiatrist and resigned at once and spoke of going into another profession; after considerable discussion in which she herself raised the question of treatment—she was completely unable to give reasons for her outburst of temper—she was persuaded to remain, partly by being asked to consider the effect of her resignation on the patient. The patient saw the psychiatrist shortly after Miss Jonathan returned to the floor and after Miss Jonathan had discussed her loss of temper with the patient. The patient's first remark to the psychiatrist was an angry insistence that Miss Jonathan should not be fired. She was completely clear and quiet, remained so and was transferred back to the convalescent ward in a few days.

At the beginning of the present study, the course of the problem was as follows: Occasionally disagreement among the nurses would become overt and this new problem would come to the attention of their superiors or even of the medical staff conference where, without exception, nothing would be decided. Under these circumstances the general frustration might be, and all too frequently was, solved by blaming the patient. The patient would come to be thought of as "extremely clever" in "driving a wedge" between members of the staff. If the patient was told this, he usually became wildly excited and frightened, aggravating the problems.

A few days after it had been discovered that an excited, confused, schizophrenic patient, Mrs. F, had been making many statements difficult to understand regarding her clothing, it was discovered that the physician and the nurse in charge of clothing had, because of a misunderstanding, been consistently making diametrically opposing statements to her regarding her clothing. When this was straightened out, the patient lost her confusion completely within a few days. Subsequently at lunch, the physician, Dr. Lewis, remarked that he thought the mechanism of the schizophrenic confusion might include administrative misunderstandings among the staff. This met with a statement by a second physician that Mrs. F might be trying to set the staff against each other. Dr. Lewis doubted this and the second physician agreed with him but repeated the interpretation twice during lunch, each time, however, agreeing with Dr. Lewis' repeated scepticism. The second physician dismissed the problem with a final remark that he thought patients should be given 15 minutes per month to complain uninterruptedly about the hospital management. Dr. Lewis remarked that the patient had made no complaint whatsoever about the hospital management in this connection, which the other doctor received with a gesture of disbelief. There was a clear implication that he thought that Dr. Lewis was misled and needed to understand the "real" problem.

An example of the effect on the patient:

A patient had been quite excited in the course of a difficulty with the charge nurse and an attendant. The attendant had threatened resignation to a senior psychiatrist. The patient had been quiet for three or four days when she was visited by the senior physician. He told her that her "manipulations" had upset the whole ward. She began to scream, "No, no, no" at the top of her voice, and, "I hate Dr. X, I hate Dr. X, I hate Dr. X," continuing long after the doctor left the floor. She was given a cold wet sheet pack, awoke in the middle of the night screaming and remained overactive in substantially this pattern for three or four days and nights. During this time she repeatedly quoted the doctor as saying she was tearing the whole hospital to pieces. Her analyst reported that no useful work was done during the subsequent week.

In addition to these problems, the study of the position of the nurse among her colleagues revealed still other regularly recurrent parts of the pattern of difficulty. The knowledge of these suggested a more reliable technique of intervention.

First, as the problem develops, the supervisors come to appear in a very patronizing light which they themselves sense. They feel that they have the responsibility of doing something to help, but their right to intervene arises only from their superior position in the social organization and not from any particular competence in this field. In general, the attitude they must take toward the nurse is somewhat similar to that of a mother dealing with an adolescent daughter in love with the wrong man. This general attitude effectively blocks whatever advice they might ordinarily be able to give and discourages the nurse from turning to them for help.

Secondly, the nurse who is involved usually moves progressively into a position of a minority of one among her colleagues. Her pleas for indulgence for the patient will, for a time, be heard with sympathy by some others, but finally even these allies begin to treat her discussions of the patient as a problem of hers and no longer agree with her point of view. Eventually all the nurses, and, as a matter of fact, many of the patients, form a silent and somewhat puzzled audience to a drama which they do not understand, but somehow sense is bad. Their reserve seems to aggravate the embarrassment.

Finally, and most important, there is always a second nurse who forms an integral part of the picture. She is generally another person in authority and her attitude toward the patient becomes the mirror image of the attitude of the first nurse, the one who is involved with the patient. The second nurse's position is much less conspicuous because she appears merely to spearhead the view held generally by the staff. Her function as a spearhead, however, is an extremely active one because in quiet ways—and almost always behind the other nurse's back—she makes derogatory remarks about the first nurse to higher authorities, to other nurses, and fairly frequently to patients. There is a certain defensiveness in her attitude also. Each nurse goes out of her way to appeal to the doctor in charge to support her particular way of handling the patient. The most characteristic fact is that the two nurses apparently always avoid the topic of their disagreement when they are together.

(The following notes from staff conference were recorded in long hand and only follow the sense of each remark. Quoted material is, we believe, nearly verbatim.)

Dr. A raised with the other doctors and supervising nurses the problem of Miss Laswell's being involved with Mr. C. He believed she put Mr. C in an unfair position. "She can't follow up her interest and affection and he can't live up to it. In a way she treats him like a baby. . . . Mr. Manning [a supervisory nurse] and Miss Laswell [charge nurse on the 8-4 shift] apparently can't handle the situation. Miss Smithson [charge nurse on the 4-12 shift] cannot go on day duty because of Miss Laswell. They apparently cannot get along. Mr. C is following Miss Laswell around like a sheep dog." Dr. A believes the attachment has been a good thing as it is the first time anyone has given Mr. C interest, but the patient is now unable to deal with other personnel. "He whines and begs things of Miss Laswell, to which she usually accedes."

Dr. B: "There is a decrease in Mr. C's dealings with other people. He is, however, more active in getting out on the grounds and in talking with Miss Laswell."

A supervising nurse stated that she didn't have good contact with Miss Laswell, and believed she, herself, had fallen down on her job and should have talked with Miss Laswell about it.

Dr. C: "Miss Laswell has a lot of enthusiasm and *joie de vivre*. It doesn't all seem to be hostility."

Dr. A agreed that she had a lot, but needed education.

Dr. D had heard nothing indicating hostility on Miss Laswell's part.

Dr. A (somewhat annoyed) believed that it would have had to be either gross selective inattention or hostility.

Dr. D: "What indicates hostility? Does she treat others that way?"

Dr. A: "She treats everyone that way. Only Mr. C accepts it."

Dr. E interrupted with a question about how to handle the problem.

Dr. A explained that he had tried to do it in the ward staff conferences: "They speak in generalities. When it becomes personal, it leads up to defensiveness, such as accounts of the way in which rules have been broken." He felt that the conferences had failed.

Dr. F: "Here is a person with enthusiasm which could be easily destroyed. It would be very easy for her to turn extremely sour. If you could say something like, 'I have been interested in your different approach,' then one could find out where her judgment is sound and where it is her own pathology."

From other sources it was learned that Miss Laswell was considered more indulgent to Mr. C than one of the supervising nurses thought proper. Disagreement had mounted to such intensity that they had to be separated on the ward and the doctor and two supervising nurses clearly sided with Miss Smithson. This occurred on another ward than the one under observation and the sequel is lost.

THE PROBLEM IN ITS SETTING

THE whole process as we see it now may be summarized as follows: Persons of either sex may play any part in the disturbance. For purposes of description we will speak of nurses, although doctors and attendants participate as frequently as nurses.

In the course of the day-to-day determination of policy regarding any particular patient, small disagreements between nurses with power to decide are inevitable. If they come to be antagonistic to each other for any reason, they tend to magnify these small disagreements and are unable to discuss and solve them; for instance, one nurse may tend regularly to stop a patient from doing something before the second nurse does. Because of the antagonism they are unable to discuss the problem and it becomes important for each to show that the other is wrong. The one who is more restrictive comes increasingly to play the role of the policeman or disciplinarian, while the other comes to play the role of the indulgent mother. The patient comes to respond regularly to each in terms of these roles. Inconsistencies arising in the course of the patient's management become systematic and, more important, the whole process in its middle stages is very, very quiet. The contrast in the patient's manner gradually draws the attention of the relatively neutral members of the group and they tend as a body to side with one or the other nurse, but also tend to remain silent. Without intervention, the nurse who has become a minority tends more and more wildly to demonstrate that she is right and begins to show signs of profound personal tension—sleeplessness, irritability, preoccupation with the single patient and relative neglect of her other duties. Shortly after she finally loses her last adherent among the staff, there is an outburst of anger directed at the patient, resignation, or a threat of resignation and a rejoining of her colleagues with considerable loss of face. In general, her colleagues do not add to her humiliation as far as we know, possibly because so many of them have suffered the same situation.

THE PATIENT

CERTAIN preliminary clinical observations have been made. Only patients of a certain type have been found to form the third party in this triangular process. In particular, patients who are markedly withdrawn have not been observed participating in this difficulty. The patient must be active to some extent, talking, and in at least partial apparent contact.

More important, in every case where the patient has been the center of attention on the ward for several days consecutively—as measured, for instance, by the relative length of nurses' reports—the patient has been found to be implicated in this process. Also in all cases where a patient has manifested a great deal of excited and conspicuous behavior for several days or more, he has been a third party in this triangular process.

The type of excitement, according to conventional psychiatric classification, has been extremely variable: manic and catatonic excitement, schizophrenic panic states, and marked agitation of a type seen in agitated depressions or so-called obsessional tension states have occurred in connection with the syndrome. Again, in every case we have seen, regardless of diagnosis, the excitement has ameliorated within 48 hours of the resolution of the process among the staff, and in all but one has disappeared completely within a few days. This rapid and profound change in the clinical course of the patients is under further study. The number of cases recorded, thirteen excitements in six patients, is inadequate for generalization, but the evidence now strongly suggests that prolonged excitements frequently require for their maintenance a covert disagreement between two persons with power to decide to some degree upon the patient's management. Perhaps this is always the case as we have found no exceptions at the time of writing.

THE MODE OF INTERVENTION

THE observation that the process is actually a triangular one, and not merely between two persons, suggested a mode of intervention which has proved reasonably adequate. In one way or another we lead the two nurses who are at odds to a face-to-face discussion of their differences, insisting that they arrive at a consensus on the professional problem of the handling of the patient.

An example will illustrate both the current method of handling the problem and our method of recording, as well as a particularly complete account of the syndrome. The following excerpts are from the nurses' routine reports and the investigators' routine records. The time covered is from May 16 to May 24. It is of interest that the psychiatrist was away from the hospital May 15, 16, 18 and 19.

May 16. Miss Bilford reports, quoting Mrs. B (the patient), "I have this terrible compulsion to run away and then I realize I have no place to go and then I want to kill myself. I just don't know what I'm going to do." (This is the first report of suicidal preoccupation in some months.)

May 17. An attendant reports that Mrs. B "has an intense and officious manner of going about things."

May 17. Miss Bilford reports, quoting the patient, "It is a matter of life and death, and death seems to be the only alternative I have." Miss Bilford continues (to other nurses) "So you might keep a little particular watch on her tonight. However, during the times she was talking about it, she didn't get desperate . . . you know, usually when she talks about things like that she gets that desperate look and gets so damned tense, but tonight it wasn't so much like that, she seemed quite comfortable."

May 18. Miss Dennis reports, "Mrs. B was very pleasant and agreeable today. When told the shopping trip would be impossible this week, remarked, 'Well, O.K.'"

May 18. Another nurse reports, "The patient became upset after reading an article which talked about schizophrenia being an organic disease. Talked about suicide and the hospital should have mercy killings for people like her."

May 19. Another nurse reports, "Mrs. B was very upset and noisy this a.m. Called the nurse 'A God-damn dirty bitch' and demanded to be taken out. Seemed very quiet and depressed this afternoon."

May 19. Investigator's note: "Miss Bilford sought out the pyschiatrist to discuss ward problems. During her talk she said, 'I have been thinking of quitting for the past week and a half.' (Not said too seriously.) 'Mr. Connolly [a superior nurse] and I don't get along. It is not what you know, but who you know around here.' "3

May 20. A nurse reports, "Mrs. B seemed very depressed and asked to see the nurse. She said, 'I am so frightened. All day I've had such horrible thoughts. I thought that if I could kill someone, I would then be killed. I can't stand going on living this way.' "

The same day, Miss Dennis reports, "Mrs. B ignored the charge nurse, saying, 'I'm angry with her.' Around 9:30 started talking to charge nurse very loud, interrupting her conversations with other patients."

May 20. Psychiatrist's note: "Last night Miss Bilford took the initiative to get hold of me. She presented a series of objections which Mrs. B had made. Miss Bilford sided with the patient against other nurses, believing them 'prejudiced' against Mrs. B. For instance, one of the other nurses had told the patient that there would be no trips available to medical and dental appointments that week, but another patient had gone shopping. Miss Bilford also mentioned that Miss Dennis did not send someone shopping with Mrs. B even though there were six people on the ward. I finally suggested that Miss Bilford apparently was in serious disagreement with Miss Dennis, at which Miss Bilford answered that I did not know the half of it. I then gave her the assignment of coming to terms with Miss Dennis. Miss Bilford went on in an apparently unrelated fashion to indicate her anger at not having adequate pack sheets. She went on to state that if something was not done about it, she was going to quit, the latter apparently semi-humorously."

May 21. Miss Bilford reports, quoting patient, "I read about murder in the papers and decided that was the way to solve my problems."4

May 21. Psychiatrist's note: "Mrs. B was deeply distressed. All the trivial objections of the past were omitted except by implication, as she complained to me of the hopelessness of it all and the fact that she did not want to live."

May 21. Psychiatrist's note: "I talked for over an hour with Miss Bonay [another nurse]. We discussed at some length Miss Bilford's feud with Miss Dennis. Miss Bonay mentioned that she sided with Miss Dennis. She stated that she had known for some time that she could not work with Miss Bilford. At this point I believe *noblesse oblige* prevented her from going into more detail, but she indicated that Miss Bilford was difficult to fight with directly, that she would give in and there would be no real meeting of minds."

It was later noted that Miss Dennis talked with Miss Bilford on May 21st about their difficulties over Mrs. B.

May 22. Miss Bilford reports: "The patient told nurse about her hour (vaguely) and how she hadn't called her analyst one name tonight. She said, 'We talked and we listened to each other. I must have delusions of grandeur.' "

May 22. Psychiatrist's note: "Conference with a senior staff member. We talked over the problem of Miss Bilford as I saw it at the time and what to do to avoid further progression of the charge nurse syndrome. The senior staff member suggested that Miss Bilford among other things might be asking for personal psychotherapy.

May 23. Miss Dennis reports: "Mrs. B was very pleasant and cooperative today."

May 24. Another nurse reports: "She seemed quite comfortable and pleasant."

There is no mention of suicide in the nurses' notes for at least several weeks.

We have increasingly put our reliance in obtaining a consensus between two staff members at odds with each other regarding the patient. This has been possible in a large proportion of cases, but there are certain technical problems which require mention. A consensus must be sharply differentiated from such pseudo-agreements as those achieved by authoritative orders, "instruction," intimidation, or defeat in argument. The first step in attaining a consensus requires the recognition of disagreement. There is frequent failure in this. Two examples will illustrate:

One physician, in speaking with another, would frequently make a statement starting with, "Since we know that . . ."; the second physician would verbally agree, but would rather regularly, over a considerable period of time, go to a third physician to whom he reported he felt he somehow had been led to say things he did not believe. He finally identified this as an automatic response of his to the above phrase, and recognized very frequently that, though he acceded, he profoundly disagreed.

Dr. A was once approached separately by two physicians, Dr. B and Dr. C, regarding an excited patient. Dr. B, the psychotherapist, stated that the patient was paranoid and that the way the patient was being handled, he couldn't get anywhere with either the patient or the administrative psychiatrist, Dr. C. Dr. C, in his turn, went out of his way to state that the patient was clearly manic-depressive, that Dr. B was nuts, but that he had handled Dr. B so that they were in complete agreement. He described in detail the way in which he had avoided overt disagreement with Dr. B's views in order not to stir up trouble. He apparently sincerely believed that he and Dr. B had a consensus and it took ten minutes for others to demonstrate to him that this was not the case.

After a disagreement has been recognized, surprisingly few difficulties have been found in its management. The direct participants often resist or postpone discussion by one means or another, but after this has been overcome, they generally solve their problems rapidly. They often note with genuine surprise that they can't find out at once what their differences really are. The change in attitude between staff members may require only a few minutes and is apparently reflected toward the patient with similar rapidity.

IMPLICATIONS

CERTAIN problems arise and remain unsettled. First, it must be emphasized that apparently no participant in this triangular process is clearly conscious of it. Secondly, attendants, nurses, and physicians carry out the pattern with quite startling fidelity, in spite of differing personalities and social status. Each actor plays his part somewhat differently than the last, and on a different stage, but the play is the same.

Even more plainly, at least some of the patient's manifestations of illness—his "symptoms"—are ways of participating in the social process within which the patient lives, and may be changed—to some extent according to plan—by altering the social environment.

Although all excited patients are involved in this process, many quiet patients may form a third party in the triangle. These other patients may become disturbed in some fashion as the intensity of the process increases, but some are only very slightly affected. The type of disturbance, when it does occur, is extremely variable. This presents an interesting contrast. While the participation of the staff seems to be quite narrowly determined in its over-all form, we have not been able to isolate any such regularity which includes all patients, except the abrupt clinical change at the termination. We assume that this may follow from the fact that the roles assigned to the staff are also more narrowly defined than the role of the patient.

PREVENTION

WE ARE on much less secure ground in speculating on the cause and prevention of the syndrome—how the play itself is written. The syndrome in any intense form has appeared less frequently upon the ward for the past several months. Many factors may have contributed to this. Increasing use of the regular nursing conference for the very early resolution of differences, increasing awareness of the importance of the differences, and the educational effect of previous difficulties of this type among the staff may all have contributed to its diminution. One may reasonably guess that the difficulty arises in some way from the character of the social organization of the institution as a whole. Any factor tending to make a consensus on management more difficult might be expected to contribute to the problem. Inadequate opportunity for discussion, unnecessary multiplication of persons with overlapping powers regarding a patient's management, and the authoritarianism implicit in the hospital tradition itself may be expected to contribute. For instance, a frequent example of inability to discuss differences is found in the young physician who has not learned that the charge nurse knows more about the patient, at least in some respects, than he, and who believes that he should write the orders without seriously considering her opinion. Very superior charge nurses, of course, expect this of young physicians and develop more or less successful techniques for manipulating the young physician into the right decision, while he believes that he is manipulating the nurse. But this is, at best, a tenuous and unsatisfactory arrangement. Under these circumstances, excitements and very profound disorganization of a whole ward are frequent.

But the role of senior physician or nurse also has vulnerabilities. With increasing experience and higher prestige, physicians or supervising nurses come to be insulated by the deference given their position which may discourage the expression of conflicting opinion. Further, the more power a person has in the hospital, the more the various reports he receives will be colored by attempts to influence him quite automatically and often unwittingly. Partly as a result of this, systematic differences of opinion between the supervisory and the floor nurses, and between physicians of comparable status, are very frequent. If this is a factor in the disturbance discussed here, however, one would expect to find evidence of tension between the floor nurses and the front nursing office, particularly at the time the triangular disturbance is occurring. This is frequently the case, but our evidence is not now adequate to demonstrate either a consistent correlation, or to suggest measures for operational validation.

SUMMARY

Close observation is reported of the phenomenon of a nurse taking a special interest in a patient, a special interest often interpreted by others as a result of a mixture of erotic and hostile sentiments. We have found that the pattern of such involvements is quite stereotyped and that it represents only the most conspicuous part of a larger, but equally stereotyped, pattern of difficulty within the group of persons concerned with the hospital ward. In each case another nurse has been found who is equally active regarding the patient, but whose attitude toward the patient is the mirror-image of the attitude of the first nurse. These two nurses consequently disagree systematically and often quite violently regarding the patient, but are unable to discuss their differences. When such a discussion is brought about—usually against appreciable resistance —the disagreement and the involvement with the patient usually evaporates with startling rapidity, often within a few hours.

All patients on the ward who have been the center of attention for more than a few days and all patients who have shown persisting excitement have been found to form the third party in this triangular process. The disappearance of the disagreement between the staff members has always resulted in a marked and often very rapid abatement of the excitement;

the evidence is therefore strong that such a disagreement between persons with power over the patient is a necessary condition, at least in this setting, for prolonged excitement.

The methods of social science are applicable to the phenomena of mental illness in a mental hospital and provide guidance for therapeutic action and research not easily available within conventional psychiatric methods of approach. A mental hospital offers an extraordinarily favorable opportunity for the testing of social science conceptions in action.

DISCUSSION

HERBERT GOLDHAMER

As a sociologist I naturally find it rather pleasing to note the emphasis in this paper on the structure of social relations in the mental hospital and the relation of this structure to the therapeutic situation.

The nurse-patient-doctor relationships discussed in the paper have, I believe, their parallels in other types of social structures. The systematic comparison and analysis of these parallel cases would probably facilitate the study of the hospital situation. I observed similar complexes of relations in the Army during the war. Here the participants were typically the senior-grade officer, the junior-grade officer and the enlisted man. The junior-grade officer develops an interest in and intervenes in behalf of the enlisted man; this precipitates tensions between himself and other officers; ambivalent attitudes develop because of the departure from officer norms and ultimate hostility toward the enlisted man may occur. The parallels between this and the doctor-nurse-patient situation could be worked out quite fully. I have the impression that the type of triadic relations discussed in the paper are most likely to occur in social structures of an authoritarian character in which inhibited hostility to authority exists.

The frequency with which nurses in these situations tend to resign or seek a transfer suggests that escape reactions had been developing well before the incidents that finally precipitate withdrawal. This suggests further that it is the nurse who is the key person in the situation. The analysis would, however, be put in a somewhat different perspective were it found that it is the patient who takes the initiative in developing the relation with the nurse, rather than the other way around. However, even in this case, the interpretation is not excluded that the patient is perceptive enough to find a nurse whose personal or psychological situation makes her an easy "prey" to the type of attachment described in the paper.

JEROME D. FRANK

The staff of the Group Psychotherapy Research Project has had an opportunity to see Dr. Stanton's paper. These remarks are based on our discussions of some of the issues raised.

It has long been recognized that many interpersonal influences besides the relationship with the psychiatrist can be psychotherapeutically help-ful or harmful. The widespread use in mental hospitals of ward activities, occupational therapy, athletics, and so on, bears witness to this recogni-tion. The great virtue of this study is that it has been able to single out and scrutinize a particular aspect of these influences. It demonstrates vividly that not only the relations of the therapeutic personnel to the patient but their relations to each other may importantly influence the patient's progress.

We have been faced with many of the same methodological problems in attempting to make sense of what happens in group psychotherapy. Like Dr. Stanton and Mr. Schwartz, we have found ourselves relying on detailed observational data which we study for regularities of pattern, especially those which appear to be modifiable, although we have not limited ourselves to these. It seems to us that although the most satis-factory validation is that of introducing planned modifications and trying to predict their effects, it may be possible to validate with some degree of probability patterns which cannot be altered. This may be done by stating them in terms of a hypothesis that when a certain defined set of conditions prevails, a certain result will follow. Then past records can be studied and future occurrences observed for the presence of this set of conditions. To the extent that the expected results do follow, the hypothesis is supported.

We wondered about the relation of the particular patient to the other patients on the ward. It would seem that the position was somewhat similar to teacher's pet or favorite child. Our experience with group therapy suggests that such a special relation with the person in charge is paid for by increasing separation from the other patients and eventually their jealous hostility. The possibility would seem worth investigating that the disturbance of the patient directly involved might be at least partly related to the attitudes of the other patients to him.

It is also possible that the self-respect of the patient involved may suffer from his realization that he is being used for the emotional satisfaction of members of the staff.

We were struck with the ease with which nurses seemed to resign after being caught up in such a situation and wondered whether perhaps the pressure to do a good job, to be psychotherapeutic, might not contribute to it. Perhaps this pressure might make them the more likely to succumb to the gratifying opportunities for tension-relieving "mothering" afforded by certain patients. That is, making a big fuss over a patient might relieve their guilt over not being psychotherapeutic enough.

Finally, I should like to emphasize how clearly the present paper demonstrates the necessity of thinking of our patients continually as en-gaging in group behavior and how useful such a relatively new way of looking at the problems of clinical psychiatry may prove. The writers are to be congratulated on this excellent piece of trail-breaking in an exceptionally important but little explored area.

HARRY STACK SULLIVAN

THIS first of what we may expect to be a series of important findings from the research unit concerned deserves far more study and thought than I can give it at the moment. Let me consider it, sketchily, from several viewpoints.

The research itself would be presumed to be an approach to the multi-disciplined pattern which now interests me greatly in terms of promising more general concepts than those which any one of the disciplines concerned could give.

It reports the findings of a pattern of relationship. Is it to be seen, at least in the larger setting of the particular ward and hospital groups? The question arises immediately: is this a pattern which is a function of the particular larger group setting, or is it one that has relatively wide validity?

In other words, how widely observable is the occurrence of this sort of pattern of relationship? Is it to be seen, at least in essential rudiments, for instance, in the stenographic and typing pool of a large office, or in comparable high school or undergraduate bodies? Is it to be seen in essential rudiments among the complement of a naval vessel, among the population of a penitentiary, in any hospital which has a relatively chronic patient population, on the wards of most mental hospitals only, or just at Chestnut Lodge?

As I read the report, I come to see this pattern as a process in which (1) a presumably impartial agent of the institution becomes closely integrated with one of the charges, or the subject-persons of the institution; (2) the dynamics of the group of such presumptively impartial agents is thus subjected to stress and the resulting strain appears in (3) another of the presumptively impartial agents becoming closely integrated with the particular subject-person—but in a way that opposes the peculiar manifestation of the initial integration. This second agent, as it were, represents the resistance of the institutional group to variation in impartiality, and thus sets up an antagonistic, anxiety-colored subintegration between the two agents with the subject-person, the patient, as a conscious, a sentient, center of the whole. At a certain stage of the process, the antagonistic motivation moves in the first instance from the subintegration of the two agents, to the first agent concerned and the subject-person: the first nurse "becomes angry at" the patient. This attentuates the force in the initial relationship, and the observable behavior of the subject-person in terms of the total group improves markedly; while the agent first involved then tends to separate herself from the group whose presumed impartiality she has been violating.

Centers of influence other than Agents One and Two and the subject-person are noted in the report and their observable contributions mentioned; the supervising nurses and members of the medical staff, for instance. The disintegrative force of embarrassment is said to come to involve all the nurses and many of the patients on the wards.

The report goes on to indicate that a resolution of the antagonistic subintegration between Agents One and Two resolves the whole pattern with "rapid and profound change in the clinical course" of the subject-person, who has, meanwhile, come to show "a great deal of excited and conspicuous behavior," perhaps growing out of an initial contrast in "improving when she [Agent One] is on duty and [being] worse than usual when she is not."

There is some uncertainty as to the adequacy of this analysis, introduced into the matter by the statement that "the contrast in the patient's manner gradually draws the attention of the relatively neutral members of the group and they tend as a body to side with one or the other nurse . . . [and] the nurse who has become a minority [presumably from the text *either* Agent One or Two can shift to this minority position] tends more and more wildly to demonstrate that she is right and begins to show signs of profound personal tension . . . preoccupation with the single patient . . . [and] shortly after she [has finally lost the support of] her last adherent among the staff, there is an outburst of anger directed at the patient . . . and a rejoining of her colleagues with considerable loss of face. . . ."

I think that this very uncertainty is of importance in considering this report. The study of courses of events in interpersonal fields—somewhat in contrast to statements of patterns of observable behavior—always includes the element of the near future, whether formulated or unclear in the sundry personal centers involved. This can often be approximated by thought about probabilities of good end-state of the energy transformations that are observable.

It is irrational to suppose that the goal of importance in the here-described pattern of behavior is the disturbance of the subject-person's, the patient's, hospital adjustment. What, then, are rational, reasonably probable suppositions about the more or less unrecognized goals of Agents One and Two? I would expect to find in the answer to this question considerable light shed on the unfortunate effect of the integration on the third element of the situation, the subject-person, the patient. I think I would expect to find two different cases to be involved: (1) that in which there was peculiar suitability on the part of the subject-person for integration with Agent One in the pursuit of the latter's (satisfactions or) interpersonal security—perhaps the 'makings' of a paranoid two-group against the world; (2) that in which there were parataxic factors in Agent Two which made the patient peculiarly suited as an object of repressive domination and thwarting; or (3) where some color of either of these cases made the situation one particularly suitable for the discharge of negative feeling between the group *and* Agent One, or Agent Two and Agent One—in other words, a situation in which the patient *was not* the primary subject-person, but in a great sense a mere unfortunate bystander *used in* internecine struggle. This third possibility I would presume to be near the basic field pattern. The generally unfortunate role of the patient in these situations would seem to reflect the complexity of the role he is called upon to play.

I must leave this analysis in this inconclusive state. I have one more point to discuss. This paper presumably concerns itself with episodes of excited and conspicuous behavior in patients who have been in residence in this hospital for some time. So far as it may be a study of the interpersonal pattern associated with the occurrence of an episode of this sort, it may also, if the analysis is pushed far enough, give a picture of at least one of the interpersonal situations associated with the occurrence of excitement before or incident to admission to the mental hospital.

ALFRED H. STANTON

The problem of the relation between this pattern on a mental hospital ward and apparently analogous phenomena occurring elsewhere is one about which we now have considerable evidence, but all of it is anecdotal in character. Apparently identical situations have been described to us, occurring in Army hospitals, general hospitals, State hospitals and in a private firm of lawyers. I am somewhat skeptical of the analogy of the situation of the teacher's pet, in that I know of no evidence that the latter is a triangular situation, but I would not be surprised to find another teacher or the child's parent taking a primarily disciplinary attitude toward the child, and not being on speaking terms with the teacher.

The evidence of hostility among the staff, as well as between the staff and patients, is, of course, overwhelming, but we have not felt that this conception was particularly helpful unless its specific type and "arrangement" were clearly enough discernible to furnish guidance toward helpful intervention. We have, of course, focussed our attention in this paper on one particular pattern which includes resignation of the nurses; this may have given the impression that resignation at the hospital is much commoner than elsewhere, a fact which we doubt. It does seem clear, however, that evidences of greater "hostility" or "tension" appear from time to time, and we are attempting an analysis of factors tending to increase and decrease such types of interaction. We certainly believe that the increase occurs at a time of generally increased disorganization, so that, for instance, the medical and nursing staffs and the patients all become tense and "upset" at the same time; but this opinion is very difficult to prove without quantitative measurement.

We are still trying to study the very early stages of the involvement we have described, to get what information we can as to whether the staff member or the patient takes the "initiative." There is evidence that at times one does and at times the other, but we are inclined to believe that really close and successful study would reveal that, in a sense, there was no "beginning," except one arbitrarily imposed on the data by the observer, for his analytic convenience.

The more detailed mechanics have not been emphasized in this paper, but are under study. Dr. Sullivan mentioned the possibility that a paranoid two-group was in process of formation, or that a situation had developed suitable for the patient to serve as an unfortunate intermediary in a conflict between two other persons. If paranoid two-group means two persons collaborating in the pretense that they are closer, different, and better than the rest of the world, against which they must struggle as allies, then our preliminary evidence suggests that both of these possibilities are combined and occur together. It is important that while it is felt that they are against the "world," one person comes to represent the "world" and is the focus of their efforts.

We believe this type of process occurs in excited patients before admission to the hospital, but we have no clear data. At least frequently when excited patients are admitted to the hospital, two other members of the family are primarily concerned and are at odds with each other. The relative accompanying the patient to the hospital has recently been very protective, but has "finally lost patience." It seems likely that the patient's admission to the hospital occurs following a situation in the family analogous to the situation described among the hospital personnel. It is possible that the family's sending the patient to the mental hospital is analogous to the patient's rejection by the nurse at the time her anger becomes apparent.

NOTES TO CHAPTER 22

1. The relevance of this observation will appear later in the paper.
2. The relevance of this observation, as in the previous example, will be developed later.
3. Up to this point the conflict between the two nurses has not come to the attention of the doctors (the quiet stage), although disturbance and suicidal preoccupations of the patient have come out clearly.
4. All the nurses have reported suicidal preoccupations except Miss Dennis, who apparently at no time sees the patient in this light.

৯৶

CHAPTER 23   The Ward Behavior

of Psychiatric Patients*

SIMON DINITZ, MARK LEFTON, JON E. SIMPSON,
BENJAMIN PASAMANICK, AND RALPH M. PATTERSON

ONE of the sociologically most relevant discussions in the Stanton and
Schwartz volume, *The Mental Hospital,* concerns the allegedly
deleterious effect of staff differences in psychiatric orientation upon the
behavior of ward patients. (3, pp. 344-345) The basic assumption underlying this hypothesis is that even the most chronically ill, disoriented, and
"back ward" mental patients are extremely sensitive to the nuances and
conflicts of their environment. (3, chap. 16) This position has also been
offered as explanation for crises in other institutional settings, such as the
current unrest in American prisons and reformatories. (4) Here it is held
that the discrepancies in the points of view of the professional and
custodial staffs are reflected in the general dissatisfaction of the inmates.

Stanton and Schwartz suggest that the behavior of mental patients is
largely dependent upon and sensitive to the social climate of the ward.
Differential ward policies and practices should be expected to be reflected
in the ward climate or milieu. It should then follow that patient behavior
will vary in accordance with these environmental differences. This extension of the Stanton and Schwartz viewpoint closely parallels the work of
sociologists on the sensitivity of non-institutionalized persons to the
atmospheres in which they live and work. (2)

It should be stressed that this paper does not presume to *test* the very
crucial hypothesis that intra-ward conflicts among staff personnel result in
therapeutically dysfunctional patient behavior (e.g., incontinence and increased anxiety). Rather the concern is with the impact of differential
ward policy as it has been observed and recorded to affect the *overt*
functioning of both patients and staff on each of five wards in a mental

* Reprinted from *Social Problems,* 6 (1958), 107–115, by permission of the authors
and the Society for the Study of Social Problems.

hospital. This paper will attempt to show that the non-structured or non-routinized behavior of institutionalized mental patients is largely the same from ward to ward despite obvious variations in inter- and intra-ward management policies. In postulating this hypothesis we are, in essence, questioning the implied "sensitivity" premise of Stanton and Schwartz; and also the often discussed hypothesis that the behavior of mental patients is merely quantitatively different from that of other persons.

METHOD

In order to obtain the necessary data detailed plans were made of all available floor space on each of the five wards at the Columbus Psychiatric Institute and Hospital. This Hospital is part of the Ohio State University Health Center and is a short-term (average stay approximately 2 months), intensive-therapy research and training institution. The Hospital is composed of five wards. These wards contain a total of 126 beds to which patients are *randomly assigned* by hospital policy. Each ward is a relatively self-contained unit consisting of all necessary facilities for the care and treatment of patients. The facilities include single, double, and dormitory rooms, recreational space in the form of one or more day rooms, treatment rooms, a nursing station, and service areas. All rooms are accessible from a corridor which runs the length of the ward.

Each ward staff consists of an administrator (i.e., chief ward psychiatrist), three or four resident psychiatrists, four graduate psychiatric nurses and a complement of an aide-clerk, aides and service personnel. In addition, each staff has its own clinical psychologist, psychiatric social worker and occupational and recreational therapists. Training personnel consisting of interns, medical students, and student nurses also are assigned to each ward.

Two psychiatric aides, one male and the other female, both with lengthy experience on the wards, were selected to record systematically the behavior of all patients and personnel on the five wards.[1] It was thought that those persons, by virtue of their familiarity with the patients and staff would interfere least with the operations of the wards. The two psychiatric aides made a series of trial recordings over a three-day period to perfect their technique and to allow patients and staff to accustom themselves to this innovation in the daily routine.

The five units were charted alternately on a pre-determined schedule. Recordings of patient behavior were made approximately every half-hour over a period of seven and one-half hours each day (i.e., from 9:00 until noon, 2:30 to 5:00 P.M., and 7:00 to 9:00 P.M.). These recordings were made for a three-week period and were designed to provide a three-fold description of patient activity in terms of whether and with whom the patient was interacting, the exact location of the patient on the ward, and the nature of the behavior observed.[2] A code system was devised to facilitate the recordings and to indicate all three aspects simultaneously. For example, a code designation of 1-1-1 meant that the patient was alone, in the day room, and in a stereotyped posture, i.e., overtly inactive.

There were 147 patients involved (97 female and 50 male). An average of 106-112 observations of all patients on each unit were recorded and this resulted in a three-week total of 11,879 patient-observations. At the same time a similar number of observations were made of the activities of ward personnel.

WARD ORIENTATION AND PATIENT BEHAVIOR

THE five wards differ significantly from one another, both internally and externally, in many respects—in the etiological viewpoints espoused, in the relative emphasis on and use of the various available therapies, in the manner in which staff members are involved in the functioning of the ward, and in the attitudes of ward administrators and personnel towards research and training. On all wards, but to significantly different degrees, the newer drug therapies, electroshock therapy, and, of course, psychotherapy are used. Four have group therapy sessions and the other does not. Three have weekly ward-wide meetings of patients and non-medical staff personnel. Patients are sent on home visits and to occupational and recreational therapy from each of the wards but the number and frequency vary perceptibly. Differences also exist in frequency, conduct, personnel participation, and discussions at morning ward meetings of staff members.

Intra-ward differences, and presumably conflict in the Stanton and Schwartz sense, were also assessed. These differences were best exemplified in the differential commitment of the various personnel on each of the wards to the usefulness of currently used therapies, and in the ward ideal as opposed to the actual utilization of therapies. Thus, interview data revealed that of six therapies rated and ranked (psychotherapy, group therapy, milieu, supportive, tranquilizers and electro-shock), intra-ward conflict was apparent in varying degrees with regard to the usefulness of each of these six therapies. The greatest intra-ward conflicts occurred over the use and effectiveness of the drug and electroconvulsive therapies. Despite these intra-ward differences there was also a more generalized ward consensus regarding psychotherapy as the most effective of the methods.[3]

These ward differences, both inter and intra, were reflected in the scheduled (i.e., prescribed) behavior of the patients on the five wards. Although there was a hospital-wide consensus on psychotherapy as the most desirable treatment measure, the percentage of patients receiving psychotherapy was found to range from 32 per cent on one female ward to 74 per cent on another female ward. Conversely no patients received electroshock therapy on this latter ward as compared with 12 per cent who did on the former. There were similar variations in the percentage of patients who received thorazine during the study period, ranging from 10 per cent on one ward to 35 per cent for the patients assigned to another ward. Nonetheless, as regards patient-time, psychotherapy sessions consumed a negligible part of the patients' 12 hour (9:00 A.M.-9:00 P.M.), seven day week—from a minimum of 0.7 per cent to a maximum of 3.4 per cent on these same wards. Even the inclusion of group therapy failed to significantly alter this picture. Total psychotherapy sessions, both individual and group, never exceeded 4.0 per cent of patient time on any unit.

TABLE 1.

Total Patient Interaction by Sex and Ward, In Per Cent

	MALE		FEMALE		
	2-E	3-E	1-W	2-W	3-W
Alone	57.7	57.7	55.6	41.1	51.3
With other patients	20.0	12.1	17.9	21.9	22.0
With staff	11.0	11.2	2.9	2.7	4.5
With visitors	2.2	1.3	2.6	1.6	.1
With therapist	1.6	1.8	1.1	2.9	4.0
a. individual	1.6	1.1	.7	2.2	3.4
b. group	—	.7	.4	.7	.6
At unit meeting	—	—	2.8	2.5	.7
With non-medical therapists	3.6	7.6	7.5	10.6	8.3
Home visit	3.3	6.3	8.7	15.5	7.4
Miscellaneous	.2	.4	—	—	—
Special care	—	.9	—	—	.7
Missing and AWOL	.4	.7	.9	1.2	1.0
TOTAL	100.0	100.0	100.0	100.0	100.0

Differential ward practices were also reflected in the number and amount of patient-time assigned to occupational and recreational therapy, group walks, and campus privileges. Total patient-time allocated to these activities varied from 3.6 per cent to 10.6 per cent. Wards providing the greatest amount of time to psychotherapy also sent the largest percentage of patients to these non-medical therapies and invested the greatest amount of patient-time in them. In addition, the average length of hospitalization and the number and frequency with which patients were sent on home visits were also found to vary by ward. At the time of the study the mean length of hospitalization varied from 37 days on one unit to 60 days on another ward.

TABLE 2.

Mean Age and Mean Length of Patient Hospitalization In Days, By Unit

	AGE*		LENGTH OF HOSPITALIZATION**	
	M	S.D.	M	S.D.
2—East	44.5	16.0	42.7	40.9
3—East	41.5	13.2	38.3	34.5
1—West	36.8	16.6	52.5	34.1
2—West	37.6	14.5	59.7	52.7
3—West	34.6	14.6	36.8	30.2

* Not significant by unit on male and female wards.
** Not significant by unit on male wards but 2-W keeps patients significantly longer than 3-W.

Another way of scrutinizing patient behavior is in terms of the therapy day (9:00 A.M.-5:00 P.M.) rather than the patient day. By eliminating evenings and weekends from consideration, a therapy day profile emerges. This profile, while more sharply differentiating the wards, in no way changes the basic relationships noted previously. Psychotherapy sessions were found to account for 2.2 per cent of patient time on one ward and 6.8 per cent of patient time on still another ward, exclusive of unit meetings. The non-medical therapy time amounted to an average of about 13 per cent of the therapy day and the time range was 6.5 per cent to 16.7 per cent of the day.

These therapy-time data would seem to indicate that unit differences do indeed affect patient activities—if only the *scheduled* activities of institutionalized patients are considered. When one contrasts the amount of patient-time allocated to medically prescribed activities as opposed to the amount of unplanned, undirected, and non-medically utilized time, the

TABLE 3.

Total Patient Interaction by Sex and Ward, Per Therapy Day, In Per Cent

	MALE		FEMALE		
	2-E	3-E	1-W	2-W	3-W
Alone	53.8	57.3	51.3	42.6	49.5
With other patients	23.9	11.4	19.1	23.7	23.6
With staff	12.1	12.0	3.7	3.1	5.3
With visitors	—	.1	—	.1	.2
With therapist	3.0	3.6	2.3	5.1	6.8
a. individual	3.0	2.2	1.3	3.8	5.8
b. group	—	1.4	1.0	1.3	1.0
At unit meeting	—	—	6.4	4.2	—
With non-medical therapists	6.5	10.6	13.4	16.7	12.3
Home visit	—	2.4	3.0	3.1	—
Miscellaneous	.9	1.5	.9	1.3	1.1
Special care	—	1.1	—	—	1.3
Missing and AWOL	—	—	—	.3	—
TOTAL	100.0	100.0	100.0	100.0	100.0

overall significance of the differential ward policies and practices seems inconsequential. Even in this short-term, intensive therapy, heavily-staffed institution (four or five psychiatrists including the unit administrator per maximum ward population of 28 patients), the physician, and the orientation of his unit, often become negligible factors in the experience of the patient and probably in his behavior as well. (1, pp. 204-225, 3, p. 73 ff.)

An average of 78 per cent of both the patient's therapy day (9:00 A.M.-5:00 P.M.), and at least this much of his week, were found to be almost wholly independent of direction and to overtly bear little, if any, relationship to the scheduled activities. Patients were alone about half of the therapy day, and with other patients 20 per cent of the time. On the men's wards they spent at least four times as much time interacting with non-medical staff members as with the medical staff.

CORRELATES OF WARD BEHAVIOR

INASMUCH as the overt activities of patients during the largest part of the day and week may be experientially as important as those derived from the medically scheduled activities, an analysis of this "leisure" time behavior is especially significant. Such an analysis revealed that (1) overt patient behavior is non-distinguishable by ward orientation, and (2) that whatever differences do exist in patient behaviors are primarily a function of patient characteristics (i.e., sex, age, and length of hospital stay) and disease entities, and not the particular and different ward management points of view. These same patient characteristics were also found to be related to the scheduled activities provided for patients.

1. SEX

UNSCHEDULED activities, in time, space and type, were found to be almost exactly the same for the male patients on both units and considerably different from that of the female patients. Male patients spent a greater part of the day alone, somewhat less time interacting with other patients and an average of three times as much time interacting with non-medical staff personnel as the female patients. Female patients spent the greater amount of time talking with other patients, over twice as much time in activities involving personal care and also devoted more time to writing and handicraft activities. Male patients made somewhat greater use of the recreational opportunities and spent considerably more time in simple physical activities (e.g., walking, pacing). The locus of the activities of the males centered in the day room and corridors, and female patients made proportionately greater use of their own rooms.

2. AGE

AGE, length of hospitalization prior to the observation period, and diagnosis were also significantly related to ward behavior. Male and

TABLE 4.

Direction and Significance of Relationships of Social Characteristics and Disease Entities with Amount of Ward Interaction and Percentage of Patients Receiving Psychotherapy and Related Therapies, by Male and Female

	WARD INTERACTION		PSYCHOTHERAPY		RELATED THERAPIES	
	MALE	FEMALE	MALE	FEMALE	MALE	FEMALE
Age						
Under 50	+	+	+	+	−	−
Over 50	−	−	−	−	+	+
X^2	73.38	16.22	−	−	−	10.30
P	.01	.01	N.S.	N.S.	N.S.	.01
Length of Stay						
Under 2 wks.	−	−	+	+	−	−
Over 2 wks.	+	+	−	−	+	+
X^2	37.11	15.99	−	−	−	−
P	.01	.01	N.S.	N.S.	N.S.	N.S.
Diagnosis						
Manic-Depressive	−	−	−	*	*	*
Schizophrenic	*	*	+	*	*	+
Psychoneurotic	*	+	+	+	*	*
Pers. Trait	*	*	−	+	*	+
Organic	N.C.°	−	N.C.°	−	N.C.°	−
X^2	17.64	157.65	−	−	−	−
P	.01	.01	N.S.	N.S.	N.S.	N.S.

* No direction indicated.
N.C.° No cases so diagnosed.

female patients aged 50 and over were the most isolated and the least active of all patients. The older male patients spent more of their interactional time with non-medical staff members and less with other patients. Elderly female patients reversed this procedure.

3. LENGTH OF HOSPITALIZATION

LENGTH of hospitalization for the male patients was positively related to the amount of inactivity and stereotyped behavior but not to the amount of interaction with other patients. On the female wards, there was also a significant relationship between length of hospitalization and amount of inactivity. Patient-patient interactions did significantly increase with hospitalization.[4]

4. DIAGNOSIS

ONLY one of the disease types, the manic-depressive psychoses with the emphasis on depression, seemed to have significance for the ward behavior of male patients. These patients were significantly more frequently inactive and stereotyped in their overt behavior than were the other diagnostic entities. The diagnostic categories were more important on the female units. Schizophrenics, psychoneurotics, personality disturbance types, depressives, and organic cases did significantly vary in their interactional patterns. Female patients classified as psychoneurotic were inactive 48 per cent of the time, personality disturbance types 57 per cent of the day, schizophrenics 62 per cent of the patient day, depressive cases 70 per cent of the time, and the organic cases 76 per cent of the time. These differences were significant at well beyond the one per cent level of significance.

TABLE 5.

Percentage of 50 Males and 97 Females Receiving
Psychotherapy by Age, Length of Hospitalization
and Disorder

	MALE %	FEMALE %
Age		
15-24		68
15-34	59	
25-34		57
35-39	53	
35-49		50
50 and over	44	45
Length of Hospitalization		
New Adm.	57	62
1-14	53	67
15-56	45	47
57-168	40	53
Disorder		
Manic-Depressive	30	50
Schizophrenic	63	50
Psychoneurotic	75	62
Pers. Disturb.	38	80
Organic	—	40

SOCIAL CHARACTERISTICS AND SCHEDULED ACTIVITIES

THESE same variables also made a difference in the scheduled activities of the patients and, in themselves, were at least as important as determinants of the therapy received as were unit orientations. Proportionately more females than males received occupational and recreational therapy. The percentage of patients, both male and female, receiving psychotherapy decreased consistently and sharply with age and with length of hospitalization.

The corresponding proportion of patients getting occupational and recreational therapy increased with age for the males, and for the females up to age 50, and with the length of hospital stay for both groups. Finally, psychotherapy also varied with disease classification. Cases classified as being of suspected organic origin least often received psychotherapy while those classified as psychoneurotics most frequently received psychotherapy. The non-medical therapies were not related to patient diagnosis.

DISCUSSION

THIS patient-observation study fails to substantiate the hypothesis that the attitudes and psychiatric policies of key staff personnel crucially affects the ward behavior of mental patients. The overt behavior of patients seems to be only slightly affected by the practices of the unit to which they have been assigned and in general is non-distinguishable from that of patients on different units. In terms of total patient time and overt experiences, the specific ward *outlook* seems to have relatively little effect. Patient activities, in time, space, and type, varied little by unit. Such differences as did exist in patient activities could be largely attributed to their social characteristics and disease classifications. The greatest differences in ward behavior were associated with the sex, age, length of hospitalization, and diagnosis of the patients. In short, these results seem to indicate that overt patient functioning or behavior, (1) because of the very structure of the hospital and its facilities, and (2) because of the disease entities themselves, is relatively constant. The unique structure and practices of any ward seem to be subsidiary in importance to the more general structure of the hospital and the disease. It is the hospital, the characteristics of the patient, and the process of institutionalization of patients and not the specific ward assignment which probably delimits, restricts, and stabilizes ward behavior.

Whether measured in terms of the more limited therapy day or the more inclusive patient day, patients were found to be "on their own" over three-fourths of the time. Most importantly, this heavily-staffed, voluntary-admission, short-term, intensive therapy institution tended on all wards to become more custodial for the patients diagnosed as being organically impaired, and for the older, less bizarre (i.e., less intriguing), longer hospitalized patients. Maximum psychotherapy time was given to the psychoneurotic, younger, more recent admission cases, regardless of ward.

LIMITATIONS

THIS study has the same types of limitations common to most investigations of patient functioning. These limitations include (1) the testing of a retrospectively formulated hypothesis with data which were not specifically collected for this purpose but which nonetheless were deemed sufficiently adequate for this purpose; (2) an additional limitation concerns the fact that these data deal only with the overt functioning of patients on the ward and not with "depth" behavior. This limitation is not as serious as some would believe since whatever significance "depth" behavior may be presumed to have should lie in its overt manifestations or it probably has very little, if any, meaning or validity.

SUMMARY

THIS study based on over 100 observation periods of the ward behavior of all patients at a short-term, heavily-staffed, intensive therapy mental hospital fails to support the hypothesis that differential ward policies and practices directly and significantly affect the ward behavior of patients. Although differential ward commitments are to some extent reflected in the medically prescribed (i.e., scheduled) activities, the nature and amount of unplanned, undirected, and non-medically prescribed behavior is not. Inasmuch as over three-fourths of the patient's day is spent in activity almost wholly independent of direction of any kind and since these activities may be experientially as important as those which are medically prescribed, the behavioral similarities among patients on different wards is highly significant.

Whereas unscheduled patient behavior was largely undifferentiated by ward, this behavior, as well as the scheduled activities, were found to be associated with such social characteristics as sex, age, length of hospitalization, and disease entity. These findings tend to focus attention upon the proposition that it is the hospital super-structure or specific characteristics of psychiatric illness which may be far more important in the determination of patient behavior and functioning than unit sub-structures as influenced by particular points of view. This hypothesis can be tested by future studies comparing patient behavior in different hospital settings. Such studies would do much to clarify the existing dilemma concerning the relative importance of the hospital as a therapeutic community.

NOTES TO CHAPTER 23

1. The authors wish to express their thanks to Mr. James Pierce and Mrs. Emily Washington, aides at the Columbus Psychiatric Institute and Hospital, for their reliable and willing assistance in the study.
2. A test of observer recording reliability indicated no significant differences in observations over time for either observer.
3. These data were collected as part of a larger study dealing with the effects of differences between real, perceived, and ideal staff relationships. Additional and more intensive analyses will be forthcoming.
4. There were no differences in patient interaction by ward when based on adjusted rates for differential length of hospitalization on the three female wards.

REFERENCES

1. Belknap, Ivan, *Human Problems of a State Mental Hospital* (New York: McGraw Hill Co., 1956).
2. Lippitt, R., "An Experimental Study of the Effect of Democratic and Authoritarian Group Atmospheres," *University of Iowa Studies in Child Welfare*, 16 (1940), 43-195.
3. Stanton, Alfred H., and Morris S. Schwartz, *The Mental Hospital* (New York: Basic Books, 1954).
4. Weber, George H., "Conflicts Between Professional and Non-Professional Personnel in Institutional Delinquency Treatment," *The Journal of Criminal Law, Criminology and Police Science*, 48 (May-June, 1957), 26-43.

CHAPTER 24   The Inmate Group in
Custodial and Treatment Settings*
DAVID STREET

P REVIOUS accounts of correctional institutions generally have portrayed
these organizations as handicapped by the informal inmate system.
This system, it has been said, invariably is built around norms and values
of solidary opposition to the official system and to staff, and its objectives
are to minimize interference and maximize accommodations from staff, to
enhance inmates' access to both official and unofficial values, to exert
vigorous control over communication between inmates and staff, and to
sanction an ideal model of behavior in which the inmate becomes a
master at "playing it cool." So far as this system succeeds, inmates released from the institution may leave more "prisonized" than rehabilitated. Such a description often has been treated as universally valid for
adult institutions,[1] and the same account appears in generally accepted
descriptions of juvenile institutions.[2]

Applicable as this image of the inmate system may be to many penal
institutions, it has several deficiencies as a general description and
analysis. First, most of the research on which it is based involves case
studies and unsystematic observation and has lacked adequate methods
to assess similarities and differences between organizations or even to
make satisfactory estimates of any variability in inmate orientations within
the single population studied. Yet, the notion that inmate attachment to
oppositional groups and culture varies has been at least implicit in much
of this research,[3] and it is clearly explicit in recent systematic research

* The research for this paper was done in close association with a study directed
by Robert D. Vinter and Morris Janowitz and supported by NIMH grant M–2104.
Complete results of this study are available in *Organization for Treatment: A Comparative Study of Institutions for Delinquents* by David Street, Robert D. Vinter, and
Charles Perrow (New York: Free Press of Glencoe, 1966).
  Reprinted from the *American Sociological Review*, 30 (1965), 40–55, by permission
of the author and the American Sociological Association.

[353]

such as the Wheeler and Garabedian studies of socialization in the prison.[4]

Second, the "solidary opposition" account fails to consider adequately the consequences for the inmate social system of changes in the larger organization, particularly the introduction of modern treatment ideology and technology.[5] Treatment programs, if they go beyond the simple insertion of psychotherapeutic counseling into the institutional program, require fundamental alterations in staff behavior toward inmates. The distinctive sociological character of the correctional institution and the deviant background predispositions of the inmates may indeed give rise to certain patterns of group development in all correctional organizations, but it is equally probable that variations in the institutional context generate changes in the inmate system.

Third, applied *a priori* to juvenile correctional institutions, the generally accepted account ignores important differences between these organizations and those for adults, including the relatively short stay and presumed lesser criminality of the juveniles and the possibility that many of the social forms that constitute severe deprivation and degradation in the adult correctional institution, where men are treated like children, may not be so degrading in the juvenile institution.

Finally, many researchers in the correctional field, lacking comparative methods, have been insufficiently sensitive to a significant theoretical question: under what organizational conditions do the members of an organization collectively become committed to or alienated from the official objectives of the organization?[6] By stressing the impact of deprivation and degradation on the inmates and the ways in which the inmates defend themselves, these researchers have developed a plausible hypothesis: that the inmate group serves the function of alleviating its members' deprivation and degradation.[7] Yet, they have failed to go farther and inquire into the effects of varying levels of deprivation or analyze the conditions necessary to stimulate, permit, and sustain the successful use of such a group solution to the problems of deprivation.

In contrast, this paper will treat inmate group patterns as problematic, bringing a comparative perspective to bear on data from several juvenile institutions. This analysis should have implications for the general proposition that the characteristics and functions of informal groups vary with the larger organizational context. Hypotheses linking the larger organization to the informal inmate system were developed by considering first, the implications of variations in goal emphasis among juvenile institutions, and second, the characteristics of the inmate group, conceived as a problem-solving system.

GOALS AND INSTITUTIONS

GOALS may usefully be regarded as the conception of the organization's tasks held by the members whose positions make their definitions of events authoritative. Their conception of task is expressed in their views of the organization's desired end product, the "materials" it must work with, the ideal and practical requirements of the task, and the organization's distinctive competencies for it. The goals imply and set limits upon the organizational technologies seen as appropriate. Thus, goals define as required, or preferred, alternative sets of social relations between staff and inmates.

Analysis of the goals of correctional institutions provides a basis for classifying these organizations along a rough custodial-treatment continuum. This classification reflects the relative emphasis on containing the inmates as against rehabilitating them. More analytically, the continuum incorporates two dimensions of the staff conception of the organization's task: the staff members' view of the actual rehabilitational potential of the inmates, and their concept of the "materials" they have to work with and the implicit "theory of human nature" they apply to these materials.[8] At the custodial extreme, major emphasis is placed on the need to protect the community by containing the inmates within the institution. The inmates are seen as simple, similar, and relatively unchangeable creatures who require simple, routine, conventional handling. To succeed here, the inmate must conform. At the treatment extreme, community and containment are comparatively unimportant, and stress is put on changing the inmate's attitudes and values by increasing his insight or otherwise altering his psychological condition. The inmate's social identity is viewed as problematic, and the inmates are seen as relatively complex beings who need complex, individualized, flexible handling—an attitude that sometimes requires such departures from conventional morality as tolerance of "acting out." To succeed here, the inmate must indicate intra-psychic change. These variations in organizational goals are accompanied by variations in the distribution of power in the organization: as institutions become more treatment-oriented, power to define events flows into the hands of a highly educated and professionalized "clinic staff."

These characterizations of the custodial and treatment types of institution are supported by a wide variety of data from the institutions we studied. The institutions were selected non-randomly to insure variation in goals and other dimensions. Each was studied intensively through observation, interviewing, analysis of documents and file data, and administration of questionnaires to virtually all staff members and inmates.[9] Two of the institutions stressed custody; the other two, treatment. Ranked from more custodial to more treatment-oriented and identified by mnemonic labels, they were:

Dick (Discipline)—a large (200-250 inmates) public institution which had no treatment program, whose staff felt no lack because of this, and which concentrated on custody, hard work, and discipline.

Mixter (Mixed Goals)—a very large (375-420 inmates) public institution with poorly integrated "mixed goals" of custody and treatment. Some treatment was attempted, but this was segregated from the rest of the activities, and for most boys the environment was characterized by surveillance, frequent use of negative sanctions, and other corollaries of an emphasis on custody.

Milton (Milieu Therapy)—a fairly large (160-190 inmates) public institution using not only individual therapy but a range of other treatment techniques. This institution resembled Mixter in its bifurcation between treatment and containment staffs and activities, but by and large the clinicians were in control, used treatment criteria, and influenced the non-professional staff to allow the inmates considerable freedom.

Inland (Individual Therapy)—a small (60-75 inmates) private "residential treatment center" in which the clinicians were virtually in complete control, allowing much freedom to the inmates while stressing the use of psychotherapeutic techniques in an attempt to bring about major personality change.

TABLE 1.

Inmate-Staff Ratios and Contacts

	CUSTODIAL		TREATMENT	
	DICK	MIXTER	MILTON	INLAND
Inmate-Staff Ratio	3.9	2.3	1.7	1.5
Inmate-Social Service Staff Ratio	125.0	45.9	22.2	15.0
Frequency of Inmate-Social Service Contact[a]	.13	.47	.76	.85

[a] Proportion of respondents to inmate questionnaire reporting two or more contacts with social service staff in the last month.

Limitations of space preclude full analysis and documentation of these differences between organizations, which in any case are presented elsewhere,[10] but some indication of their nature may be conveyed by data on staff-inmate ratios and contacts (Table 1), and by data from the staff questionnaire (Table 2). Higher ratios of staff, especially social service staff, to inmates, and higher inmate-social service contacts characterize the treatment institutions. The questionnaire results show that in the more treatment-oriented institutions staff members are more likely (1) to see the organization's goal as producing change in attitudes, values, and insights; (2) to value treatment programs more highly than custodial considerations; (3) to believe that inmates can be rehabilitated; and (4) to believe that adults can have trusting, close, and understanding relations with inmates, the development of such relationships being part of the staff's task. In contrast, staff members in the more custodial organizations are more likely (5) to stress order, discipline, and the use of powerful negative sanctions; (6) to insist on inmate conformity to institutional rules, including immediate response to staff members' demands; (7) to believe

TABLE 2.

Perspectives of Staff Members, by Institution[a]

PERCENTAGES OF STAFF WHO:	CUSTODIAL		TREATMENT	
	DICK	MIXTER	MILTON	INLAND
1. Perceive the executive's view of organizational purpose as bringing change in inmate attitudes, values, and insight.	10	19	38	51
2. Say they would approve of sacrificing custodial security in order to introduce a new treatment program.	41	53	76	80
3. Say you can change most inmates.	56	39	72	78
4a. Believe you can trust and have close relationships with delinquents (3-item scale).	68	53	79	78
4b. Think staff are expected to develop close relationships with inmates.	19	23	46	54
4c. Say understanding is important in working with delinquents (3-item scale).	16	32	63	83
5a. Think staff must keep order at all times.	58	45	13	14
5b. Believe delinquents need much discipline (5-item scale).	76	67	34	15
5c. Say they would invoke strong sanctions for a wide variety of inmate misbehaviors (5-item index).	61	68	24	10
6a. Believe the best way for an inmate to get along is "don't break any rules and keep out of trouble."	58	46	8	3
6b. Believe inmate must do what he is told and do it quickly.	92	75	44	16
7. Believe all inmates should get the same discipline for rule-breaking.	85	50	30	30
8a. Believe informal inmate groups always or usually have a bad influence.	96	26	4	5
8b. Believe inmates should keep to themselves.	40	38	15	3
Number of Respondents	(57-62)	(115-170)	(105-108)	(37-40)

[a] Differences in proportions between staff of the two custodial and two treatment institutions are statistically significant at or beyond the .05 level on every item.

in universalistic application of rules; and (8) to have negative attitudes toward informal relations among the inmates, believing that the inmates should keep to themselves. Such attitudinal differences between institutions hold up among cottage parents and in other groups when the respondent's staff position and his education are controlled,[11] and, further, the implied differences in behavior toward the inmates are confirmed by observations made in the institutions of the use of physical punishment, for example. To see how these different institutional environments affect the inmates, let us consider the inmate social system.

THE INMATE GROUP

INFORMAL group structure grows out of primary relations among inmates in all institutions, and it can be assumed to have a significant role in socializing and relating the inmate to the institution, in defining informal norms of inmate behavior and approved sets of values and beliefs, and in defining and allocating valued objects (e.g., contraband) among the inmates. Given the inmate group as a system potentially oriented toward ameliorating its members' deprivation, two major environmental factors could condition its response: (1) variations in the balance of gratifications and deprivations, and (2) variations in the conditions under which the group must attempt to solve its problem—that is, in the patterns of control and authority that the staff exercise over inmate action and behavior.

1. Variations in the balance of gratifications and deprivations. By limiting the available supply of rewards and thus creating a high ratio of deprivation to gratification the institution sets the stage for the development of a system for obtaining and distributing scarce values, both licit (e.g., choice job assignments) and illicit (contraband). Development of such a system presupposes that some inmates have access to values in short supply, and that inmates are sufficiently interdependent to set up a system of allocation and stabilize it in role expectations. Continuing access to the valued objects, and various forms of mutual aid, require a division of labor, which in turn is likely to produce a leadership structure reflecting differential power with regard to values within the system. Norms of reciprocity are likely to develop, to limit the advantages of those powerful enough to monopolize scarce values, but the latter nevertheless form a leadership cadre in which power is relatively highly centralized. To the extent that the system is deeply involved in the secretive and illicit transactions of contraband allocation, these leaders may have, at least covertly, very negative attitudes toward the staff and institution. Such leadership cadres might influence the group and make it more hostile to the official system than it otherwise would be.

2. Variations in staff patterns of control and authority. Rigid and categorical practices of control and authority are likely to facilitate the inmates' recognition of a common fate and their potentialities for collective problem-solving. Differences in authority, general status, age, and often social class, between staff and inmates, generally lead inmates to see each other as members of the same category in all institutions, but the authority structure and its impact vary among institutions. Frequent scheduling of mass activities in the company of other inmates, group punishment, and administering physical punishment before groups of inmates enhance the probability that inmates identify strongly with one another against staff. When, in addition, staff maintain domineering authority relationships and considerable social distance, inmates further perceive themselves as members of a group opposed to staff, and divergent interests between these groups are more fully recognized.

Staff patterns of control and authority also limit inmate association and group elaboration. Thus at the same time that rigorous practice of control and authority stimulate recognition of a common problem and the use of group solutions, they also make such solutions more difficult to achieve. Although only extreme techniques, such as keeping the inmates locked in separate rooms, effectively prevent the emergence of social relations among the inmates,[12] rigorous control could severely limit and structure opportunities for interaction and group formation—particularly the formation of groups covering the entire institution. In this situation, group activities must be conducted on a covert level, involving norms of secrecy and mutual defense against the staff.

HYPOTHESES

THESE two dimensions, gratification-deprivation and patterns of control and authority, link the institutional goals with the responses of the inmate group; both vary between the custodial and treatment settings. On the first of these dimensions, treatment institutions place much less emphasis on degradation ceremonies, the use of powerful sanctions, and denial of impulse gratification, and much greater emphasis on providing incentives, objectives, and experiences that the inmates consider desirable. On patterns of control and authority, treatment institutions place much less stress on surveillance, control over inmate association, restrictions of freedom, rigid conformity to rules, and domination and high social distance in authority relations. The simultaneous effects of these dimensions on informal groups in each type of setting should be as follows:

The Custodial Setting. Because of the high level of deprivation, the group is organized to allocate legitimate and illicit values and provide mutual aid. These functions reflect and generate relatively negative and "prisonized" orientations toward the institution and staff. Although staff control and authority practices increase the need for inmate group solutions, they also handicap interaction and group formation, so that integration and solidarity are relatively underdeveloped. The leaders, highly involved in illicit and secret activities, tend to have a negative orientation toward the institution.

The Treatment Setting. The inmate group is organized more voluntaristically, around friendship patterns. Since the level of deprivation is lower, mutual aid is less necessary, and any ameliorative system tends to lose its market. The group is involved in the allocation of values among its members, but these are positive rewards, more consonant with staff definitions of merit. Staff gives much freer rein to inmate association, so that primary group integration and norms of group solidarity are at a higher level than in the custodial setting. This cohesiveness does not necessarily imply opposition to staff, however, for the inmate group emphasizes more positive norms and perspectives and greater commitment to the institution and staff. Leaders' orientation is also more positive.

Finally, the more positive character of staff behavior toward inmates and the positive orientation of the inmate group generates more positive attitudes toward self among the inmates of treatment institutions than among those in custodial organizations.

Data are not available to test all features of the foregoing contrasts, but a reasonably satisfactory test can be made of the following specific hypotheses:

1. In the custodial institutions, the dominant tone of the inmate group will be that of opposition and negative, "prisonized" norms and perspectives with regard to institution, staff, and self; in the treatment institutions, positive, cooperative norms and perspectives will dominate.
2. Inmate groups in the custodial institutions will display somewhat lower levels of primary relations and weaker orientations of solidarity than will groups in the treatment institutions.
3. Relatively uncooperative and negative leaders will emerge in the inmate groups of the custodial institutions; relatively cooperative and positive leaders will emerge in the treatment institutions.

FINDINGS

THE hypotheses will be tested here by analyzing results of the inmate questionnaire. The inmates' responses, shown by institution in Table 3, convey the dominant tone of inmate group norms and perspectives.[13]

Findings on all but one of these items support the hypotheses.[14] Inmates in the treatment-oriented institutions more often expressed positive attitudes toward the institution and staff, non-prisonized views of adaptation to the institution, and positive images of self change. The exception is that on the index of "ratting to staff" no difference between custodial and treatment institutions appeared.

TABLE 3.

Inmate Perspectives, by Institution

PERCENTAGE OF INMATES WHO:	CUSTODIAL		TREATMENT		STATISTICAL SIGNIFICANCE[a]
	DICK	MIXTER	MILTON	INLAND	
Score high positive on summary index of perspectives on the institution and staff.[b]	42 (209)	44 (364)	58 (155)	85 (65)	p < .01
Score high on cooperation with staff on summary index of "ratting."[c]	54 (209)	46 (364)	49 (155)	54 (65)	N.S.
Gave a "prisonized" response to question about the best way to get along.[d]	74 (202)	73 (348)	55 (151)	45 (60)	p < .01
Gave a "prisonized" response to question about ways to receive a discharge or parole.[e]	59 (187)	47 (352)	27 (140)	13 (65)	p < .01
Score positive on self-image index.[f]	38 (188)	42 (327)	51 (143)	79 (60)	p < .01

[a] Significance refers to the difference between the inmates of the two custodial institutions combined and those of the two treatment institutions.

[b] The specific items summarized by this index were (paraphrased): (1) Is this a place to help, send, or punish boys? (2) Rather be here or in some other institution? (3) Summary: Did you think this would be a good or bad place, and what do you think about it now? (4) Agree that the adults here don't really care what happens to us. (5) Agree that the adults are pretty fair. (6) Agree that adults here can help me. (7) How much has your stay here helped you?

[c] The specific items summarized in this index followed a presentation of hypothetical situations, and were (paraphrased): (1) Should a boy warn an adult that boys plan to rough up his friend? (2) Should he warn an adult that inmates plan to beat up a staff member? (3) Would you tell an adult which boys were stealing from the kitchen, when group punishment was being used? (4) Would you try to talk a boy out of running?

[d] The question was "Regardless of what the adults here say, the best way to get along here is to . . ." ("stay of the way of the adults but get away with what you can" and "don't break any rules and keep out of trouble" were classified as "prisonized" responses, and "show that you are really sorry for what you did" and "try to get an understanding of yourself," as "non-prisonized").

[e] The question was "*In your own words,* write in what you think a boy has to do to get a parole or discharge from here" (responses of conformity, avoidance of misbehavior, "doing time," and overt compliance were coded as "prisonized").

[f] Those classified as "positive" on the index of self-image said that they had been helped by their stay a great deal or quite a bit and that the way they have been helped was by having "learned something about myself and why I get into trouble," rather than having "learned my lesson."

TABLE 4.

Percentages of Inmates Positive on Index of Perspectives on Institution and Staff, by Selected Background Characteristics and Institution[a]

	CUSTODIAL		TREATMENT	
	DICK	MIXTER	MILTON	INLAND
Seriousness of major offense[b]				
Less serious	38	52	57	82
	(66)	(75)	(67)	(45)
More serious	42	43	60	90
	(140)	(286)	(84)	(20)
Number of offenses				
Less than 3	42	52	51	87
	(161)	(40)	(43)	(54)
3 or more	40	43	60	73
	(48)	(307)	(112)	(11)
Number of times returned to this institution[c]				
None	44	47	62	84
	(156)	(283)	(135)	(63)
One or more	31	38	29	100
	(52)	(78)	(17)	(2)
Previous institutionalization of any kind[d]				
None	42	48	61	94
	(191)	(295)	(118)	(16)
Some	33	33	50	83
	(15)	(66)	(34)	(6)
Age				
Under 16	34	50	56	85
	(94)	(204)	(121)	(41)
16 and over	47	40	62	83
	(114)	(160)	(34)	(24)
Race				
White	43	47	62	82
	(181)	(245)	(104)	(55)
Non-white	24	40	48	100
	(25)	(116)	(48)	(10)
I.Q.[e]				
90 and below	30	45	58	80
	(44)	(120)	(41)	(5)
91 and above	37	43	64	85
	(38)	(203)	(56)	(55)
Family situation				
Intact, no problems	46	49	62	80
	(95)	(204)	(42)	(39)
Not intact, or problems	36	40	56	92
	(111)	(157)	(108)	(26)

TABLE 4. (*continued*)

	CUSTODIAL		TREATMENT	
	DICK	MIXTER	MILTON	INLAND
Rural-urban origin[f]				
"Rural"	41	50	55	100
	(208)	(126)	(107)	(3)
"Urban"	—	43	64	85
	(0)	(235)	(45)	(60)
Occupation of father or other head of household				
White collar	22	71	63	78
	(18)	(21)	(8)	(18)
Blue collar or not in labor force	42	44	58	85
	(179)	(330)	(141)	(34)

a Data were obtained from institutional files. The index of perspectives on institution and staff is described in Table 3.

b The "more serious" category includes arson, forgery, sex offenses, breaking and entering and crimes of violence, but excludes truancy, "incorrigibility," "maladjustment," theft, and vandalism.

c The Milton figures underestimate the actual number of returnees to some unknown degree because ordinarily only those who are re-committed to the institution, after having been supervised for several months following release by another state agency, are entered in institutional records as returnees. Others, returned during the period of supervision, generally are not so classified.

d Information on the majority of cases at Inland was missed due to coding error.

e The majority of inmates at Dick were not tested.

f "Urban" inmates are from counties with at least one city of 90,000 or more; "rural" inmates come from counties that do not have such a city.

Background Attributes and Length of Stay. Question immediately arises as to whether these differences in perspectives on the institution and staff, adaptation, and self might not reflect variations in inmates' predispositions rather than variations in the institutional setting. A careful analysis of the impact, by institution, of delinquency history, past institutional record, age, race, IQ, family situation, urban-rural background, and social class indicates a negative answer to this question.[15]

Table 4 shows that the direction of the effect of each of the background variables on perspectives varies from institution to institution, and that the custodial-treatment differences in perspective hold up when background attributes are controlled. In nearly every instance, the inmates of both treatment institutions were more likely to have positive perspectives on staff and institution than the inmates of either custodial institution. The three exceptions to this predicted pattern were: (1) among those with fewer offenses, Mixter inmates (51 per cent positive) did not differ from those in Milton (50 per cent positive); (2) disproportionately few (29 per cent) of the Milton inmates classified as returnees had positive perspectives; and (3) a disproportionately large number of positive responses came from Mixter inmates with white-collar backgrounds.

The first of these exceptions suggests that a portion of the relatively negative over-all response at Mixter may be a result of its heavy recruitment of inmates with many offenses. But this would not explain why those with three or more offenses are so negative compared with similar inmates at Milton and Inland. The second exception is probably a result of the fact that the Milton returnees, as indicated in the note to the table, are not directly comparable with the others, apparently constituting an especially "hard core." The last exception may simply reflect the small number of "white-collar" inmates at both Mixter and Milton. Altogether, these exceptions do not challenge the conclusion that these background attributes cannot explain the observed differences between types of institution.

Similarly, inter-institutional variations were not simply a reflection of the fact that the treatment institutions usually keep their inmates longer. Data on this point may also be used to assess the degree to which the prisonization model or one of its variants "fits" these institutions.[16] Figure 1, graphing positive perspectives on the institution and staff against length of stay, indicates that differences between types of institution cannot be accounted for by differences in average length of stay. Inmates of the treatment institutions are more likely to express positive perspectives at almost every point in time. Within the custodial institutions, the over-all trend is for the proportion negative to increase with length of stay. Although this tendency toward increasing negativism in the custodial institutions is akin to what one would predict under the prisonization model, attitude changes in the treatment institutions are in the opposite, positive direction. In these institutions, the proportion expressing positive perspectives increases rapidly over time in the early months and, after a downturn, increases further in the later months.[17]

Effects of Primary Group Integration on Perspectives. Data on integration into the inmate group provide a more adequate test of the hypothesis about the dominant tone of the inmate group if one assumes that when those who are better integrated express more positive perspectives, it is because their group exerts a positive influence, and when the better-integrated are more negative, it is because their group exerts a negative influence. Operationally, the better-integrated inmates are those who said they had two or more friends in the institution.[18]

The findings clearly indicate that positive attitudes are more closely associated with primary group integration in the treatment institutions than in the custodial institutions (Table 5). Results on the four indices significantly related to integration consistently display the predicted pattern. Thus integration into the inmate group was more strongly associated with positive perspectives on the institution and staff in the treat-

---

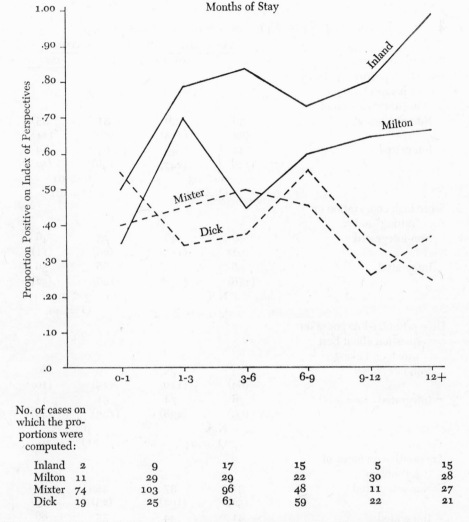

No. of cases on which the proportions were computed:

	0-1	1-3	3-6	6-9	9-12	12+
Inland	2	9	17	15	5	15
Milton	11	29	29	22	30	28
Mixter	74	103	96	48	11	27
Dick	19	25	61	59	22	21

FIG. 1. LENGTH OF STAY AND PERSPECTIVES ON INSTITUTION AND STAFF

ment setting than in the custodial environment. Further, despite the fact that custodial and treatment settings did not differ wih respect to scores on the "ratting" index (see Table 3), integration and cooperation with staff are positively associated in the treatment but not in the custodial setting. (This finding principally reflects the strong positive association in Milton; in Inland and in both custodial institutions, it was relatively weak.) Finally, in the treatment institutions integration was inversely associated with the prisonized view of adaptation and positively related to a positive self-image, while in the custodial institutions there was little or no association with these indices.

TABLE 5.

Inmate Perspectives, by Integration Into the Inmate Group[a]

PERCENTAGES OF INMATES WHO:	CUSTODIAL		TREATMENT	
	DICK	MIXTER	MILTON	INLAND
Score high positive on index of perspectives on institution and staff				
Non-integrated	36	36	31	**55**
	(62)	(115)	(26)	(11)
Integrated	44	49	64	89
	(146)	(247)	(126)	(52)
	p < .05		p < .01	
	Q = .22		Q = .61	
Score high cooperation on "ratting" index				
Non-integrated	48	48	23	46
	(62)	(115)	(26)	(11)
Integrated	56	44	55	56
	(146)	(247)	(126)	(52)
	N.S.		p < .01	
	Q = .01		Q = .49	
Give prisonized response on question about best way to get along				
Non-integrated	73	73	72	60
	(62)	(110)	(25)	(10)
Integrated	76	74	51	44
	(139)	(238)	(123)	(48)
	N.S.		p < .05	
	Q = .04		Q = −.39	
Are positive on index of self-image				
Non-integrated	31	37	35	44
	(52)	(101)	(23)	(9)
Integrated	41	44	55	86
	(135)	(225)	(119)	(49)
	N.S.		p < .01	
	Q = .16		Q = .50	

[a] Kendall's Q is used to measure the association between integration and the score or response indicated.

An analysis of the joint impact of integration and length of stay on these attitudinal measures indicated that variations in length of stay did not account for these variations in the relation between integration and attitudes.

Levels of Inmate Primary Relations and Solidarity. A variety of findings consistently support the second hypothesis, that inmates in the treatment setting have more highly developed primary relations and stronger orientations of solidarity (Table 6).[19] Inmates of the treatment institutions more frequently reported "hanging around" with other inmates, having several friends, and (reflecting the difference between Mixter and Milton) wanting to see other inmates again after release. In addition, the treatment inmates more frequently indicated a willingness to talk with other boys about a personal problem and more often rejected the view that you "have to be pretty careful what you say or do" around other inmates.

TABLE 6.
Inmate Social Relations, by Institution

PERCENTAGES OF INMATES WHO:	CUSTODIAL		TREATMENT		STATISTICAL SIGNIFICANCE[a]
	DICK	MIXTER	MILTON	INLAND	
Hang around with three or more boys	59	71	78	91	p < .01
Have three or more close friends (integration index)	70	68	83	83	p < .01
Want to see all or most inmates again after release	27	14	35	27	p < .01
Would talk to other inmates about a personal problem	58	50	66	76	p < .01
Say you don't have to be careful around the other boys	14	18	21	27	p < .05
Are high on index of solidary orientation	27	28	31	55	p < .01
Numbers of Respondents	(202-208)	(356-363)	(152-155)	(62-64)	

[a] Refers to differences between the custodial and treatment organizations.

Finally, scores on an index of solidarity orientation, here defined as emphasis on general loyalty to the group beyond primary ties with particular others, show a similar pattern. In the treatment settings, especially Inland, inmates were more likely to express such an orientation than were those in the custodial institutions. In neither setting was solidary orientation related to a statistically significant degree to perspectives toward the institution and staff or to scores on the "ratting" index.[20]

Leadership. Data bearing on the third hypothesis, that the attitudes of inmate leaders would be relatively positive in the treatment setting and relatively negative in the custodial environment, also tend to follow the predicted pattern. Boys who were nominated four or more times as having the most "influence" in the institution were classified as leaders.[21] On three attitudinal indices, statistically significant differences between leaders and non-leaders were found in either the custodial or treatment setting (Table 7). Leadership is more strongly associated with positive perspectives on staff and institution in the treatment environment than in the custodial setting, reflecting the strongly positive association at Milton. The same finding emerges on the self-image index—again the Milton leaders are highly positive. On the index of "ratting," leadership and cooperation with staff tend to be negatively associated in all institutions, but the association is stronger in the custodial than in the treatment institutions. Thus, findings on all three indices support the hypothesis that leaders have more positive perspectives in the treatment environment.

TABLE 7.

Leadership and Perspectives Toward the Institution and Staff[a]

PERCENTAGES OF INMATES WHO:	CUSTODIAL		TREATMENT	
	DICK	MIXTER	MILTON	INLAND
Are positive on index of perspectives toward the institution and staff				
Non-leaders	42	45	53	83
	(177)	(318)	(130)	(48)
Leaders	37	48	80	88
	(32)	(46)	(25)	(17)
	N.S.		p < .01	
	Q = −.005		Q = .52	
Are highly cooperative on index of "ratting"				
Non-leaders	56	47	51	56
	(177)	(318)	(130)	(48)
Leaders	38	37	44	47
	(32)	(46)	(25)	(17)
	p < .01		N.S.	
	Q = −.26		Q = −.14	
Are positive on index of self-image				
Non-leaders	39	41	47	75
	(162)	(287)	(120)	(44)
Leaders	32	53	74	87
	(25)	(40)	(23)	(16)
	N.S.		p < .01	
	Q = .09		Q = .53	

[a] Q measures the association between leadership and the score or response indicated.

A separate analysis indicates that these differences among leaders characterize both "integrated" and "non-integrated" leaders. And other data, on inmate perceptions of leadership in general, support the characterization of leaders in the treatment settings as having more positive attitudes.[22]

These and the other findings reported here indicate a difference between the two treatment institutions, Milton and Inland. On the one hand, data on inmate perspectives, effects of length of stay, and social relations clearly indicates that inmates have more positive attitudes and more highly developed primary relations at Inland. On the other hand, group involvement, as measured by integration and leadership, was more closely associated with positive perspectives at Milton than at Inland. Milton is a "milieu" institution; perhaps this finding reflects its conscious attempt to manipulate the inmate group.

Data from Additional Institutions. Data on inmate groups in three other institutions for juvenile offenders, studied less thoroughly than the four organizations just analyzed, shed additional light on the custodial-treatment differences I have reported. The first of these units, *Maxwell* (Maximum Security) was a geographically and administratively separate part of Mixter, established to handle the "most difficult" inmates of the parent institution shortly before the end of our field work. The other units, *Regis* (Religious) and *Bennett* (Benign), were small private institutions that were "open," sending their charges away from the institution every day for ordinary public or parochial schooling. In their goals and in the staff's behavior toward the inmates, these two open institutions seemed to fall between the custodial and treatment types; their goal might be characterized as "training." The inmate is viewed as changeable, but such simple techniques as altering skills and habits are considered appropriate. Within this training model, Regis stressed constant work and recreation activities along with indoctrination and enforcement of obedience and religiosity, while Bennett emphasized the creation of a home-like environment with staff serving as parental surrogates.

Results from these three units are represented by findings on the association between integration into the inmate group and responses to four attitudinal items (Table 8). These data, together with those from the major institutions (Table 5), show, first, that integration is negatively associated with positive perspectives on the institution and staff, cooperativeness with staff in "ratting," and self image in Maxwell but not in the custodial or treatment institutions, and that a direct association between integration and "prisonized" response to the third item occurs only at Maxwell. Second, patterns in the two open institutions are generally inconsistent: Regis resembles Maxwell on the first two items, Bennett resembles the treatment institutions on all items, and in both institutions the

TABLE 8.

*Inmate Perspectives, by Integration into the Inmate Group,
in Maximum Security and Open Units*[a]

PERCENTAGES OF INMATES WHO:	MAXIMUM SECURITY	OPEN	
	MAXWELL	REGIS	BENNETT
Score high positive on index of perspectives on institution and staff			
Non-integrated	64	84	36
	(11)	(19)	(11)
Integrated	54	63	91
	(33)	(38)	(23)
	Q = −.19	Q = .17	
Score high cooperation on "ratting" index			
Non-integrated	45	47	27
	(11)	(19)	(11)
Integrated	21	32	35
	(31)	(38)	(23)
	Q = −.51	Q = −.15	
Give prisonized response on question about best way to get along			
Non-integrated	60	72	60
	(10)	(18)	(10)
Integrated	73	71	45
	(33)	(38)	(22)
	Q = .28	Q = −.14	
Are positive on index of self-image			
Non-integrated	56	40	33
	(9)	(15)	(9)
Integrated	60	58	71
	(30)	(31)	(21)
	Q = .09	Q = .49[b]	

[a] Q measures the association between integration and the score or response indicated.
[b] Difference in proportions significant at the .05 level.

association between integration and self-image is positive, as it is in the treatment institutions.

These findings and other results suggest that in Maxwell—which, with its stringent security regulations, resembles the traditional adult prison more than any of the other institutions—the "solidary opposition" model fits the inmate group reasonably well. Only in this institution was the relation between scoring high on the index of solidary orientations and strong opposition to staff on the "ratting" index statistically significant ($p < .05$ and $Q = .75$). Our data collection took place only three months after the unit was opened, however, and after several crises of organizational birth, when the inmates may have had a special *esprit de corps* because they were the first group considered incorrigible enough to be sent there. We have no evidence, therefore, that the "solidary opposition" model will continue to fit inmate groups in this type of setting.

Despite the fact that Regis and Bennett were open, allowing their inmates considerable freedom away from the institution, this milieu did not consistently generate as positive a response as did the closed treatment setting. On the other hand, the fact that on some dimensions, e.g., self-image, the association with integration is positive, and as strong as in Milton and Inland, suggests that a relatively benign, open environment might make it possible to achieve some of the benefits of treatment without the expense of a treatment program.

DISCUSSION

THESE findings generally support hypotheses about differences between custodial and treatment settings with regard to inmate norms and perspectives, social relations, and leadership and therefore clearly challenge the general applicability of the "solidary opposition" model of the inmate group, at least to juvenile institutions. Variation in organizational goals gave rise to differences in inmate orientations and characteristics of the inmate group, and only in the limited data from a new maximum security unit was there any consistent indication that the "solidary opposition" model was appropriate. By treating the balance of gratification and deprivation and patterns of staff authority and control as variables affecting the inmates, I have replaced the assumption that inmates form solidary and oppositional problem-solving groups with the assumption that under different conditions, different patterns of orientations, social relations, and leadership occur among the inmates. This more open perspective should be applicable to the study of adult institutions, too.

Although we were unable to obtain comparable data on recidivism for the various institutions, our findings indicate tentatively that both custodial and treatment organizations tend to accomplish their proximate goals. By stressing covert opposition and "playing it cool," the custodial inmate group encouraged behavior consistent with the custodial goals of containment and conformity. Thus, the level of "prisonized" orientations was higher among the custodial than among the treatment inmates. Similarly, the treatment inmate group seemed to produce in its members an orientation consistent with the goal of achieving change. Evaluating outcomes with reference to goals is more difficult in the treatment case, of course, for the nature of the most appropriate technology for rehabilitation is undiscovered. Under the current treatment technologies, however, a minimally positive orientation toward the agents of change, e.g., the counselors, is clearly a necessary pre-condition to successful rehabilitation. The inmate groups in the treatment settings more frequently encouraged a positive orientation, and less often encouraged the development of a negative self image, apparently, than in the custodial institutions.

Finally, this research suggests that the study of correctional institutions would be substantially improved if researchers more frequently recognized the generality of the concept of social control and the variety of devices used to maintain control. All correctional organizations exercise a great deal of control over their inmate members, but while custodial organizations emphasize formal and severe sanctions directed at ordering and containing the inmates, treatment institutions are more likely to rely on informal, personal sanctions and incentives directed at behavior perceived as relevant to inmate change. The implementation of a treatment program in a previously custodial environment implies a shift not to less control, but rather to *different types of control* exercised on the bases of different criteria. As numerous writers have pointed out, humanitarian pressures have already limited severely the use of the most repressive (and perhaps most effective) custodial techniques in American juvenile institutions, even though most of them still are predominantly custodial. Under continuing humanitarian pressure, and faced with evidence that custodial techniques are incompatible with other organizational goals, these institutions are very likely to alter their patterns of authority and control in the coming decades. Researchers interested in the question of implementing successful rehabilitation programs in correctional settings might do well to consider and investigate more fully a variety of combinations of different social control and rehabilitation techniques. Perhaps the treatment model represented in this research is the only really viable model, or perhaps other models, e.g., some form of the "training" model, could combine order-keeping and rehabilitation successfully and in a manner more compatible with the budgets and present commitments of most institutions today.

NOTES TO CHAPTER 24

1. For example, Sykes and Messinger, reviewing over 35 studies of correctional organizations, conclude that "Despite the number and diversity of prison populations, observers of such groups have reported only one strikingly pervasive value system . . . [which] commonly takes the form of an explicit code . . . The maxims are usually asserted with great vehemence . . . and violations call forth a diversity of sanctions ranging from ostracism to physical violence . . . The chief tenets . . . [include] those maxims that caution: *Don't interfere with inmate interests,* which center of course in

serving the least possible time and enjoying the greatest possible number of pleasures and privileges in prison. The most inflexible directive [is] *Never rat on a con* . . . The prisioners must present a united front against their guards no matter how much this may cost in terms of personal sacrifice." (Gresham M. Sykes and Sheldon L. Messinger, "The Inmate Social System," in Richard A. Cloward, *et al., Theoretical Studies in Social Organization of the Prison*, New York: Social Science Research Council, 1960, pp. 5-8).

2. For example, Lloyd E. Ohlin and William C. Lawrence, "Social Interaction among Clients as a Treatment Problem," *Social Work*, 4 (April, 1959), pp. 3-14. Similar treatments of the inmate group in juvenile correctional organization are found in Richard A. Cloward, "The Correctional Institution for Juveniles: A Discussion of Selected Problems," paper read at the New York School of Social Work seminar on juvenile institutions, 1956; and George P. Grosser, "The Role of Informal Inmate Groups in Change of Values," *Children*, 5 (January-February, 1958), pp. 25-29. Other analyses suggesting that the inmate system is these institutions operates principally to oppose or circumvent the organization's aims include Howard Polsky's study of a cottage in a treatment institution, reported in "Changing Delinquent Subcultures: A Social Psychological Approach," *Social Work*, 4 (October, 1959), pp. 3-16, and *Cottage Six—The Social System of Delinquent Boys in Residential Treatment*, New York: Russell Sage Foundation, 1962; and Lloyd Ohlin's observations on a training school for girl delinquents, "Reduction in Role Conflict in Institutional Staff," *Children*, 5 (March-April, 1958), pp. 65-69.

3. Variation in inmate attitudes and behavior underlies the whole notion of prisonization. See Donald Clemmer, *The Prison Community*, New York: Rinehart, 1958, and the various studies of social types in the prison, for example, Clarence Schrag, "Social Types in a Prison Community," unpublished M.A. thesis, University of Washington, 1944, and his "Leadership among Prison Inmates," *American Sociological Review*, 19 (February, 1954), p. 42, in which he writes of "a number of dissentient minorities [which] resist, at least to some extent, the dominant influence of the typical leader group."

4. Stanton Wheeler, "Socialization in Correctional Communities," *American Sociological Review*, 26 (October, 1961), pp. 697-712, and Peter C. Garabedian, "Social Roles and Processes of Socialization in the Prison Community," *Social Problems*, 11 (Fall, 1963), pp. 139-152, and "Legitimate and Illegitimate Alternatives in the Prison Community," *Sociological Inquiry*, 32 (Spring, 1962), pp. 172-184. See also the discussion of the inmate society as made up of three subcultures dependent on latent identities, in John Irwin and Donald R. Cressey, "Thieves, Convicts, and the Inmate Culture," *Social Problems*, 10 (Fall, 1962), pp. 142-155, along with the contributions by Wheeler, Schrag, and Donald L. Garrity to Donald Cressey (ed.), *The Prison: Studies in Institutional Organization and Change*, New York: Holt, Rinehart, & Winston, 1961.

5. The major empirical works directly addressing the problems of the inmate group but taking exception to the general view of it are studies of treatment-oriented camps for young offenders by Oscar Grusky, "Organizational Goals

and the Behavior of Informal Leaders," *American Journal of Sociology,* 65 (July, 1959), pp. 59-67, and Bernard Berk, "Informal Social Organization and Leadership among Inmates in Treatment and Custodial Prisons," unpublished Ph.D. dissertation, Univerity of Michigan, 1961. Other writings deriving from the same study as the present report, and directly relevant to many parts of it, include Robert Vinter and Morris Janowitz, "Effective Institutions for Juvenile Offenders: A Research Statement," *Social Service Review,* 33 (June, 1959), pp. 118-131; Mayer Zald, "The Correctional Institution for Juvenile Offenders: An Analysis of Organization 'Character,' " *Social Problems,* 8 (Summer, 1960), pp. 57-67, and "Comparative Analysis and Measurement of Organizational Goals: The Case of Correctional Institutions for Delinquents," *Sociological Quarterly,* 4 (1963), pp. 206-230; Rosemary Conzemius Sarri, "Organizational Patterns and Client Perspectives in Juvenile Correctional Institutions," unpublished Ph.D. dissertation, University of Michigan, 1962; Juvenile Correctional Institutions Project, *Research Report,* Ann Arbor: University of Michigan, 1961; and David Street, "Inmate Social Organization: A Comparative Study of Juvenile Correctional Institutions," unpublished Ph.D. dissertation, University of Michigan, 1962.

6. After considerable study and discussion, informal groups have come to be viewed as neither wholly reflective of the larger structure nor wholly determinative of it; rather, the role of these groups in the attainment of organizational ends varies according to the organizational context. Students of industrial plants generally have stressed the negative impact of informal groups on productivity (for example, see the classic discussions of informal relations and structures in F. J. Roethlisberger and W. J. Dickson, *Management and the Worker,* Cambridge: Harvard University Press, 1941, and Orvis Collins, Melville Dalton, and Donald Wray, "Restrictions on Output and Social Cleavage in Industry," *Applied Anthropology,* 5 (1946), pp. 1-14), while sociologists who have studied military organization have traced the positive functions of such groups (Samuel A. Stouffer, *et al., The American Soldier,* Princeton: Princeton University Press, 1949, Vol. II, pp. 130-49; Edward A. Shils, "Primary Groups in the American Army," in Robert K. Merton and Paul F. Lazarsfeld (eds.), *Continuities in Social Research: Studies in the Scope and Method of "The American Soldier,"* Glencoe, Ill.: Free Press, 1950, pp. 19-22; and Edward A. Shils and Morris Janowitz, "Cohesion and Disintegration of the Wehrmacht in World War II," *Public Opinion Quarterly,* 12 (1948), pp. 280-315). For a recent conception of this problem in general terms, see Amitai Etzioni, *A Comparative Analysis of Complex Organizations,* New York: Free Press of Glencoe, 1961.

7. The inmate system is seen as providing new, deviant standards that allow the inmates to assuage guilt by "rejecting their rejectors" (Lloyd W. McCorckle and Richard Korn, "Resocialization within Walls," *The Annals,* 293 (May, 1954), pp. 88-98), to achieve compensatory status and to benefit from contraband and illegitimate activities (Ohlin and Lawrence, *op. cit.*), and to defend against aggression and exploitation by other inmates (Sykes and Messinger, *op. cit.*). The latter authors, even though they seem to assume that the inmate group is inevitably cohesive and opposed to official goals, also suggest that the extent of deprivation and degradation might predict the inmate group's response (p. 19).

8. On the theory of human nature, see Erving Goffman, "On the Characteristics of Total Institutions: Staff-Inmate Relations," in Cressey, *op. cit.*, p. 78.
9. Here I shall report findings principally on the four "closed" institutions studied intensively in the juvenile corrections project. Near the end of this paper I shall refer to findings on three additional institutions, not as directly comparable for the problems discussed here. For details of questionnaire administration and other research techniques, see Street, *op. cit.*, pp. 198-202.
10. See especially Juvenile Correctional Institutions Project, *op. cit.*
11. *Ibid.*, chs. 7 and 9.
12. Even this technique is not necessarily effective. See Richard McCleery's account of an adult maximum security unit, "Authoritarianism and the Belief Systems of Incorrigibles," in Donald Cressey (ed.), *The Prison: Studies in Institutional Organization and Change, op. cit.*, pp. 260-306.
13. Indices were derived partly from the results of a factor analysis of inmate responses. For details of this analysis and of the construction of indices, see Street, *op. cit.*, pp. 213-224.
14. I have used statistical tests of difference between groups of respondents heuristically, to help decide whether to deny predicted differences between the custodial and treatment types of organization. Although the non-random selection of institutions, the clustering of all respondents in four organizations, and the sampling of entire institutional populations make use of the word "test" in its strict sense illegitimate, no more appropriate bases for decision-making are available. Note, too, that because the tests (as well as the measures of association presented below) combine the data for each of the pairs of institutions, to highlight the differences between the custodial and treatment types, the results may obscure differences within pairs. Important within-type variation will be discussed in the text.
15. Street, *op. cit.*, pp. 75-83.
16. Clemmer, *op. cit.*, Wheeler, "Socialization . . . ," *op. cit.*, and Garabedian "Social Roles . . . ," *op. cit.*
17. Institutional records shows that average stay before release is: Dick, 10 to 11 months; Mixter, 7.5 months; Milton, 15 months; and Inland, 11.5 months, with an average of 18 months for those who complete the institution's program.
18. The question was: "How about *close* friends? Some boys have close friendships with other boys here and some boys don't. How many of the other boys here are close friends of yours?" We assumed that a respondent who reported one or no friends was not really integrated into the group, having at best only a single "buddy." While this definition of integration is subject to questions regarding the probable reporting error and the relation of this "primary relations" interpretation to other meanings of the concept, it provides an empirically profitable starting point for analyzing the consequences of integration.
19. The specific questions asked were: (1) "Do you usually hang around here with several guys, a few, mostly with one boy, or with none?" (2) The integration question (see note 18); (3) "How many of the boys you have met here would you like to see again after you get out?" (4) "Suppose you had

been feeling sad for several days and are very upset about a personal problem. Are there any *boys* here you would go to and talk with about the things that made you sad?" (5) "Some boys say that you have to be pretty careful about what you say or do around the other boys here, or else they may give you a rough time. What do you think about this?" (6) Summary of responses to "How much of the time do you think most of the boys here really stick together, and are loyal to each other?" And "Regardless of how much the boys actually do stick together now, how much do you think they *should* stick together?" Respondents who answered both questions positively were scored high on the solidarity orientations index.

20. That these differences in social relations actually follow from organizational control practices is suggestion by responses to a question asking for agreement or disagreement with the statement that "You have to be careful about the boys you get friendly with around here. To stay out of trouble with the adults you have to keep to yourself." Considerably higher proportions of inmates rejected this statement in the treatment setting (79 per cent in Inland and 52 per cent in Milton) than in the custodial institutions (30 per cent in both Mixter and Dick).

21. The specific question was "What three boys are best at getting other boys to do what they want them to do—that is, which three have the most influence among the boys? Think of the boys that you know in your cottage, in school, and in the work program, or recreation."

22. Street, *op. cit.*, pp. 116-119.

Section IV

THE FUNCTIONAL COMPONENTS

OF INSTITUTIONS

ॐ

INTRODUCTION

SOCIAL scientists posit a small set of organizing principles that characterize all durable human groups.[1] According to Homans,[2] the analysis of a social system reveals two fundamentally distinct problems:

1) What are the procedures a group undergoes in attaining its goals within a social environment?

2) What are the operations for maintaining satisfying and efficient cooperation among the members of a group to enable it to carry out its goals?

In other words, every durable functioning social system has a concrete job to get done; at the same time it must promote loyalty among its members and commitment to the goals of the group. This distinction between task-performance and system-maintenance underlies every social system.

The aggregate of tasks that must be carried out by any system to maintain itself are what Parsons and Bales refer to as "functional imperatives." If any of these four tasks, or functions, fails to be executed at some minimum level, the entire system is upset and in danger of collapse. The functional imperatives consist of:

1) *Adaptation.* Adaptation is the process whereby the group organizes to meet the requirements of the larger social system in which it is located. The adaptational task is that of properly perceiving and carrying out the formal rules and informal expectations of the larger society. In order to do so, a certain amount of cooperation or enforced order must be imposed on the group. The fulfillment of the adaptational requirements often leads to frictions and dissatisfactions in group members' relations with one another.

2) *Goal Attainment.* Like adaptation, goal attainment is an external system imperative. It refers to the task of articulating and carrying out the purposes and autonomous goals of the group. Groups attract and hold members because they attain goals that individuals alone cannot.

[1] See the articles by Fallding and by Polsky and Claster, in Section I.
[2] George C. Homans. *The Human Group.* New York: Harcourt, Brace, 1950.

3) *Integration.* Integration is a feature of the internal system, whereby the group develops a satisfying social and emotional climate among its members. It refers to the necessity for groups to reduce the tensions and strains incurred in executing goals and meeting adaptational requirements, as well as those stemming from individual personality problems.

4) *Latency.* Latency is the interlude between meeting institutional requirements and attaining goals. It consists of providing emotional support for members so that they can carry out the activities connected with goal attainment and adaptation. In essence, the latency sphere concerns individual psycho-dynamics; its management is an attempt to prevent personality problems from disturbing the effective functioning of the group.

The articles in this section highlight institutional issues in each of the four functional spheres and the inter-dependence of spheres. They illustrate how a change in one functional component of the system reverberates throughout the whole system. Similarly, some of the articles will point out how neglect of one of the system imperatives influences other system functions, thereby affecting the operation of the entire institution.

ADAPTATION

As "no man is an island unto himself," similarly, no group is so self-sufficient that its needs and purposes are not in some part directed toward the larger community or surrounding social system. Adaptation refers to the process whereby a group mobilizes to meet the requirements and expectations of the external system. Often this is a rather unpleasant task, in that the demands may restrict members' latitude of acceptable behavior.

The article by Dentler and Mackler describes quite cogently the pressures that the larger system, the staff of a well-known school for retarded children, exert upon their charges in socializing them to acceptable modes of institutional behavior. The most frequent method used to accommodate children to regulations was endless repetition of cues, consisting of simple commands like: "Don't make noise," "Don't get into fights," "Don't get in trouble," "Just be quiet." Another technique to insure obedience was deprivation of privileges and seclusion. Also, since the adaptational sphere is heavily stressed and staff members have few privileges to give out, they try to convert gratifications that children customarily expect into privileges. This was a third way the staff used to socialize the children. A fourth was the staff's capacity to delegate authority to children who were able to successfully conform to regulations. The success of these socialization techniques is reflected in the children's appraisal of one another. Initially, it was found that boys with the highest sociometric choice status received the most frequent disciplinary restrictions. At that point, apparently, group integration was achieved as a result of emphasis on the custodial function. In the second month after arrival, however, after the group had become socialized to adult norms, the status structure changed radically; the boys who gained the greatest reduction in frequency of discipline had the highest status.

Adaptation is not only a problem for the smaller social system that is forced to conform; it poses problems for the larger system that imposes the requirements as well. Mouledous agrees that "if an egalitarian approach is held, the administration relinquishes control of the total penal environment and allows for the development of an inmate social system which gradually dominates the environment and becomes the main reference for inmate standards and behavior." His solution assumes that. . . . "If administration maintains control of the penal environment by developing an authoritarian rather than egalitarian approach, the inmate behavior and standards can be oriented to those of administration." To implement such an approach, Mouledous suggests that the administration maintain its power by "distributing to the inmates various material resources and freedom of movement in exchange for their cooperation." His approach to the custodial problem, then, is to replace the threat system with an exchange system as a prize for inmate accommodation to the demands of the administration. This "solution" is not the only alternative, of course. Grosser (in the following sub-section on goal attainment) discusses a similar problem in adolescent training schools. He prefers using the inherent resources of the inmate group as a resocializing agent, rather than neutralizing the effectiveness of the inmate group, as Mouledous suggests.

Ryan is impressed with the proclivity of patients in a closed ward of a psychiatric hospital to prefer this structured custodial atmosphere. This preference may be regarded as antithetical to the tendency of many modern mental hospitals toward increased freedom and individualization. On the closed ward, patients adhered to a strict routine. They ate and went to bed at a specific time. Rules were firmly enforced except for the sickest patients, and even they were encouraged to conform as much as possible. In this very structured and protective environment, Ryan reports that 93 per cent of the patients felt a sense of comfort and security. Many of those who had led lonely and isolated lives were able to make contact with other people and develop a sense of identification with the patient group. In social system terms, Ryan is suggesting that strict enforcement of rules and tasks frees the patient from the need to make decisions and plan his own goals. For this reason he conforms easily to the structure and integrates comfortably with peers.

A view opposing custodial emphasis is contained in the article by William Deane, a sociologist. He spent a week as a participant observer in a

mental hospital. Two features of the hospital impressed him most unfavorably—the overly supervised routines for major activities like eating,
sleeping and jobs; and the absence of a purposeful program of leisure
activities. While leisure time makes up a considerable portion of the
hospital routine, there is relatively little to command the patient's attention or interest when he is free from the demands of his schedule. Deane
describes vividly the extreme discomfort and anxiety, leading to depression and psychotic symptoms, which he himself developed under these
conditions.

GOAL ATTAINMENT

WHILE it is true that each of the functional imperatives must be maintained if the system is to survive, in some respects the goal attainment
sphere may be regarded as the fundamental aim of the social system.
Whether fully aware of the fact or not, individuals enter into group interaction because groups can attain goals satisfying to their members which
the members cannot attain separately. In this sense, the group's goal orientation and accomplishments are not only the major payoff for group
membership, but actually its *raison d'être*.

This rationale is rather clear for informal groups, where common motives often lead consciously to the formation of a group. In informal
groups, neophytes enlist and veterans depart as the group's goals shift
from one interest to another. But for total institutions, where residents are
often committed against their wishes and assigned to resident units (cottages, hospital wards, cell blocks, etc.) without being consulted about
their preferences, peer group dynamics have to be re-conceptualized.
One distinguishing feature of institutional groups stands out: ". . . among
inmates in many total institutions there is a strong feeling that time spent
in the establishment is time wasted or destroyed or taken from one's life;
it is time that must be written off. . . . This time is something its doers
have bracketed off for constant conscious consideration in a way not
quite found on the outside."[1] Unless the inmate can be stimulated to
develop meaningful goals, he will persist in thinking of the total institution as a place of internment, not as a place where learning and resocialization are possible. Without motivating the inmate's interest in his own
autonomous development, rehabilitation is impossible.

The first article in this section, by Hyde and Solomon, indicates one way
of helping patients to develop autonomous goals in the total environment
of residential institutions. The article describes an experience at Boston
Psychopathic Hospital in which psychiatric patients developed a system
of self government. From group interview sessions, in which patients

---

[1] Erving Goffman. *Asylums*. Garden City, N.Y.: Doubleday, 1961, pp. 67-68.

recommended changes in ward conditions and made other requests of the administration, there emerged a democratic system with a constitution drafted by patients, elected officers, and most important, patient responsibility for carrying out many activities, with appropriate limitations, on their own. The essential factor for the success of such a program, the authors feel, is a responsive hospital staff which trusts patients enough to share some authority with them.

Grosser, in the next selection, points out how training school administrators have created a situation which makes it virtually impossible for resident groups to develop socially approved group goals. To begin with, these schools set up a status hierarchy which placed the resident in such a low position that spanning the distance from resident status to one of respect and acceptance from the administration is nearly impossible. Second, the administration's restricted definition of acceptable behavior is not shared by the resident group. Furthermore, the inmate group is not encouraged to develop autonomous goals; in the eyes of the administration, the inmate group is an unavoidable disability of inmate confinement.

Thus the administrative view is self defeating: by deprecating the capacity of the inmate group to work toward constructive goals, the administrators discourage development of healthier modes of adjustment which they in fact consider desirable. Feeling thus rejected, the inmate group in turn rejects the goals of the administration and turns toward its own membership for support, affection and respect, in a word, for a sense of identity. To counteract the patients' militant, anti-rehabilitation aims, Grosser proposes that the administration utilize the resources of the inmate group to develop goals both gratifying to the inmate group and approved by administration.

A program to assist psychiatric patients in developing their own goals for recovery, both inside the hospital and in the community after release, is presented in the next paper. Through coordinating services in the hospital as well as stimulating volunteers from outside, McCullough helped patients to feel accepted as part of a group. With acceptance the patient is better able to accept himself, a tolerance he extends in turn to others. Finding others in the group have similar problems, he has less need for defensive attitudes and can then devote more attention to developing new autonomous perspectives about his life situation.

The proper climate for developing and carrying out comprehensive and improved hospital services depends upon an insightful, flexible administrator, according to the next article. In effect, Clark sees the good administrator as one who pays adequate attention to all the functional spheres of the hospital's social system. He is the pace-setter; he approaches the "right" personnel with skills needed for carrying out a particular program (adaptation), he sees that good morale prevails so that staff can work harmoniously (integration), he locates the personnel in the hospital most resistant to change (the blocks to goal attainment), and he reassures them and induces their support (latency management). Successfully coordinating these functional spheres creates an atmosphere which maximizes the goal of improving hospital service.

INTEGRATION

A SPIRITED rapport—the feeling of well-being among group members who hold similar interests and accept one another as important—is essential to group interaction if the members are to apply themselves to the group's tasks. In this sense integration, like goal attainment, is both an attraction and a payoff of group membership. The level of group integration serves as a barometer of the functional quality of the other system spheres. When the other functions are adequately met and the aims of the group carried out, group cohesiveness seems to be automatically engendered.

Maxwell Jones's pioneering therapeutic community, at Belmont Hospital in England, illustrates the central role of the function of integration. Jones's unit stresses the importance of interpersonal relations by encouraging free communication among staff and patients, while playing down status differences. For example, it was felt that the uniforms usually worn by hospital staff and patients symbolize these differences; to promote freer contact both patients and staff at Belmont Hospital wear street clothes. Jones's work is not explicitly couched in social system terms, but its emphasis on patient and authority roles in the institutional setting, and its awareness that system functioning depends on the structure of the relations, lays the groundwork for more explicit system formulations.

An article by Boyd, Kegeles and Greenblatt illustrates how social system strains can lead to a breakdown of integration. The authors interviewed staff and patients after a destructive gang incident on a psychiatric ward. An analysis of the factors related to the incident revealed that there was a lack of harmonious integration of patients on the ward. On the same ward were aggressive paranoid patients who had been referred from the courts for purposes of diagnosis, as well as more severely disturbed treatment cases. The court-referred patients organized themselves into a delinquent clique. They were more socially perceptive and better organized than the treatment patients, and manipulated the latter for their own antisocial purposes. Integration was also strained on the ward because of staff resentment against court-referred cases for taking up bed space without paying for it and for neglecting staff directives. Nursing staff loyalties and favoritism toward certain patients impeded the already poor communication between administration and patients, and increased the resentment and frustration of patients on the ward. Finally, failure to provide outlets for frustration and boredom led directly to the destructive incident. On a week-end, when the staff-patient ratio was lower than during the week, the patients went on a rampage.

McCorkle has followed Grosser's suggestion, discussed above, by employing the social resources of the inmate group in resocialization. In guided group interaction the major emphasis is on the group and its development, rather than on analysis of individuals in the group. The rationale for this technique holds that the delinquent will benefit from peer social experiences where "he can freely discuss, examine and understand his problems without the threats that have been so common in his previous learning experience." New insights into his own behavior may induce the inmate to give up self-defeating peer roles.

The article by Caudill and his colleagues demonstrates how patient integration develops in a social setting where the opportunities for goal-attainment are underdeveloped and the custodial orientation is not strict enough to incur "natural" group solidarity through opposition. "The patients felt that many of the ordinary conventions and social gestures of the outer world were made temporarily meaningless by hospital life." Among his peers, each patient constructs a role which is nominally functional to the informal patient group and enables him to identify with it. Moreover, the group assists newcomers in this process. In one case, for example, the group found roles for two of its members as preparers of the evening snack because they realized that the social facility of these two patients was rather limited. By fulfilling such functions, the informal group gains control over patient life.

LATENCY

AT ONE level a social system is a consolidation of norm-directed individuals, and at another, a matrix of conflicting intra-psychic processes. The latency sphere links these two levels; group functioning is generally facilitated by successful reduction of its members' psychic or status conflicts.

Individuals characterized by considerable intra-psychic conflict are severely impeded in employing adequate social skills. They tend to project their motives and conflicts onto other individuals. Among problem children, projective behavior stems from the child's belief that others pose threats to instinctual demands. Such a belief leads to a highly stereotyped defensive attitude which prevents the child from responding when he is removed from his home to a nurturant treatment environment. In order to reduce these defensive "vigils," Bettleheim and Sylvester, at the University of Chicago's Orthogenic School, provide the problem child from the start with a stable, undemanding structure. The staff members are highly permissive of deviant behavior and make minimal demands; they attempt to satisfy generously the infantile needs of the children, and to induce positive relationships between children and themselves. Since the staff members remain consistent and non-threatening, defensive attitudes are reduced, making successful social behavior appreciably easier.

In working with latency problems of residents in total institutions, the practitioner must be clear about the implications of his therapeutic approach. McCorkle and Korn maintain that "the impulse to help has become confused with treatment and seems to require defense as treatment." The humane handling of inmates—for example, permitting them to set up their own expectations for such routines as labor—has failed as badly as the more punitive techniques of the past. This is because prison officials have tended to use the inmate power structure as an aid to prison administration for maintaining order. They have not realized that in manipulating the inmate structure they are in turn allowing themselves to be manipulated. Under this method of "least-effort," prison administration has surrendered to the distorted realities of inmate pressures instead of demanding a more realistic and therapeutic work situation. By relinquishing custodial demands to inmate pressure, the prison administration reinforces the inmate power structure and thereby prevents rehabilitation.

Gilbert and Levinson look at latency tension management in another way. They describe differences in attitudes toward mental illness that prevail among staff members in a psychiatric hospital. They then proceed to show that these attitudes reflect general approaches to life problems, related to deeper personality dynamics. The authors conceptualize two ideal types of staff ideology. "Custodial ideology has important psychic functions for authoritarian hospital members. . . . [For] the person who has a great defensive need to displace and project aggressive wishes concerning authority figures to those who can be regarded as immoral, custodial ideology has special equilibrium-maintaining value through its justification of punitive, suppressive measures. . . . Humanistic ideology has corresponding functions for its adherents. By supporting a critical attitude toward the established order, it permits many equalitarian individuals to express generalized anti-authority hostilities in an ego-syntonic form. The principle of 'self-control through self-understanding,' applied in the treatment of patients, often serves to maintain and consolidate the intellectualizing defenses of equalitarian personnel." In this sense the mental patient's opportunity for developing autonomous and meaningful goals depends largely upon the personal qualities of staff personnel with whom he comes in contact.

Powelson and Bendix, the former a psychiatrist and the latter a sociologist, see a similar bifurcation of custody and treatment among prison staff, but they attribute it to role rather than personality differences. The agents of custody, the guards and the warden, think of prisoners as aspiring above all else to get out of prison by any means available and so to escape their "just punishment." Once the prisoner is termed as "justly confined," in their view, any means of punishment or control becomes defensible.

Psychiatrists and social service workers, on the other hand, are agents of rehabilitation. They look at the inmate's present behavior, not as an indication of his moral depravity, but as an outgrowth of a maladjusted personal history. Thus, they emphasize the need for treatment rather than punishment. Yet it is the custody agents who have the power. They supervise prisoners' activities day by day so that a "smooth operation" results, at the cost of conditions conducive to rehabilitation.

Adaptation

৯৯

CHAPTER 25   The Socialization of
Retarded Children in an Institution*

ROBERT A. DENTLER AND BERNARD MACKLER

INTRODUCTION

IN GOFFMAN's terms, a state hospital and training school for mentally
retarded children is one type of "total institution": A residential institution within which specially defined persons are grouped or aggregated
for special purposes, and where customary divisions between the sleep,
play and work patterns common to non-institutional life in communities
are reorganized into scheduled uniformities. As Goffman notes,

> Total institutions . . . are social hybrids, part residential, part formal organi-
> zation, and therein lies their special sociological interest. There are other reasons
> . . . for being interested in them, too. . . . Each is a natural experiment . . . on
> what can be done to the self.[1]

This paper reports on the manner in which aides in one state hospital
and training school for retarded children socialize newly arrived children
toward the adoption of institutionally acceptable patterns of behavior. By
socialization is meant the process by which the children are trained toward
compliance with the demands made by agents in a particular environment.
The analysis is restricted chiefly to the period covered by the first two
months after entry into the institution. It is also restricted to consideration
of what will here be defined as socialization toward compliance with
management and interpersonal, in contrast to academic and medical,
routines. Both sociologically and practically, the problem of institutional-

* This research was supported in part by a grant from the Graduate Research Fund
of the University of Kansas. The authors are indebted to Leland Miller, Max Siporin,
Robert Sommer, Bernard Farber, Joseph Spradlin, Ross Copeland, and Charles War-
riner for their comments and suggestions.
Reprinted from the *Journal of Health and Human Behavior*, 2 (1961), 243–252, by
permission of the authors and the American Sociological Association.

ization is "a most crucial one because it bears not only the problem of the effects of environmental change on performance and potential but on one of our society's major ways of handling . . . mental retardation."[2] The main questions addressed in this report are: (1) What routines of management are emphasized by aides in the institution, and how are these implemented? (2) What are some of the effects of institutional socialization on the interpersonal relations of children?

RESEARCH PROCEDURES

STATE School was selected for investigation for two reasons. First, State School is regarded by experienced practitioners in this special domain as a relatively "optimal" institution. Its physical plant, the qualification of its staff, its aide training program, and its research program, have gained national attention for their excellence. Few state institutions for retarded children in the nation are considered superior to State School by the practicing professions. This provided some basis for assuming that, while no single institution could be representative of others, practices of aides at State School could not be attributed in some judgmental fashion to limited resources or "poor" standards. Secondly, the arrival of a group of new children, all assigned to a newly constructed cottage managed by experienced aides, offered a novel opportunity to study institutional socialization.

The 29 new boys, inhabitants of Cottage X, arrived at State School within a few days of one another. They ranged in age from six to 12, with a mean of 9.6 years. Their mean IQ was 56, and all were classified tentatively by the staff as educable. Four fifths of the boys were diagnosed as exhibiting no noteworthy central nervous system pathology.

The boys and aides in Cottage X were observed by the authors for three weeks. Every hour of the day was observed, with emphasis given to the waking periods. The authors stationed themselves in corners of rooms, tagged along to meals, to the playground and the gymnasium. Most of the boys ignored the observers after the first two days, but about one-third of them persisted with efforts to involve the "non-participating" observers in reading or writing mail to parents, in sharing in games or secrets, and in unelaborated physical contact. Thus the informal social relations of the boys were not left untouched or unaffected. A code for classifying observations was adapted from the scheme developed by Spiro,[3] who studied children in an Israeli Kibbutz. But observation was only partially systematic. Unique incidents, unanticipated types of interaction, and general insights were tape recorded together with as exhaustive a report on mundane matters as could be recalled immediately after leaving the cottage scene. More exact observations were also secured. These are reported elsewhere.[4]

To investigate the question of the effect of institutionalization on the interpersonal relations of the children, the authors devised sociometric tests that these children appeared capable of taking. Each child's photograph was mounted on a large but portable board with pins. The photographs were arranged randomly in six rows of five columns. At the close of their third week of observing, the authors established rapport with each child, one at a time, and administered the following questions in the privacy and comfort of a cottage bedroom:

Which boys would you most like to play with in the Day Hall?
Which boys would you not like to play with in the Day Hall?
Which boys would you most want to be (like)?
Which boys would you most like to work with in cleaning up the cottage?

The children responded with pleasure and apparent understanding to these questions. A minimum of *three* choices were elicited on each criterion.[5] Two weeks later, these sociometric questions were administered again. The arrangement of the pictures was changed and the tests were administered not in the cottage but in the hospital research unit.

ORGANIZATIONAL CHARACTER

STATE School may retain children against their will; yet, unlike state mental hospitals, State School is subject, under varying legal conditions, to the continuing agreement of parents or guardians. The terms of entry and release are more flexible than those common to institutions for adults. Children at State School may be released temporarily to vacation at home or undertake treatment or education elsewhere. A few are allowed access to the surrounding community. This flexibility is somewhat limited by the fact that, under law, entering children are defined as incompetent minors. This status naturally intensifies the custodial responsibility of State School.

The primary, manifest functions of State School are management, treatment, rehabilitation and education. As studies of other types of total institutions have demonstrated, these functions are somewhat incompatible.[6] Efficient custodial care, for instance, militates against achievement of educational objectives. State School has changed during the last decade from a relatively single-purpose custodial hospital for adult epileptics to a multiple-purpose institution. In the course of improvements in physical plant, reduction in patient load from one thousand to about three hundred, and of changes in external relations between the institution and the state, State School staff members have given increasing priority to rehabilitative and educational goals. In spite of this marked change, as Zald has noted about other institutions:

The actual degree of dominance of one goal over another is not wholly determined by the chartering agents. Even if they were to specify quite precisely the relative emphasis upon goals that were to be expected, the organization might not be able to realize this goal ratio. Depending upon its resources,

structure, personnel, and clientele, the institution might be more or less successful in attaining its goals. . . . The existence of the two major goals of custody
and rehabilitation heighten the possibility of conflicting occupational role groups
and the development of conflicting policies.[7]

The organizational dilemma of incompatible goals is complicated by the
contrast between bureaucratic structure (or what Goffman refers to gen-
erically as formal organization in total institutions) and informal relations
as these emerge wherever aggregates of persons eat, work, play and sleep
in close extended proximity. State School constitutes a bureaucratic structure. It operates within a legally and administratively prescribed context
of specialization, a hierarchy of authority, a system of rules, and with
relative impersonality. Defined as patients, children at State School are
expected to learn to behave in terms of rules established by the leadership within this structure. Blau has observed that:

Bureaucracy, then, can be defined as . . . an institutionalized method of
organizing social conduct in the interest of administrative efficiency. On the
basis of this definition, the problem of central concern is the expeditious removal
of the obstacles to efficient operations which recurrently arise.[8]

Other functions are performed at State School but the primary task of
the institution is the maintenance of efficient, safe routines for the management of patients defined as incompetent minors. State School has little
if any difficulty achieving this objective at the level of the staff. The
physical plant is relatively adequate, communication facilities are excellent
and lines of authority established. From the point of view of the institutional functionary, the critical obstacles to efficient operations are various
behavior patterns of patients.

Patients may be treated by nurses, psychologists and physicians, educated by teachers and ministers, and rehabilitated by a variety of therapists, but their day to day and night to night behavior is managed by
residential cottage aides. The *initial* task of the aides is to prepare the new
patient for accommodations to the institution. From the point of view of
the professional staff, rehabilitation becomes possible principally when
this accommodation has been achieved. Initially, therefore, virtually all
interaction between staff and children is mediated by cottage aides. When
a child in Cottage X was diagnosed by a psychologist, for example, the
psychologist's secretary telephoned an aide at the cottage. The aide made
an appointment note and, at the appropriate hour, called the child from
his room, the cottage lounge or the play area, and walked him to the hospital office of the psychologist. After his hour in the hospital, the child
was picked up by an aide and returned to the cottage. Later in his institutional career, the same sequence of events occurs, but the child is directed
to make his own visit and return from the hospital to the cottage.

The managerial responsibility of the cottage aide during the first two to
three months after a child's arrival is very extensive. It includes all aspects

of the management of sleep, play, eating, participating in cottage cleaning and limited work routines, toilet and bath and dress habits, assistance with communications between child and family, discipline and superficial medication. Administrative regulations embrace these domains of responsibility, and the department of nursing bears the burden of maintaining periodic as well as emergency supervision. Exclusive of scheduled contacts with individual staff professionals and the preparation of meals, however, the context of life in the early months is totally established and managed by cottage aides.

ROUTINES AND SOCIALIZATION

DURING the period of socialization, only a very few persons other than aides entered or left the cottage X. Nurses made periodic rounds. All but one of the nurses concentrated exclusively during the visits on the paper reports, prepared by the aides, on tap at the aide desk inside the entry hall of the cottage. The one nurse paused sometimes to interact with the children. A recreation therapist stopped at the cottage to pick up groups of children for trips to the gymnasium. And on four occasions during three weeks, older boys from other cottages entered Cottage X to carry out housecleaning assignments. Excerpts from the notes convey an impression of the nature of the daily routine:

Two aides were on duty at all times. They woke the children, who sleep two to a bedroom and four to a bedroom in some cases, at 5:50 a.m. From 6:00 to 7:00, the aides helped the children wash, toilet, dress, and make their beds. At 7:00, the aides lined the children up in pairs at the front door of the cottage and directed them at a casual pace to the cafeteria. Shifts at the cafeteria are so arranged that no more than two cottage groups eat together. Inside the cottage, aides directed the boys into the television lounge, where they watched cartoons.

Between 9:00 and 9:15 a.m., the aides opened one of the toy closets in the day hall. Eight of the 29 boys moved out of the TV lounge and into the day hall. There was much drifting of boys between the two rooms. Infractions were frequent at this time; and individual boys were disciplined by being sent to their bedrooms. The drifting within the cottage continued until 10:00.

The chief aide assembled the boys in the day hall at 10:00. Each boy was told to take a chair at a table. The aide said, "Now it is time to have a talking session. Who remembers what we learned yesterday at the talking session?" M's hand went up. The aide said, "No, M told us what we learned the last time I asked. Who else knows?" G made a stab at an answer. Aide said, "No, that's not right." (I had attended yesterday's Talk Session but could not recall what had been learned, either). J tried. Aide said, "No, that's not right."

Four more children tried answers. Aide then outlined what we had learned: "First we learned no kicking and no pushing. Then, we learned we shouldn't go into the rooms of any other boys or bother their belongings. These are what we learned. Now we will have some cookies, because IC got some in the mail."

LB got a box out of the toy cupboard. Aide opened it and LB moved about the room giving each boy a cookie. The waste basket was set by aide in the center of the room. Aide said, "Take one piece and say thank you to L as he comes past."

The boys sat quietly at the tables. Aide said, "Ah, that is good. You are all learning to sit nicely and quietly in here. Now we will have our new thought for today. Our new thought is that we should have no wrestling or playing in the television room. We should play only in the day room. Can you remember that?"

The second aide entered and removed four boys, "For Music." They were sent to the department of music therapy. At 10:10, the chief aide said, "Keep in your seats and be quiet now. We've got about four minutes left. Sit down there now. This lasts until 10:15. Now who can tell me what we talked about that is new this morning?" The procedure described was repeated identically.

At 10:15, aides directed the boys to the TV room. The set was turned on, this time to a soap opera. Drift between TV room and Day room continued and much disciplining was necessary. Non-conformers were punished by being sent to their bedrooms again. (On some days the children were allowed out of doors at this time in the morning to play on bikes, wagons and scooters.)

At 11:30 the children washed and dressed for lunch. They got ready for and walked to the cafeteria just as for breakfast.

After lunch, from 1:00 to 4:00, activities were diversified for the first time. Some children were sent to professional departments for evaluation, treatment, or classification. Others took naps for two hours, then played perfunctorily around the cottage.

At 4:30 the boys got ready for dinner. They washed up, toileted, then sat and watched TV or played in the play room. At 4:50, they walked (casually) in pairs to the cafeteria, eating and returning to Cottage X at 5:45. They took showers and assisted in cleaning the cottage rooms from 6:00 until 8:00. They sat in the Day room or watched TV for 45 minutes. Then they were seated at tables in the Day Room and given crackers and milk.

Contacts during the day with non-Cottage personnel included: three nurses on their rounds, one minister who came to observe for an hour, recreation therapist and cafeteria food servers.

HOW SOCIALIZATION IS CONDUCTED BY AIDES

THE critical demands of the institution, during the initial phase of socialization, were for conformity to routines, fulfillment of instructions from aides, and minimization of conflict with peers.

Management involves physical protection and "time filling." As the outline of the schedule suggests, blocks of time each day are unoccupied during the first three months after arrival. One task of the aide is to occupy this time. As Goffman has observed,

In the inmate group of many total institutions there is a strong feeling that time spent in the establishment is time wasted or destroyed or taken from one's life; it is time that must be written off. It is something which must be "done" or "marked" or "put in" or "built" or "pulled." . . . As such, this time is something that its doers have bracketed off for constant conscious consideration in a way not quite found on the outside. . . . Harshness alone cannot account for this quality of life wasted. Rather we must look to the social disconnections caused by entrance and to the usual failure to acquire, within the institution, gains that can be transferred to outside life—gains such as money earned, or marital relations formed, or certified training received.[9]

Young children with mental ages between two and ten do not define their life situation this way. The children did not "mark time." Some had been separated from their parents with the expectation that they would be going to school, and as unintentional school failures in their communities, this was a powerful incentive. But for two months, no classroom experience was presented. One boy faced each day with the remark, "Today I go to school." Two or three times daily he would attempt to leave the cottage. Retrieved, he would explain, "I am going to school."

For the aides, who attended to the clock closely in scheduling events for the children and in waiting for their changes in shifts, management was a matter of socializing the children toward increased control. The cues employed were simple. They were repeated endlessly. Summed up they were, "Don't make noise, don't get into trouble, don't get into fights, just be quiet."[10] In achieving these controls, the primary techniques were *deprivation* and *seclusion*. If a boy did not "mind the aide," he was deprived in accordance with the extent of the deviation. Toys were taken away and locked up for a fixed period of time. Or the child was sent to his bedroom, or placed on a chair in a corner of an unoccupied lounge, or made to sit or stand on the "Naughty Bench," a stone settee that ran along one wall of the TV lounge. When a child was disciplined, the particulars of his infraction and the discipline taken were written on pink slips, to be circulated among staff departments and then filed in the child's records. Here are excerpts from the pink slips filed by aides:

8:10 p.m. H restricted to his room for 30 minutes for pulling down S's pajamas. Taken off restriction at 8:40.

One day restriction: L would not stay in his room during nap time. D was crying and L went to his room and told him to shut up. Aide warned him several times, but L ignored this. D was crying for his mother.

B was told to stay on a restricted walk while on wheel toy. When he disobeyed, B was taken to room and kept there for 20 minutes. After release, B slipped out of cottage without coat and cap, was brought in and set (sic) on chair for 15 minutes.

The most severe technique was placement in the "psychiatric unit," a closed ward for "disturbed children," for a fixed period of time. For example, "M was placed in psychiatric unit at 5:30 P.M. for putting water in O's hat, then throwing this water all over O's bed and floor."

In addition to deprivation and seclusion, physical directives were used. For example, children described in their medical records as enuretic were wakened periodically about every hour and a half throughout the night and escorted by an aide to the toilet. According to a night aide, "No matter how careful we are, darn it, two or three of them wet or soil their beds anyway."

Rules were abundant and closely enforced. As Sykes[11] has noted of guards in prisons, aides have but a small number of privileges to mete out. Thus they tried to make privileges out of gratifications children customarily take for granted. Watching television was thus defined as a privilege in Cottage X. Efforts were made to limit periods when the set would be turned on. If the noise level seemed too high in the cottage, the set was turned off. Eating crackers and milk was made into a privilege, as was receiving the mail, playing with the wagons and bicycles, and listening to the phonograph.

To increase their stock of privileges, aides also *delegated authority*. Boys were chosen to sweep the hall, run messages, go to get the mail, and so forth. This was the aide's most powerful resource. But, only one fourth of the boys in Cottage X were capable of completing "trustee-type assignments," and these tended to be the boys least in need of socialization. Some aides employed physical affection as a reward. Conforming children were spoken to, hugged, petted, or played with briefly. This tactic became confused insofar as the children differed greatly in their degree of affective dependency. Demonstration of affection was difficult to ration selectively. Some children took it from aides by hanging close by or pressing close, others got it by provoking reactions. Others avoided these forms of aide contact. Finally, aides regarded *drugs* as control agents. Aspirin as well as thorazine and other "tranquilizers" were believed to improve greatly the chances of developing a quiet, well behaved cottage. Upon the agreement of the professional staff, children in Cottage X were not placed on drugs during the course of our observations. Toward the close of the second week, aides began to resent this agreement. They felt their capabilities for improving control had been reduced substantially. Indeed, observation was cut short by a request from the medical department that drug programs be introduced at once.

To convey something of the quality of socialization in action, two fragments of observations are presented:

At 7:00 p.m., the children finished cleaning up the cottage, clean-up being the primary privilege extended on Home Night. The aides directed all but seven of the children to the TV lounge and to seats along the walls. Soon, individual children took chances at entering the center floor area of the lounge. They were controlled from the aide's desk. Aide C would call out, "Get back in your chair," "Get your feet off the chair, you," "Get back in your chair," "Go stand in the corner—you know you must stay in your chair," and so forth. Three corners of the lounge were used as punishment centers. At 7:40, one child, G, began to slump into sleep in his chair. The aide called out, "G, you get up here and go out and wash your face with water and wake up. It's not bedtime yet."

At 6:50, the aide said, having seated the children around the walls in the TV lounge, "If everyone is quiet now, we'll watch a little television." There was a brief uproar of glad approval from the boys. The aide walked to the set, hesitated till a silence came over the group, and then switched on the last ten minutes of a western, "The Rebel." For the next half hour, no more than four boys watched the TV screen at any one time. All other boys spent their time watching one another or the aide at the desk. At 7:05, child M came over and touched my mouth and chin and throat very gently and looked carefully at me. Aide C interrupted this at once: "Get back to your chair, M, at once!" M returned to his chair and began to cry loudly. Some of the boys around him began to mock his crying.

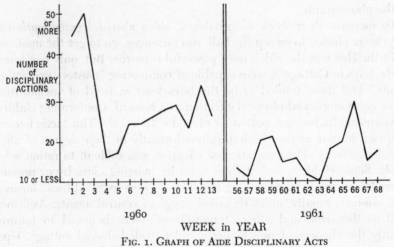

FIG. 1. GRAPH OF AIDE DISCIPLINARY ACTS
PER WEEK, INITIAL PERIOD (1960)
AND LATER

Figure 1 illustrates an aspect of the process of socialization through disciplinary action. Aide's pink slips reporting infractions of children and disciplinary action for two comparable time periods were summed in units of weeks for the 26 out of 29 boys who remained in State School for more than one year. The first period comprises the first thirteen weeks after the 26 had entered Cottage X. The second period consists of thirteen weeks in a comparable season of the following year. The points on the graph reflect dual behavior; namely, violations of cottage rules and disciplinary acts. Disciplinary acts by aides were not always responses to misconduct, however, as aides could define behavior as deviant or ignore it. Certainly, the two events were mutually interactive. The graph is interpreted here as representing trends in *degree of pressure* exerted by aides in maintaining control.

Pressure was most extreme during the first three weeks. In the fourth week, drug programs were initiated, and pressure was relaxed. This initial degree of pressure was never reintroduced, but the trend from the eighth to the thirteenth week suggests that disciplinary pressures were intensified periodically. An equilibrium was never achieved, but the data from the 1961 period suggest that sufficient control was established so that the degree of pressure became consistently lower. After one year, a level of control was realized under which most children appeared quiet, subdued and conforming. In the initial phase, for example, one boy received more than 13 per cent of the total number of pink slips, and the mean was 7 per child. A year later, two boys among the 26 received 47 per cent of all the pink slips, although the mean declined to 3 per child. There is some consistency over time in which individual boys were and were not disciplined. The correlation between ranked totals for the first and second periods is .34 ($p < .05$). Among the four boys disciplined most frequently in the second period, however, only one received more than average punishment in the initial period.

INTERPERSONAL RELATIONS AMONG CHILDREN

How were the socialization processes and the social behavior of the children in Cottage X interrelated? What were the social consequences for the children of adaptation to this new life situation? The instrument for exploring this question was sociometric choice. It was assumed that the status structure of any group is indicative of the values endorsed by the group; that structure is built around a reward system for conformity to norms; and that the choice status of individual members may be used as an index of social acceptance and of what is valued by the members. These assumptions echo the theory developed by Riecken and Homans.[12]

In a previous report, the authors presented an analysis of the correlates of individual sociometric status.[13] It was found that, initially, the boys with highest choice status among the children received the most frequent disciplinary restrictions. In the second month after arrival, however, the status structure changed. The boys who gained most in status were those who showed the greatest reduction in frequency of disciplinary action. The evidence from analysis of individual choice status supported the conclusion that the boys in Cottage X adapted progressively to institutional life through incorporation of the norms imposed by cottage aides. Rewards of status from peers were given increasingly to those boys who conformed with all routines or rather who stayed out of trouble. As these were the boys with minimal capabilities for effective action, that is, the most apathetic and retarded, the correlation between mental ability and declining status was extremely significant.

Friendship ties or mutual preferences are, like choice status, meaningful indicators of interpersonal relations. The emphasis on who is over or underchosen, however, is replaced with an emphasis on the degree to which individuals are contained in or excluded from one or more sub-groups and the degree to which a network of social sentiments has developed. A greater than chance number of reciprocal choices suggests that a group has developed solidarity. A lower than chance number suggests that barriers to interaction exist which reduce exchange of sentiments among members.

FIG. 2. SOCIOGRAM OF COTTAGE X, FIRST MONTH

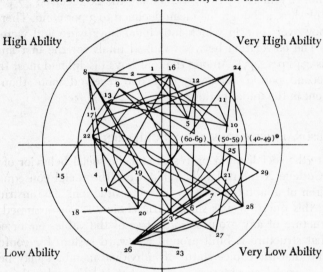

High Ability   Very High Ability

Low Ability   Very Low Ability

°Normalized Scores on Choice Status

In Figure 2 is presented a target type diagram of the sociometric structure of mutual relations between the 29 boys in Cottage X in the *first* month. The quadrants of the target contain boys grouped by level of functioning ability. The three bands of the target reflect level of individual choice status, with the most overchosen boys located in the inner circle and the most underchosen in the outer circle. Figure 3 is an identical diagram based on sociometric responses in the *second* month. In both figures, the lines represent mutual ties or reciprocal choices between individuals.

The single most important datum of this study consists of the extreme contrasts between the structure of interpersonal preferences in the two time periods. Using the three criteria of playmate, work mate, and identification preferences in a composite fashion, 45 mutual preferences occurred in the first month and three in the second.

Using the probability model recommended by Katz and Powell,[14] Cottage X boys appear to have developed interpersonal ties in the first month that were greater than would be expected by chance. Figure 2 thus depicts a group structure that approximates a statistically expected structure. Figure 3, using the same model, is .02 points distant from the most extreme deviation from chance obtainable under conditions set by the choice questions. The extent of interpersonal reciprocation, in other words, is extremely close to the absolute and to probabilistic minima. There are fewer reciprocal choices than would be expected by random choosing alone.

FIG. 3. SOCIOGRAM OF COTTAGE X, SECOND MONTH

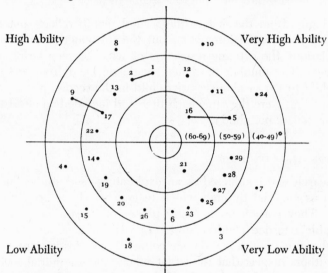

*Normalized Scores on Choice Status

The contrast may be interpreted as evidence of *avoidance learning*. This process underlay the socialization practices and was witnessed frequently. The development of friendships depends on opportunities for social interaction. For sentiment to develop, activities must be shared. Under the conditions imposed by aides, such activities became, over time, occasions for deprivation and seclusion. For example, here are illustrative excerpts:

A new aide replaced Mr. Y this evening. While he was being introduced to a nurse and to the other aide, several boys, noting that the aides were not in direct control, began to wrestle playfully and teasingly near the TV lounge. P, who initiated this play, was observed by the old aide and placed for ten minutes in a corner of the lounge with his face to the wall.

J and R were sitting on a couch watching TV. W was sitting with O nearby. J began to talk to R. Aide N said, "Hey, hush up." S and K were also seated together. On TV a western film was showing. About half the boys were watching it. Whenever any boy talked, Aide N said, "All right, guys, get quiet." J got up and came toward O. Aide N said, "OK J, get up on the naughty bench and don't say a word." M had already been assigned to the bench. Soon J began to try to play with M. Aide N said, "I told you to get up there so you would stay out of *trouble*—and there you go again."

K and G were playing, talking and giggling in the hall. Aide N said to them, "Keep still now." S and SY began playing with two small rubber balls that S brought out of his room into the corridor. They bounced them cautiously up and down for a moment. Aide N said, "You don't play ball in here. You know that." The activity stopped at once.

B moved across the TV lounge and talked to me. Thereupon, Aide B told him to sit down, face forward, and "put your feet on the floor."

The change from the first to the second month reflects not the total absence of preferential interaction but the introduction of caution into social relations, the extreme restriction of what Moreno terms *social* expansiveness. The number of choices made declined from 308 or about 10 per child to 101 or about 3.5 per child in the second phase (although the instructions were the same each time and included an effort to obtain at least 9 choices per child).

DISCUSSION AND CONCLUSION

This research was conducted as an exploratory field study; findings are intended as material through which to generate hypotheses for further research. They pertain to the early phases of institutional socialization, to educable retarded children under 13 years of age, and to what was observed and measured in only one cottage in one institution.

The authors suspect that the latent function of the initial socialization process is to reorganize the self of the newly arrived patient. Through severe initial control over interpersonal relations among the children, the social responses brought in as part of the presenting culture are broken down. The result is a child obliged to accept peer as well as adult relations on terms specified completely by the institution, at which point the *colonized* patient may be rehabilitated.

From observing "Old Boys" briefly, the authors speculate that the system succeeds in fulfilling its objectives. The basic routines, once established, especially among the educable patients, are maintained indefinitely. Patients generally are prepared to re-enter the outside world with improved manners and greater independence in the tasks of eating, bathing, and the like. Furthermore, between the years from 13 to 21, academic education and vocational training are added to the patient's repertoire.

Through job training, which was observed, "Old Boys" develop job-centered attachments to peers. In the matrix of a work group, the adult social self begins to develop and gratification is increased. The ideal end-product, the social outcome, we suspect, is a quiet, well mannered, even subdued young adult, demonstrably independent and able to earn a living.

The reorganization of a new patient is functional not only because it leads to colonization and thus guards against rebellion. The "stripping away" of older response sets is probably also *economical*. Goffman has demonstrated that this is the case in mental hospitals.[15] To move aggregates of persons through elaborate schedules across long periods of time, it is important that mechanisms be devised that are certain to reduce individual differences. Efficient, economical control may be obtained by increasing the stability or predictability of behavior. The mechanisms discussed are ones that assist in the reduction of differences, just as colonization leads toward uniformity of perception among the patients.

Whether individual potentialities would be realized more completely under a different process of socialization is a question that this report seems to pose rather sharply. This much of the question perhaps can be answered: the character of this total institution is incompatible with the goal of maximum fulfillment of individual potentialities. It is not incompatible with efficient management and rehabilitation toward limited participation and adult subsistence in the outer community.

NOTES TO CHAPTER 25

1. Erving Goffman, "Characteristics of Total Institutions," in *Symposium on Preventive and Social Psychiatry* (Washington, D.C., Walter Reed Army Institute of Research, Medical Center: Government Printing Office, 1958), p. 48.
2. Seymour Sarason, *Psychological Problems in Mental Deficiency* (New York: Harper & Brothers, 1959), p. 626.
3. Melford E. Spiro, *Children of the Kibbutz* (Cambridge: Harvard University Press, 1958).
4. Robert A. Dentler and Bernard Mackler, "Effects of Sociometric Status of Institutional Pressure to Adjust Among Retarded Children," submitted to *Child Development;* and Robert A. Dentler and Bernard Mackler, "The Porteus Maze Test as a Predictor of Functioning Abilities in Institutional Retarded Children," *Journal of Consulting Psychology,* in press.
5. As a small internal check, we included the picture of a boy who did not live in Cottage X. Each child was asked to point to the picture of the boy who "Does not live in your cottage." Three-fourths of the children identified this picture correctly. Incidentally, children were invited to point to their choices, eliminating the problem of unscrambling a verbal response.
6. Erving Goffman, *op. cit.* See also Gresham Sykes, *Society of Captives*

(Princeton: Princeton University Press, 1958), Mayer Zald, "The Correctional Institution for Juvenile Offenders: An Analysis of Organizational 'Character,'" *Social Problems*, 8 (1960), 57-67; and Ivan Belknap, *Human Problems of a State Mental Hospital* (New York: McGraw-Hill, 1956).

7. Mayer Zald, *op. cit.*, pp. 58-59.
8. Peter M. Blau, *Bureaucracy in Modern Society* (New York: Random House, 1956), p. 60.
9. Erving Goffman, *op. cit.*, pp. 62-63.
10. That silence is valued at other state schools is suggested by a fictional yet documentary autobiography of a cottage aide in a state training school for the retarded. Martin Russ, *Half Moon Haven* (New York: Rinehart, 1959), p. 27.
11. Gresham Sykes, *op. cit.*, pp. 53-54.
12. Henry Riecken and George W. Homans, "Psychological Aspects of Social Structure," in Gardner Lindzey, ed., *Handbook of Social Psychology*, Vol. 2 (Cambridge: Addison-Wesley, 1954), pp. 786-832.
13. Robert A. Dentler and Bernard Mackler, *op. cit.*—first paper named in reference 4.
14. Leo Katz and James H. Powell "Measurement of the Tendency toward Reciprocation of Choice," *Sociometry*, 18 (1955), 659-664.
15. Erving Goffman, *op. cit.*

ॐ

CHAPTER 26   Organizational Goals and

Structural Change: A Study of the Organization of a

Prison Social System*

JOSEPH C. MOULEDOUS

T HE RELATIONSHIP of the inmate and his keeper has been of vital interest to students of penology. As early as 1920 Frank Tannenbaum,
under such titles as "Psychology of Prison Cruelty" and "Prison Democracy,"[1] described the prison as being composed of two mutually exclusive
worlds, worlds separated by such intense contempt that association between the prisoner and his keeper was almost impossible, except as it expressed itself in dominance. Recently the writings of McCleery,[2] Wheeler,[3]
Goffman,[4] and others, have shifted the perspective to the elements of
accommodation and compromise as the predominant condition, and consensus rather than force as the main basis of control. McCleery forcefully
states this position when he writes that "the illusion that control rests on
instruments of force rather than procedures for creating consensus is a
rich source of error for inexperienced scholars or officials."[5]
 While the problem of inmate-staff relations and the basis of control has
been most dramatically revealed in penitentiaries, it is not limited to that
world but is part of the broader problem of "handling men" which has
been brought so sharply into focus by the development of vast bureau-

* This paper is a revised version of a paper read before the annual meeting of the
Southern Sociological Society, Louisville, Kentucky, April 1962. It is based on material
from the writer's unpublished master's thesis entitled "Sociological Perspectives on a
Prison Social System," Louisiana State University, 1962. The data on which it is based
consists of historical sources, statistical reports, personal documents, interviews, and
participant observation while the writer was employed by the Louisiana State Peni-
tentiary, Angola, Louisiana, from 1957 to 1960. Appreciation is expressed to Drs.
Frederick L. Bates, William Haag, Rudolf Heberle, Walfrid A. Jokinen, and Vernon J.
Parenton, who read this paper and/or the writer's thesis.
 Reprinted from Social Forces, 41 (1963), 283–290, by permission of the author and
The University of North Carolina Press.

cracies. Litwak,[6] Melman,[7] Bendix,[8] Sykes,[9] and others, have discussed
the problem and it is to this literature that we add the following exploration of the Louisiana State Penitentiary.

The significance of the Louisiana State Penitentiary lies in the fact that
it provides concrete historical examples of how essentially contradictory
social relations have been coordinated to achieve organizational goals.
Furthermore, the fact that two grossly different methods of coordinating
behavior have been used at the same time, and that these gave rise to
significantly different social structures, has importance to those of us who
are concerned with the manner in which men are handled.

In Louisiana, shortly after the turn of the century, a newly created
penal administration inherited from the numerous plantations, levee and
road camps, and from an obsolete urban prison, a predominantly servile
Negro inmate population which was relocated on 18,000 acres of rich
river-bottom land. There this population was divided into eight semi-
autonomous and separate camps—two white male, five Negro male, and
one mixed female—to farm the surrounding acreage. Originally, rehabilitation was expressed as a goal of administration and a staff of more than
150 was employed to maintain order, supervise work and rehabilitate
the inmate. These goals grew out of demands—as most clearly expressed
by the Prison Reform Association—to correct the evils of the previous
"lease system" by inaugurating a true prison rehabilitative system. At the
same time other elements of the greater community, including officials
of the state and the governor, conceived of using this mass of inmate labor
to provide the state with a source of income through farming and to contribute to the communities surrounding the penitentiary by maintaining
and expanding their road systems. To achieve these economic goals the
legislature refused to legislate monies for penal operations and insisted
that the penitentiary be self-sustaining. The penal staff was reduced to a
supervisory staff of less than 50 employees, who, while being underpaid,
were permitted to live with their families in residences on the periphery
of the camps they supervised, and who were permitted to supplement
their meager cash incomes with the products, goods, services, and labor
available in the camps. By this method, explicit goals of the administration
which were primarily concerned with production, and the personal interest
of each staff member, that is to say, his economic interest, were intertwined. A staff member could not approach his job as simply an appointed
task, nor simply as a duty he had to perform as long as he held that position. Rather, he approached his task in a much larger, more total perspective, for his income, status, and prestige rose and fell as a result of the
manner in which he "handled his men" and made a good crop.

Thus it was required that the inmate be perceived as a worker, and the
main problem which this undermanned staff faced was to devise a means
of handling them as workers: that is, to insure that they would produce.

Two separate methods were devised: one was a threat system, the other an exchange system. The threat system fitted the demands of non-mechanized, unskilled farming when the land to be farmed was exceedingly rich, and the supply of labor virtually unlimited, and which also coincided with the dominant ideology of the southern whites toward their servile rural Negroes. Specifically, they inaugurated a threat system in which men were punished for failing to meet their quotas or to keep up with the pace. For example, there existed a common practice of placing each man on a row of cane, cotton or some other crop that required weeding or harvesting. The job would then begin like a foot race: 50 or more men each with his own row to work. The last five to reach the far end of the row were whipped. Under this system, the inmate was not encouraged to assume individual responsibility for the efficient performance of his job, nor were there built into the work area positive rewards which the inmate could strive to achieve. Rather, the inmate, as an inmate, was held to have a duty and an obligation to provide the penitentiary with hard labor—as the court had specified when passing sentence—and he was threatened with corporal punishment if he failed adequately to provide this labor.

While the non-mechanized, unskilled, easily-supervised farm jobs permitted the development of a coercive system, the administration, being grossly understaffed, was faced with the problem of using inmates for jobs normally performed by lower staff members. With a total staff of less than 50, and with eight camps to supervise, each camp was normally supervised by four officers: a captain-in-charge, a field foreman, a yard-dormitory supervisor, and a night officer. Such jobs as gun-tower guard, farm-line guard, gate man, maintenance worker, blacksmith, medical orderly, clerk, bookkeeper, butcher, baker, cook, and so forth, were all performed by inmates and it was necessary to devise a method whereby these inmates would be responsible for and responsive to the demands of their jobs; that they would not, in Veblen's terms, "withdraw their efficiency."

The method devised was startlingly simple, but it differs markedly from the familiar penal pattern, and in effect virtually erases the American definition of a penitentiary.[10] Those inmates who assumed the individual responsibility to perform the duties of an inmate guard or of a skilled trusty worker were given a small income, relieved of custodial requirements in that they did not have to stand count, permitted to traverse freely the entire penitentiary and even to leave the grounds for limited visits to nearby communities or home, given unofficial permission to have conjugal visits with their wives, and some were even allowed to eat and sleep, in a word, live at their job sites. Thus the administration superimposed upon a brutally coercive threat system as exchange system with a vast range of positive rewards which the inmate could strive to achieve. The inmate, in exchange for his skills and his assuming of the burden of responsibility for control, output, and efficiency, could achieve the ultimate position of being an inmate by legal definition only, or he could gain any number of lesser rewards.

The effect of this dual treatment of the inmate was to divide the inmate population into two broad classes: gunman and inmate guard-trusty. The typical gunman, that is, men who worked under the gun in farm lines, normally lived and worked in a world sharply divided and isolated from the officials, a world in which hostility to staff was the expected pattern and such norms as "not talking to screws," "being a right guy," and so forth, supported the need for mutual aid to one another and hostility toward staff. Membership in the gunman group and membership in groups of inmate guards or inmates holding responsible jobs were largely, but as we shall see, not entirely mutually exclusive. And as Blau and Scott remark, "in the absence of overlapping memberships . . . conflict tends to split a community into two hostile camps with little communication between them."[11] At the same time, among the gunmen there always existed a number of inmates who held expectations that they would soon be permitted to leave this extremely deprived inmate body, to secure a job and share in the privileges attached to that job. Having such expectations they had a definite interest in quelling the simmering hostility and preventing the threat system from breaking down into overt conflict. Their influence lay in the fact that they expected to be promoted into the privileged ranks where they would have access to goods and services and become centers of communication, and this expectation of such roles introduced into their existing role of hostility, norms of compromise ("play it cool," "do your own time").[12]

In each gunman camp there were always a minority of inmates, generally mature men with long sentences, who held responsible jobs with access to goods and services and with direct communication with staff members. In many ways such jobs were identical with those performed by responsible trusties or inmate guards, with the exception that the occupant performed them directly under a gun, or in the case of gunman-riskies, with short periods of freedom from the gun.[13] Such jobs within the gunman compound as medical orderly, barber, cook, storekeeper, required that the occupant assume individual responsibility for the efficient performance of his job, develop norms of cooperation with staff, trusties, and inmate guards, and perform roles that were responsive to their interests. Such occupants, therefore, moved out of the center of the gunman population to a point on the periphery, or in Parsons and Bales's terminology, at the boundary,[14] where they were required to express norms of compromise and cooperation with two hostile populations: gunmen and staff. Similarities between these positions and those of the industrial foreman and military sergeant are striking, and it has been noted that such positions, being exposed, are vulnerable; but it is appreciated that they fill important functions of siphoning off conflict, alleviating hostility, and encouraging compromise. Furthermore, in the schema developed by Bates, it is these individuals who, in their interaction with members of groups other than their own, form the links, or interstitial groups, which cohere separate and possibly antagonistic populations.[15]

Inherently weak, these positions were made strong by an administrative policy of permitting all gunmen to enjoy illicit privileges within their residential environment, after the day's work had been completed: cooking, gambling, drinking, handicrafts, homosexual unions, all were permitted behind the closed doors of the dormitory at night, as long as it did not interfere with work performance, and fights were kept to a minimum. In view of the deprived and coercive work environment, such residential privileges were intensely desired, and it was through those inmates who held responsible jobs within and without the camp that the materials were provided to facilitate such privileges. The jobs, then, were virtually essential to the gunman's residential privileges and they strongly supported them. Subsequent strength was gained from the condition that most of these jobs were held by a single occupant, who gained from them economic rewards, as well as prestige and power, through the control of goods, services, and information. Thus it was to the interest of the individual occupant to embody and in some manner "work out" the interests of his job, the interests of the administration, his personal interests, and the interests of the gunman inmates with whom he lived. In this sense a great deal of role conflict could be tolerated as long as it was to the "self-interest" of the occupant. Furthermore, since these positions were important links, points of interaction between staff and gunmen, they became the major source of informal communication between the two groups. For the staff they provided information on the behavior occurring in "the guts of the camp," and for the gunmen they supplied information on the attitudes and plans of staff. They, in effect, created an image of each for the other.

From this sketch the penitentiary is pictured as a vast achievement system in which men, both staff and inmate, are motivated to increase their material rewards through efficient production. In areas where the conditions of work are easily manageable and skills and individual responsibility are not required, staff assures high production by the use of the most brutal, coercive methods. In areas where the conditions of work require skills and individual responsibility, staff develops a sensitivity to the needs and interests of the inmates and develops material rewards and privileges of freedom from custodial restrictions to satisfy such needs and interests. These conditions are comparable to the findings of D. C. Pelz. Pelz found that in "uniform," repetitive work areas authoritarian methods produced greatest motivation and results, while in "non-uniform" work areas motivation and results increased with the employee's control of the environment.[16]

Furthermore, through the cooperation of these privileged inmates, staff officially provides illicit privileges to gunman farm workers, in their residential environment, which helps alleviate their deprivations, quell their hostility, as well as lend strength to the position of privileged inmates. The result is that the administration achieves its production goals; it also elicits from a sizeable number of inmates behavior that manifests individual responsibility, cooperation, successful handling of conflicting roles, and sensitivity to and tolerance of interests other than their own, which is all that any rationally planned rehabilitative program can hope to achieve. However, it is equally likely that since labor and responsibility provide, so remarkably easily, an immediate access to high social status and power in the penal environment, the inmate may gain unrealistic expectations of the positions he can gain in the greater society through a similar quality of labor and responsibility.

Thus, a number of basically antagonistic and hostile groups are welded together into a prison social system by the cooperative, responsive interaction of staff and inmate in numerous "interstitial groups," as they act to achieve distinct goals: staff, inmate, and personal goals, and goals inherent in the groups. The strength of such groups, and thereby the strength of the social system, arises from the "self-interest" each occupant has in successfully achieving its goals, as well as the elements of power and prestige these groups possess through the control of goods, services, and information.

In the past decade, the old penal administration has been replaced by one led by federally trained, professional penologists, and a philosophy of rehabilitation has been introduced as the basic goal of administration. An adequate budget has been appropriated by the legislature, old camps have been torn down and a new centralized plant built, staff has grown to approximately 400, departments of education, vocational training, and classification have been developed, farm jobs have been greatly mechanized, an industrial program has been introduced, rules and regulations specifying the conduct of inmate and staff have been published, staff is presently employed and promoted according to rules specified by a State Civil Service, and staff and their families have been moved from their old homes—where they could come into frequent and informal interaction with inmates—to a newly constructed housing area set apart from the prison plant. In a word, a bureaucratization of the penitentiary has largely occurred and impersonal formal relations are replacing the informal personal methods of the old order.

In effecting these changes and in pursuing rehabilitative goals, the new administration held that "inmates were sentenced *as* punishment, not *for* punishment," and that staff had a duty to provide these inmates with the services necessary for their rehabilitation. Administration opposed the inequalities in privileges provided by the old regime, and took immediate steps to eliminate them and to create a system whereby all inmates would be granted essentially the same privileges, unless they overtly misbehaved, and under such conditions privileges would be temporarily rescinded.[17] Thus there developed a situation almost identical with that described by Sykes: the administration makes an initial grant of all rewards and then threatens to withdraw them for overt misbehavior; the inmate comes to expect such rewards as their inalienable rights, not something to be earned, and thus the whole system of rewards and punishments collapses as an effective means of handling men.[18]

For staff a related development occurred. Through written rules and regulations, controls were placed on staff which attempted to eliminate the material rewards they could gain from the job areas they supervised and the goods and labor they controlled. Since wages had increased and were now adequate, and "fringe benefits" existed in the form of inexpensive housing and free vegetables, administration felt that competent men could be employed. Unquestionably this was a correct premise, but as Bendix points out, there is a significant difference in motivation between men who pursue their economic interests and men who perform their appointed tasks.[19] And when these tasks involve the handling of prisoners, with a deficient system of rewards and punishments, the element of motivation becomes extremely important.

The effects were varied and interesting. On farm jobs, controls over the men disintegrated badly. Punishment, if legitimately enforced, meant a week to ten days in "isolation," which was considered a "vacation" from odious farm labor, and loss of "Good Time," which was normally restored after a period of good behavior. Punishment applied by the officials in violation of penitentiary rules meant a clubbing or beating in the fields or in the isolation cell, but this could cost an official his job. Still it was used, and most frequently on Negroes. The major reward developed by farm supervisors was the recommending of good workers for better jobs, and this source of power was drastically cut into by the development of rational methods for filling vacancies by the classification department. It is not surprising, then, that in spite of the vast mechanization of farming methods and an increase in acreage farmed, farm production never attained the level established in 1942, and only slightly surpassed 1921 production. Furthermore, in this area of interaction, behavior on the part of staff ranged from apathy and withdrawal for those staff members who simply put in a day's work, to frustrated hostility for those who attempted to handle their men and achieve production goals with deficient controls. Norms of inmate conduct varied from letting the apathetic "boss man" alone or "shooting the breeze" with him to help pass the day, to agitation and overt hostility toward the "pusher."

In maintenance, clerical, and similar work areas which required skills and a degree of efficiency on the part of the inmate worker, in spite of the fact that he was directly supervised by a staff supervisor, and which normally had a quantity of work far more than any one or two employees could handle and thus required the assistance of inmates, illicit privileges were widely introduced. Staff brought gifts of cigarettes, candy, fruit, etc.; staff permitted cooking, allowed the inmates to use work materials and work time to make personal items, and, until classification interfered, seriously considered inmate recommendations when replacements were needed. Staff achieved the freedom to allow such illicit activities by involving other members of staff, such as custodial officers who could make inspections, in illicit relationships, such as, repairing automobiles, building items of furniture, supplying materials, and so on. In this way staff exchanged the labor, goods, and services of their unit for a type of protection. Thus, inmate-staff interaction still elicited norms of cooperation and accommodation, but these were colored by the fact that such behavior involved conniving on the part of staff, conniving to insure that the inmate workers would not withdraw their efficiency. While such behavior on the part of staff did not basically differ from behavior of staff members of the old regime pursuing their economic interest, the significance lay in the fact that the old regime approved, supported, and considered it the proper way to manage the penitentiary, while the present regime opposed it. Thus, the norms of cooperation which arose did not grow out of a sensitivity to and tolerance of the interests of others while one pursued his own interests, but rather, they arose from staff's weak position which required that they enter into illicit relationships with the inmates. A dominant criminal attitude, that is, that society has many "holes,"[20] or the criminal pattern of pursuing material goals by illegal innovations,[21] was reinforced, and this is not what a rehabilitation program hopes to achieve.

Furthermore, contemporary administration, through the equalization of privileges and the reduction of the motivating factor of self-interest, which led to the development of illicit privileges and conniving, not only relinquished its material and coercive basis of power, but also lost whatever respect it previously may have had. The result is that the penal social order which is developing is largely based on and oriented toward conditions inherent in the inmate environment. Coercion as a basis of power residing in inmate cliques, or individual toughs, is a growing condition and has been given great impetus by the new centralized prison plant. Status as a basis of power has shifted from the status derived from one's position within the privilege system to a status largely inherited from the criminal reputation brought to the penitentiary, especially the range and quality of criminal contacts and future criminal plans, as well as criminal knowledge and skills. Material wealth or privileges, as a basis of power has been undermined by the equalization of privileges, not the least of which is the incentive pay program which allows all inmates to earn at least two cents per hour. This small income, combined with the illicit privileges provided on the job, and the free tobacco, shaving equipment, library privileges, nightly television, weekly movies, recreational equipment, and leisure time provided by the administration, creates conditions of privilege which, while being minimal, are satisfactory. The redistribution and inequalization of this material wealth which is passed out to the inmate population now becomes the activity of cliques and toughs who coerce, "hustle," or in some manner appropriate this wealth for themselves and their buddies. Power has been usurped by the inmate population and labor has become an inmate threat, a threat to withdraw or to provide the efficiency and responsibility which many supervisors still need.

Our study supports the generalization that if an egalitarian approach is held, administration relinquishes control of the total penal environment and allows for the development of an inmate social system which gradually dominates the environment and becomes the main reference for inmate standards and behavior. If administration maintains control of the penal environment by developing an authoritarian rather than an egalitarian approach, behavior and standards can be oriented to those of administration. I say *can be,* because if administration primarily aims coercively to control the inmate population, a totalitarian approach, it essentially rejects that population and places insurmountable barriers between itself and the inmates, and again behavior and standards will become oriented toward the inmate population. If, on the other hand, an authoritarian administration maintains its power by also involving inmates in various activities, by distributing to them various material resources and freedoms of movement in exchange for their cooperation, administration then becomes the orientation of inmate behavior and standards.[22] Furthermore, through such an approach administration fragments the penal population into numerous interest groups which not only helps prevent the development of an inmate social system but also helps minimize and solve conflicts when they arise.

NOTES TO CHAPTER 26

1. Frank Tannenbaum, "Prison Cruelty," *Atlantic Monthly,* Vol. 125 (1920), pp. 433-444, and *Wall Shadows: A Study in American Prisons* (New York: G. P. Putnam's Sons, 1922).
2. Richard McCleery, *Policy Change in Prison Management* (East Lansing: Government Research Bureau, Michigan State University, 1957), and "The Governmental Process and Informal Social Control," *The Prison,* ed. Donald R. Cressey (New York: Holt, Rinehart & Winston, Inc., 1961).
3. Stanton Wheeler, "Role Conflict in Correctional Communities," *The Prison,* pp. 229-259.

4. Erving Goffman, "Characteristics of Total Institutions," *Identity and Anxiety,* ed. Maurice R. Stein (Glencoe, Ill.: The Free Press, 1960), pp. 449-479.

5. McCleery, "The Governmental Process . . . ," *loc. cit.,* p. 153.

6. Eugene Litwak, "Models of Bureaucracy Which Permit Conflict," *American Journal of Sociology,* LXVII (1961), 177-184.

7. Seymour Melman, *Decision Making and Productivity* (New York: John Wiley and Sons, Inc., 1958).

8. Reinhard Bendix, *Work and Authority in Industry* (New York: John Wiley and Sons, Inc., 1956).

9. Gresham M. Sykes, *The Society of Captives* (Princeton: Princeton University Press, 1958).

10. Historical examples of prison systems which devised methods grossly different from those found in the typical American penitentiary can be found in the German concentration camps, to a lesser degree in the French concentration camps, and in certain penal systems in the southern region of the United States. In these prison systems there existed a variation of the ruler-ruled dichotomy which consisted of delegating official functions to a segment of the inmate population, which then performed, in effect, roles generally considered the property of official personnel. See the following: Elie A. Cohen, *Human Behavior in the Concentration Camp* (New York: W. W. Norton and Co., 1953); Raul Hilberg, *The Destruction of the European Jews* (Chicago: Quadrangle Books, 1961); Arthur Koestler, *Scum of the Earth* (London: Collins & Hamish Hamilton, Ltd., 1955); Eugen Kogon, *The Theory and Practice of Hell* (New York: Farrar, Straus and Cudahy, Inc., 1950); and Lord Russell, *The Scourge of the Swastika* (New York: Philosophical Library, Inc., 1954).

11. Peter M. Blau and Richard W. Scott, *Formal Organizations* (San Francisco: Chandler Publishing Co., 1962), p. 199. This volume has a bibliography containing more than 800 items. It should be noted that their concept *cui bono* applies to our discussion.

12. This concept of role is derived from Frederick L. Bates and Robert K. Merton. See: Frederick L. Bates, "Position, Role and Status: A Reformulation of Concepts," *Social Forces,* Vol. 34 (1956), pp. 313-321; and Robert K. Merton, "The Role Set: Problems in Sociological Theory," *British Journal of Sociology,* VIII (1957), 106-120.

13. Within each gunman camp were a small number of men called "riskies." In performing their duties these men would be permitted to work in areas outside the surveillance of guards. A risk was taken by staff, and the term "risky" developed.

14. Talcott Parsons and Robert F. Bales, *Family, Socialization, and Interaction Process* (Glencoe, Ill.: The Free Press, 1955).

15. Frederick L. Bates, "Institutions, Organizations, and Communities: A General Theory of Complex Structures," *The Pacific Sociological Review,* Vol. 3 (1960), pp. 59-70.

16. Litwak, *op. cit.,* pp. 178-179, refers to an unpublished paper by D. C. Pelz, entitled "Conditional Effects in the Relationship of Autonomy and Motivation to Performance" (August 1960, mimeographed).

17. Throughout this paper we use a framework which is similar to Erving Goffman's. Goffman perceives "total institutions" as privilege-deprivational systems structured around residential-work areas to which the inmates develop certain adaptive patterns: situational withdrawal, conversion, colonization, rebellious line, and secondary adjustments. The similarity of Goffman's typology with that of Robert K. Merton's is striking.

18. Sykes, *op. cit.*, pp. 51-52.

19. Bendix, *op. cit.*, p. 14.

20. Harry M. Shulman, "The Family and Juvenile Delinquency," *Annals of the American Academy of Political and Social Science*, Vol. 261 (1949), pp. 24-31.

21. Robert K. Merton, *Social Theory and Social Structure* (Glencoe, Ill.: The Free Press, 1957), pp. 141-149.

22. These terms are derived from Barrington Moore, Jr., *Political Power and Social Theory* (Cambridge: Harvard University Press, 1958).

ॐ

CHAPTER 27   The Therapeutic Value
of the Closed Ward*

JAMES H. RYAN

INTRODUCTION

MATERIAL collected from interviews with 100 mental patients at time of discharge is presented to evaluate therapeutic factors operating in a closed-ward hospital. Surprisingly, a large percentage of these patients indicated that certain hospital practices generally considered to be unfortunate necessities of hospital care actually have therapeutic value.

Since the Second World War the tendency in modern mental hospitals has been toward increased freedom and individualization of the patient. Maxwell Jones, for many years concerned with the need to increase the patient's participation in his own recovery, has developed a concept he has called the "therapeutic community" (6). Main believes that ego strengthening can occur only in a setting which permits the de-socialized patient to experience social demands in a realistic situation. The conventional mental hospital does not provide such a setting (7). Wilmer described success in his experience in a Navy hospital after an atmosphere of freedom and sociability was created on the ward (12). Stanton and Schwartz described a hospital where permissiveness and democracy were considered to be essential for proper care (10).

Certainly these developments represent progress in the humane treatment of mental patients. We are impressed, however, with the response of some patients to "old-fashioned" hospital techniques, and are now concerned that some of these older practices, which have great therapeutic value, may be discarded by some hospitals in the hope of gaining an undemonstrated therapeutic advantage.

* Reprinted from *Journal of Nervous and Mental Disease*, Volume 134 (1962), pages 256–262. Copyright © 1962, The Williams & Wilkins Co., Baltimore, Maryland 21202, U.S.A. By permission of the author and The Williams & Wilkins Co.

PATIENT SELECTION AND METHODOLOGY

THE Bronx Veterans Administration Hospital is a large general hospital with a 172-bed psychiatric wing. Patients are admitted to the service from the general hospital, or as transfers from other general or psychiatric hospitals, or as new patients. On admission, patients are routinely placed on one of the two closed wards for an average period of 59 days. When their condition permits, they are transferred to one of the two convalescent wards. Here they are allowed to receive visitors and to go out on pass, yet they remain in an essentially protective, highly controlled environment.

Ninety-three per cent of the patients are discharged into the community after an average total hospitalization of 117 days. The remaining seven per cent must be transferred to a chronic hospital. For economic and personnel reasons it is seldom possible to attempt to bring about characterologic changes in these patients through psychotherapy. The primary goal is symptom relief and anxiety reduction. Patients are returned to the community and to their vocations when they feel well enough to leave and when the doctor believes they are able to make a new effort to adapt to the outside environment. Twenty-three per cent of these patients are returned to hospital within one year of discharge, a substantial indication of failure to bring about a lasting improvement.

Patients on the closed ward are isolated from the community. Ward routine is strictly enforced on both the closed and the convalescent wards. Patients must eat together at specified times. They must go to bed and get up at certain times. Rules of behavior are firmly enforced except for the sickest patients, who are encouraged to conform as much as possible. Patients participate in occupational, educational and recreational therapy at specified times during the day.

Brief psychotherapy is available to all. In the study group, the patients were seen an average of 1.3 times per week, with an average duration of interview of 26 minutes. Thirteen patients received electric shock therapy, and nine were treated by insulin coma. Two patients received both therapies.

Diagnostic categories on discharge were: 56 per cent schizophrenic, 19 per cent psychotic depression, seven per cent anxiety reaction, five per cent chronic brain syndrome, four per cent involutional depression, and nine per cent undetermined. Many of the patients in the psychotic depression, the anxiety reaction and the undetermined groups might have been diagnosed in other hospitals as schizophrenics of the "borderline" or "pseudoneurotic type." Only occasionally is a clearly defined neurosis seen in this hospital.

Interviews were arranged with one hundred patients on the day of discharge from the hospital. Using an interview protocol, the author questioned the patients about various aspects of their hospital experience.

Patients were urged to express their attitudes toward their therapeutic regimens and the program of activities, *e.g.*, physical therapy, social service, that had been available to them. They were asked to indicate what factors they felt to be most important in their improvement. These interviews lasted thirty minutes or longer and patients' responses were recorded verbatim.

The study group contained only male ex-servicemen, 32 of whom suffered from service-connected disabilities for which they received compensation. They would be classified by Hollingshead and Redlich's criteria in a Class 4 or 5 socioeconomic grouping. Few could afford private psychiatric care. Their attitudes toward hospitalization and the experimental interview may have been influenced by their earlier military training as well as by their socioeconomic class. In some interviews the author noted a submissiveness of responses possibly stemming from the patient's military training.

Certain measures were taken to promote free, unguarded communication, and to overcome the patient's natural inclination to tell the interviewer what he might believe the interviewer wanted to hear. The patient was told that the investigator had no clinical or administrative duties, and no authority or interest in altering discharge plans. The investigator was described as interested in finding out what the patient thought about the hospital, and not simply what he was supposed to think about it. An informal, open atmosphere was thus created. Patients were encouraged to elaborate or even to ramble on as much as they cared to. Most patients responded in an open, unguarded fashion; a few responded with suspicion. Such responses, when observed, were commented on by the investigator in a humorous way, and the patient was invited to a true sharing of his experience. This potential source of error is believed to have been held to a minimum.

After interviews were completed, all reports (100) were examined by the author, who found that the primary responses generally fell into several categories. Here again, a limitation of the experimental methodology is observed. Every effort was made to be aware of and to eliminate conscious feelings on the part of the author-interviewer which might prejudice the results. The goal was not the defense of a particular type of hospitalization, but rather the determination of those events during hospitalization which might have been helpful.

PATIENT RESPONSES

Protection: Twenty-six of the patients indicated that the protective quality of the hospital was its chief therapeutic advantage. At the time of admission they had felt they were no longer able to deal with the complications of life and the hospital offered them a refuge, protecting them from the worries and threats of their life situations. Typical statements: "Here I had no worries about the rent. I didn't have to compete." Also: "My wife was divorcing me and I was always worrying what to do. Here I was removed. I didn't have to do anything. It's like a vacation from worries so you can figure out what to do."

Some implied that they were protected from internal as well as external threats; one said, "I hit my wife and the kids. I was afraid I might hurt them."

These responses indicate that the limitation of freedom serves not only to protect the community from the patient, but also to limit community access to him. The patients reported a sense of comfort and security as a result of the efforts of the hospital to protect them from the real or imagined dangers both outside the hospital and within themselves.

Routine: Nineteen per cent of the patient responses indicated that hospital routine was the most therapeutic influence. Outside the hospital they had felt unable to organize their lives with meaningful, goal-directed behavior, and their failure to utilize external or internal controls had created anxiety. The hospital provided a structured pattern of space and time which reduced their need to cope with decisions and change. One patient said: "Here it was like normal living. I got up and went to bed on time. It's not like outside." Another: "Outside I'd just sit around. I'd never eat or go to bed on time."

The hospital can create an organized pattern of living for the patient who cannot do it for himself. These patients reported that this patterning of behavior was most effective in their improving.

Friends: Fourteen patients reported that the major factor in their improvement was the opportunity available in the hospital to be with people again. Most had led lonely, isolated lives, and described the anxiety and depression produced by inability to make contact with another human being. Typical statements from this group: "Outside everyone is too busy. I was left alone." Also: "Here I became associated with a group. I went where everyone else went. I didn't sit by myself. It gave me someone to associate with. Outside I was afraid to talk to people."

In the evaluation of this kind of response two separate aspects of this "friendship" pattern appear. For many of these patients the most important factor was merely the re-establishment of human contact. Having someone to talk to, or just someone to be with, can relieve to some degree this painful sense of loneliness. Indirectly, however, these comments contain another implication. Some patients reported a sense of relief from being admitted to the patient group, or from being recognized as a member of it. On becoming a member of the group many patients reported feeling a new sense of identity. They became "patients" and "sick persons"—but also members of a group and human beings.

Stainbrook (9) and Parsons (8) describe the significance of the "sick role" to a patient. One affected by the bizarre, frightening sensations of mental illness often does not see himself as a sick person, but as "different" or "strange." He feels removed from other men, and becomes frightened. Not until the community agrees to accept the patient's behavior as "sick," and the patient, on his part, accepts the community's decision, can the patient feel again that he is a human being who is simply ill.

This group reported that the hospital permitted them not only to be with people again, but also to regain a sense of identity with the human race by becoming a member of the patient group.

The Physician: Eleven patients reported that contact with their doctor was felt to be the most helpful experience in the hospital. Patients so reporting were seen individually by their doctors on an average of 1.5 times a week, as compared to 1.3 times a week, the average for the entire group, a difference which is not statistically significant. However, the average duration of interview was 39 minutes for these eleven men, compared to 26 minutes for the group as a whole, a difference which is statistically significant.

Some of these patients appeared to have increased intellectual understanding of their problems, but no substantial characterologic changes were observed by the author at this time.

These patients seemed to be reporting a "transference cure." They described a sense of security gained by forming a dependent relationship with a strong, authoritarian figure, and often felt relief after being given the opportunity to ventilate emotionally charged material to a non-punitive, respected physician. Typical statements from this group: "My doctor was interested in me here. I had faith in him. If he tells you to take a treatment and you have faith in him, it helps." Also: "My doctor took a real good interest in me so I never felt alone. She always had time for me."

The Staff: Ten of the patients indicated that the combined staff effort was responsible for their improvement. They said that the feeling that the nurses, attendants and doctors were there to help gave them tremendous support. Typical statements: "In many ways the hospital has gone all out. They tried. They made an all-out effort to help." Also: "You feel here that people are fighting for you."

These patients seem to benefit from the opportunity to experience friendly, interpersonal relationships, much as did those, above, who spoke of the value of social interaction with other patients. However, for this group the dependency gratification derived from contact with people in positions of authority is more important than the gratification derived from a contact with peer group. Despite the limited patient-staff interaction, these patients reported that it was of the greatest significance in their improvement.

Outside Change: Five of the patients said that, since admission to hospital, the conflictual situation outside had been resolved. They were grateful for the part the hospital had played, directly or indirectly, in this resolution. One reported that his wife had changed, that since she had come in to see the social worker she no longer nagged him. Another reported that his wife listens to him, now that she knows he has serious problems.

Manipulation of the environment brought about by hospitalization was described by Wood (13). For such patients the hospital serves not only as a refuge from attacks and fears, but also as a tool to gain control over a member of the family. The social service department actively tries to alter social factors which may have contributed to the patient's illness; in this sense, the hospital supports the patient's efforts to manipulate his environment by seeking admission to the hospital.

Random Responses: The remaining 15 patients will be discussed here as a single group. Five reported no improvement and saw no therapeutic potential in the hospital, although the judgment of the interviewer was that their condition was at least slightly improved. No evaluation of their responses was feasible.

One patient was hyperactive and euphoric on discharge; he felt everything was wonderfully therapeutic, and his response could not be evaluated. Four indicated that their medication was of the greatest benefit. At one time or another during their hospitalization, all of the patients in the study group had been on drugs, usually Thorazine or Librium. Most patients felt that the medication had been helpful, but only four attributed major therapeutic results to the drugs, these four reporting that the drug decreased their anxiety and allowed them to feel more comfortable in the hospital.

Although 24 patients received electric shock or insulin treatment, none reported these treatments to be of primary importance. (Certainly the therapeutic effect of these agents was clearly observed by the staff in most cases.) That these patients neglected to give primary importance to the organic treatments may be attributed to the following factors: The patient had no clear memory of the treatment or of the events surrounding it. He was unable to discuss what happened with any clarity. Also, these organic therapies have an uncanny, impersonal quality, and we suspect that such therapies tend to reduce the patient's self-esteem. The patient wants to feel responsible for his psychic reintegration, thereby regaining self-esteem and a feeling of control. Admission of the therapeutic value of the organic therapies makes him feel he has had no part in his own recovery, and that it was brought about by an exogenous and possibly disruptive force which will give only temporary relief. In any case, these patients did not appear to be interested in discussing these treatments.

Two patients discussed the gratification resulting from learning a skill in the hospital (1). Patients often utilize hospital facilities to acquire mastery of new techniques and thereby to develop increased self-esteem. One young patient who wrote poetry received encouragement and praise:

"I won first prize and the grown-ups said my poetry was good. I missed that when I was a kid." An older patient, with an involutional melancholia: "In O.T. I discovered I can still work. When I played cards I found out my mind was still good. Before, I was afraid I couldn't."

In this study we were unable to evaluate the significance of "social learning" in the treatment program. The relearning of social roles and positions through feedback from other patients, as described by Caudill and Redlich (3), must have some therapeutic merit, but in most patients these responses would be unconscious and not available for study with the interview methodology.

Two other patients stated that the hospital gave them an opportunity to play. Their comments suggested that the hospital had permitted these two men enough freedom from outside worries to rediscover a capacity for pleasure. One (a patient with a colostomy) had been afraid to become involved in playful social relationships, but in hospital had been encouraged to. The other patient had led a pleasureless existence, totally involved in his business. A partial regression in hospital had helped him to participate in less meaningful but more pleasurable activities, which provided him with a measure of relaxation and fun. One patient, a dependent-psychopathic young man, reported that the hospital situation scared him: "I didn't want to work so I thought I had found a haven. But I saw how sick everyone is here and I want to get out."

DISCUSSION

THE relative advantages or superiority of the open ward over the closed ward cannot be determined from this study. An open-ward control group and long-term follow-up would be needed to determine the prolonged effect of the treatment. Nevertheless, the rapid relief of symptoms in 93 per cent of the patients here reported, suggests that closed-ward treatment does have therapeutic value. This study explored certain aspects of hospital care by using the patient as an observer, but the patient-observer and patient-interview methodology has serious limitations. Many patients have difficulty in describing their hospital experiences, and few are sensitive observers. Also, the prejudices of the interviewer can bias results. By seeing a great many patients and attempting to avoid personal bias, we tried to reduce error to a minimum.

The largest group of patients (26) described the advantage of the protective atmosphere of the hospital, pointing out that their primary need on admission was for safety. The hospital served as a protective parental figure for these patients, guarding them, like a parent, against the hazards of life. In this sense the hospital became a substitute ego: it allowed the patient to utilize the hospital organization as an adaptive defense against the world and against his own feared impulses. (Perhaps, too, the hospital serves certain superego functions, in that hospitalization may be seen by some patients as a punishment for unacceptable impulses.)

Eissler (4) described the danger inherent in prolonged treatment: the satisfying of masochistic attitudes in patients who seek hospitalization. The patients however, felt that this protective quality of the hospital was significant in reducing anxiety and relieving symptoms. For most, the reduction of anxiety permitted the ego to reintegrate and to regain a measure of its capacity to repress unconscious conflicts. Ninety-three of our patients were again willing to attempt to function outside the hospital, utilizing as best they could their reintegrated ego strength.

Fromm described the anxiety of modern man, living in a structureless world and lacking sufficient ego maturity to create patterns of behavior for himself (5). In the closed hospital, as in the fascist state, the burden of choice is removed from the patient. He must go where and do what he is told. In some patients, such an atmosphere inhibits any potential for psychologic growth, but for many it seems to offer immediate symptom relief.

Of this study group, 19 per cent reported that the enforced routine was the major therapeutic advantage. Here also the hospital became a substitute ego, organizing the patient's life in a meaningful way. This group found that the loss of choice brought immediate relief: they experienced a gratifying reduction in anxiety and, in most cases, their symptoms disappeared and they were again able to attempt a new adaptation outside.

These two groups, 45 per cent of the study population, gave evidence indicating that the closed or highly structured hospital ward is an effective means of dealing with the acutely anxious patient. Of the remaining 55 per cent, the largest group referred to the therapeutic usefulness of an interpersonal relationship—with friends in the hospital (14 per cent), with their doctor (11 per cent), or with the staff in general (10 per cent). This type of hospital interaction has been studied and described extensively in the literature (2, 11, 13), and we will make no attempt here to elaborate on this work, other than to point out the possible effect on such interaction of a closed-ward as compared to an open-ward situation.

On the closed wards the patients are in constant intimate contact with one another. They must participate in organized activities together. They are to a large extent *forced* to form relationships with other people, whereas an open-ward patient is free to avoid many of these contacts. Even though at times friendship groups may be formed to provide a defiant, mutually protective resistance against the authoritarian hospital, they may still serve a useful purpose. Friendship patterns on closed and open wards should be the subject of further study.

In general, these patient-reports indicate the need for more thorough examination of therapeutic approaches to in-patient care. Specific questions emerge from this study: 1) What type of patient profits from closed hospital care? 2) Is the limited goal of symptom-relief economically and psychologically more practical in large institutions than prolonged in-patient care with intensive psychotherapy? 3) What kind of out-patient treatment can be utilized to maintain the reintegrated patient in the community? 4) Do the patient observations agree with observations made by ward personnel and outside observers?

This study suggests that certain "old-fashioned" techniques of hospital care—*e.g.*, isolation and control—are effective in the treatment of acutely ill, psychotic patients. Further studies should be carried out, utilizing a control group and long-term follow-up, before possibly useful management techniques are discarded.

SUMMARY

ONE hundred hospitalized mental patients were interviewed at time of discharge, to determine, from the patient's point of view, what therapeutic factors are offered by closed and semi-closed wards. Forty-five per cent of the study group indicated that protection from the community and super-imposed control of their lives were the two factors most significant in their recovery. The effect of interpersonal relationships with staff and other patients is discussed briefly. This report suggests that the positive therapeutic effect of isolation and control be studied further before these techniques are discarded in favor of the open hospital.

REFERENCES

1. Bateman, J. F. and Dunham, H. W. The state mental hospital as a specialized community experience. Amer. J. Psychiat., 105: 445-448, 1948.
2. Brody, E. B. and Fishman, M. Therapeutic response and length of hospitalization of psychiatrically ill patients. A. M. A. Arch. Gen. Psychiat., 2: 174-181, 1960.
3. Caudill, W. and Redlich, F. Social structures and interaction processes on a psychiatric ward. Amer. J. Orthopsychiat., 22: 314-333, 1952.
4. Eissler, K. Limitations to the psychotherapy of schizophrenia. Psychiatry, 1: 381-391, 1943.
5. Fromm, E. *Escape From Freedom*, p. 305. Farrar & Rinehart, New York, 1941.
6. Jones, M. *The Therapeutic Community*. Basic Books, New York, 1953.
7. Main, T. F. The hospital as a therapeutic institution. Bull. Menninger Clin., 10: 66, 1946.
8. Parsons, T. Illness and the role of the physician: A sociological perspective. Amer. J. Orthopsychiat., 21: 452, 1951.
9. Stainbrook, E. The community of the psychiatric patient. *American Handbook of Psychiatry*, I: p. 150. Basic Books, New York, 1956.

10. Stanton, A. and Schwartz, M. *The Mental Hospital.* Basic Books, New York, 1954.
11. Wadeson, R. Friendships among psychiatric patients. A. M. A. Arch. Gen. Psychiat., 2: 694-700, 1960.
12. Wilmer, H. A. Toward a definition of the therapeutic community. Amer. J. Psychiat., 114: 824-834, 1958.
13. Wood, W. C., Rakusin, J. M. and Morse, E. Interpersonal aspects of psychiatric hospitalization. A. M. A. Arch. Gen. Psychiat., 3: 632-641, 1960.

ॐ

C H A P T E R 2 8   The Reactions of a Non-Patient

to a Stay on a Mental Hospital Ward*

WILLIAM N. DEANE

I N this report I shall tell of my experiences during one week as a "patient" on one of the rehabilitation wards utilized by the Vermont
Project for the Rehabilitation of Chronic Schizophrenic Patients.[1] In many
respects, the characteristics of ward life painted here are no longer
typical of the particular ward where I stayed, for there have been many
changes in routine and patient activity since that time, designed to enrich
the patients' lives and to reduce to a minimum their long periods of idleness. However, this picture may continue to be reasonably typical of ward
life in many situations. This paper will, after some preliminary description
of the setting, present my reactions to my stay, as I wrote them down during the three days after I left the ward. This section is essentially a first
draft; I felt that allowing it to stand as first written would convey the
sense of urgency which the experience had for me and the deep impression which it made on me.

On Sunday, December 8, 1957, at approximately 7:30 P.M., I became a
volunteer "patient" at the Vermont State Hospital in Waterbury. It was
agreed that I would live on 1 South, the rehabilitation ward, and that my
routine would be that of the patient in all regards, including medication
three times daily. To make the experiment more real, the date and time of
my release were not known to me. I had reason to believe that I would
probably not spend much longer than seven days in the hospital, but not
knowing the exact time of my release was perhaps the most significant
factor in making me feel that I was truly sharing the patient role. Since
I was the sociologist attached to the Rehabilitation Project for Chronic
Schizophrenic Patients, I was well known to the patients on 1 South.

* Reprinted by special permission of The William Alanson White Psychiatric Foundation, Inc., and the author from *Psychiatry*, 24 (1961), 61–68 (copyright by the
Foundation).

About half of these attended my weekly group therapy sessions; others were known to me through interview contacts and the routine of daily duties. Many other male patients in the hospital were also known to me.

The conditions surrounding my stay made it clear to the patients on 1 South that I was not "sick." They were told that I wished to come into the hospital and live as a patient in order to better understand the patient. In my group therapy session and at a meeting which I attended with all the members of 1 South, notice of the stay was given two days before my arrival on the ward and was warmly received.

I was "released" from the hospital at about 8:45 A.M. on Sunday, December 15. Thus, my stay in the hospital was a little less than seven full days.

During this time, I did not attempt to conduct formal interviews or to keep detailed notes on my observations. At some time during the evening, I would compile a few notes on the more noteworthy events of the day. While occasionally I asked the patients questions about themselves and their views on certain aspects of hospital life, I did not do this systematically.

I entered into the industrial therapy program of the hospital, being employed in the laundry folding clothes. This particular job was selected for me by the Project Director of Industrial Therapy because more Project rehabilitation patients work in the laundry than anywhere else in the hospital. Folding clothes also offered the best vantage point for observing the patients.

I was not told what my medication was and, at the time of the original writing, I was unaware of its exact composition and amount.[2]

SOME CHARACTERISTICS OF PATIENT LIFE

RATHER than describe in close detail the actual activities of the ward, many of which will emerge in the next section of the report, I shall attempt to characterize patient life in terms of a few convenient descriptive categories.[3] First of all, a ubiquitous routine and sameness characterize most days. All major activities follow a close and nearly invariable schedule. The ward arises almost as one man at 6 A.M., and proceeds through a series of activities including housekeeping, eating, working, taking medication, and so on through the remainder of the day. There are, of course, individual variations of activity—particularly in work assignments, since the thirty ward members are employed at many different places in the hospital industrial plant. But the job to which each patient goes generally requires the same sort of routinized, scheduled activity that other major areas of his life require.

Second, there is considerable supervision of patient activities. Indeed, the routine life is enforced by supervision. This is not heavy-handed or

unfriendly and does not operate too obviously. Yet it is perfectly clear
that "paid help" are always present to insure an orderly existence. In
addition, patients are always accompanied by attendants and others when
they go from one section of the hospital to another. But it must be underscored that in most situations supervisors do not direct every move the
patient makes, nor repeatedly tell him what to do. It is rather that various
supervisors are always at hand to see that the day's activities proceed
systematically. However, these people often render very real help to
patients in many practical ways.

The entire routinized life is regulated by clear-cut expectations and
rules. Few of these are explicit, or written down, but most patients are
perfectly clear about them. These rules affect not only the major areas of
patient life, but also such matters as when and where one can smoke; how
many cigarettes one is entitled to as payment for his employment
(patients are not paid in money); how often one may take a bath or
obtain a clean sheet or towel; where one may sit in the dining hall; what
wards one may visit; and so on.

The above considerations per se do not make hospital life different
from life outside the hospital, since few members of the community
escape routine, supervision, and various regulations of activity. The
difference is in the greater inclusiveness of routine and regulation in the
hospital, and in the further fact that the patients themselves have very
little part in determining their own routine, supervisory needs, or regula-
tory conditions. These are imposed at the convenience of the staff in the
interest of efficient, economical management with minimal risk and must
be observed by the patient whether he sees any sense to them or not.

In spite of the brisk and inclusive regulation of patient life, leisure time
constitutes a fairly large proportion of the waking day. There are always
bits of time during the day, ranging from a few minutes to an hour or so,
when patients have nothing required of them. Most evenings represent
unscheduled blocks of time, as do Saturday afternoons and Sundays for
most patients. Also, in a good many of the industries the work is irregular with long periods of idleness interspersed here and there. On the other
hand, the ways in which leisure time may be utilized are limited. The
ward has some magazines and paper-backed novels, but there are not very
many of these nor are they systematically available. One would have difficulty reading a serial article in a particular magazine because some copies
would be missing. Some days there is a morning newspaper, some days
not. There are a few decks of cards, a cribbage board or two, a television
set which brings in only one channel clearly, and one or two radios. In
short, when the patient is free from the demands of his schedule, there
is relatively little to command his attention or interest. Should he be
interested in reading or playing cards, for example, his interest might soon
be threatened by the lack of variety of the literature or the limited capabilities of the other patients for playing cards.

Again, the difference between hospital and community life is not so much in the fact of large amounts of leisure time existing in the hospital. Leisure time is a prominent commodity of many people in all American communities. It is rather the greater dearth of possible outlets for the use of this time in the hospital which makes the difference. Moreover, for many citizens leisure time may be accompanied by greater freedom from restrictions, in comparison to their employment hours. For the patients on 1 South this is less true. Regulations concerning smoking, taking baths, moving freely about the hospital, and so on, hold relatively constant for all points in the day. Therefore, leisure time occurs within the framework of limited recreational outlets and continued rules and regulations.

These are some of the characteristics of life on one ward in one mental hospital. Others could be noted, and, indeed, a different observer might be more impressed with other aspects of life than those covered here. These characteristics are mentioned because they were the most apparent to me, and because when patients "griped" in my presence about hospital life, these represented the areas of major complaint. On the other hand, it is perfectly true that some patients, particularly the "old settlers," like hospital life largely because of the characteristics I have been describing.

MY REACTION TO THE PATIENT ROLE

THE following description of my reactions was written during the three days following my release.

My reactions toward being a "patient" varied considerably during the seven days. In fact, mood swings became apparent before my entrance into the hospital. The idea of living on the ward came to me about three days before my stay began. At that time, my reactions to the idea were those of exhilaration and a sense of adventure. Within twenty-four hours after discussion of the idea with George W. Brooks, Director of the Project, all arrangements for my entrance and the conditions of my stay had been worked out. From this point on, I developed a growing sense of apprehension, which abated frequently and was replaced by the familiar feeling of adventure. The emotion of apprehension was distressing in terms of the ostensible reasons for it. I discovered that I had some actual fear of living with "crazy people," that beneath the façade of my consciously enlightened attitude toward mental illness there existed an emotional acceptance of popular folklore about the "madman." Also, although I was familiar with the hospital and knew that it was a well-run and humane state institution, the stereotype of the "snake pit" lurked in the back of my mind. These fears were not too pronounced in terms of stark detail, but the fact that they existed even inchoately was in itself a shock and a disappointment.

It must be admitted that at the time of my arrival in the hospital, these fears had largely subsided as explicit ideas. However, the first night my sleep was poor. I awoke innumerable times. Ernest Jordon,[4] who slept in the same dormitory, against the wall opposite from me, was having a restless night. I was constantly aware of his turning and thrashing. Toward morning (it must have been shortly before 6 a.m., when the day shift comes on), I became aware of the cars entering the driveway. A bay window juts out from the dormitory in which I slept, and I found the car lights flashing into the window and cutting across the ceiling extremely annoying, as I did on other nights if I was having difficulty sleeping.

The first day in the hospital passed rather uneventfully. Since I was doing everything for the first time, I was not conscious of too much boredom except during the long lulls when there were no clothes to fold. I was somewhat self-conscious, feeling distinct and different from the patients. The patients, as a whole, however, seemed to be well aware of my coming, and all who expressed themselves to me felt that it was a good idea.

I felt somewhat tired and sleepy during the day, but whether this was due to the medication, which was begun in the morning, poor sleep the night before, or self-consciousness was not clear to me.

On the second day, I became aware of a sense of huge boredom. The day dragged endlessly. On the other hand, I slept very well during the night. My appetite was keen. I was definitely sleepy and listless and began to feel some depression. I began to worry about when I would be released and became conscious of a slight dread that I might actually become psychotic and not be released. I began to feel a closer identification with the patients.

By the third day, my depression deepened markedly. This may, in part, be explained by the fact that I was scheduled to spend that day in Occupational Therapy. On the night before, I had been looking forward to it, but on Wednesday morning I discovered that men who were to go to OT did not leave the ward until 9 a.m. My spirits sagged during the hour and a half of waiting to go. By the time 9 a.m. came, I didn't much care if I went or not.

Upon arriving in OT, I saw Miss Elizabeth Lowe, the hospital and Project occupational therapist. I work with her daily. I was naturally glad to see her. However, she was "playing the game according to the rules," it having been agreed that no doctor, staff member, ward attendant, or other paid employee of the hospital would treat me any differently than patients are treated. This meant that I was to be addressed as "Mr. Deane" or "Deane" and shown no familiarity.

Miss Lowe's friendly but nonfamiliar treatment of me disturbed me even though I understood it, and I began to feel a sense of resentment toward her which I quickly generalized to all staff members and "paid help" in the hospital. This feeling did not abate during the week; if anything, it increased. However, it did not extend to the attendants on 1 South, toward whom I had a warm and friendly feeling even though they were scrupulous in avoiding any show of favoritism toward me.

Miss Lowe suggested that I compile an inventory list for her. She told me that if I got tired of this, I could work with Jean LaSorda, a 1 South patient who was typesetting some parole cards. I had difficulty developing an interest in the typesetting and quickly gave it up. I told Miss Lowe that I would work with Jean but that I wanted to smoke first. She told me that I would have to wait until 10 a.m. to do this. This irritated and frustrated me. I am a relatively heavy cigarette smoker and was having difficulty budgeting my cigarettes to five or six a day. Here was a new frustration, because in the laundry you can smoke any time you choose. This is also true of the ward up until 8 p.m.

I walked over to look at what Jean was doing. Miss Lowe had asked him to help me. I know Jean well, since he is a member of my therapy group. I took a look at the type and lost all interest in it. I felt confused and tired. I felt that it was an effort to move. I said to Jean, "Look, I can't learn that. I feel lousy. I'm tired and sleepy. My head feels funny." He tried to encourage me to try the work, explaining that it wasn't hard. Miss Lowe came over and began arranging type and explaining each step. I said, "Look, I can't learn this. Let me go back to the laundry and fold clothes."

Eventually 10 o'clock came and I had a smoke. I spent the rest of the morning watching Jean but doing nothing. Finally, at 11, we returned to the ward. After dinner, I was scheduled to return to OT. Again I had to wait until 1 p.m. before I could go. I had the same feeling of endless time, although the wait was not more than 45 minutes. On arriving at OT, I discovered Jean was not there. Mr. Eastman said that I had better wait until Miss Lowe came over at 2 p.m., as he wasn't sure where the paper was for running off the print Jean and Miss Lowe had arranged. I said to him, "Well, in that case, why don't I go back to the laundry?" He offered no objection and let me out. I went over to the laundry with a sense of relief and felt somewhat better the rest of the working day.

The evenings passed routinely. I didn't, in general, feel the same sense of boredom and depression at night as I did during the day. My schedule was about the same on any given night. I played cards with the patients much of the time. I read some, although the things that I read—magazine articles and one paper-bound novel—I would not under normal circumstances be interested in at all. I watched television, but with less interest than usual, although I am not too interested in many television programs at any time. Some time during the evening I compiled a few notes on the day's activities. I found that this took considerable effort and was especially fatiguing. On virtually all nights, I went to bed around 8:30, half an hour before the 9 p.m. ward curfew. Not being able to smoke seemed to create the philosophy in my mind that I might as well sleep and get the night over with as soon as possible.

On Thursday my spirits were reasonably good during the morning. I was looking forward to group therapy in the afternoon and was anticipating the interesting experience of being a member of the group which I normally led. Also, I knew that I would see my wife, Hope, briefly, since the therapy group met in one of the rooms of the female OT and Hope is a volunteer worker in female OT on Tuesdays and Thursdays. So, with these anticipations in mind, my morale was good.

However, after dinner, there ensued the long wait of nearly an hour and a half until it was time to go to group therapy. During this interval, my enthusiasm drained out. I didn't much care whether I went or not. Moreover, I began to develop some anxiety about Hope and the children. I was afraid that I might find her unwell, or that she would tell me the children were sick, or have some sort of bad news to report. I also knew that she, along with Dr. Brooks, knew when I was to come home. I knew that she wouldn't tell me this, because I had made her promise to withhold that information from me, but I began to resent the fact that she knew. I also recalled that Dr. Brooks had gone to New York, and I resented the fact that he wasn't around.

When we got down to OT, I saw Hope for just a minute before going into the

meeting. I asked her several times if everything were all right. She assured me
that it was, but I had difficulty believing this.

In the group therapy meeting, I felt very depressed. It appeared that Dr.
Grant had not brought any hospital cigarettes, and one of the things I had been
looking forward to was the opportunity to smoke two or three extra cigarettes.
Isaac Myers launched a discussion on hallucinations, which had been a topic
the group had agreed to take up a week earlier. I noticed during this discussion
that Gino Russo, who had been hearing voices all week, was mumbling to himself and shaking his head back and forth. Dr. Grant told Isaac that under certain conditions anyone can be hallucinated. I began to describe the hypnagogic
hallucination, which is a common occurrence with me. Marius Ramazotti stared
at me intently. I did not use the words "hypnagogic hallucination," but Isaac
spoke up and said, "I read in a psychology book once about the hypnagogic hallucination." I told him that this was what I had been talking about. Richard
Heath asked how he could overcome fear of the dark. He had been explaining
this fear to me when we had been smoking earlier on the porch. I was relieved
to hear Dr. Grant tell him much the same thing that I had told him—that fear
of the dark is but a specific aspect of a more generalized type of fear and that
self-understanding is the only way to really overcome it. At this point, Dr.
Grant received a telephone call and had to terminate the meeting. He gave us
the pack of cigarettes that he had with him.

Originally, the group had planned to stay after the meeting and join some of
the female patients in practicing Christmas carols. This session was set for 3:30.
However, as our group had finished its meeting quite early, Mrs. Longe, one of
Miss Lowe's assistants, decided that we should return to the ward and come
back to OT at the appointed time. As we were filing out, she stopped me and
said, "I want you to stay here." The purpose of this was to give me more time
to talk with Hope.

I felt somewhat guilty about remaining, as though it were an act of favoritism
shown me. On the other hand, it was Thursday afternoon, one of the visiting
days, and it was between one and four, the visiting hours. Hope and I went
into one of the side rooms to talk. I felt strange and tense. I was unable to relax.
I questioned her all over again about her week. She told me that things were
fine, but I still retained some gnawing doubts. I could tell that she was a little
concerned about me and how I felt. I tried to reassure her, and yet I more or
less deliberately wanted to convey the impression that I was having a hard time.
I was ambivalent of mind, wanting on the one hand to reassure her, and yet
wanting her to understand that I was not having a pleasant experience. She
wanted to know how long I felt that I should stay in the hospital, from my point
of view. I told her that I thought seven days would do it. This would give me a
complete unit of time. Having said this, I set my mind, for the rest of the week,
on getting out some time on Sunday. I figured that I would leave Sunday night,
but my anxiety about possibly having to stay longer increased as this idea took
form.

After a few minutes, Hope had to get back to her patients. I said that I would
see her at 3:30. I could tell that she was not altogether happy about me, that
my ambivalence and tension had been conveyed. Yet I either couldn't or
wouldn't go further in my attitudes and behavior toward reassuring her.

I returned to the ward alone. Shortly after I got back, a call came from female OT that the rehearsal had been postponed. I felt desolate and guilty about my behavior in front of Hope and worried about this the rest of the week.

On Thursday night, I decided to go to the movies which are shown twice a month to patients. I wasn't much interested but felt that I should go on the grounds that I should see and do as much as possible in order to get the flavor of patient life. One of my major reasons for not wanting to go was the fact that I wouldn't be able to smoke during the movie. I was not then aware that one could smoke after returning from the movie, so it seemed to me that there would be an unbearable period of time betwen about 6:45 p.m., the time of the movie, and the next morning, during which I couldn't smoke.

On arriving at the movie, I saw one of my fellow folders across the hall. He waved at me in a cheery fashion. The main feature was preceded by a short cartoon. Then the movie got under way. I maintained a reasonable interest in it. However, since the film was showing on one camera only, there were frequent interruptions for reel changes. This annoyed me far out of proportion to the short interval of time involved.

Sitting at my left during the movie was a large, rawboned patient who constantly repeated several complicated movements. He would clench his hands together, unlock them, cross his arms and grip his sides, and bring his hands together over his mouth, making strange sucking sounds. He would then drop his hands and begin the whole sequence again. He seldom stopped these motions, and they were invariable. This had no effect upon me, however. I was not annoyed by it, but only interested in slyly observing the stereotyped motions.

It was a relief to me on returning to the ward to have Mr. Byrd, the attendant, explain that I could have one smoke if I wanted to. Parenthetically, on the subject of smoking, I did not realize until Monday night, my second night, that one could not smoke after 8 p.m. Sunday night I had brought no cigarettes with me and steadfastly refused offers of them from the patients. Karl Russell, a patient, had tried to give me "three or four to tide you over to morning." On Monday night, I asked Mr. Byrd for a light at 8:15. For a moment he looked a little embarrassed, and then said, "If you want me to really treat you like a patient, I can't let you smoke after 8 p.m." Interestingly enough, I felt no resentment toward him at all.

My attitude for the rest of the week continued resentful and depressed. Two or three times patients either asked me for cigarettes or I offered them. This reduced my precious supply and was a source of anxiety. I debated asking the ward attendants to reimburse me these cigarettes, but couldn't bring myself to do it.

The feeling of identity with the patients and social distance from the staff began to increase. However, I still continued to feel warm toward the ward attendants. I became noticeably more restless both in the laundry and on the ward. I paced the corridors from time to time, and once, in the laundry, I undertook a complete inspection tour of the place, looking intently at all the machines and gadgets, but actually having no interest in any of it. I would take several long walks to the drinking fountain, although on none of these trips was I thirsty. I would speculate a good deal about the sociological implications of hospitalization, but frequently these ideas would be interrupted by lengthy indulgences in fantasy. Indeed, fantasying definitely increased as time wore on. I found that the rhythmic, simple, unthinking motions of folding clothes seemed to stimulate this.

I continued to have a good appetite and to sleep well until Friday. I had observed in the dining hall that the way to assure yourself of a good meal was to eat the first serving as rapidly as possible and then return for seconds. First servings were quite meager, but second servings were very generous. I also ate large quantities of bread slabbed heavily with butter. I consumed as much tea and coffee as possible by drinking each cup rapidly and sticking my cup out for more whenever the pitcher was brought to our table. On Friday, I began to take less interest in food. I found that one helping was sufficient. I ate much less bread but still continued to drink as much tea and coffee as possible.

Friday evening my whole emotional state underwent a sudden change. That evening, Raymond Craft, from 7 South, a manic who was steadily swinging into a "high" mood,[5] came down to visit me. In fact, Raymond had shown a proprietary interest in me all week and had made it clear that he was going to see that I "got a fair shake." We had played two games of cribbage earlier in the week, and each of us had won one game. He suggested that we go up to 7 South and play a rubber. I got permission and went up there. Raymond bustled around and introduced me to everyone. I began to feel benevolent and gay. I talked with all the men, who were extremely friendly and complimentary toward my stay. A patient named John Holton said he felt that all the doctors should do this. I agreed heartily, taking sardonic delight in the idea.

I stayed for an hour, successfully befriending two patients named English and Montroy. Then I went back to 1 South. I felt elated but restless. A patient named Hunter was on the ward. I had worked with Hunter and eaten at the same table with him all week. He is a very "high" manic. I had found him wearying but now I talked with him eagerly and had a great fellow feeling with him. His incredible ramblings seemed to make more sense than before.

However, I still went to bed at 8:30 in spite of the elated mood. I went to sleep directly but slept poorly. I awoke several times in the night and was conscious of bad dreams. I generally dream every night, but this had been the first night that my dreams had taken on a vivid and rememberable color.

On Saturday, I felt quite depressed and hopeless. My mood stayed fixed at this level for the rest of the time. At one point on Saturday, Henry Jarrette, one of the 1 South men, told me that he had heard that I was going to stay ten days. I thought that this might be true, and I began to feel very sorry for myself. I began to talk more about how bad I thought life was in the hospital. If the men asked me how I felt, I would say, "Lousy." This seemed to bring forth a combined reaction of amusement and sympathy.

I continued to show less interest in eating throughout the day. During the morning, I had looked forward to watching the football game on television, since I didn't have to work on Saturday afternoon, but I actually didn't enjoy watching it when the time came. Normally, I thoroughly enjoy professional football on television.

On Saturday night, I went to bed with a definite sense of inner tension. I felt as though I were shaking inside and as though my muscles were going to start spasmodic jerking. I had a series of nightmares which seemed to be continuous. One I still recall very vividly. I was sitting at a table. My middle son, Gordon, aged eight, was sitting at my left, and Dr. Brooks was sitting directly across the table. I was much older and very tired. I kept dropping my food and spilling my milk. Gordon kept telling me about it and urging me to stop doing this, but I couldn't seem to prevent it. Gordon's face became indistinct, and he looked lumpy like clay. Then I wasn't sure whether he was Gordon or Thatcher, my three-year-old son. I put my hands over my face and, in some strange way, made a square out of them. I realized that I was undergoing an acute schizophrenic reaction. I started to cry in despair. Dr. Brooks looked at me and laughed. I awoke alarmed. One of the patients, Stanley Morgan, who occupied a single room across the hall, was crying out in his sleep. This was the only time I heard anything like this. I could hear some stirring on the ward and decided to get up. It was 5:45. This was the only morning that I got up before 6 a.m.

I decided that I would go to church on Sunday morning. The ward attendant wanted to know which service I wished to attend. I said that I didn't care, but that if I had to make a choice, I would go to the Catholic service. I am a Protestant in upbringing, but was conscious of being hostile toward Protestantism and feeling very warm toward Catholicism. I was anxious to see a priest in his ecclesiastical attire. The attendant said, "You can go to both if you want to." I said I would do this.

I then began to get anxious about how to behave at a Catholic service. I sought out Marius Ramazotti and asked if I could sit with him. He agreed readily and got the prayer book to show me what I was supposed to do. Looking at it increased my anxiety. Before we had gone very far with this, the group assembled for the Protestant service. I went to the service and all through it felt very emotional, as though I wanted to cry.

When it was over and we came back to the ward, Dr. Brooks was there and asked to see me. He said he thought I should go home. I agreed and began to get ready. I recalled that I owed a cigarette to Wilson Wood and one to Karl Russell, so I paid them back. I had three cigarettes left, and I gave these to Jack Sherring, who was pacing the hall. I shook hands with all the men and had difficulty holding back tears.

Once outside of the hospital, I actually broke into sobs for a few seconds. I walked across the street to my house. I almost cried again when I greeted my wife and children. All that day, I was restless and tense. I drank innumerable cups of coffee and smoked endlessly. Sunday night I slept badly and was bothered by nightmares. In fact, at the time of this writing, which is now over two days after my return, I still feel considerable tension and a rather intense desire to move restlessly about and do exciting things. My sleep is still somewhat disturbed, and my dreams are of a nightmare quality.

Looking back, it seems as though it were ages ago that I left the hospital. The unpleasantness of the experience is already subsiding, and I recall more clearly the pleasanter side of the stay.

There are one or two subtle aspects of my emotional reactions that should be touched on in concluding this account. For one thing, I observed that familiar parts of the hospital which I had seen many times, such as the laundry, the tunnel, the OT departments, and 1 South, appeared different to me than they had before my stay [or have since]. This is in no sense a perceptual distortion. It is rather a condition of seeing things through a "different set of eyes" which has the effect of making the familiar appear unfamiliar. I noticed this in walking through the tunnel more than at any other time. Indeed, this experience became apparent to me between the time of forming the idea of living on the ward and arriving there, but was more intense after my stay began.

The second aspect has to do with speech changes that I experienced. This was a very subtle thing that could be demonstrated only through a series of tape recordings of my normal speech patterns before or after the stay, as compared with recordings of about the middle part of my stay. It seemed to me that I developed a mode of speech which omitted many connecting words, that I tended to speak explosively and faster than usual, and yet in a lower and softer register. I became more conscious of having done this after it ceased to exist than I was during it. It seemed to be a phenomenon of transitory duration, taking place around the third or fourth day. It perhaps represented some sort of a psychogenic contagion in which I borrowed speech patterns from several of the men.

One of the most apparent reactions to my ward stay was that I took on in mild form some of the symptomatology of certain of the patients. For example, there was some withdrawal from active participation, as shown by my early retiring, frequent drowsiness, and indulgences in fantasy. There was considerable projective hostility directed toward the staff and my wife. I was hostile, also, about rules and regulations, particularly those pertaining to smoking, and I resented certain activities in which I was asked to participate, particularly those in OT.

I used work as a protective shield, escaping to the laundry in order to avoid the typesetting activity in OT. Fantasy and autistic thinking tended to grow during the week. My mind was flooded with an almost childish preoccupation with the sensory deprivation I was undergoing. There was a great concern and anxiety about cigarettes and a huge desire for coffee. What scheming to beat the system I attempted was designed to reduce sensory deprivation—to eat fast and get more food, to drink my coffee quickly and get another cup, to go to group therapy and get some extra cigarettes.

I felt some depression, which was associated with idleness and with my speculations about going home. Anxiety was very pronounced and attached itself to a host of things, as the report suggests. Anxiety also appeared in my dreams. This affect appeared to be, in part, a reaction formation against the hostility I felt toward the staff and my wife. There was also some regression shown in my elated moods, overidentification with manic patients, and patronizing attitudes toward some of the patients, as for example, the 'befriending' of Montroy and English. Mild dissociative reactions are suggested by the experience of "seeing things through a different set of eyes."

All of the above mental states are associated with some mental patients. They reflect the reactions of many patients on 1 South, but by no means all. The fact that I experienced these in a milder way, yet in a more intensive form than is normal with me, does suggest that some of the symptomatology of mental patients may be due to the effects of hospitalization, and not to the fact of mental illness per se.

On the other hand, hospitalization may also serve to make existing personality traits more intense, to bring them out in more florid fashion. My over-all responses seemed to be enlargements of those characteristic of a person with strong superego development. A person more psychopathic in nature, for example, might have responded quite differently in the same situation, reacting in ways which would have represented in milder form the symptomatology associated with another type of patient.

NOTES TO CHAPTER 28

1. Office of Vocational Rehabilitation, Special Projects Grant #180.
2. Mild amounts of meprobamate and pedanticine were taken orally three times daily and twice daily respectively.
3. Observations in this section pertain specifically to ward 1 South and to its members who worked in the laundry. Significant differences may obtain for other wards and workers.
4. Patient names are fictitious. Staff identification is actual.
5. Raymond is a member of my therapy group by his own choosing. He is not a rehabilitation patient. He was transferred to 2-B, a disturbed ward, on Saturday because of his manic state.

Goal Attainment

ಕ಼

CHAPTER 29   Patient Government:

A New Form of Group Therapy*

ROBERT W. HYDE AND HARRY C. SOLOMON

Patient government is a method of self-government to permit the patients to participate in the administration of the hospital, express themselves in an organized fashion and contribute to their own care and comfort. It is the latest step in the humane movement first highlighted by Pinel's casting the chains off the mentally ill and freeing them from punishment, progressing through periods of autocratic control to paternalistic management and overprotection to reach this point of freedom of expression and self-determinism.

In patient government the patients can:

1. Develop constitutional government with bylaws and regular meetings and elect officers to positions of leadership and responsibility which are recognized by both patients and hospital authorities. These leaders can assist the administration, occupational therapists, nurses, attendants and volunteer workers through consultation in planning and assignment of tasks.
2. Vote on complaints and suggestions and present them to the hospital authorities as the collective desire of the patient body rather than of one individual.
3. Organize and assign their own ward rules.
4. Recommend changes in ward rules.
5. Arrange, organize, conduct and assume responsibility for social activities.
6. Originate, plan and carry through a variety of special activity

* The authors wish to acknowledge the assistance received from Catherine F. Hurley, Charles R. Atwell and Francis MacCumber.

Reprinted from the *Digest of Neurology and Psychiatry*, 18 (1950), 207–218, by permission of the authors and the *Digest*.

programs such as painting projects, mural paintings, writing and editing the hospital paper.

7. Form committees and elect leaders to engage in any program of hospital betterment approved by the hospital authorities.

These accomplishments lead to release from the onerous burden of rules and regulations arbitrarily imposed by others with resulting acquisition of a new freedom, a fuller life, an increased feeling of personal responsibility, of being able to contribute to their own recovery, of gaining experience in service to others, of democratic living and toward acquiring more versatility in social skills. These accomplishments depend upon the trust of the hospital staff, recognition of the ability and competence of the patients. It requires the relinquishment of some authority by the hospital administration leading to a more democratic sharing of authority with the patients.

Patient government is a new and effective form of group therapy, a form which has proved to have many positive advantages in its three years' experience at Boston Psychopathic Hospital. It corresponds closely to student government, the value of which is recognized in many schools.

It is the natural outgrowth of our basic attitudes of providing a hospital atmosphere wherein the patient is encouraged to creativity which will give him a sense of satisfaction, appreciation and socialization. Perhaps the highest goal to be achieved in socialization is to permit the patients to govern themselves, to learn the give and take of mature social relations, to learn to create for themselves a congenial social atmosphere. It was thought that this experience would give the patient a better education for everyday life, a greater interest in his fellow man and an improved ability to cooperate with others.

An early description of a form of self-government is found in Charles Dickens "American Notes"[1] in which he records his impression of the South Boston Asylum which he visited in 1842:

"They have among themselves a sewing society to make clothes for the poor, which holds meetings, passes resolutions, never comes to fisticuffs or bowie-knives as some assemblies have been known to do elsewhere; and conducts all the proceedings with the greatest decorum. The irritability which would otherwise be expended on their own flesh, clothes and furniture is dissipated in these pursuits. They are cheerful, tranquil and healthy."

Experiences of other hospitals with patient government have not been completely reviewed but appear to be rare. A literary club at Worcester State Hospital[2] has been described which developed almost spontaneously on the part of the patients, fostered by a doctor, and was an endeavor having many of the characteristics of a self-governing body.

The success of a self-governed social club in a public mental hospital in England[3] was described. It differed from ours in that five members of the staff took active and dominating part and that its activities were primarily social.

There is mention of it at Winter Veterans' Hospital[4] "the therapeutic community" mentioning "teamwork among patients, athletic teams by wards, carefully scheduled games, self-government is stimulated by having patients elect ward committees to promote orderly behavior and transmit ward gripes to authorities."

OUR EXPERIENCE WITH PATIENT GOVERNMENT

PATIENT government came about in this hospital in a singular way. In October, 1947, Miss Emily Hatch, psychiatric social work student from Simmons College School of Social Work, in preparing a thesis[5] entitled "The Attitudes of Patients in Convalescent Wards of Boston Psychopathic Hospital Toward Their Entire Hospital Experience," interviewed 100 patients to find out their attitudes toward their hospital experience. She found the best manner of interviewing them was in small groups of 2 or 3 in which they felt freer to express themselves than when interviewed separately. The patients' answers were frank and informative, ranging from criticism of the coffee to appreciation of the special social activities of the hospital. After talking with this social worker the patients on the female convalescent ward (Ward 5) began to discuss ward conditions and wrote out a list of the things they thought were wrong with the ward which they felt should be corrected. This list was forwarded to the Assistant Superintendent and received immediate attention. Criticisms such as enforcement of the rest period were referred back to the patients themselves and they were advised to apply their own social pressure to enforce the rest period. A request for a group therapy session was acted on by asking them what time and hour they would like to see a doctor for this purpose and a regular group therapy session was initiated which has run from December, 1947 to the present time.

A head nurse (Mary Knell, R.N.) was sent to Ward 5 at this time, partially in response to the patients' request for the assignment of a head nurse to the ward. She was told that the patients were discussing their ward problems and planning remedies and that it would be worthwhile to encourage this attitude. The patients worked with her telling her what they needed on the ward. Together they planned their work, their parties and entertainment. Gradually the informal organization of the patients of Ward 5 developed to a more formal one designated as patient government in January, 1948. At this time officers elected were: president, vice president, secretary and treasurer.

Patient government ran successfully for several months on the female convalescent ward before it was started on the male ward. We waited for it to develop spontaneously on the male ward from the example set by the increased pleasure and democratic living of the female patients. After the female patients had invited male patients over for tea and told them that they had arranged this and other social events themselves, the male patients established their own organization which became fully as active and successful as that of the female group. For a time the two groups functioned separately, each electing their own officers but soon they began to hold some of their meetings together. Then they came together as one "Patient Government Body" with only one set of officers.

The growth of patient government throughout 1948 was not without difficulties. Two attendants who had spent many years on the female convalescent ward rebelled, saying "What are we here for anyway? They (the patients) won't let us to anything, we can't set out the food or do the cleaning. We feel useless. We'll quit if you don't take us off the ward or put a stop to letting the patients run everything."

Many of the officers elected by the patients to govern the organization progressed rapidly to recovery and departure from the hospital. Frequently several of the leaders left the hospital in a week's time, changing the organization from one which had been exceedingly active to one of inactivity. As a corrective measure four ward representatives and a recording secretary were added to the list of officers.

Difficulties arose in selecting hospital personnel to attend patient government meetings and perform a liaison function between the government and the hospital. Often a person selected for this duty started with quite non-directive method but slipped into an authoritarian rôle.

One feature that was maintained throughout was that of sending a written report of meetings to the Superintendent of Nurses, Assistant Superintendent of the hospital and the Head Occupational Therapist. Prompt action was taken in bringing about either corrective action to the liking of the patients or giving a detailed explanation of why such action could not come about. The spirit of the organization appeared to depend to a great extent on this feeling that their wishes could be heard and that they could accomplish things.

Patient government took final form in May, 1949, when a committee of patients and an interested nurse, Howard Holland, R.N., and attendant Thomas McEneaney drafted a constitution, incorporating in it those features which had proved successful and adding measures to correct difficulties which had been encountered.

The constitution is not included here for it follows the form of constitutions of other organizations and perhaps here lies much of its merit. The patient has in patient government an experience similar to that which he would have in any active club or governing body.

The constitution states the object of the organization, the eligibility of all patients to membership, the officers and their duties, the manner of election, the time of meetings, the regular committees and their duties, the appointment and function of the hospital staff advisor, the order of business, parliamentary authority and method of amendment. The objects of the organization as stated in the constitution are:

"(a) By self-government to provide the members with an opportunity to gain experience and education in democratic living.

"(b) To promote the unity of patients in order to develop mutual help in improving environmental conditions, inter-patient and hospital staff-patient relationships."

Following the adoption of the above constitution the organization has made many impressive developments and encountered few difficulties. The greater number of officers, nine rather than the previous four, has reduced the probability of simultaneous loss of all officers through recovery and discharge. The addition of ward representatives served to bring about more interest and activity on each ward between the general meetings as well as to furnish steps toward the higher positions. It also brought about the incorporation of the entire patient body in the government, bringing in the patients from the acute wards who were able to attend the meetings.

Since the constitution went into effect there have been weekly meetings open to the whole membership. The activities of the body were so many that business could not be completed with less frequent meetings. These weekly assemblies have become one of the most important social events of the patients of the hospital, competing in popularity with patients' dances, bingo parties, variety nights, etc.

No difficulty is now encountered with the coordination of the patient government with the rest of the hospital organization. The liaison personnel selected by the hospital are changed frequently so that they do not get possessive or autocratic in attitude. At present the position is rotated through four different departments: occupational therapy, social service, psychology and nursing, thereby bringing all these departments into close relationship with the patient government.

ACCOMPLISHMENTS OF PATIENT GOVERNMENT

ALTHOUGH a complete study of patient government has not been made, a presentation of some of the more obvious accomplishments serves to justify its existence, to demonstrate how it functions, and to reveal its importance as a new group therapy method.

Perhaps the most important accomplishment is the patient's experience in the democratic process itself, centering largely about patient participation in patient government meetings. Such participation encourages patients who are withdrawn or depressed to express themselves. It also succeeds in guiding the domination of overactive patients. Altogether the patients gain the experience of working together toward a constructive goal and develop a knowledge of socialization, organization and effective group leadership. They learn to explore the reality situation and analyze their own needs. A sample of this is offered in a report of the liaison officer of a meeting of July 27, 1949.

"When the patient asked for any new business, Mr. A. (Psychosis with Epidemic Encephalitis, with depression, paranoid ideas and a marked tremor) got up and said: 'Why don't we go on a beach party some day?' They all laughed and got a big kick out of it. Mrs. Catherine Lambe, O.T.R. (liaison officer) got up and said that plans were being formulated for a beach party the next week and if they wanted to vote on a beach, that would be good. Mr. A. said: 'Why don't we go to the Cape, I have a place down there.' Some one else suggested Revere. Mrs. B. (General Paresis with grandiose features) suggested Lynn. Mrs. Lambe got up and said they had been near Lynn previously, that they had been at Nahant and got a private beach. They they took a vote on it. No one voted for the Cape, 6 voted for Revere and 9 for Nahant. After the voting was over Mr. C. (Manic Depressive-Manic, aggressively overactive and domineering) walked in and said he thought Revere was where they should go and wanted a re-vote. Miss D. (Manic Depressive-Manic) got up and said, 'How about Nantasket?' Mr. C. said that was even better. He said he could constitutionally ask for a re-vote. There was a re-vote and 19 voted for Nahant, 3 for Revere and 7 for Nantasket.

"Mr. C. got up and said he had more knowledge than anybody there, he was an older man and better educated and that he had forgotten more than any of them ever knew. That started a controversy. He then said, 'I'm going to appeal the whole matter to the doctors.' The patients all started to get up and talk. Mr. E., secretary, (Dementia Praecox, paranoid and withdrawn) was first and said the majority had voted on Nahant and that what the majority of patients wanted was where they should go. Mr. C. got up again and said it was still legal for him to appeal it. Another patient got up and said the majority had voted for Nahant. Mr. E. was up and down all the time and one time said Mr. C. had no idea of what their preference was and if that was what they wanted, they should have it. Miss F. (Dementia Praecox-Catatonic, young and usually shy) got up and said quite dramatically, 'You may be an older man and know more than we do but you still don't know what our preference is.' Mr. C. interrupted all through and told them they were full of hot air and he was going to appeal it to the doctors. Mrs. Lambe got up and said that inasmuch as she was a liaison officer, she knew the doctors had nothing to do with it and if the majority of patients wanted it, an appeal could not be handled.

"Mr. G. (Involutional Psychosis-Melancholia with agitation, restlessness and depression) got up and said Mr. C. was out of order, that it was a majority vote and should hold. Mr. C. said he would bet five dollars we wouldn't go to any beach. Mr. H. (Dementia Praecox-Other Types, with ideas of reference and delusions of persecution) got up and said, 'I'll take that bet.' Miss I., president, (Dementia Praecox-Paranoid, with delusions of persecution and grandeur) said the patient government did not permit betting. Mr. C. said, 'Let's take another vote.' Miss I. agreed but the patients didn't want to. They took another vote and everybody but Mr. C. voted for Nahant. Mr. C. said, 'Let's call the Metropolitan District Commission and ask them what beach we should go to.' Mr. E. said they had nothing to do with it, that it was a majority vote. During this discussion Mrs. J. (Involutional Psychosis-Melancholia) turned to Mrs. Lambe and said, 'I certainly understand why a lot of people are here.'

"When Mrs. K., ward 5 representative, (Manic Depressive-Mixed, with depression and suspiciousness) got up to give her report, Mr. C. interrupted her. She sat down and said, 'I thought I had the floor but apparently I haven't.' He begged her pardon and sat down. She got up and continued her report but he interrupted her again. She went up to him and very dramatically pointed to the porch and said, 'Get out! We have had enough of your exhibitionism.' When she finished her report and sat down, everybody clapped."

In this meeting the patients resisted the domination of aggressive members and carried through social action to completion. The domineering (manic) patient, Mr. C., who failed in his effort to dominate other patients, had a wholesome therapeutic experience. He was quieter, better organized in his thinking the following day and apologized to the officers of the patient government for his behavior. The satisfaction of many of the more timid and fearful patients in their success at not succumbing to domination was considerable.

Ward housekeeping became an interest and concern of the patients through patient government. At one time all work details were assigned by the patient government. Later they changed the policy by permitting the attendant or nurse on the ward to set up the duty roster but having the ward representative check it and advise as to any inequitable distribution of work. The reason for changing to the latter procedure given by the patient government was that the attendant was especially trained in the requirements of ward housekeeping and could do it better than they could except for occasional assignments when patients felt hurt by too much or too little work.

Improvement of ward conditions has always been an important concern of the governing body. Many projects came about which the occupational therapy department could not arrange themselves. For example, the female patients of Ward 5 painted the walls and ceilings of their toilet and dressing room, converting a small writing room into a dressing room and decorating it. They brought about fuller use of dining rooms by adapting them into writing and card rooms when they were not being used for eating. They noted deficiencies in ward supplies, details which the overworked attendant had not been able to care for adequately. They brought about improvements such as the quality of their coffee and the initiation of evening snacks. These they arranged through meetings with the dietitian.

They have been very concerned with some of the ward rules, many of their suggestions being in the direction of instituting certain enforcements such as requiring the rest period after lunch. These suggestions were turned back to the patient government for their own enforcement which they did successfully. This resulted in a growing understanding on the part of the patients of the reasons behind hospital rules and routine so that they became no longer arbitrary dictates but reasonable organizational principles.

The patients had asked several times for a television set and as there was no money available to purchase it, they started campaigning for funds and within two weeks they had raised enough money for two sixteen-inch screen television sets.

Three of the evening programs of the hospital have been conducted by the patient government for some time. The first of these was the Saturday evening coffee hour with a varied program of card playing, singing and dancing arranged by the patients of the female convalescent ward. Psycho Pops, a semi-classical record program of musical appreciation, though not instituted by patient government, ran for over a year entirely managed by the patient's music committee which arranged all of the selections, printed the programs and conducted the sessions. Another evening activity instituted in July, 1949, was that of a variety night. In spite of the fact that it is a difficult program to arrange as it means canvassing the patients of the hospital for talent—the talents being dancing, singing, recitations, playing musical instruments, arranging small plays, etc.—it has been a very successful event. The patients have been able to uncover more talent among themselves than the occupational therapy department had found.

The hospital has, every day, several volunteers from Gray Ladies, Boston Psychopathic Hospital Auxiliary, Volunteer Service Bureau and miscellaneous sources. It became the practice to have new volunteers with special talents introduced to the recreation committee of patient government so that they could work out together how the patients' needs could best be served. For example, one volunteer became social advisor to the patient government and worked directly with it to obtain orchestras and arrange programs for special seasonal dances. These events for which patients worked with plans, decorations, etc., became the most impressive and spirited which the hospital has seen.

This direct relationship between patient government and the hospital volunteers proved exceedingly valuable in bringing about a smooth introduction of new volunteers to the hospital. They had an opportunity to discuss directly with the patients their needs, and overcome any timidity and confusion regarding their rôle by these first hand contacts. This made any volunteer program one which was sponsored by the patients from the start rather than something forced upon them.

Throughout the summer of 1949 the government did much of the work of planning picnics away from the hospital and arranging many details which were conducive to maximal morale and minimal danger. Several plays have been put on by patient government assisted by volunteers who made arrangements directly with the patients. These have been important events giving variety and stimulus to the total social program of the hospital. The last play to be put on was written by the patients.

One of the important features of patient government from the first was its effect upon patient-personnel relationships. Here was a part of hospital treatment in which the nurses and attendants played the dominant role. The enthusiasm of patients was conveyed to nurses, attendants and vice versa. Patients discussing projects and problems of patient government between meetings would often talk their plans over with an attendant or nurse on their ward. The nursing personnel were thereby directly included in many of the developments of patient government. This spontaneous relationship has never been one in which the attendants and nurses dominated the situation but rather one in which they felt satisfaction in being included. Actually many came to function as non-directive leaders. This was early demonstrated by an arrangement made by an attendant interested in patient government whereby male and female patients from the convalescent wards had dinner together over the week end, a time when hospital activity is at its lowest point.

The increased recognition and understanding of patient government by the hospital staff as a whole has been an impressive development. This came about in several ways. The patients tell their doctors what they are doing in patient government. The minutes of the patient government meetings are printed weekly in the Psycho News, the hospital weekly newspaper, thereby coming to the attention of all the personnel of the hospital. As the Psycho News has an extensive mailing list to friends of the hospital, trustees and other interested parties, it brings the problems and accomplishments of patient government to the attention not only of the hospital staff but many other community resources. This brings about many direct responses from friends of the hospital to patients' needs.

At one noon staff conference, September 27, 1949, three officers of patient government made an hour presentation of the organization, its activities, accomplishments and problems. One of these patients summarized their work as follows:

"Patient government is desirable. This is the type of hospital it should be worked out in. It has worked out fairly well here. We hope we can get contributions for our television set so we will have it for Christmas. We would like to have something done to create a board of governors (ex-patients) to have meetings once a month."

The board of governors mentioned here is a new project originated by patient government to get ex-patients together for monthly meetings, to organize in a way that they can present the needs of the mentally ill to the public and to work with patient government to further any of its activities.

The major accomplishment of patient government is the improved morale among the patients. The ability to join in a group and make suggestions as an organized unit rather than as an individual in itself enhances the hospital spirit. The fact that such suggestions are seriously considered and acted upon also has a part in producing a feeling of well being. As a side accomplishment improved patient morale is reflected in improved general hospital morale.

DISCUSSION

A STUDY of the hour-by-hour life of the patients in the average mental hospital often gives a most unhappy picture. Not infrequently it shows a combination of idleness, inactivity, boredom and regimented uselessness. Such a situation is certainly not conducive to recovery and can create a "prison psychosis." Somewhere in the treatment of the mentally ill is a place for providing those opportunities for choice, expression and creativity that are so prized in democratic society.

Patient government is a logical and effective means of permitting the patients to assist themselves in providing a more creative and wholesome hospital life. The skills of social expression break down the social anxiety, fear and ineptness which are so much a part of most mental illnesses.

The fact that various forms of group therapy are coming into vogue raises the problem as to just which methods of group therapy are indicated in which situation. Many approaches fail to consider the hospital community which is already a form of group therapy, good or bad as the case may be. Patients are assigned to live a well-defined and organized type of life in a ward group under the leadership of doctors, nurses and attendants. This is the therapy group which already exists. Patient government is an attempt to utilize this existing group situation to best advantage.

Explaining the success of patient government is difficult because of the variety of opportunities it offers. Patients given an opportunity for expression and encouraged by each other are able to function at a higher level than any of them could individually. It is impressive to see a patient who is deluded, suspicious and fearful on the ward preside over a patient government meeting in a calm, self-assured, competent manner and then see the decrease on the ward of his previous abnormal symptoms.

The opportunity offered here for patients to help each other brings in some of their deepest motivation, that of compassion, love and identification with others suffering as they are or have recently. The thoughtfulness of each other demonstrated at patient government meetings is notable. One patient comes to the support of another who is making a painful effort to present a point. Here the government provides a stage for constructive action requiring group cooperation which stimulates the thinking and feeling of the group members.

One notable accomplishment of the organization was that of providing a creative outlet for many of the patients who found little interest in the usual occupational therapy opportunities, that is, patients who had a particular need for planning, administrative and organizational work.

An opportunity is provided in the patient government for the dynamic experience of expressing hostility toward authoritarian figures (doctors, nurses, attendants, etc.) without incurring punishment or rejection. Sometimes the hostility is masked as joking aggression and dramatized in plays but is still quite evident.

One appraisal of the organization was given by a graduate theological student who worked closely with the officers of patient government both to study the organization, and to determine the rôle of counsellor to it. His statement was: "Not only was patient government an important factor in giving the patient a direct opportunity to alter his own living conditions and have a direct part in managing his own activities but it also gave the patient the feeling of being more at home because he was 'guiding his own destiny' through this very difficult period of his life."

Altogether patient government appears to be an effective method of providing the patient with a hospital experience which has therapeutic value. It calls upon personal resources of cooperation, initiative and expressiveness which have been dormant throughout his illness and perhaps were never adequately developed.

All this is accomplished without any increase in personnel, a particularly impressive point at a time when all our institutions are suffering from inadequate staffing. In fact, with patient government, ward personnel find their duties lightened due to the increased creativity of the patients. What is required to establish patient government is not additional personnel but a special attitude on the part of personnel which recognizes the validity of the patients' suggestions, the importance of all their efforts, and which maintains a desire to bring about constant improvement of the patients' total hospital life. The staff must be willing to relinquish authority and share credit for both hospital management and patient recovery with the patients themselves.

SUMMARY

WE HAVE described an experience with patient government at Boston Psychopathic Hospital, outlining its development, the problems encountered, and their solution. The accomplishments of patient government were varied and impressive, far beyond anything that was expected.

It is hard at this time to analyze its broader therapeutic implications but its value is amply demonstrated in improved morale, better ward management, greater activity promotion and better personnel-patients relations. This evidence shows that patient government gives the patients an opportunity to learn the social skills of democratic living. It appears to be a special type of group therapy adapted directly to the patients' needs and the existing hospital environment.

As very little personnel time was involved in initiating and carrying on this venture, it appears to be a method which can be utilized even in hospitals greatly handicapped for personnel. We feel that it is applicable to any mental hospital. In the larger hospitals it might have to start in a ward or building at a time.

The prime requisite of successful patient government appears to be the willingness of the hospital administration to be receptive to suggestions coming from the patients. Without the basic attitude that the patients' ideas of their hospital experience are valid, nothing can be accomplished.

REFERENCES

1. Dickens, Charles: "American Notes," Leipzig, Bernhard Tauchnitz, 1842, p. 52.
2. Blackman, Nathan: "Experiences with a Literary Club in the Group Treatment of Schizophrenia," Occup. Therapy, 19:293-305, 1940.
3. Bierer, J., and Haldane, F. P.: "A Self-Governed Patients' Social Club in a Public Mental Hospital," J. Ment. Sc., 87:419-426, 1941.
4. Deutsch, Albert: "The Menningers of Topeka," Survey Graphic, September, 1947, p. 475.
5. Hatch, Emily: "The Attitudes of Patients in Convalescent Wards of Boston Psychopathic Hospital Toward Their Entire Hospital Experience." Thesis submitted in partial fulfillment for degree of Master of Social Work at Simmons College School of Social Work, 1948.

ð

CHAPTER 30   The Role of Informal Inmate
Groups in Change of Values*

GEORGE H. GROSSER

THE GROUP nature of much delinquency is an important point from
which to examine the treatment process in training schools for delinquent youth. It reminds us that the behavior of individuals is strongly
influenced by their group membership and by the interplay of the various
groups to which they belong.

Such a paucity of research data is available from the field of corrections
that what I have to say can be presented only as suggestive of research-
able hypotheses. My theoretical propositions are drawn largely from
experiments carried on in the fields of industrial relations, group dynamics,
and small-group research, rather than from the field of corrections.

An individual's adherence to social norms is determined not only by the
initial internalization of values but also by interaction with other individuals adhering to the same values. The group, in other words, has a definite
effect on the persistence or change of norms which complements the
psychodynamic forces working within the individual.

In a training school for juvenile offenders, most of the residents are
adolescents. While they are there because of having violated the law,
they nevertheless share a large part of the values of society or at least of
society's subcultures. Their delinquent behavior encompasses only a
small range of their total behavior. The training school exercises a custodial and reformative function and, regardless of its philosophy, provides
an authoritarian setting. That is, the administration does not exist by or
depend on the consent of the residents and is the sole determinant of
policy for the institution.

* "Inmate" is a word generally avoided in reference to children and adolescents.
The author uses it in this article to distinguish those for whom the institution exists
from those who run it.
    Reprinted from *Children* (U.S. Department of Health, Education, and Welfare,
Social Security Administration, Children's Bureau), 5 (1958), 25–29, by permission of
the author.

Within the training school an interaction of two groups, the administration and the inmates, is constantly taking place. Between these groups is a line of cleavage defined by a differentiation in status, which is reinforced by the difference in status between delinquents and representatives of the law outside the institution. The integration within one social system of two such different groups, as in an institution, contains many facets not found elsewhere in a democracy:

1. The inmates and the administration are so separate in status that rising from the lower to the higher is an impossibility.
2. While the administration has a specific task orientation, the inmate population does not share this nor have any specific task orientation of its own. Predominantly membership- or group-oriented, the inmate population has no group goal which the young people recognize as valid and achievable through their own coordinated efforts. Moreover, both administration and inmate population maintain networks of informal organization among their memberships.[1, 2]

This informal group structure arises out of needs generated within the institution and within the subcultures from which the young people have come. It is based on:

1. Adolescent needs for peer-group relationships, generated by the conflicts that adolescent status in our society produces.
2. The normal tendency for people spending extensive amounts of time together to cluster into informal groups on the basis of affective ties.
3. The need of persons in the same boat for support from one another. In this sense, the inmate social system has many of the aspects of a minority group under stress.
4. The adolescent need for friends of one's own sex in a culture in which heterosexual relations in childhood and adolescence are generally frowned upon.[3]

THE ROLE OF INFORMAL GROUPS

THE informal groups tend to maintain their identity, their norms, and their cohesiveness for, since they serve the needs already mentioned, their persistence is consciously and unconsciously striven for by the membership. Some of their mechanisms for survival explicitly threaten or violate discipline in the institution; others do not and therefore are often considered not particularly noteworthy. On the whole, however, the self-maintenance of the group is synonymous with the maintenance of the value system of its members. This fact tends to defeat the reformative aims of the institution. This is so even when the groups conform in large measure to the demands of the institution.

Among the mechanisms of group control which these informal groups share with other groups under stress are:

1. Recruitment and screening of membership and transmission of the institutional lore to the newcomer.
2. The development of social norms and rituals—characteristic institutional slang, ritual forms of interaction, the sharing of secrets with respect to illicit activities, and the establishment of a definite hierarchy of leaders and followers.
3. The application of sanctions to violators of the group code, ranging from gossip and ostracism to outright violence.
4. The development of loyalty and group ties.
5. The constant reinforcement of the separateness of the group through an attempt to create an orthodoxy of beliefs. This is done by informal communication, the spreading of news through the grapevine, and biased interpretation of the administration's policy, especially where it concerns the fate of particular group members.

OBSTACLES TO CHANGE

As INDICATED, the informal groupings in training schools for juvenile delinquents not only fulfill many of the inmates' basic needs but tend to become self-perpetuating with the development of mechanisms of group control and group maintenance. They militate against change in the delinquent's value system and against true rehabilitation of those individuals who throughout their stay remain attached to this type of social organization. In the absence of reliable research data, the author, from personal experience in training schools, would estimate this group as comprising from 30 to 50 percent of the inmate population.

While the obstacles to change differ from person to person, depending upon past experience and character formation, these informal groups in general present conditions which are often hampering to the best efforts of individual therapy. Psychological and sociological research has shown that the stabler the frame of reference of an individual, the more resistant is he likely to be to a contradictory frame of reference, and that the stability of a frame of reference depends not so much on the individual's own experience and reality testing as it does on group consensus and reinforcement.[4, 5, 6] This reinforcement of an existing frame of reference makes it extremely difficult for an individual to change even when he has considerable ambivalence in his feelings toward his group. The group always has mechanisms for displacing intragroup hostility onto outsiders.

It is, then, not surprising that so many failures occur among training-school alumni. To blame this on the environment to which the delinquent is sent after release is begging the question, for he will select those associations which are congenial to his character and values. It is likely that in many cases the individual, unchanged by his training-school experience, seeks out a delinquent environment upon release.

THE TASK OF CHANGE

THE accumulating evidence that persistence and change of norms are not solely a factor of the individual's own personality structure, but also depend on successive group affiliations and on the resolution of conflicting loyalties in these affiliations is of crucial significance for training schools. What seems to work so effectively in the maintenance of antisocial values could, if the theoretical assumptions are sound, also work in the opposite direction. Evidence that the group can effectively change the individual's value system has been produced by a variety of social-psychological experiments in laboratories and a number of studies in actual life situations.[7, 8] The common element in all these studies is that the individual's frame of reference, attitudes, and value system experience a change under group influence if the individual desires acceptance in the group with which he has been brought into contact. Most delinquents who enter training schools want to be accepted by their fellow inmates.

Therefore, if we wish the young person upon his release from the training school to become integrated into a peer group that pursues constructive aims and does not violate the law, we must somehow prepare him in the training school for such group affiliation. A mere environmental change, such as a foster home, will not be sufficient if the individual emerges from the training school unchanged.

Bringing about change, therefore, would require producing within the institution an informal peer group which is not focussed on hostility to the administration and to law-abiding society and to let such a group influence the newcomer. How is such a group to be molded? Can psychotherapy, for instance, achieve this goal?

PSYCHOTHERAPEUTIC METHODS

TRADITIONAL individual therapy is essentially a dyadic relationship. As such, it rests on the transference of the patient's affectional feelings and excludes others from this relationship. The incentive to change which comes from the patient's relationship to the therapist is purely individual. Therefore as far as a group is concerned it constitutes a divisive element. It arouses jealousy and antagonism, suspicion and mistrust.

There is considerable evidence in the literature on institutions that the informal social group distrusts and resents individual therapy and that this resentment is in direct proportion to the strength of the group's hostility towards the administration and of the need for social cohesion aroused by its members' defensiveness. The effect of intensive individual psychotherapy is to separate the patient from the informal group, since a motivation stronger than group influence has set in and the identification with the therapist replaces identification with group members and leaders. Such a relationship seems to be achieved more successfully with individuals whose group loyalty to the informal inmate organization is not particularly strong to begin with, and who, because of specific neurotic problems, have always moved on the fringes of the informal group. With those group members who maintain a very strong loyalty to their informal peer group, individual therapy is very often, though by no means always, ineffective.

In general, individual therapy tends to weaken the informal organization and atomize its membership. Since it cannot be effectively provided to all, partly because it promises no success in some cases, partly for economic reasons, it cannot be expected to change group values.

As limitations of individual therapy have become recognized, group therapy has been called upon to fill in the gaps. However, it too has its limitations.

The beneficial effects of group therapy on withdrawn individuals, some types of alcoholics, and other isolates, have raised expectations for this type of treatment which, in the case of juvenile delinquents, have not as yet been fulfilled. The most important misconception of the applicability of certain forms of group therapy seems to lie in the failure to understand that in the case of many a delinquent the need is neither to foster his integration into his peer group nor to help him overcome a sense of isolation. Indeed, the average individual in a State training school, whatever his personality difficulties, shares a value system and considerable degree of intimacy with like-minded individuals. It is, perhaps, precisely for the sake of this sharing that he has entered into delinquent activity. Therefore, the traditional form of group psychotherapy, which is supposed to effect reorientation of an individual to his society, misses the mark, creates a conflict between the members of the informal social group, and tends to isolate the patient rather than help him integrate into nondelinquent society.

A more hopeful version of the process, called guided group interaction, has been tried out by McCorkle, Bixby, and others.[9] Its aims and mode of attack seem more likely to satisfy the conditions necessary for changing group, and hence individual, values. How effective it can be is not as yet clearly apparent, but very likely with a group of selected individuals, on a very small scale, as in the current Highfields project, it can succeed. At Highfields, an experimental institution in New Jersey, the individuals are there for such a short time that they hardly have time to become strongly attached to an informal group structure. While this experiment may ultimately be of use, the method is not practicable within the framework of most training schools as set up now.

While efforts at both individual and group psychotherapy can be useful within institutions, their effectiveness is limited by the institutional setting and the varieties of individual personalities it includes.

CARRIERS OF CHANGE

HISTORICAL and experimental evidence amassed during the past few years points to the potentialities of the social group as an effector of change in values. Evidence from industrial relations, the armed forces, religious sects, and small-group research indicates a way to the development of hypotheses suitable for testing in correctional settings. The following are only a few of the propositions that seem particularly relevant:

1. Changes in the attitudes and values of group members are directly related to the needs that can thereby be fulfilled. Therefore, if recognized needs can be envisaged as better met by a change in group goals or values, the group is likely to change.
2. Such changes are the more effective the more the members have participated in formulating and discussing them.
3. Value changes in organized groups are more effective if the group is definitely task-oriented and if clear-cut communication and understanding exist concerning the goal to be reached and the means whereby it is to be reached.
4. Change in values of group members is positively correlated with a lack of competitiveness and conflict within the group.
5. Change is related to the degree in which each individual sees that his effort is needed for the achievement of the common goal or the maintenance of his standing within the group.
6. Changes of attitudes and values are more likely to occur through group goals set through the group's own motivation rather than imposed from outside the group, and are less likely to occur through goals dictated by an out-group with which the in-group is in conflict.

STEPS TOWARD CHANGE

AMONG the suggestions for training schools that can be derived from these propositions are the following:

1. Ways might be explored for making the institutional population's informal organization, as well as the individual, more task-oriented. In other words, attempts might be made to discover what other goals, especially group goals, aside from the goal of release from the institution, can be explicitly fostered and achieved by the population of the training school. This is an exceedingly complicated problem but one well deserving of exploration, for the aimlessness of life in many an institution contributes many undesirable features to the informal social organization.

The possibilities of task orientation are not exhausted by industrial work or work in the ordinary sense of the word. These possibilities include well-defined group goals and an array of means to their achievement. General goals enunciated by the administration as, "We are here to learn to live together," or, "We should learn to get along with our fellow man," are not task-oriented in the sense referred to here. Parenthetically, task orientation among adolescent groups in general is a pressing need in present-day society, and if made part of a delinquency prevention program might well have strong beneficial effects.

2. Since the breaking up of informal organization is difficult to achieve, and even when achieved may not be very beneficial because of the resulting individual isolation, means might be explored for lessening the social distance between the administration and the informal social groupings.

If the adolescent in a training school is eventually to live as part of law-abiding society he must be able to see himself in a role accepted by law-abiding society. The greater the distance between administration and institutional population the less likely are the young people's groups to change in a desirable direction.

The process of reducing social distance between administration and institutional population is not as difficult in respect to adolescents as to adults. Even the delinquent adolescent leans toward accepting the leadership and ascendancy of older persons because he has his dependency needs and because general cultural patterns tend in this direction. For the administration to share experiences with the informal organization and to recognize its position may be one way of lessening social distance.

3. Reward systems might be developed for group rather than individual performance. Group incentive will become easier to stimulate as a more task-oriented group life is developed in institutions. The present system of individual rewards tends to foster isolation and to leave the more antagonistic group members untouched.

4. Use of the existing group leadership to foster change within the group might also be explored. Leaders are generally considered troublesome because the direction in which they assert their leadership more often than not runs counter to the aims of the administration. However, just as informal groups are part and parcel of any large-scale organization, so are informal group leaders. Since they play an important part in maintaining group cohesiveness and fostering group identification they can be key figures in an attempt to utilize the group for effecting change of individual values.

5. Finally, since many group members might be amenable to therapy, informal groups might be made the units of therapy rather than artificially formed groups based on individual selection. While Slavson and others have suggested that the usual type of group

therapy is counterindicated for certain types of character disorders,[10] a more directive form, such as guided group interaction, utilizing the informal grouping might be helpful in changing group goals. This could be followed up by a more traditional type of therapy, group or individual, for some persons.

IN SUMMARY

IT SEEMS, then, that the informal groups which emerge in a training-school population might be made to serve important retraining functions if properly utilized. This suggestion is based on the observations that much delinquent behavior is group behavior and that the social group is a crucial agent in the maintenance or change of the value systems of its constituent members. A better understanding of the group dynamics within a training school may serve to make it a more effective agency in the retraining of juvenile offenders.

NOTES TO CHAPTER 30

1. Clemmer, Donald: The prison community. Boston: Christopher Publishing House, 1940.
2. Hayner, Norman S.; Ash, Ellis: The prison as a community. American Sociological Review, June 1939. (Pp. 362-369.)
3. Buxbaum, Edith: Transference and group formation in children and adolescents. *In* Psychoanalytic study of the child, Vol. I, New York: International Universities Press, Inc., 1945.
4. Sherif, Muzafer: The psychology of social norms. New York: Harper & Bros., 1936.
5. Asch, S. E.: Effects of group pressure upon the modification and distortion of judgments. *In* Group dynamics: research and theory. Cartwright, D.; Zander, A., editors. Evanston, Ill.; Row, Peters & Co., 1935.
6. Newcomb, T. M.: Attitude development as a function of reference groups: the Bennington study. *In* Readings of social psychology. Swanson, Guy E.; Newcomb, T. M.; Hartley, E. L., editors. New York: Henry Holt & Co., 1952.
7. Lewin, Kurt: Group decision and social change. *In* Readings in social psychology. Swanson, Guy E.; Newcomb, T. M.; Hartley, E. L., editors. New York: Henry Holt & Co., 1952.
8. Stouffer, S. A., et al.: The American soldier, Vol. II. Princeton, N.J.: Princeton University Press, 1949.
9. Bixby, F. Lowell; McCorkle, Lloyd W.: Guided group interaction in correction work. American Sociological Review, August 1951. (Pp. 455-459.)
10. Slavson, S. R.: The practice of group therapy. New York: International Universities Press, 1947.

$\sim$

CHAPTER 31 Report of an Integrated
Therapeutic Program: A Three-Year Ward Experiment*

WILLIAM E. McCULLOUGH

WHY SHOULD a special report on a ward experiement oriented to group psychotherapy be of special interest, now that this psychiatric technique is no longer news?

Because, in the writer's opinion, group psychotherapy is somewhat like the textbook study of physics or chemistry. From group psychotherapy, one learns the principles which motivate us; the dynamics of our personalities. But the verification of these principles and their application to the business of daily living, take place largely outside the class.

It may, therefore, be that the patient to whom group psychotherapy is available in an institutional setting, shares an exceptionally favorable environment. In addition to offering insight into his problems and offering intellectual understanding of himself and others, such a group situation offers, with help and guidance, a laboratory in which to practise the application of the knowledge gained.

This report concerns itself with an integrated therapeutic program; a ward experiement conceived in terms of mass-treatment techniques, which became an actuality in the spring of 1949 at Camarillo State Hospital in southern California.

The ward on which this program matured and operates is A-1, which, when the program began, became an open and 100 per cent working ward for women patients who were believed able to benefit from psychotherapy. There was equal emphasis on therapeutic work and social activities.

From its inception to the end of the planned three-year experimental period on April 1, 1952, there were 675 admissions of participating patients.

* At Camarillo State Hospital, Camarillo, Calif.

Reprinted from *The Psychiatric Quarterly*, 29 (1955), 280–309, by permission of the author and the *Quarterly*.

[456]

I. BACKGROUND OF THE EXPERIMENT

DURING 15 years of private psychiatric practice in greater New York, during part of which time the writer served as consulting neurologist to a state hospital staff, he became increasingly interested in taking part in an experimental therapeutic program in a state hospital or other controlled environment.

With the interest and encouragement of the late Dr. C. C. Burlingame of the Hartford Retreat, some tentative ideas were developed. In 1948, Dr. Thomas Haggerty, superintendent of Camarillo State Hospital, was approached with the general proposal. He saw the possibilities for expanded horizons in institutional therapeutics, and made available the hospital facilities and a service for experimental purposes. At Camarillo in December 1948, with a general go-signal for the plan, two closed wards, F and F-1, having a total of 310 women patients, were first used. Here, the infancy and pre-adolescence of the techniques eventually adopted were worked through.

These wards were practically unclassified; they had everything! One ward had a large percentage of custodial and chronic patients, as well as involutional paranoid patients; and few of them were able to assume work responsibilities. The other was called a working ward, but only about half the patients were actually able to work.

The first efforts were directed toward clearing the classification jungle. Both wards became work detail wards, and many patients were transferred. In the course of reclassification, every patient was interviewed, with particular attention to her apparent susceptibility to some form of psychotherapy—at that time an innovation at Camarillo on any mass basis. The writer's evaluation included considerations of disposition, type of illness, intelligence, and so on.

It was evident that there were too many patients and that the task was too great for any consistent form of individual psychotherapy. The only alternative was some type of group treatment.

The project was approached without experience in group psychotherapy, but familiarity with the general literature. The trial period—during which the undoubted effectiveness of this technique was learned through experience—largely preceded establishment of the experimental ward. Full operations were ready when A-1 became an open ward for women patients, all to receive group psychotherapy, on April 1, 1949.

II. THE HOSPITAL AND WARD A-1

CAMARILLO was the largest and newest of California's state hospitals and averaged about 5,400 resident patients during 1951. Patients on Ward A-1 averaged 86, with a ward capacity of 100; and, therefore, comprised less than 2 per cent of the patient population, and occupied an exceedingly favorable place in the general picture of 20 per cent excess population for the hospital as a whole. (Figure 1.)

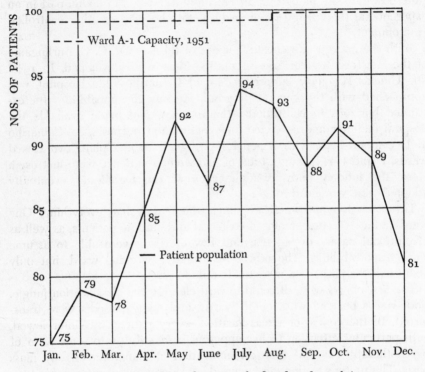

(Patient population figures are for first day of month.)

FIG. 1. WARD CAPACITY AND PATIENT POPULATION: YEAR ENDED DECEMBER 31, 1951
(1951 AVERAGE PATIENT POPULATION—86)

Drawing on the sprawling Los Angeles area for a majority of its patients, Camarillo is located about 65 miles north of the metropolis, just inland from the coast. Its attractive tiled white stucco buildings of modified Spanish architecture occupy a winding, irrigated valley in the midst of 1,650 hospital acres. About half that land is under cultivation, and the institution is partially self-sufficing in farm produce.

Ward A-1 shared with other services and hospital facilities an L-shaped building unit, forming two sides of a large landscaped and unlocked court. Other units completed the enclosure. The larger part of A-1 occupied the second story of the L, and included two dormitories with a total capacity of 71. Other facilities included a day hall, a classroom and a dozen smaller rooms of various sorts.

The downstairs space of this ward occupied only part of the first floor and consisted of a 28-bed dormitory, a day hall, and several miscellaneous and service rooms. The upstairs office served both ward units. No attendant was stationed downstairs where only the more responsible patients were assigned. The total ward capacity was 99 beds until the addition of one more in 1951, brought it to 100.

III. THE STAFF

THE PERSONNEL administering the ward program had, from its inception, received continuing formal and informal training in orientation, motivations and techniques, from the therapist and others. During the three-year period, the ward personnel consisted of a psychiatrist, a psychiatric nurse, a charge attendant, one day attendant, and one night attendant, all permanently assigned. There were other assisting or substitute attendants. For six months, a resident clinical psychologist was a valuable adjunct to

These are some of the characteristics of life on one ward in one mental the ward program, but it was not possible to replace him when he left the hospital service.

The modest size of the staff should be underscored, in light of the intensive program that was undertaken and pursued without interruption. The significant contribution made by the attendants was, in large measure, due to the opportunity to select the most promising and interested of those concerned with the first tentative developments on F and F-1. Specialized personnel serving the entire hospital was called upon freely: social service workers, state rehabilitation officers, and so on. It was a continuing policy to use all resources to the utmost.

A disruptive factor during 1951—although it was indicative of ward personnel standards—was the loss of the pioneer charge attendant and two successive psychiatric nurses to advanced supervisory or training posts.

IV. THE PATIENTS

PATIENTS on Ward A-1 were carefully classified, although of widely divergent diagnoses. Guiding principles both for their selection and for the treatment program were established and operating when A-1 became entirely an experimental psychotherapy ward, and comprehensive statistical records were maintained.

Cited here to illustrate this report, the 1951 calendar year, as a base statistical period, yields data fairly representative of any of the three experimental ward years. In certain fields, notably social therapy, it reflects a relatively mature and stable program. Such vital ward programs as the Alpha Club, and its expansion of chapters in communities served by the hospital, were gradual, planned developments.

Table 1 shows data on age, education and marital status of patients on the ward over 30 days, who were served by the integrated work-social-psychotherapy program during 1951, including carry-overs from 1950.

TABLE 1.
*Age-Group, Education and Marital Status of All Patients on Ward
Over 30 Days, Year Ended December 31, 1951*

AGE ON ADMISSION*			EDUCATION**			MARITAL STATUS		
AGE—GROUP	NO.	PER CENT	YEARS OF SCHOOLING	NO.	PER CENT	STATUS	NO.	PER CENT
			Grades					
17-19 years	7	2.6	Under 8 years	12	4.5			
20-24 years	24	9.0	8 years	17	6.3	Married	113	42.5
25-29 years	33	12.4	9 years	10	3.8			
30-34 years	46	17.3	10 years	33	12.4	Single	63	23.7
35-39 years	43	16.1	11 years	22	8.3			
40-44 years	58	21.8	12 years	108	40.6	Divorced	55	20.7
			College					
45-49 years	31	11.6	1 year	10	3.8			
50-54 years	17	6.7	2 years	22	8.3	Widowed	11	4.1
55-59 years	5	1.8	3 years	7	2.6			
60-61 years	2	0.7	4 years	23	8.6	Separated	24	9.0
			Postgraduate					
			2 years	2	0.8			
All patients	266	100.0	All patients	266	100.0	All patients	266	100.0

* Median age: 36 years.
** Median education: Completed 12th grade (high school graduation).
Number of high school graduates: 172 (64.7 per cent of 266 patients).
Number of college graduates: 25 (9.8 per cent of 266 patients).

Age. With few patients having disorders of a chronic, custodial or "incurable" type, the average age tended to be lower than on a majority of the wards. The median age of A-1 patients was 36, with almost 90 per cent in the 21 to 49 age-group.

Education. Median education was the twelfth grade level (high school graduation), with 65 per cent in this group; and 10 per cent of all patients, college graduates.

Marital Status. The 1951 group included 32 per cent married, 24 per cent single, 21 per cent divorced, 9 per cent separated, and 4 per cent widowed.

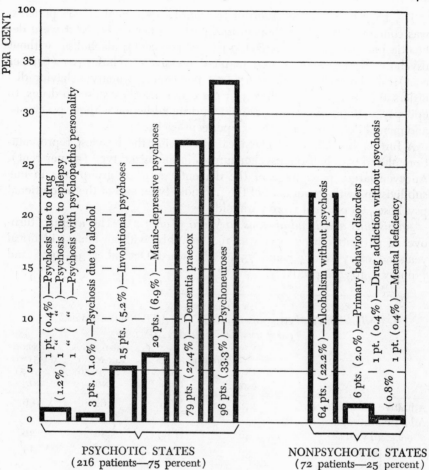

FIG. 2. GROSS DIAGNOSTIC CLASSIFICATION* OF ALL PATIENTS (288) ON WARD, YEAR ENDED DECEMBER 31, 1951

* Classifications: American Psychiatric Association, 1945 rev., slightly modified by California State Department of Mental Hygiene.

Of interest, though not strictly comparable, are United States Bureau of Census figures on the marital status of females 14 years old and older (1949): 63 per cent married, 20 per cent single, 2 per cent divorced, 3 per cent separated, and 12 per cent widowed. Even with the heavier weighting of the census figures in the lowest and highest age-brackets, something of the disruptive effect of mental and emotional disturbances on marriage may be seen by the comparison.

Gross Diagnostic Classification (Figure 2). The classification used is that of the American Psychiatric Association code (revised 1945), slightly modified for California State Department of Mental Hygiene use.

The largest diagnostic group of the ward's 1951 total of 288 patients, was composed of the psychoneuroses, 96 (33.3 per cent). Next were dementia praecox (schizophrenia), 79 (27.4 per cent); alcoholism without psychosis, 64 (22.2 per cent); manic-depressive psychoses, 20 (6.9 per cent); involutional psychoses, 15 (5.2 per cent); primary behavior disorders, 6 (2 per cent); alcohol, 3 (1 per cent); psychoses due to drugs, to epilepsy, with psychopathic personality, drug addiction without psychosis, and mental deficiency, 1 each (0.4 per cent each).

A further breakdown of classifications having the heaviest representation, placed over half the psychoneuroses in the mixed type (54 per cent). An even larger percentage of the dementia praecox group was in one subdivision, with 57 per cent of the paranoid type; and of the involutional psychoses, 66 per cent were paranoid.

Admissions and Readmissions to Ward (Table 2). The average turnover of patients during 1951 was 19.5 monthly, with an almost identical year-end carry-over; 74 and 75 on the ward December 31, 1950 and January 1, 1952 respectively.

TABLE 2.

Admissions and Readmissions to Ward: All Patients on Ward,
Year Ended December 31, 1951

TYPE	TOTAL		ADMISSIONS ON WARD 12-31-50	ADMISSIONS 1-1-51 TO 12-31-51
	NO.	PER CENT	NO.	NO.
Admitted once only	248	86.1	62	186
Admitted more than once, all years	40	13.9	12	28
All patients	288	100.0	74	214
Single admissions (on ward once only)	248	79.5	62	186
Readmissions on ward one to three times, 1951)*	64	20.5	21	43
All admissions	312	100.0	83	229

* Breakdown of 64 readmissions by 40 patients: 18 patients were on ward once only during the year ended December 31, 1951; 20 were on the ward twice; two, three times.

Patients on the ward—for all periods whatever—during the year totaled 288. Of these, 248 (86.1 per cent) were admitted once only, during all the years covered. Patients who had ever been on the ward before, plus the 1951 first admissions returning during the year, totaled 40—with the total readmissions of these 40 reaching 64 during 1951. There were 18 readmissions who were on the ward once only during 1951; 22 who were there twice; and two, three times. The carryover and 1951 admissions for 288 patients totaled 312.

TABLE 3.

Type of Admission and 30-day Observation Period: First Admission or Readmission, All Patients on Ward, Year Ended December 31, 1951

PATIENTS	FIRST ADMISSIONS OR READMISSIONS DURING 1951	
	NO.	PER CENT
Type of admission		
Voluntary	70	24.0
Commitment	218	79.0
All patients	288	100.0
30-day observation period:		
On ward over 30 days	266	92.0
On ward under 30 days	22	8.0
All patients	288	100.0

Type of Admission (Table 3). The 1951 first admissions and readmissions for 288 patients included 218 (76 per cent) committed through the courts or public health officers, and 70 (24 per cent) admitted on a voluntary basis.

Not acceptable to California state hospitals on a voluntary basis, are chronic alcoholics and drug addicts without psychoses, mental defectives, and certain other diagnostic groups which were not represented on A-1.

Observation Period (Table 3). An observation period of 30 days was routine, with the patient usually assigned to ward duties during this time. All members of the ward team took special note of special problems, characteristics and capacities of the new patient, and pooled observations for the purpose of treatment needs and plans.

Patients remaining on the ward less than 30 days were in general those who became acutely upset, were found not to be qualified for an open ward, or who escaped. Certain detailed statistical data, primarily of personal or social nature, were not recorded for this short-term group.

During the year, 266 of 288 patients (92 per cent) remained on the ward beyond the observation period, with 22 (8 per cent) transferred, granted indefinite leave, discharged or escaped during their first 30 days.

Movement of Patients (Table 4). Of 288 patients, 196 (68 per cent) came to A-1 directly from the receiving ward, with the remaining 92 (32 per cent) transferred from other treatment wards. Of the 1951 readmissions, 17 (71 per cent) were from the receiving ward, and seven (29 per cent) were from other wards, totaling 24.

Of 237 total separations from the ward in 1951, 219 were of first admissions, and 18 of readmissions.

Of first admissions, 170 patients (78 per cent) left the hospital under favorable circumstances; 123 (56 per cent) on indefinite leave, and 47

TABLE 4.
Movement of Patients, Year Ended December 31, 1951

MOVEMENT	FIRST ADMISSION		READMISSION		TOTAL	
	NO.	PER CENT	NO.	PER CENT	NO.	PER CENT
On ward December 31, 1950	62	—	12	—	74	—
Entered ward during 1951 (all admissions)	288	100.0	24	100.0	312	100.0
From receiving ward	196	68.0	17	71.0	213	68.0
From other treatment wards	92	32.0	7	29.0	99	32.0
Separated from ward during 1951	219	100.0	18	100.0	237	100.0
Indefinite leave from hospital	123	56.0	6	33.0	129	55.0
Discharge from hospital	47	22.0	3	17.0	50	21.0
Unauthorized leave from hospital	14	6.0	5	28.0	19	8.0
(Separated from hospital)	(184)	(84.0)	(14)	(78.0)	(198)	(84.0)
Transferred to other wards	35	16.0	4	22.0	39	16.0
On ward January 1, 1952	69	—	6	—	75	—

(22 per cent) discharged. Unauthorized leaves in the group leaving the ward numbered 14 (6 per cent), and 35 patients (16 per cent) were transferred to other wards.

Of 18 readmissions separated from the ward, six (33 per cent) received indefinite leave; three (17 per cent) were discharged; five (28 per cent) took unauthorized leave; and four (22 per cent) were transferred to other wards.

Although 20.5 per cent of the 1951 admissions were of patients who were on the ward more than once (readmissions, all years), the percentage of individuals readmitted was 13.8.

Reflecting hospital and state-wide trends, alcoholics (22.2 per cent of the 1951 ward patients) accounted for a disproportionate number of readmissions to the ward. They accounted for 40 per cent of all 1951 first admissions of patients who had been on the ward previously in any year; 41 per cent of all second readmissions; and 50 per cent of all third.

Alcoholism and Other Diagnoses Related to Off-Ward Movement (Table 5). The difficult problem of the alcoholic patient emerges clearly also, in considering the relationship between diagnosis and off-ward movement. It is especially evident in the high incidence of alcoholic patients taking unauthorized leave.

Of a total of 33 patients leaving A-1 in 1951 during their first 30 days, 19 left with official sanction—indefinite leave, discharge or transfer to other wards.

Unauthorized leaves accounted for the remaining 14, of whom 11 (79 per cent) were alcoholics without psychosis. Of the five unauthorized leaves by patients after the 30-day period, only one patient was alcoholic.

The only other diagnostic groups than the alcoholic that contributed more than one AWOL patient were: psychoneuroses, three, and involutional psychoses, two.

Effective late in 1951, a hospital directive provided that patients committed for alcoholism without psychosis should remain on closed wards during their first month. Despite obvious advantages in reducing the number of unauthorized leaves, there are drawbacks from the therapeutic angle. With limited psychotherapy available in the hospital as a whole, and with A-1 operating the only integrated work-social-psychotherapy program, many eligible alcoholics now tended to remain on the ward of original assignment. The number of alcoholics benefiting from the A-1 program dropped sharply.

It is the author's observation that committed alcoholics in general have no great degree of insight into the fact that their difficulty is symptomatic of a deeper maladjustment. They, therefore, seek psychiatric help less readily than other nonpsychotic groups. Assignment of the alcoholic to psychotherapy from the beginning of hospitalization would seem to offer more promise than any degree of reversion to the old physical-custodial

TABLE 5.

Diagnostic Classification: All Patients Leaving Ward During 30-Day Observation Period; All Taking Unauthorized Leave, Year Ended December 31, 1951

DIAGNOSIS	OFF WARD FIRST 30 DAYS			TOTAL (AWOL)		UNAUTHORIZED (AWOL) AFTER 30 DAYS
	TOTAL	OFFICIAL	UNAUTHORIZED (AWOL)	NO.	PER CENT	
Involutional psychosis:						
Melancholia	1	1	0	2	10.5	2
Psychoneurosis:						
Psychasthenia, compulsive states	1	1	0	0	—	0
Reactive depression	2	2	0	0	—	0
Mixed type	4	4	0	2	10.5	2
Character neurosis	1	0	1	1	5.2	0
Manic-depressive psychosis:						
Manic type	5	4	1	1	5.2	0
Dementia praecox						
Catatonic type	1	1	0	0	—	0
Paranoid type	4	4	0	0	—	0
Other types	1	1	0	0	—	0
Alcoholism without psychosis	11	0	11	12	63.4	1
Primary behavior disorder:						
Simple adult maladjustment	2	1	1	1	5.2	0
Total patients	33	19	14	19	100.0	5

type of care. That type has proved, in the writer's opinion, of little long-term benefit to most alcoholics.

In spite of the fact that alcoholic patients accounted for 63 per cent of all 1951 unauthorized leaves from A-1 (12 out of 19), 82 per cent of the 64 alcoholics on the ward remained for the usual three-month hospitalization required of that category. Several remained voluntarily for longer periods for additional psychotherapy.

V. ACTIVE TREATMENT PROGRAMS

Group Psychotherapy. Participation in group psychotherapy, from the inception of Ward A-1 and its inclusive treatment program, has been required of all patients. Each attends a weekly class meeting, a minimum of one and one-half hours, under psychiatric leadership.

Throughout 1951 there were five groups, each composed of patients having similar or related mental or emotional problems or symptoms. Classification lines were not followed with absolute rigidity, as a consistent attempt was made to meet individual needs.

Group psychotherapy may be defined simply, as a technique for re-education in terms of attitudes, values and other emotional components of the personality, in a social setting; with group identification and interchange a vital part of the learning process. Group psychotherapy has cardinal values of its own, besides being an effective substitute for intensive individual psychotherapy. From a hard-pressed administrative standpoint, it multiplies the number of doctors.

The writer's earlier service was a proving ground for several types of group psychotherapy procedure before the form followed by all classes in the three-year A-1 program was settled upon.

The pioneer groups had met in small classes; 10 to 12 patients of mixed diagnoses—psychoses, psychoneuroses, personality behavior disturbances, and so on. There was early emphasis on younger patients only as promising material, but the groups soon included a much wider age-range. These early meetings followed no particular form, but consisted generally of informal and free discussion of personal problems by the group, with the therapist not injecting himself too much into the discussion. With this nondirective pattern, however, it was soon evident that some patients participated little or not at all. Evaluating alernatives, seeking means to insure participation by all members, the biographical method went into effect with the opening of A-1.

Under this method, the patient was required to write and submit her life story, presented in terms of her reactions to events—her feelings about the things which had happened to her. The form was concise enough to allow a story to be read aloud in about 15 minutes; approximately 750 to 1,000 words. (It is perhaps significant that a general high level of writing seemed to result from this simple form of reporting deep emotional experience; a level often far superior to the patient's usual apparent capacity for written expression.)

At first, life-stories were unidentified, and the discussion did not refer to the author. Soon, however, class members were willing to identify themselves with their stories and participate in direct discussion of them. Reaching this point, they invariably expressed willingness to answer related questions. Considering the relative unsophistication of a majority of patients, and the intimate and often painful nature of material honestly presented in a life-story, it was interesting to note that less than 10 patients of the several hundred who participated in the ward experiment requested to be transferred in order to avoid group psychotherapy.

This method of group psychotherapy is of the directive type, dictated largely by the size of classes. With an average ward population of 86 in 1951, classes ranged from 16 to 20 members.

The major topic of most sessions was thus a biography or life-story of a class member. After the reading, each member asked questions to bring out additional significant material. Then, on the basis of reading and discussion, each member was encouraged to discuss briefly the factors which might have contributed to or influenced the patient's difficulties, or which might have been causative in her illness.

The therapist then summed up the discussion in simple explanatory terms, sufficiently broad to apply to similar or related problems.

Additional insights were gained from scheduled question and free-discussion periods, periodic blackboard demonstrations and simple lectures on the dynamics of mental and emotional illness.

The five classified groups functioning throughout 1951 were:

Class A—Chronic alcoholism and drug addiction. Very few members of this group had been diagnosed as psychotic or deteriorated, though many exhibited psychoneurotic symptoms aside from those of an addictive nature.

Class B—Undifferentiated diagnostic group characterized primarily by age (17 to 25 or 30), by immaturity in psychological development, and by relative unsophistication. Behavior problems such as are encountered in simple adult maladjustment, were shared by a majority of Class B members.

Class C—Psychoneuroses. A majority in this group had diagnoses of mixed psychoneurosis; but other major types included reactive depression, hysteria, psychasthenia, hypochondriasis and anxiety. This group requested, and had approval for, an extra group psychotherapy session one evening each week, under their own moderator. One and one-half hour meetings were held for discussion of personal and group questions and problems of their own choice, in their own way. The group held 26 successive and successful extra meetings, achieving strong group identification. This extracurricular activity seemed to accelerate group and individual progress in the regularly-scheduled classes.

Class D—Dementia praecox (schizophrenia). Almost 60 per cent of the members of class D had a paranoid type of personality disturbance. Of the remainder, most fell into the simple or catatonic types. A majority had received electric shock treatment, either in Camarillo or elsewhere. (Table 6.)

TABLE 6.

Previous Hospitalization and Electric Shock Treatment of 266 Patients on Ward Over 30 Days, Year Ended December 31, 1951

	PATIENTS	
HOSPITALIZATION	NO.	PER CENT
Previous to current hospitalization	126	47.0
No previous hospitalization	140	53.0
All patients	266	100.0
Electric shock treatments:		
EST before admission to ward	73	27.0
EST before admission and while on ward	12	4.5
EST on ward only	4	1.5
(Total patients receiving EST)	(89)	(33.0)
No EST	177	67.0
All patients	266	100.0

Class E—Manic-depressive and involutional psychoses. The largest diagnostic groups in Class E, about equally divided, were manic-depressive-manic and involutional paranoid; with manic-depressive-depressed accounting for most of the balance.

REQUIRED ATTENDANCE

REGULAR group psychotherapy class attendance was required of all patients, who at every other reasonable time were permitted to have vistors —these taking precedence over work assignments and other hospital or ward activities. Only genuine illness or other real emergency was acceptable as excuse for absence from class. Equally strict adherence to the class schedule was self-imposed by the therapist and the psychiatric nurse, who assisted at each meeting by reading the story and participating in the discussion. Full notes of the discussion were taken and later transcribed.

Duration of Class-Attendance (Coterminal with Residence on Ward) (Figure 3). As every patient attended weekly psychotherapy class throughout her stay on the ward, data on the number of classes attended serve also to indicate the length of time spent on A-1.

PATIENTS   NUMBER

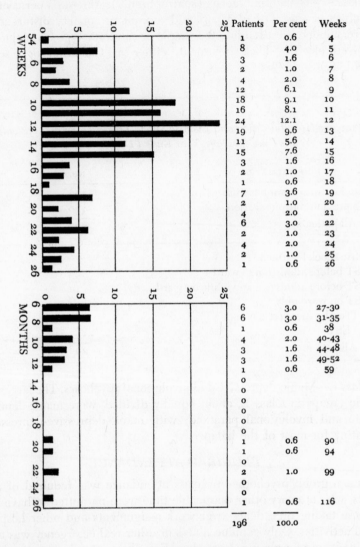

Patients	Per cent	Weeks
1	0.6	4
8	4.0	5
3	1.6	6
2	1.0	7
4	2.0	8
12	6.1	9
18	9.1	10
16	8.1	11
24	12.1	12
19	9.6	13
11	5.6	14
15	7.6	15
3	1.6	16
2	1.0	17
1	0.6	18
7	3.6	19
2	1.0	20
4	2.0	21
6	3.0	22
2	1.0	23
4	2.0	24
2	1.0	25
1	0.6	26
6	3.0	27-30
6	3.0	31-35
1	0.6	38
4	2.0	40-43
3	1.6	44-48
3	1.6	49-52
1	0.6	59
0		
0		
0		
0		
1	0.6	90
1	0.6	94
0		
2	1.0	99
0		
0		
1	0.6	116
196	100.0	

FIG. 3. NUMBER OF WEEKLY PSYCHOTHERAPY CLASSES (EQUAL TO TOTAL WEEKS ON WARD): 196 PATIENTS ON WARD OVER 30 DAYS, SEPARATED FROM WARD IN YEAR ENDED DECEMBER 31, 1951. THE UPPER PART OF THE FIGURE COVERS CLASSES (AND WARD RESIDENCE) FROM THREE TO 26 WEEKS; THE LOWER PART SHOWS CLASSES ATTENDED BY PATIENTS IN RESIDENCE FROM SIX TO 26 MONTHS.

Median No. of classes (meeting weekly, one and one-half hours): 13 ....

A total of 196 patients, who had remained over 30 days, were separated from the ward in 1951. This group may be taken as representative of the length of exposure to group psychotherapy and the integrated ward program.

The median number of classes was 13 (19.5 hours), including the observation period—thus 13 weeks on the ward was median residence.

Though the number of classes varied, for the individual, from four to 116, 12 to 18 classes were attended by 115 patients, or 59 per cent of the total. Less than 15 per cent attended as many as 26 classes (six months).

Individual Psychotherapy. Office interviews with the ward psychiatrist were an integral part of the planned program. The doctor's door was never closed. A fairly long and early initial interview with each patient was supplemented by later interviews with the therapist.

Every patient was encouraged to write down disturbing feelings and reactions, however trivial the precipitating incident may have seemed to her. This kept the therapist informed as to her general and specific difficulties, and also afforded her some emotional release through the writing itself. Many patients wrote voluminously, all with the assurance that the material would be read by the doctor, and much of it formed the basis for subsequent interviews.

The therapeutic team of Ward A-1 (the psychiatrist, psychiatric nurse and charge attendant) conducted both formal and informal interviews with all patients, depending upon specific problems, the momentary or long-term needs of the patient, and personality considerations. Each member of the team saw every patient in at least one extended conference during the observation period, followed by many planned series of additional interviews.

During 1951, the ward psychiatrist conducted an average of 19.5 initial interviews monthly, matching the intake of patients—with 49 additional personal interviews of varying duration, not including narcosynthesis or collateral conferences.

Previous Hospitalizations (Table 6). Of the 266 patients on the ward during 1951 who remained over 30 days, 126 (47 per cent) had histories of previous public or private hospitalization. Some of this number had been patients at an earlier date in Camarillo or other state hospitals, but the figure does not include those having been on other wards during their current hospitalization. No previous hospitalization was reported by 140 patients (53 per cent).

Electric Shock Treatment (Table 6). Patients requiring extensive series of electric shock treatments were transferred or sent as "guests" to the shock ward, usually returning to A-1 on completion of the series. An occasional patient needing very limited shock treatment had EST while remaining on the ward; with only 16 such patients in 1951.

Of 266 patients on the ward during that period, 73 (27 per cent) had received EST at some prior date, either at Camarillo or elsewhere, and received none while on the ward; 12 patients (4.5 per cent) had received EST both prior to ward residence and while on A-1; four patients (1.5 per cent) received EST only while on the ward. A majority, 177 patients (67 per cent) had received no EST at any time. The common diagnostic classifications among EST patients were dementia praecox, manic-depressive and involutional psychoses.

Narcosynthesis. In selected cases, averaging seven a month in 1951, the psychiatrist, assisted by the psychiatric nurse, conducted sodium-amytal or sodium-pentothal interviews, with an aim of facilitating the expression of suppressed or disturbing material.

Carbon-Dioxide Inhalation. A more recent innovation in the ward therapeutic program was CO_2 therapy, primarily used in the treatment of the more deep-seated and severe psychoneuroses. The therapeutic goal is similar to that of narcosynthesis, but the patient tends, in dreams experienced under CO_2, to abreact rather sharply and directly. Subsequent verbalization varies.

CO_2 treatments require much less time than narcosynthesis (an average of 15 minutes as against 75 or so); and, while the two are by no means entirely interchangeable, CO_2, in cases offering a choice, has advantages for mass treatment. Another advantage is the immediate return of the patient from CO_2 to full consciousness and functioning, with no aftercare involved.

An insufficient number of CO_2 series has so far been given, to permit conclusions of any real validity. However, several patients have shown definite improvement in insight and adjustment after only a few treatments.

General Medical Program. Sedation is rarely authorized, and patients are encouraged to an awareness of the psychosomatic nature of many functional disorders. Psychotherapy class lectures on the dynamics of mental and emotional disturbances emphasized conversion hysteria and other defense mechanisms.

Medications prescribed routinely on the ward included vitamins for the alcoholic patients and others in whom a deficiency was known or suspected; dilantin for epilepsy; stilbesterol for the more acute menopausal difficulties; and other more or less standard medications as required.

Surgery, dentistry and special diets are routine services where indicated.

Work Therapy. All Ward A-1 patients had regular work assignments (or "details"), always suited as nearly to the individual's needs, capabilities and experience as was possible in an institutional situation. Hours of work ran from about 25 a week to almost a full 40-hour work week in a few cases. The average was between 25 and 30 hours.

Approximately 21 patients were detailed to the ward itself, and were responsible for a general high standard of ward housekeeping, and for operation of the clothing, shoe and linen rooms, and for handling personal effects and ward maintenance equipment. New patients were usually assigned to the ward detail for their first few weeks, both for more rapid orientation and for purposes of closer observation.

Off-ward work details were of many types, ranging from routine jobs, such as typing, filing, clerking, waiting on tables, etc., to highly skilled work, such as technical assistance in the recreational, music or occupational therapy departments, medical secretarial work, research, library work, and the like.

Several factors effected a generous contribution of skilled A-1 workers to the general hospital program. All A-1 patients were sufficiently stable to be on an open working ward; most were in the age-groups of highest productivity (median age, 36); and the level of education (median, twelfth grade) was comparatively high.

An example of work assignments used as a psychotherapeutic aid may be seen in the case of a psychoneurotic patient who had a conscious fear of, and aversion to, children, reactions never overtly expressed, but strongly experienced and intellectually recognized and deplored.

The patient and therapist traced these reactions to a specific incident during the patient's fourteenth year. Armed with this awareness, and with the therapist's support, she was able first to assist the director of the children's occupational therapy program with office and materials work; then, to some degree, with the children themselves. While an entirely spontaneous and relaxed relationship with children is hard to achieve, this patient at 43 approaches normal reactions. A new field of emotional experience had opened and her hitherto sternly suppressed maternal instincts were accepted by her and attained favorable expression in general interpersonal relationships.

Social Therapy (Table 7). With an accepted principle of psychotherapy recognized as the development and strengthening of healthy personality traits in the mentally or emotionally disturbed patient, assignment of social responsibility suited to the capacities of A-1 patients was part of the original ward plan.

A balanced program of social and other ward activities operated from the beginning, but in the early days often originated with members of the ward team who also gave much actual leadership.

Inspired by experimental gestures toward self-government elsewhere, but more importantly, by the desires of increasingly group-conscious ward members, the Alpha Club was formed in March 1950 to assume all ward social and educational activities, and a considerable part of the disciplinary and housekeeping responsibilities.

With the active support of the therapist and the ward team, the Alpha Club almost immediately became a potent force in actual ward self-government by patients. As a city council is limited by laws on several

TABLE 7.

Co-ordinated Ward Activities—Psychotherapy and Social Therapy, Year Ended December 31, 1951

MONTH	FORMAL PSYCHOTHERAPY CLASSES (WEEKLY) (5 GROUPS)	INFORMAL GROUP THERAPY MEETINGS (WEEKLY)			ALPHA CLUB ACTIVITIES (SOCIAL THERAPY)			ALPHA CLUB CHAPTERS (FORMER PATIENTS OUTSIDE HOSPITAL) MEETING (TWICE MONTHLY)
		EXTRACURRICULAR PSYCHOTHERAPY CLASS "C"	SUNDAY SESSIONS	ALPHA A.A. GROUP	CLUB MEETINGS*	SOCIAL FUNCTIONS	ADULT EDUCATION CLASSES	
January	23	—	4	5	2	4	32	—
February	17	—	4	4	2	1	26	—
March	22	—	4	4	3	2	25	—
April	20	—	5	4	2	3	28	—
May	25	—	4	5	2	5	46	1
June	20	—	2	3	2	4	73	2
July	24	4	5	5	3	3	53	2
August	29	5	4	4	2	2	33	2
September	20	4	2	4	2	5	49	2
October	23	4	4	3	3	3	75	2
November	20	3	2	3	2	2	47	2
December	15	3	2	3	2	4	30	4
Total	258	23	42	47	27	38	517	15

* Attended by all members. Board committee meetings, not included, averaged 10 a month.

[474]

levels, so the Alpha Club was limited by broad ward and hospital regulations, but wide scope for action remained to the executive body. In some cases, the club was instrumental in obtaining modification of general regulations.

All A-1 patients automatically assume club membership on entry into the ward, and, with membership, its responsibilities. The organization—with constitution and by-laws, elected officers, a board which serves as a steering committee, and appointed committee chairmen—operates along usual parliamentary lines. A majority of its bi-weekly meetings, except in details of subject-matter, would be undistinguishable from those of any typical women's organizations. Staff members are usually not present, though invited.

Among major activities, now routine and smoothly operating, are: a trained hostess service to welcome new members; orientation of new members to the therapeutic purposes of the ward; consideration of suggestions and grievances; an extensive program of patient-taught adult education classes; maintenance of a common fund or treasury to assist new patients and others without funds to obtain small necessities, and to provide refreshments for ward parties; and provision of leadership for a well-rounded program of ward parties, invitation dances and special events and programs such as the annual Ward Open House.

Ward housekeeping functions are performed through the "O.D." Committee which, in 1951, made a detailed efficiency study, report and recommendations on hours and standards of work, and on the personnel necessary to perform the ward housekeeping job. These recommendations were adopted *in toto* by the club and approved for reorganization purposes, by the ward team. Spearhead of the committee in routine operation is the officer of the day, chosen in rotation from among ward workers.

This committee also has authority to deal, through impartial action, with habitual offenders against the flexible housekeeping and the social behavior standards of the club—short of behavior problems symptomatic of illness. Observation of rest hours; the use of radio, piano and record-player; responsibility for proper use of books and magazines; reasonable decorum on and off the ward, are all subject to enforcement through committee action, with penalties usually in the form of extra work stints. Serious or dangerous infractions of rules are brought to the attention of the ward staff.

Liaison relationships with other hospital services in connection with club activities are handled directly by patients delegated through officers or the chairman: arrangements for cut flowers or plants through the nursery; arrangements for special materials or services by the recreational, occupational or music therapy departments; and such matters.

Club action has modified the hospital's general 6:30 A.M. reveille to a permissive 7:30 on Ward A-1, and has extended the generally prevailing

8:30 P.M. curfew to 10 o'clock. With the aid of the therapist, it has been so arranged that ward members are no longer compelled to go to breakfast at the women's cafeteria, but may remain on the ward to use the kitchenette for light breakfasts, if they choose.

Such little freedoms greatly ease the rigors of institutional life, help new members to adjust in a minimum of time to the requirements of group living, and promote an atmosphere favorable to the highly desirable group identification as a therapeutic goal.

Club adult education classes are an important and continuing part of the program, with the range of subjects and the number of classes dependent on available qualified teachers and on demand. During 1951, an average of 10 classes a week met in the large classroom, equipped with blackboard, the leader's desk and comfortable chairs. These classes were usually scheduled in the evening. A year's major subjects included shorthand, sewing, singing, dancing, charm, exercise, Spanish, French, English and spelling, games, book discussion and drama.

Classes meeting regularly when this paper was written included choral-drama (an original choral-pageant for the 1952 Open House), shorthand, English, current events, community singing, and handwork such as knitting and crocheting.

There is an average of four organized social affairs each month, including several Saturday night ward parties, and an invitation dance, with the hospital orchestra and with refreshments provided by the hospital. Ward parties are varied: programs with member-talent or invitation performers from outside; folk-dancing and games; bingo; dress-rehearsal parties; farewells and other special-occasion celebrations, such as birthdays or anniversaries.

All social affairs, including liaison with off-ward offices and outside organizations, are handled through committees in a manner typical of any well-run active organization. The club also serves as a valuable public relations organ, obtaining the friendly interest and assistance of outside groups and individuals, for the benefit of the ward and the over-all hospital program.

When it is recalled that the median time on the ward of patients leaving it in 1951 was only 13 weeks, the achievements of the Alpha Club will compare more than favorably with many outside organizations of considerable community status. Neither club members nor ward staff—who would invite such comparison—would ask for any handicap because the club members also happened to be patients in a hospital.

Sunday Sessions. Another ward activity tending to strengthen group identification and transference, is a popular Sunday Morning Session conducted by a talented charge attendant. In 1951, all members of the ward attended these "free-for-all," informal, non-directive group psychotherapy sessions—which encompassed a wide range of hospital, ward, group and personal subjects and problems. They lasted from one to well over two hours.

Alpha Alcoholics Anonymous Group. The Alpha AA Group, all patients committed for alcoholism or other addictions, meets weekly. Following the usual AA procedure, serious talks and discussions are often concluded with coffee-and-doughnut therapy.

Contributing three general secretaries to head the Camarillo Hospital AA Group during 1951, Alpha AA members participated actively in hospital-wide meetings.

The ward organization achieved sufficient status to be listed as the Alpha AA Group in the 1952 International AA Directory.

Special Ward Services. An informative evening was conducted once each month with Jean Paul, hair stylist of a leading Hollywood salon, who regularly volunteered his services to Alpha members. Devoting several hours on the ward to practical instruction in make-up, hair-styling and other essentials of personal grooming, he occasionally brought professional friends as helpers. In addition to this direct assistance for strengthening weak egos, Mr. Paul, a gifted painter and ceramist, gave informal discourses on the principles of aesthetics. From the psychiatric point of view, such freely-given service is excellent therapy.

Another ward service is a newly-instituted occasional presentation of rather special movies on the ward, in addition to the weekly hospital movies.

General Hospital Services. Hospital services of a social, recreational or cultural nature that are generally available include music participation and appreciation; concerts; organized and informal games; weekly movies and dances; handicrafts; such performances as plays or dance programs by outside groups; a library; and a well-equipped beauty shop.

The ward usually contributes talent for special observances and programs such as the Easter cantata, the Fourth of July "county fair," and the Christmas program. News for an "Alpha Antics" section of the hospital monthly paper is an Alpha Club responsibility.

A-1 patients are invariably among workers staffing the canteen and store, both nonprofit activities for the convenience of patients, staff and visitors.

Among other freely-utilized hospital services are consultations with the Catholic and Protestant chaplains, and church services, including provision for Jewish patients.

OUTGOING SERVICES

Vocational Rehabilitation. The ward has taken maximum advantage of vocational rehabilitation services available to outgoing patients through the California State Department of Education.

The Education Department program assists "handicapped persons, including those with mental impairment," to enter suitable employment. Services most commonly benefiting A-1 patients are: job training or retraining, usually in schools, on the job or by correspondence; maintenance and transportation, if necessary, during rehabilitation; equipment and licenses; suitable job placement; and follow-up.

Former ward members now "out on rehab" include a number in beauty, secretarial and art schools. Several patients still on the ward are scheduled for junior college, trade and craft schools on leaving.

This program is a happy supplement to an all-out ward program. It offers a relatively secure transition service to appreciable numbers of untrained outgoing patients and patients needing to regain vocational self-confidence.

PROGRAM FOR FORMER PATIENTS: THE ALPHA CHAPTERS

PERHAPS the most gratifying fruition of the A-1 experiment was inauguration, in 1951, of a continuing program for patients who have left the hospital.

The writer had long hoped to establish ward alumnae chapters to offer supportive group psychotherapy and social therapy, and to be of service to the ward and outgoing patients.

The first outside the hospital, the Santa Barbara Area Chapter, held its maiden meeting in June 1951. Since then, other chapters have been formed in Los Angeles and Ventura, with a healthy and active membership.

Alpha chapters, all of whose members are former A-1 patients, formulate their aims as (1) continuing group psychotherapy in order to hold, consolidate and increase individual gains; (2) assisting Alpha Club members of the chapter area as they leave the hospital, and (3) giving assistance to the ward Alpha Club and to the hospital generally.

Groups usually meet one evening monthly with the therapist, and once with their own moderator, rotating the meeting place among members' homes. Plans are under way to form several chapters in the extensive Los Angeles area. As yet, a comparatively large membership meets in a single group, but provides for transportation and for informal subgroup meetings through area committees.

Material benefits have accrued to the ward from these chapters, in addition to a strong feeling of support and to the enrolling of understanding friends outside. Chapters have provided sewing supplies, cosmetics, Alpha Club letterhead stationery, clothing, food snacks, cigarettes, modest cash gifts to the treasury, and outings for girls having few or no visitors.

It is the writer's conviction that such chapters can, not only fulfill their stated aims, but can also, through strong group support, keep some borderline patients from relapsing and going back into the hospital.

The Los Angeles Chapter has already performed this service for a patient whom the writer had fully expected to see back on the ward some time ago. This patient was a gifted and intelligent woman on the upper border of middle age. She faced a double problem on discharge: to obtain immediate employment and to find sufficient emotional support outside the hospital to bolster her meager self-confidence. Fearful that she would make no move to leave the hospital, though she was a voluntary patient, the writer decided to put the metropolitan group to the test.

Through the chapter president and others, the patient was not only chauffered, bag-and-baggage, from the hospital to a week-end haven with friends; she not only had the loan of a member's vacant apartment for a few weeks; and received spontaneous doses of encouragement by phone and in person; but she has found a reasonably satisfying job for which she feels competent.

This sort of thing is repeated in a variety of guises, not only for the outgoing patient, but also for alumnae chapter members themselves who encounter stormy emotional weather.

A byproduct of the alumnae chapters is increased solidarity and a sense of status within the mother-group on the ward. The active and practical friendship of outside chapters seems also to moderate anxiety about any stigma which might result from state hospitalization.

CONCLUSIONS

STATISTICAL assessment of results obtained by multiple therapies in mental or emotional illnesses is often difficult or impossible. Clear-cut, readily demonstrable conclusions more frequently follow highly selective, controlled experimental subjects and environments.

An experiment such as the three-year Ward A-1 program does not readily admit of a control for purposes of comparison, a public institutional unit providing a wide variety of treatment and activities for a changing population totalling many hundreds of patients.

Conclusions are, therefore, presented on the evidence of the A-1 experimental unit alone. The aim is to present them dispassionately and conservatively and, whenever possible, with other qualified judgments sought.

With a median of only 13 psychotherapy classes, or 19.5 hours of formal group psychotherapy, the writer did not expect patients to show dramatic gains in insight.

However, the classes were a sound foundation to which were added individual interviews by the therapist and others, special psychiatric and medical treatment, training or re-training in group adjustments, and the vital emotional support afforded by an integrated work and social therapy program.

Many patients thus exposed to a "total push" showed marked improvement in both insight and group adjustment.

TABLE 8.

Gross Evaluation* of Insight, Before and After Psychotherapy: 196 Patients Separated from Ward, Year Ended December 31, 1951

INSIGHT BEFORE PSYCHOTHERAPY			CHANGE: INSIGHT AFTER PSYCHOTHERAPY					
			NEGLIGIBLE		MODERATE		DEFINITE	
EVALUATION	NO.	PER CENT	EVAL.	NO.	EVAL.	NO.	EVAL.	NO.
Very poor	58	30.0	Poor	28	Fair	27	Good	3
Poor	88	45.0	Poor	5	Fair	53	Good	30
Fair	50	25.0	Fair	7	Good	43	—	—
Total	196	100.0		40		123		33
Per cent	—	100.0		20.0		63.0		17.0

* Gross standards in evaluating patients' insight:
Very poor or poor: Little or no recognition or understanding of the illness.
Fair: Some recognition of illness; some understanding of root problems.
Good: Clear recognition of the illness; considerable understanding of dynamics, of basic problems and conflicts within the personality.

Table 8 presents gross evaluation of insight, before and after psychotherapy, for 196 patients separated from the ward in 1951. Evaluations were reached in conference, on the basis of personal interviews, group psychotherapy classes, case histories, and the combined reports of all trained personnel dealing therapeutically with the patient.

Of these patients, making up the total 1951 separations, 20 per cent showed little or no gain in insight; 63 per cent, a moderate gain; and 17 per cent, a definite or marked gain.

A further use of rough evaluations for the same group is presented in Table 9: gross evaluation correlated for insight, ward and work adjustment. In general, the success of ward and work adjustment appears closely related to the degree of insight possessed by the patient.

Table 10 presents gross evaluations separately for insight, ward and work adjustment.

With 80 per cent of the evaluation group showing moderate-to-definite gains in insight; with 72 per cent rating good in ward adjustment; and 71 per cent good in work adjustment, the picture of total improvement is still incomplete. One must add the marked gains made by a majority of patients in their relationships with those outside the hospital during their course of treatment, gains observed by members of the therapeutic team and testified to by patients, families and friends.

TABLE 9.

Gross Evaluation Correlated for Insight, Ward and Work Adjustment:
196 Patients Separated from Ward, Year Ended December 31, 1951

INSIGHT ON LEAVING WARD		WARD ADJUSTMENT		WORK ADJUSTMENT	
EVALUATION	NO.	EVALUATION	NO.	EVALUATION	NO.
		Poor	16	Poor	15
				Fair	1
				Poor	1
Poor	33	Fair	11	Fair	9
				Good	1
				Poor	1
		Good	6	Fair	2
				Good	3
				Poor	1
Fair	87	Fair	25	Fair	16
				Good	8
				Poor	3
		Good	62	Fair	6
				Good	53
		Fair	3	Good	3
Good	76	Good	73	Fair	2
				Good	71

Though these two tables may seem to attempt the measurement and correlation of factors and qualities too elusive for conclusive evidence, they, nevertheless, possess sufficient validity to give some support to the writer's own general conclusions.

The writer is convinced that an integrated ward program can provide both direct and supportive therapies to assist the patient most effectively in meeting the immediate need for social recovery and, further, can project both influence and services beyond the hospital to help the patient continue progress toward a reasonably well-adjusted and rewarding life.

If most mentally and emotionally disturbed people are "suffering an

TABLE 10.

Gross Evaluations of Insight, Ward and Work Adjustment; Shown Separately

INSIGHT	NO.	PER CENT	WARD	NO.	PER CENT	WORK	NO.	PER CENT
Poor	33	17.0	Poor	16	8.0	Poor	21	11.0
Fair	87	44.0	Fair	39	20.0	Fair	36	18.0
Good	76	39.0	Good	141	72.0	Good	139	71.0
Total pts.	196	100.0		196	100.0		196	100.0

acute pain in their interpersonal relations," as the late Harry Stack Sullivan said, then the Ward A-1 program is attacking the problem at its source; using psychotherapy as a base for intensive emphasis on group learning, living and loving.

In essence, with the aids of an integrated program, a patient may come to feel accepted by, and feel a part of, a group—to be at home with people; to have a less parochial outlook, deeper understanding and broader tolerance. And with acceptance, one becomes better able to accept one's self, a tolerance reflected out to others. Thus the patient is freed, at least to a degree, to make constructive effort to modify those personality traits and reduce those conflicts which may have caused maladjustment and acute distress.

Further, the program is one of relative simplicity and is readily adaptable to wide institutional use. It operates with a minimum staff; requires no unusual skills, facilities or equipment; and, in the writer's opinion, gives sufficiently clear-cut favorable results to be worth broader application and further development.

CHAPTER 32 Administrative Therapy:
Its Clinical Importance in the Mental Hospital*

D. H. CLARK

PSYCHIATRY today is becoming steadily more specialised, and the day of the old-time medical superintendent who was master of all possible trades within the asylum has passed. He was at once senior psychiatrist, consultant physician, medicolegal expert, morbid pathologist, and general practitioner to the resident staff. Today no-one is called upon to exercise all these skills, and there is a chance to examine afresh the work and role of the medical superintendent and see what therapeutic possibilities they offer. From my attempt to study this I have emerged with a concept of Administrative Therapy—the art (perhaps some day to be a science) of treating psychiatric patients in a mental hospital by administrative action. Group therapy developed from individual therapy; administrative therapy is treatment of a much larger group, the hospital. It draws on the knowledge and skills of psychiatry and group psychotherapy, the experience of the professional administrators, and the accumulating contributions of the social anthropologists.

THE ADMINISTRATIVE ROLE

WHAT does the role of medical superintendent mean to the doctor who undertakes it? What limitations and obligations does it place on him? Every psychiatrist cherishes a fantasy of what he would do if he were medical superintendent of his hospital; the essence of this fantasy is the delusion that the medical superintendent is omnipotent and can do anything he wishes. A doctor who becomes medical superintendent soon finds

---

* Based on an address to the psychotherapy and social-psychiatry section of the Royal Medico-Psychological Association on Oct. 9, 1957.

Reprinted from *The Lancet*, 1 (1958), 805–808, by permission of the author and the journal.

out how limited he is; there are so many things that he cannot do or that take a long, long time. There are the obvious limitations which block his programme—shortage of money, ancient buildings, overcrowded wards, shortage of nurses, not enough doctors, conservatism of those long in office, limitations of Treasury finance, and the tremendous difficulty (in the complex organisation of the National Health Service) of getting any new idea accepted. All these things are well known and understood. Underlying them all is the inertia of any large human organisation, which is the sum of the unwillingness of many people to change their ways.

More limiting than the things he cannot do, however, are the things he must do. Every administrator must carry out a number of ritual public actions which can be performed by no-one else; they may be disturbing, frustrating, or merely boring, but he must do them. It is in this context that the word "role" which we use so glibly approximates most closely to its theatrical meaning, for the leader of any organisation has to perform certain acts which are prescribed for him and for which he may personally have little taste. He is the figurehead, the spokesman, and at times the voice of conscience; these duties take up time which he often feels to be wasted, for they give him no feeling of achievement and certainly none of "proper work."

As figurehead he must function on public occasions, making speeches, setting forth the principles of the organisation, proposing votes of thanks graciously; he must offer public congratulations; he must make presentations to the employees who have been a long time in the hospital; he must speak at nurses' days and at the opening of new buildings. At all these times he must express the feelings of the staff and the patients and yet at the same time draw out unifying themes and suggest future goals. He must act as chairman of certain essential coordinating committees within the hospital, where departments are in conflict and only he can mediate. It is only reasonable to hand over some of these tasks to others, but he must beware how often he does this; he must remember that there is always a loss of definition when he does.

There are aspects of the role which may be frankly repugnant, especially to a sensitive psychotherapist. Promotion must be made; every time one person is gratified by promotion several are dissatisfied or even embittered. When someone breaks the rules, the administrator must not shirk the unpleasant duty of seeing the errant offender, cautioning him, and if necessary discharging him. Much can be done to obviate social disturbance by fair dealing, by constant self-scrutiny, and by willingness to admit mistakes; but there comes a time when someone must pronounce the community disapproval of an individual's actions, and the leader of the community forfeits its confidence and weakens it if he is not prepared to do this.

The administrator should not actively seek transgressors; seeking transgressors is an antitherapeutic activity best left to those whose task it is, such as auditors. If communications are free, malpractices soon come to light; if an irregular procedure gives no-one cause for complaint, then there is little need to seek it out. If an administrator spends his time checking his juniors, he conforms to the traditional asylum stereotype of fault-finding authority and soon paralyses the hospital. His task is the more difficult one of seeking out and encouraging initiative and therapeutic development.

The doctor who becomes medical superintendent will learn some of the lessons and pains of administration. He will find folklore and fantasy condensing about him whatever he does, so that he will be credited by some with magical prescience and wisdom, and by others with malignant cruelty and foolishness. He will find injustice and even tyranny exacted in his name. He will learn the gratification of seeing a change, long fought for, produce the desired result, and the bitterness of espousing and effecting a change only to see it fail because of flaws he had not perceived. He will learn how long it takes to bring about a change; how change imposed is of little value; how patience and a sense of timing often achieve more than enthusiasm.

The role of medical superintendent, like every other worth-while role in life, will have a moulding effect on him. To the characteristics developed by years of medical responsibility will be added characteristics of the wielder of power—the cautious utterance, the guarded promise, the ready excuse that saves the need of self-scrutiny, the specious justification, the growing pomposity and intolerance of criticism, the diminution of scientific detachment. All these will come, and his friends and colleagues will commiserate with his wife as they become more obvious.

MEDICAL OR LAY?

THESE are some of the experiences and problems that face any administrator. Is a doctor, a psychiatrist, the person to undertake them? Administration of general hospitals is carried out by non-medical professionals in England (though not in Scotland); some of them have pressed strongly that the mental hospitals would also be better out of the hands of the doctors—though they state this as an altruistic desire to "free the doctors for their proper work." The debate often reaches a high pitch of acrimony as the well-organised and vocal groups battle for privilege and power; many of the arguments are specious, transparently self-interested, and valueless except as debating points. But the question must be considered. A bad administrator is a disaster for any hospital, be he medical or lay— and examples of both are easy to find in English hospitals. Their faults are different but equally pernicious. The bad lay administrator is a petty-minded bureaucrat, ruled by regulations, frightened of responsibility, and insensitive to human needs; the bad medical administrator is a patient-centred doctor who regards administration with contempt, who lacks the ability to plan and think ahead, the courage to face group situations, and the imagination to understand the problems of non-medical professional groups.

Any doctor who undertakes to be an administrator must accept what that means. He must be prepared to learn something of administration; he must have an interest and ability in handling, leading, and uniting people. He must be tolerant of the status systems of professions other than his own, and understand that coming in by the front door, or wearing a collar, may mean as much to someone as the right to a long white coat once did to him. He must learn a smattering of many jargons. He must lend an interested ear to the catering officer, the engineer, and the garden manager, and must understand what pains them. He must, too, be ready to think seriously about the structure of authority and organisation; it is not enough to rely on traditional modes of direction.

Doctors do not generally make very good administrators. All their training has been away from this, and if a doctor is a good administrator it is because a talent for handling groups and an interest in working with them has survived his medical training. Throughout the medical training, skill is developed towards a two-person situation, and a very special two-person situation—the handling of a patient who is often socially and intellectually inferior to the doctor, and, if he is not, is unmanned by anxiety, pain, and fear of death. The doctor is the expert whose words are weighty and powerful; his verdict is the utterance of a judge. The psychiatrist and the psychotherapist are further trained to think of the individual patient and his good, but seldom of the good of the community or the group.

The doctor with experience of group or social therapy comes to administration with an advantage. He has learnt to think in terms of the group rather than the individual; he has already begun to swing away from the exclusive one-patient orientation of the traditional doctor and traditional psychotherapist. This is of great value when he comes to administration, where every decision has to take into account the needs of a number of individuals. In his group therapy he has acquired an ability to handle the group situation, which again is valuable. Many medical superintendents never acquire this: when they are alone with a patient or with a junior doctor they are competent and powerful; when faced by a group they become anxious, secretive, and fear-ridden. A group therapist, however, should have worked through this. He can sit among a dozen other people, watch what they are doing, listen to what they are saying, and contain the anxiety that arises in him when heavy hostility or pressure is directed against him; he can feel what is happening, engage in the interaction, and yet keep sufficiently apart to observe it and wait his time for joining in.

The psychiatric administrator has to take part in one group which is an entirely new experience to him—the management committee. Here he is not the leader, the therapist doctor, the omnipotent expert; he is not even a member of the committee, he has no power to vote, he is merely an official. The determination of policy is in the hands of the committee.

This role comes hard to doctors, for they are accustomed to being experts, and the experience of working with lay committees can be peculiarly disturbing for them. Perhaps for the first time since he entered medical school the doctor meets laity who may not be much impressed by his statements and can say so; who do not credit him with omniscience. Those fascinating and admirable people who give constant and assiduous voluntary service on committees have limited respect for experts of any kind, including doctors. They themselves are magistrates, town councillors, and aldermen; accustomed to judge the affairs of their fellow men and make decisions affecting the lives of others. They have often heard experts explain with specious technical jargon why certain courses must be followed, and they are no longer to be taken in. They have seen through borough surveyors, have deflated headmasters, and have goaded medical officers of health into action; they are little impressed by oracular certainties. If the medical superintendent wishes to carry the management committee with him he must learn to justify his policies on sound well-based grounds of the general good. They will allow the doctor his full meed of expert knowledge but if he wishes to spend more public money, he must show good reason why.

THE FABRIC OF HUMAN RELATIONS

THE third report of the World Health Organisation's Expert Committee on Mental Health[1] said that the most important single factor in the efficacy of the treatment given in a mental hospital is "an intangible element which can only be described as its atmosphere." They gave in detail some of the elements which make up that atmosphere, and went on to say:

"As in the community at large, one of the most characteristic aspects of the psychiatric hospital is the type of relationship between people that are to be found within it; the nature of the relationships between the Medical Director and his staff will be reflected in the relationships between the psychiatric staff and the nurses and finally in the relationship not only between the nurses and the patients but between the patients themselves."

This is a challenging statement, and contains the kernel of administrative therapy—which may be defined as the manipulation, modification, and constant scrutiny of the relationships spreading out from the administrator, with the aim of controlling their effect on the patients.

Administrative therapy is in much the same state as psychotherapy was in the 1880s. At that time many doctors, neurologists, and alienists were talking to patients about their lives and their problems and helping them; some were exhorting patients to follow different modes of behaviour and by that exhortation were improving their adjustment to life. There was, however, no awareness of what they were doing, no insight into the factors concerned, and such instructions as they gave were based on self-evident principles. Then Freud showed how much more went on between the doctor and the patient, and interpersonal reactions began to be explored. After fifty years we are now at last beginning to understand something of the dynamics of the two-person therapeutic situation. Administrators at present tend to handle their organisations with as much insight as Charcot used with his hysterics; they proceed from intuition, self-evident deductions, and political theory, their only guide being catchwords and slogans. We need to study how actions and activities of the administrators finally affect the patients, and (more important) learn how to alter these actions therapeutically. In this way we shall develop some knowledge of administrative therapy.

The fathers of institutional psychiatry had no doubt in their minds about the importance of administrative therapy though they called it "moral management." One has only to read Tuke's *Description of the Retreat*[2] or Pinel's *Treatise on Insanity*[3] to see the importance they give to the management of the house; both stressed how unimportant formal medicine is and how useless drugs, bleeding, and purgation. Both of them discussed with admiration the work of the men who ran their hospitals; Pinel rapturised about Pussin, Tuke soberly praised the skill and consideration of Jepson; both devoted large sections in their books to describing just how the asylum should be organised and the rules that should be laid down for the life of the patients.

In each generation reformers arose, like Kirkbride in America and Simon in Germany, who restated some of the principles, occasionally with an individual twist of their own; they were heard for a time, and then they were forgotten and dropped away. The W.H.O. report sets out the principles yet again, and they are very similar to those of Tuke and Pinel. Patients are to be trusted and given as much freedom and responsibility as possible; their individualities must be preserved, and the life in hospital made as much like that outside as possible, particularly by providing regular planned and sustained activity and employment.

FOUR PRINCIPLES

WHEN a psychiatrist decides to become a medical superintendent how can he look at his job? What are the principles that he is to follow? There are four main facets of administrative therapy:

1. Organisation of the patient's life
2. Staff organisation
3. Medical organisation
4. Community leadership

These are, of course, interlinked, and maladroitness in one affects the others; but they are in some degree separate. Of every action one must ask the dynamic questions: How was it done? Did it have the effect desired? What other side-effects did it have? Did it help the patients?

PATIENT'S LIFE

THE first is perhaps the easiest of the four, for a great deal is known about it. The ideas of moral treatment and the principles put forward by the W.H.O. report give a start. It would take several years' work in any hospital to get these accepted as a fundamental way of life. The abolition of restraint, seclusion, locked doors, and over-sedation is the first move. Proper segregation into wards each with a definite function is of great value. Diligent organisation of a full work therapy programme for all patients in the hospital takes time and it must include a proper system of rewards and payments. These first essentials can be fairly easily achieved over a few years, though a close guard must be kept against the custodialism which is forever creeping back under the guise of economy and "efficiency." Next comes the development of self-government for the patients and experiments in communal living—group therapy, discussion groups, play-reading, hospital magazines, and mixed units.

STAFF ORGANISATION

To organise a therapeutic staff is more difficult. The staff in any mental hospital has been trained for years in custodial attitudes; they were trained to count patients and to watch stock, they learnt that an escape was the most awful sin—worse even than a suicide or an accident—and they have acquired whole series of custodial and often punitive reflexes that are not easily abandoned. In most hospitals, too, there is a rigid hierarchical system with orders passed down from above and a severe blockage on the flow of information upwards; there are usually rigid status barriers between the different categories of staff. The administrative therapist must decide what to tackle first. He cannot just plunge in naïvely with the ideas of making everybody democratic; if he endangers the security of senior staff, he himself may be extruded.

The emphasis should be first on communication. Meetings should be held with various groups of staff and they should be encouraged to bring forward ideas; through such meetings new channels of communication can be laid down. It is a grave mistake to come to the conclusion that some person or other is nothing but a bar to all progress and to attempt to "drive him out." If your patients are to have human dignity, your staff must have it too. The only correct assumption is that everyone has something to contribute and that given the chance he will do his best.

Questions of responsibility and authority are central and must be constantly studied. In most mental hospitals there is scope for far wider devolution of responsibility.

MEDICAL ORGANISATION

THE administrative therapist must give special thought to the organisation of the doctors. They may have little interest in his abilities as a social therapist, but they wish to believe that he can practise their art of clinical psychiatry at least moderately well. The medical superintendent should continue to see his own cases and have cases within the wards, otherwise he will no longer understand his colleagues' problems. The relations of the administrative therapist with the consultant psychiatrists are a difficult and testing point. At present there is much pain and bitterness about this in English mental hospitals. Some medical superintendents still think in terms of the pre-1948 situation, when the medical superintendent was personally responsible for the treatment of every patient. Today the consultant psychiatrist has full responsibility before the Law and before society for the treatment of his patients, and there can be no excuse for the medical superintendent interfering in the treatment prescribed. But the issue goes deeper. The consultant psychiatrists are the only group of peers whom the medical superintendent meets; the only group who share his professional training. Many consultant psychiatrists despise administration and do not think much of administrative therapy or social psychiatry. What they want to do is to treat individual patients in the one-doctor/one-patient relationship; this they think of as the highest good. The administrative therapist's task is to provide a milieu in which everyone may do his chosen job to the best of his ability without interference, and this is as true of the consultant psychiatrist as of humbler people in the organisation. If an administrative therapist does his own job well and takes the same care to avoid trespassing on another doctor's patients that is standard throughout medicine, his relations with his consultant staff should be good. If he can provide them with the facilities they need to do their work, free of the more vexatious hospital irritations, he will gain their gratitude and respect.

The medical organisation will vary with the size of the hospital. It has been suggested that the best size of unit for administrative therapy is about 300 beds; it is still just possible to administer 1000 beds as a unit. With larger hospitals, however, the span becomes too great and it is necessary to split the hospital into "firms" running self-contained units with a consultant and senior nursing officer in charge. The only difficulty with this is that differing cultures develop in the self-contained units; if they differ too much, it is hard for patients and junior nurses to understand that one institution can have such different units within it, and they may find the passage awkward from a liberal environment to a restrictive one.

COMMUNITY LEADERSHIP

IF ANY human organisation is to work well, it should have confidence in itself, it should have a policy, and it should have good morale. The administrative therapist must give these to the hospital as best he can. The hospital policy must be clearly formulated. In the past the cries have been "non-restraint" and "full activity"; recently it has been "open doors." The policies of the W.H.O. report must be worked into the structure of the hospital and embodied in slogans which can be understood by the most uninterested staff member. They must be repeated again and again until they really have meaning and until the words "therapeutic community" mean not just the bee in the superintendent's bonnet but a way of living and acting.

Relations upward are always difficult, and it is in this sphere that some social therapists fail sadly, while some autocratic medical superintendents have often been quite successful. The hospital management committee decide the policy of the hospital; if an administrative therapist is going to change the whole life and way of a hospital he must carry the management committee with him. They are mature and tend to conservatism; they are dubious about the enthusiasms of youth and many have much previous experience of the hospital. They must be won to new policies which must be put to them in terms of the humanitarian gain to the patient, for in this they are always interested. Beyond them the policy must be carried to the public; it is no use opening your doors if the local public and the police shout to have them locked again. In this the co-operation of the local press is vital and the administrative therapist must work with them. Cheerful reports about the hospital will dispel criticism, will build up the morale of the staff, and will do much to allay public anxieties.

IN AN N.H.S. SETTING

WITHIN the National Health Service there is constant work to do. Though new buildings do not produce good psychiatric treatment, some new equipment is needed for the hospital; and the hospital which feels that it gets the last handout of everything may become dispirited. The administrative therapist as leader of the hospital and spokesman for its policy must be prepared to argue policy up the various tiers of the National Health Service; this involves knowledge of local power relationships and a willingness to explain again and again things which seem crystal clear.

It needs patience and self-control to put over an idea, which is of great personal importance, to a committee who are perhaps uninterested or committed to the needs of another hospital, and to carry conviction so that the needed money is granted.

There is also a constant defensive battle to be fought; ever busy within the fabric of the National Health Service are those white ants, the auditors, nibbling away and eroding the fabric of human relations and good feeling. They are employed to peer through every hospital attempting to prove that everyone is dishonest and that no-one can be trusted; given their way they would multiply the regulations until the hospital was bound in a cocoon of red-tape, all in the name of "efficiency." They must be watched unceasingly and every claimed advance in efficiency scrutinised with great care to see it does not harm the human relations of the hospital. Luckily they too are only servants, and the masters are the hospital management committee, the representatives of the public; if an administrative therapist is worth his salt he can carry the point against the auditors and show that the welfare of the patients and the trust and happiness of the staff are first essentials.

But the most important task of the administrative therapist is to establish the atmosphere of the hospital. And this, the most important, is the task most difficult to describe. He needs openness, consistency, respect for everyone's human dignity, and a welcome for everyone's contribution; a belief that everyone wishes to help and that no-one is past recovery— neither the most demented patient nor the most stupid nurse. For one thing is certain: as he treats his staff so will they treat the patients.

*   *   *

These are some of the aspects and personal meanings of the art of Administrative Therapy as they strike one new to the field, but there is so much to learn. Studies like those of Stanton and Schwartz[4] point the way to an understanding of the dynamics and the effects of administrative action. By such means, knowledge may gradually replace intuition until the art becomes a science.

NOTES TO CHAPTER 32

1. World Health Organization. Third report of the Expert Committee on Mental Health. Geneva, 1953.
2. Tuke, S. A Description of the Retreat. York, 1813.
3. Pinel, P. A Treatise on Insanity. London, 1806.
4. Stanton, A., Schwartz, M. The Mental Hospital. London, 1955.

Integration

ફ≥

C H A P T E R 33   The Concept of a
Therapeutic Community*

MAXWELL JONES

APPLIED to a psychiatric hospital the term "therapeutic community" implies that the responsibility for treatment is not confined to the trained medical staff but is a concern also of the other community members, *i.e.*, the patients. How far can patients usefully participate in the treatment of other patients and how will this participation affect them? How far can they in turn be helped by other patients?

The importance of staff tensions as they affect treatment have long been recognized and the work of the Chestnut Lodge group has had a profound effect on the thinking and practice of psychiatric nursing and we hope of psychiatrists themselves. This subject has been ably discussed in the recent publication by Stanton and Schwartz (1). Relatively less attention has been paid to the social life of patients when staff are not present and the therapeutic possibilities this social interaction may have. Attention has been drawn to this subject by the interesting experiences of Caudill, a social anthropologist, who was admitted to a mental institution for 2 months as a patient in order to study the social situation from the patients' point of view. He states (2):

While the staff exercised control over the patients, they did not give recognition to the patient world as a social group, but rather, they interpreted the behavior of the patients almost solely in individual dynamic-historical terms. The patient group, thus lacking an adequate channel of communication to the staff, protected itself by turning inward, and by developing a social structure which was insulated as much as possible from friction with the hospital routine. Nevertheless, such friction did occur, and the subsequent frustration led to behavior on

* Read at the 111th annual meeting of The American Psychiatric Association, Atlantic City, N.J., May 9-13, 1955.

Reprinted from the *American Journal of Psychiatry*, Volume 112, pages 647–650, 1956, by permission of the author and the *Journal*.

the part of the patients which, although it overtly resembled neurotic behavior arising from personal emotional conflicts, was, in fact, to a considerable extent due to factors in the immediate situation.

If a therapeutic community with active patient participation is to be established in any psychiatric treatment unit a drastic revision in existing staff and patient roles and role relationships will be called for. It is clear that the changes that might be attempted will depend on many factors, including the type of patient, the treatment goals, the previous training of the staff, the degree of self-determination and freedom of action granted to the center, the culture of the adjacent hospital, if any, the culture of the wider community, economic factors, etc. In this presentation, however, we are assuming positive sanctions from higher authorities, complete freedom shared by staff and patients alike to organize the community, and a single therapeutic goal, namely the adjustment of the individual to social and work conditions outside, without any ambitious psychotherapeutic program.

Detailed description of all the role changes and social reorganization which, in our experience, are necessary cannot here be undertaken (7); however, certain main points can be discussed. The psychiatrist has, like all doctors, been given and accepts many of the qualities of the witch doctor. His greater knowledge is assumed in all treatment situations whether individual or group. The patient understandably enough wants to feel that the doctor knows what he is doing and by his attitude contributes to what is often an illusion. The doctor maintains many of the symbols of his office even when they have no immediate usefulness, *e.g.*, the traditional white coat, prominent stethoscope, and, in the U.S.A., the peculiarly ugly framed official qualification found in most doctors' offices. Moreover, in America the status of psychiatry is higher than its proved usefulness merits. How far do factors such as these create barriers to free communication between doctors and patients? How honest are we in admitting our limitations to our patients, nursing staffs, etc., and how readily do we turn to them for help? To give a simple illustration, how often is the wrong patient sent from an open to a closed ward in an attempt to resolve a tense ward situation? The fact is that we do not know and unless we attempt to analyze the disturbance we cannot find out. Such an analysis will usually involve the whole ward community and may be difficult or impossible to carry out without free communication between patients and staff and between the individual members in both groups. If, however, it is possible to institute a ward meeting and to achieve some degree of communication it may be possible to learn a great deal about the patients' feelings, their attitudes toward the staff, and so on. It has been our conscious aim to develop the freest possible communication between patients and staff and this has necessitated a reorganization of the doctors' timetable. Increasingly less time has been spent in individual interviewing and proportionately more in group and community meetings so that at present ⅓ of the day is spent in the former and ⅔ in the latter. A group meeting usually comprises about 10 patients, a psychiatrist, and several members of the nursing staff. These meetings are run on analytic lines but techniques vary with the personality and training of the psychiatrist. Every patient attends his group meeting (one hour) daily. By a community meeting we mean a discussion group involving the entire population of the unit (100 patients of both sexes, 4 psychiatrists, 1 psychiatric social worker, 1 psychologist, 1 social anthropologist, 4 workshop instructors, and a nursing staff of 15).

A community meeting epitomizes the function of a therapeutic community. The aim is to achieve the freest possible expression of feeling by both patients and staff. This is a departure from the usual role of staff members in the familiar therapeutic group of 8 to 12 persons. In the latter it is the patients only who verbalize their feelings and the staff use such communications as seem therapeutic but do not reveal (at least not intentionally) anything of their own feelings. In a community meeting the staff are free to verbalize their own anxieties where they relate to the community, *e.g.*, the growing hostility of the hospital authorities and local residents to the drunken behavior of certain patients. This threat may have been unknown to the patients but is now fed back to the total community by the staff. The community is thus faced by a social problem which has meaning for everyone. It has taken us 8 years to arrive at the point where the patients no longer attempt to sidestep their responsibility in tackling both the therapeutic and administrative aspects of such a problem in collaboration with the staff. The meaning of the individuals' need to turn to alcohol is the major problem and can be discussed as a current event with the other patients who participated in the outing. This can be implemented by further communications from the patients' own doctors, the P.S.W., members of their groups, and so on. Moreover, the timing of a particular alcoholic "binge" can often be seen in response to some current tension, say a general feeling of antagonism to the supposedly authoritarian behavior of certain staff members or to a state of unresolved tension in the staff members themselves. This in turn may uncover some of the deeper feelings of antagonism toward parental figures and highlight some of the transference or counter-transference difficulties. Thus the emphasis may be on uncovering therapy, on group dynamics, on education, or it may become clear to some staff members or patients that at least one factor in the situation is a response, often unconscious, by patients to unresolved staff tensions. In the latter eventuality the current practice is to postpone discussion of this tension to a later staff meeting, but we feel that a time may soon arrive when such discussion will constantly occur in the presence of the patients themselves. Already we are aware of the extraordinary sensitivity of some patients to such tensions and the probable advantages in accepting their participation, as we do in dealing with patient problems. We have already gone some way in this direction by admitting freely that the staff frequently display neurotic defenses and have casualties luckily only of a minor kind. These neurotic manifestations are usually commented on by the patients and when my own emotional difficulties begin to get out of control the patients show a most touching solicitude and desire to treat me, or an obvious pleasure in my discomfiture, depending on the particular patient! Someone will probably be heard to say that it is time I talked about my difficulties or more specifically that I have a work problem! In addition, the patients are fully aware that we have frequent staff meetings to deal with our own group and interpersonal tensions. Thus we are patently at one with them in constantly needing treatment. The only reason for separating the two treatment areas (patients and staff) is to give the patients the feeling that our difficulties refer to immediate problems particularly in the field of learning, *e.g.*, the training of new staff members and are not of such magnitude as to warrant the term "illness." Clearly patients want to feel that the staff can cope with their own problems, if they are going to be able to treat them competently, so it is probably better to hold staff groups separately until such time as community techniques have reached the point of perfection when patients can safely be told the whole truth.

The community meeting is a sort of general feed-back and clearing house for current problems from both patients and staff. A problem relating specifically to a particular subgroup, say a workshop or a ward, may be left for later discussion by the particular subgroup. More often, however, it will touch off a more general problem and lead to an immediate discussion. Sometimes the community's current anxiety centers around a particular patient and the whole hour is spent in discussing this patient. It may be that the patient is acting out in so disturbing a way that a decision must be made about his possible transfer to a mental hospital where there are adequate facilities for the supervision of individual patients.

Take the case of an adolescent behavior problem in a girl who has been resorting to excessive amounts of Benzedrine by eating the contents of inhalers that she can buy in any chemist's shop in England. In addition to this, she set fire to a roller towel in the kitchen of her ward. The cause of the fire was at first unknown and it was only as a result of various group meetings that the factors became known and could be fed back into the community meeting. In working through many aspects of this girl's problem—her early rejection, her illegitimacy, orphanage upbringing, the development of her criminal activities, etc.—the whole community became involved and informed about her problem in some depth. She was able to say why she wanted to burn down the hospital and needed to take Benzedrine; that she hated her doctor and could not communicate with him in individual interviews because he reminded her of the magistrate who had sent her to a corrective institution. Moreover, it soon became clear that no matter how kind the community might be the only real friends she had ever known belonged to the criminal fringe and she felt almost as strong a desire to return to them as to get well.

This type of problem involving adaptation to a new set of values and the whole concept of health is probably best handled in the community where many other patients are preoccupied with similar problems bearing on social values.

The constant verbalization of problems and working them through in daily group and community meetings lead to the development of a rather sophisticated and articulate community. Visitors are constantly surprised by the patients' understanding and insight in handling their problems in collaboration with the staff. Social attitudes come in for frequent discussion, *e.g.*, such problems as informing, discipline, etc., which have such sinister associations for patients—many of whom have been in prison— and have obvious importance in relation to the establishment of free communications, as do the various attitudes patients adopt toward the general topic of "treatment." How many patients in psychiatric hospitals have clear ideas on this subject? One is tempted to ask the same question in relation to hospital staffs. To staff members who are prepared to recognize this problem we can recommend the advantages of discussing the topic in community with the patients. A surprising amount of mutual education can result. The trained staff member is forced to review some of his traditional attitudes and is unable to retreat to his safe position of omnipotent silence. For instance, in most psychiatric hospitals sedatives are used in large amounts. Stimulated by the frequently occurring problem of drug addiction and the tensions produced by the "acter-outers" in demanding sedatives from the night staff, we have found it necessary to discuss this problem on many occasions. The community has slowly changed its attitude until it is now accepted by everyone that our previous practice of giving sedatives was in the main a defense against difficulties (both patient and staff) which were much better dealt with by verbalization or other forms of acting out in the group or community meetings. Little distinction is made by the patients between the use of sedatives and of alcohol. The latter is seen in the main as a regressive symptom of the patient whereas sedation is seen as a symptom in this case not only confined to the patient but frequently involving the staff as well. The staff's need to give sedatives has been freely discussed and was seen to reflect the anxieties of doctors and nurses at least as much as it was used as a

specific therapeutic procedure. I know of only one other hospital where
the use of sedatives has been discontinued and this again was the result
of a careful analysis of the staff motivations in prescribing drugs.

We have developed another community technique which gives us some
insight into the patients' attitude toward treatment and the unit generally.
Every Friday morning we have a 2-hour seminar with any professional
visitors who care to attend. The majority of the staff is present and the
patients are represented by 8 different volunteers each week. The average
number of visitors is 20 and we avoid any temptation to structure the
meeting. The usual pattern is that the patients start talking about their
current tensions or seek information about the visitors, their particular
professions, reasons for studying the unit, and so on. As the visitors are
drawn from the social science and medical fields they may well touch off
some controversy, *e.g.*, between probation officers and patients with an
antisocial background. The patients are frequently openly hostile to the
unit or staff members; this draws the staff into the discussion and the
situation becomes very similar to the daily community meetings. Usually,
however, at some point the visitors' need for specific information leads
the patients to express their own views about treatment, the social organization of the unit, and similar subjects. In this way we learn a great deal
from the interdisciplinary seminar and not only can test the patients'
concept of the unit culture but can learn something of the reaction of
trained outsiders.

There is nothing particularly new in the concept of a therapeutic community. John Wesley had something like this in mind when he formed his
"bands" some 200 years ago. The field of juvenile delinquency has produced experiments like those of Aichhorn (3), Bettelheim (4), and
Redl (5), and it is not pure chance that our own recent experience has
been largely in the field of "adult delinquents" or the "acting-out disorders." I feel strongly that we psychiatrists have largely failed to meet
the treatment challenge of the antisocial patient, whatever his classification. These patients need specially trained staff and a therapeutic community if their antisocial attitudes are to be modified. To the best of my
knowledge the social rehabilitation unit at Belmont Hospital is the only
one of this kind with the possible exception of some prison communities.
I have deliberately left any mention of the antisocial patient to the end
and avoided writing specifically about this problem, as there seems to be
an equally good case for the application of the general principles of a
therapeutic community in most, if not all, psychiatric hospitals.

Thanks to the courtesy of Professor Bob Matthews, I was able to spend
the month of February 1954 visiting the department of psychiatry at
Louisiana State University, and also several of the state mental hospitals.
This experience has been reported elsewhere (6) but briefly it helped
to confirm my impression that many of the principles of a therapeutic

community are equally relevant to a psychiatric hospital and social rehabilitation unit such as ours.

BIBLIOGRAPHY

1. Stanton, A. H., and Schwartz, M. S. The Mental Hospital. New York: Basic Books, 1954.
2. Caudill, W., et al. Am. J. Orthopsychiat., 22:314, 1952.
3. Aichhorn, A. Wayward Youth. New York: Viking Press, 1935.
4. Bettelheim, B. Love is Not Enough. Glencoe, Ill.: Free Press, 1950.
5. Redl, F., and Wineman, D. Controls from Within, Glencoe, Ill.: Free Press, 1952.
6. Jones, M., and Matthews, R. A. Brit. J. Med. Psychol. In Press.
7. Jones, M. The Therapeutic Community. New York: Basic Books, 1953.

ॐ

CHAPTER 34 Outbreak of Gang Destructive Behavior on a Psychiatric Ward*

RICHARD W. BOYD, S. STEPHEN KEGELES, AND MILTON GREENBLATT

INTRODUCTION

PSYCHIATRIC journals seldom report ward life problems handled unsuccessfully, especially instances of the destruction of property and assault upon personnel. It is true, nevertheless, that these "disintegrative" ward events occur often enough to be of serious concern to personnel in staff conferences.

The paucity of reports of disturbed psychiatric wards may result from the paucity of investigation of the mental hospital ward as a system of human action: only a few studies are available in which the ward as a social system is considered. An analysis of those social factors associated with "good" and "poor" social interaction among patients formed the basis of this investigation (1). A study of the social clique membership on a female acute psychiatric ward as a function of a hospital social system was completed recently (3). Stanton and Schwarz discuss, from a clinical viewpoint, the manner in which cleavages between administrative and practicing psychiatrists result from "stereotype" decisions regarding the social life of the patient (5).

The present report, continuing an emphasis similar to those just mentioned, investigates the influence of a severe disruption of the social life on an acute psychiatric ward on both the patients and personnel. The value of a sociological view of the event, and the techniques of analysis the viewpoint affords, are related to the solution of the problem.

* The authors are indebted to Robert W. Hyde, M.D., Asst. Supt. at BPH and Harriet M. Kandler, R.N., M.S., Director of Nurses at BPH, for encouraging this study.

Reprinted from *Journal of Nervous and Mental Disease,* Volume 120 (1954), pages 338–342. Copyright © 1954, The Williams & Wilkins Co., Baltimore, Maryland 21202, U.S.A. By permission of the authors and The Williams & Wilkins Co.

METHODS AND PROCEDURES OF THE INVESTIGATION

PRESENTLY a full description of the episode is given; meanwhile, the basic facts are offered as follows: between a Friday afternoon and the following Monday morning, on a 24-patient male acute psychiatric unit, there occurred a series of disturbances on the ward including destruction of hospital property, and in one instance, assault by a patient upon a staff person. On Monday morning at a staff conference a discussion resulted in an invitation to a few members of the research department to investigate the social conditions of the disturbed ward and to provide an analysis, if possible, of factors responsible for the events.

METHODS

THE choice of method was determined by the following objectives of the investigation: 1) the location in the ward system structure of the person-to-person associations, and especially to define the "clique" on the ward, with its "leaders," "members," and "sphere of influence;" 2) appraise the effect on the conscious feelings of the patients of the disturbances and outbursts of atypical social behavior; 3) assess the personnel method of analysis of the situation, and the techniques obtaining from this analysis. The three methods adapted to these objectives were: 1) observational sociometry, 2) open-end interviews with patients, and 3) interviews with key personnel and evaluation of the discussion of the events at the Monday staff conference for the assessment of personnel attitudes related to their analysis and treatment of the ward situation.

Observational sociometry, known also as the "clumping technique" (2; 4) consists of periodic, half-hour observations on the ward continuously for an eight-hour period. Observation is made of the contacts among patients. Each patient received two scores: (a) a "proximity" score, or the sum of the times the patient was seen in the company of another patient or patients, and (b) a "sphere of influence" score, or the sum of patients throughout the eight-hour period which a given patient contacted. Clique "members" were defined as the patients observed together most often; clique "leaders" were defined as patients of widest "sphere of influence" and highest proximity to other patients.

Open-end interviews with the 24 patients on the ward were conducted by a social scientist who asked each patient the following questions:

(1) When did you enter the ward?
  (a) How did you feel about the ward then?
  (b) How do you feel about the ward today?
(2) What caused your change (or lack of change) of attitude?

(3) What do you feel could be done to make the ward a better place for you?

The interviewer urged the patients to answer as fully as possible, and with some patients, "probed" for answers until satisfied he had as full as possible an answer. The interviewing required eight hours.

Interviews with personnel were conducted by a social scientist, who talked informally with staff persons about the disturbances on the ward, and recorded, with the factual information, personnel feelings about those events and suggestions for preventing a recurrence of ward disturbance. On Monday notes were taken by the social scientist of the comments by personnel at the staff conference.

PROCEDURE

A RESULT of the staff conference was an invitation to the investigators to study the ward under discussion. The purpose of this study was to provide sociological analysis of "causes" and "effects" of the disturbances on the ward. One investigator made sociometric observations, and the other investigator interviewed patients and staff persons. A nursing supervisor was trained to observe and to make some observations; so that the ward was observed for the entire eight-hour period of investigation.

THE EPISODE OF WARD DISTURBANCE

THE period of severe ward disturbance began suddenly Friday with an outburst as a series of atypical social events, including destruction of hospital property and assault upon personnel, and ended as abruptly as it began, Monday noon, when the ward was again "quiet." The disturbance on the ward, personnel said, "was brewing Friday," "came to a head Saturday morning," and persisted Saturday night and Sunday, with events of increasingly severe destructiveness, to Sunday night, and therefrom to subside until Monday morning. Reports did not establish a precise sequence of events, but all informants agreed to the following as a list of consequences of the disturbed behavior on the ward (6):

1. Sinks pulled off the wall in the toilet room.
2. The toilet room flooded on two occasions.
3. The outer hallway flooded.
4. Windows in the toilet room broken.
5. An estimated 40 window panes broken on the ward.
6. Chairs in the sunparlor and on the ward broken and overturned.
7. Magazines and newspapers strewn throughout the ward, the sunporch area and the grounds below the ward.
8. Toilet tissue littered on the toilet area and adjacent hallway.
9. A table broken, a radio put out of operation.

10. Beds of the ward overturned and/or stacked upon each other in corners of sleeping areas.
11. Dishes broken.

Also, a patient assaulted an attendant, and another "psychopathic-paranoid" patient attempted what personnel termed "sham suicide" by exposing himself to gas from an oven, and again, by attempting theft of a lethal medicine ampule.

The disturbance on the ward insinuated itself into the community environs when the shouting of patients calling "Help!" awakened neighbors, who summoned police officers to the hospital area. The police met hospital administrative officers, who related the causes of the "disorderly conduct," and the officers reported this information to the citizens.

Initial attempts to control the patients on the disturbed ward included the following administrative decisions:

1. Order was given to *restrict* the "high" (violent) patients to the ward area, thus limiting their privileges.
2. Order given to *detain* the violent patients from the weekly "movie" entertainment.
3. A patient, whom nurses and attendants reported to the executive officer on duty as the "ringleader," was *secluded*.

The reason given for secluding the "ringleader" was "to protect him from the other patients who were about to gang up on him."

Staff persons' perceptions were not limited to the facts of destruction but included "intuitions" about the rise of tension on the ward and the probable leaders or "gang" associated with the destruction. However, personnel were unable to organize their facts and intuitions to prevent the breakdown of the ward social structure.

FACTORS RELATED TO THE EPISODE OF DESTRUCTIVENESS

FOLLOWING is a discussion of the discernible factors contributing to the outbreak of aggressive and destructive behavior on the ward. The serial order does not intend either importance or contiguous relation among the factors.

CONCENTRATION OF PARANOID-AGGRESSIVE PATIENTS

AT THE time of the disturbance, the ward had an unusual complement of aggressive and paranoid patients, diagnosed "psychopathic personalities." Most of these individuals were young. They were admitted to the hospital by referral from the courts, which requested study by psychiatrists of their anti-social behavior, emotional instability and possible paranoid schizophrenic tendencies. These patients continued in the hospital the aggressive behavior which had rendered them misfits in society. They endangered the ward equilibrium because of this aggressive behavior and because, as socially perceptive persons, they organized themselves into a goal-directed clique (sociometrically defined) or "gang" which, when motivated, easily enlisted cooperation from less perceptive and less socially integrated patients. At least, the "power" concentrated in the aggressive "gang" dominated the other patients, who could neither prevent the destruction nor refuse the gang tacit approval of their tyranny.

CLIQUE RESENTMENTS OF WARD AND HOSPITAL ADMINISTRATION

To BEGIN with, the clique members were resentful of the "justice" which put them into a mental hospital, which, for their part, was tantamount to a prison. The insult added to their injury was the feeling that they were discriminated against, as shown by their detainment from social activities permitted to "treatment" patients or "non-court" cases. The court cases, as those patients are called, are considered diagnostic problems and stay in the hospital but a short period, after which they are returned to the courts for disposition. Staff persons were aware of these facts, and were less interested in establishing personal relationships with these patients than with the "sicker" "treatment case" patients. The staff persons' want of relationship with the court case patients is heightened by the fact of resentments against them for taking bed space in a *psychotic* patient hospital, and because the bed space used for court cases is not paid for by the patients or their relatives. The hospital is not reimbursed. Further resentment by personnel may develop because the court case patients are admitted by a judge, whose order takes priority, so far as admission to the hospital, over any and all psychotic persons, no matter how acute or perilous their illness. Thus, an objective of the hospital, as treatment of the sick, is to an extent curtailed by the inflow of patients from the court.

This discrimination is translated into administrative orders which prohibit certain social privileges to court case patients. For example, they do not go on picnics outside the hospital, and often they are detained from movies, and are prevented access to O. T. facilities, the use of recreational facilities and freedom of the grounds. Specifically, the clique group members resented "cold food" and the regulation of their social privileges. Thus, resentments toward patients extended into resentments toward the hospital administration. Then resentment to hospital authority was directed to those beds and desks and sinks which stood for it, and which symbolically, therefore, were destroyed.

POOR COMMUNICATION BETWEEN PERSONNEL

THIS was manifested in two ways. First, attendants and some nursing staff members felt that trouble was brewing but failed to alert administration to the problem. Second, personnel were divided in their loyalties to different patients. They disagreed in identifying the main instigators and the factors responsible for the outbreak. Instead they kept their loyalties and identifications largely to themselves and failed to reach common understanding. Notes taken from a staff conference showed clearly the existing antipathies among personnel:

1. "The movies left all the disturbed ones back on the ward. . . . There was too small a coverage with the disturbed patients." (Nursing Supervisor.)
   "The ward was pretty good during the movie." (Psychiatrist.)
2. "They (the destructive patients) didn't ask to go back to the ward." (Male Supervisor.)
   "They did ask to go back to the ward." (Head Nurse.)
3. "Blank (a patient) likes to disconcert the staff." (Head Nurse.)
   "No, he doesn't." (Male Supervisor.)

A few examples of the communication difficulties may be quoted from individual interviews with personnel:

"There was a weekend blowup because the personnel's views are not known. . . . There is a need for more communication from the upper levels to nursing people." (Head Nurse.)

Personnel had conflicting analyses of the causes of the difficulties; for example:

1. "They (the destructive patients) need more help, more individual attention." (Psychiatrist.)
2. "We should send the food up to the ward later so that it does not cool off so soon." (Attendant.)

THE WEEKEND SLUMP

DURING the weekend the size of the ward staff is reduced by at least 2 out of 5, giving a lower staff-patient ratio. One O. T. worker carries the load of 4 regular O. T. staff persons. Thus, O. T. and recreational activities are relatively discontinued. Patients are left very much to their own devices. They are not offered interesting or distracting activities. Their resentments and aggressions grow.

THE SOLUTION OF THE PROBLEM

AT THE height of the disturbance on the ward administrative officers took steps to solve the problem through established psychiatric techniques: the ringleader of the group was secluded and given somatic treatment; some patients were sent to occupational therapy or to physiotherapy; and other patients were taken to the yard, leaving the most disturbed patients on the ward with the diminished ward personnel team to look after them. On Monday morning psychiatric decisions made on Friday (before the outbreak) were carried out; one of the most disturbed patients was transferred to another hospital; another patient began treatment; and another was transferred to a different ward in the hospital. In addition to these administrative decisions, emergency steps were taken to separate the active members of the "gang" by prescription for one patient to have physiotherapy (where he could take out his aggression on a punching bag), and for another to begin his somatic treatment.

DISCUSSION

OUTBREAKS of violence in psychiatric wards are very familiar. Usually they involve one individual who acts out psychotic content in some aggressive manner. These are often catatonic, paranoid or turmoil schizophrenics. Their outbreaks, often unpredictable, can be very disturbing to the whole social system but do not generally involve a gang action. Gang action among disorganized schizophrenics is relatively rare; but gang action among better organized paranoid schizophrenics and psychopaths occurs not uncommonly. Sometimes manic patients are able to bring other ward citizens into aggressive destructive group activity (7).

Clique formations are not rare in psychotic wards. Kegeles has shown in repeated sociometric studies that cliques are always to be found (3). Well-preserved psychopaths living among psychotic patients may dominate the group (3).

Our study points up the stress which arises when mental hospital personnel have underlying resentment against any group of cases—in this instance psychopathic individuals hospitalized on wards meant for psychotic patients. Personnel do not regard them as true "treatment" cases. They do not form positive identifications. Administration resents the loss of bed space and the Department of Mental Health gets no financial return for their hospitalization.

Stanton and Schwarz have adequately described the disturbances which patients manifest in triangular situations, that is, where personnel are at odds as to their identifications, loyalties and ideas of management. This was very much the case in the present situation (5).

One problem arises when an attendant attempts to indicate to the physician his feeling that the ward is in a potentially explosive state. The physician is slow to take the attendant seriously, first, because attendants are often overly anxious in their relations with patients, and second, because the attendant's anxiety often contributes to the outbreak. The physician is in the position of wishing to allay the attendant's anxieties, without closing his eyes to serious realities which the attendant may be the first to recognize.

Attention has been called to the weekend "slump" as one of the major defects in hospital treatment. It is uneconomical and perhaps at times even dangerous to patients' lives and welfare. The weekend slump in a mental hospital is greatly aggravated by the fact that many of the "non-court" patients go on visits, leaving behind patients who may become resentful, disturbed or depressed. The whole treatment pattern is crudely interrupted by absence of key therapeutic personnel and by a complete break in wholesome social distractions.

As to the handling of the disturbance, it is clear that personnel resorted to the time-honored method of dealing with gangs, namely, separating the members involved. A variety of means were used—seclusions, distracting by O. T. therapy, intensive individual therapy and transfer or discharge. These methods are apparently adequate, but unfortunately were applied after the clique had run its anti-social course. It is to be hoped that such outbreaks might be avoided by preventive measures without damage to the ward society. This might be accomplished by increasing personnel's awareness of existing cliques and of their goals, by better communication, and by reducing weekend breaks in social-therapeutic activities. Perhaps most important of all would be a better understanding at the policy level with respect to the management of so-called court-cases in a mental hospital primarily devoted to intensive treatment of psychotic maladjustments. In large mental hospitals where the "court case" problem occurs only infrequently, there remains the problem of gang aggressive behavior due largely to "neglect" of patients whose energies need to be diverted to constructive types of occupational activities.

REFERENCES

1. Boyd, R. W., Baker, Thelma, and Greenblatt, M.: Ward social behavior: an analysis of patient interaction at highest and lowest extremes. *Nurs. Res.,* 3:77-79, 1954.
2. Kandler, H., Behymer, A. F., Kegeles, S., and Boyd, R. W.: A study of nurse-patient interaction in a mental hospital. *Am. J. Nurs.,* 52:1100-1103, 1952.
3. Kegeles, S. S., Hyde, R. W., and Greenblatt, M.: Social network on an acute psychiatric ward. *J. Group Psychotherapy, 5:* Nos. 1-3, Apr.-Nov., 91-111, 1952.
4. Kegeles, S.: Methods of sociometric analysis in a mental hospital, (MMS in preparation.)
5. Stanton, Alfred H., and Schwarz, Morris: Medical opinion and the social context in the mental hospital. *Psychiatry, 2:* No. 12, 1949.
6. Information quoted here and in following parts of the paper was drawn from three sources: interviews with patients, notes from a staff meeting, and interviews with three persons intimately acquainted with the facts in the case, e.g., a psychiatrist, a charge nurse, and an attendant.
7. From discussion with Dr. H. C. Solomon, Superintendent of Boston Psychopathic Hospital and Professor of Psychiatry in Harvard Medical School.

ॐ

CHAPTER 35   Guided Group Interaction
in a Correctional Setting*

LLOYD W. McCORKLE

THE INITIAL application of group therapy to the treatment of offenders
was largely a phenomenon of World War II. The need for manpower
resulted in the armed forces' willingness to accept experimentation in the
treatment of offenders. In addition to providing a correctional climate
where group therapy could be applied, it also enabled civilian correctional administrators serving in the armed forces to come in close contact
with these programs. The most extensive experiment with group therapeutic techniques for military offenders developed at the Fort Knox
Rehabilitation Center. There, under the leadership of Dr. Alexander
Wolf, a comprehensive group therapy program that embraced all aspects
of institutional living was initiated. This program was further implemented by the work of Dr. Joseph Abrahams and the present author.
This program has been described and its effectiveness has been evaluated.[1]

After the war a number of correctional institutions developed group
activities which they referred to as group therapy. In a survey conducted
in 1950 of 312 penal and correctional institutions, 39 responding institutions reported having a "group therapy" program. In addition several
indicated a willingness to include one in their treatment efforts. However, the same survey revealed that correctional institutions apparently
responsive to the universal tendency to be fashionable had merely re-
designated social and other types of group activities as group therapy.
This was clearly indicated in the responses: 75 per cent of the institutions incorporated group therapy into such activities as occupational
therapy, activity and orientation programs. Only 25 per cent of the institutions reported that group therapy as such was considered a part of

* Reprinted from the *International Journal of Group Psychotherapy*, 4 (1954), 199–
203, by permission of the author and the *Journal*.

the general psychotherapy program. Also in correctional institutions 58 per cent of the therapists or leaders were trained as teachers, occupational therapists, counselors, and educational directors. In general, correctional institutions rely on a lecture-discussion method, and only 9 per cent reported a psychoanalytic approach.[2]

In the development of the New Jersey group therapy programs at the training school and reformatory level it was felt advisable to differentiate clearly between group activity and other forms of group psychotherapy. In the first presentation of the New Jersey experiment in 1948, it was pointed out that "to avoid confusion with the use of group psychotherapy as practiced by psychiatrists, and to avoid any implication that all inmates are mentally abnormal and unbalanced, we decided to call the application of group therapy principles to inmates 'guided group interaction.' "[3] As this title suggests, the therapist is active in the discussion, especially in the initial sessions, and plays a critical, supportive, guiding role throughout the course of the group history. Also implied in the title is the fact that the major emphasis is on the group and its development rather than on an attempt at analysis of individuals in the group. "Guided group interaction," like all correctional techniques, makes assumptions about the kinds of socializing experiences delinquents need and can use, if they are to achieve their usefulness as responsible citizens. It assumes the delinquent will benefit from social experience where, in concert with his peers and the leader, he can freely discuss, examine and understand his problems of living, without the threats that had been so common in his previous learning experiences. It further assumes that the mutual "give and take" of group discussion stimulates the delinquent to some understanding of the relationship between what takes place in this learning situation and his immediate problems of living. Therefore, the relationships encountered, and the material discussed, must be felt by the participant as making some contribution to his critical struggle for adjustment.

If participants are not degraded or excluded from the group because of their impulsive, aggressive behavior, the "group climate" must be lenient, accepting and structured to give support to all. Freedom must exist for each participant to evolve his own role in the group, to learn to understand his present role, and opportunities must exist to develop new roles. This type of group activity requires an easy informal atmosphere where members are equals and where democratic social controls evolve out of interaction and increased understanding. It is inevitable, if these goals are reasonably achieved, for free emotional expressions to follow with the characteristic modes of adjustment of all participants exposed to one another and the therapist. In this process the participant's conception of self and others as well as the historical origin of these concepts are, through group discussion, related to his modes of adjustment. Groups of this type do not suddenly come into being because some person decides to form them. Rather, as a result of interaction and communication, members develop ways of relating to one another which makes possible the analysis of behavior patterns.[4]

The above description suggests some of the major difficulties involved in the establishment of "guided group interaction" program in the unique correctional environment. When the outside community and the correctional community are compared as the immediate external situations for group therapy, certain striking differences appear. An analysis of these differences, especially in terms of their negative aspects, would appear essential prior to the setting up of therapy groups in the controlled social ferment which constitutes a correctional institution. It is a universal observation that therapeutic changes in the personality are accompanied by increased anxiety and tension. In the various stages of the group history the individual is subjected to experiences increasingly threatening to his established self-image. The deep-rooted defenses of the inmate are pierced and he frequently emerges from the sessions in a temporarily "crippled state" produced by the destruction of a previously important prop of the self.

At this point, the striking difference between the correctional institution and the external community as a setting for group therapy is seen. The patient emerging from the therapist's office on the outside can, in a sense, lose himself in a multiplicity of noncritical interpersonal situations. Thus the more "anonymity" the external community provides, the greater are its shock-absorbing potentials. For the person outside there are more places to hide and lick wounds, and more ways to distribute compensatory reactions to the inevitable initial feelings of personal devaluation. One of the supportive conditions of group therapy on the outside is the patient's ability to escape from the group. In the correctional institution, the inmate cannot really leave the group. He is involved in numerous other activities and living experiences with the same people with whom he has shared intimate revelations, frequently against his will and in spite of all attempts at control and disguises. These individuals include his peers, his competitors, his enemies, or friends of his enemies— persons continually on the watch for signs of weakness or vulnerability.

The inmate, especially one of high status—and the higher the status the greater need for the emotional breaking down in most cases—has one of two unhappy alternatives at this point. The more healthy of these alternatives is to abandon his compensatory defenses and accept the more realistic image of himself. But this ideal alternative has many difficulties in correctional institutions where the wearing of socially appropriate masks is frequently the condition of personal survival. The individual who has committed himself to an aggressive leadership role has inevitably made enemies of those aspiring to a similar role and, like the despot in a feudal society, he can abandon his status only at his peril. Yet, these individuals are at the same time the most appropriate targets of an ambitious therapy program, since they form the major psychological supports of the antisocial inmate community.

This condition almost inevitably predisposes the inmate of high status under therapeutic attack to adopt a less healthy but more immediate comforting adjustment of aggressive compensation. This adjustment is full of danger to other inmates to whom the inmate now feels it necessary to reassert his threatened role. Another aspect of this situation is presented by the previously low-status inmate who has gained strength from the group experience as a result of measuring himself against the high-status figure under attack. Where the latter is confronted with the painful prospect of a world to lose, the former is powerfully tempted by the prospect of a new world to win.

In this way, the therapeutic group in the correctional institution, if it is effective, must take the risk of becoming a manufactory of human projectiles let loose in a social situation which already has all the aspects of a human arsenal. It is therefore the moral obligation of the therapist to consider very carefully the serious question of the adequacy of the control elements in the institution, and the extent to which these are able to cope with the multiple tensions which will be generated. Failure to anticipate the effects of this added source of instability in an already inherently unstable situation will defeat the objectives of the program.

What are the gains for delinquents who participate in "guided group interaction" sessions? To find some answers to this question a research program was established in 1950 to evaluate the import on young offenders of a program oriented around guided group interaction.[5] Although this study will not be completed for several years, the results to date seem encouraging. In a preliminary report on the sentence completion records of twenty-five boys exposed to "guided group interaction," an investigator's tentative findings can be summarized as follows: On the post-test the records reveal less blocking, less suspicion and distrust, less dependence on platitudes, greater ego strength, increased ability to carry conflicts into consciousness, more realistic in the appraisal of self, more hopeful of the future, but there was some increase in depression. The answer to whether or not this will be reflected in improved relationships with authority in general and the law in particular must await the final report of this research.[6] It should also be borne in mind that the above results were obtained in a highly unusual correctional situation, more similar to the freer external community than to the rigid compressed human environment in conventional correctional settings.

NOTES TO CHAPTER 35

1. Abrahams, J. and McCorkle, L. W.: "Group Psychotherapy on Military Offenders." *Am. J. Sociol.*, March 1946; *idem:* "Group Psychotherapy at an Army Rehabilitation Center." *Dis. Nerv. System*, February 1947.

2. McCorkle, L. W.: "Present Status of Group Therapy in United States Correctional Institutions." *This Journal,* 3:79-87, 1953.

3. Bixby, F. L. and McCorkle, L. W.: "A Recorded Presentation of a Program of Guided Group Interaction in New Jersey's Correctional Institutions." *Proceedings of the Seventy-eighth Annual Congress of Correction of American Prison Association,* 1948.

4. McCorkle, L. W.: "Group Therapy in Treatment of Offenders." *Federal Probation,* December 1952.

5. Bixby, F. L.: "A Plan for Short-Term Treatment of Youthful Offenders." National Probation and Parole Association Conference, Atlantic City, New Jersey, April 27, 1950.

6. Weeks, H. A.: "Preliminary Evaluation of the Highfields Project." *Am. Sociol. Rev.,* 18, June, 1953.

CHAPTER 36   Social Structure and Interaction
Processes on a Psychiatric Ward*

WILLIAM CAUDILL, FREDRICK C. REDLICH,
HELEN R. GILMORE, AND EUGENE B. BRODY

THE INDIVIDUAL who enters a mental hospital finds himself placed in a number of new social situations, all of which influence his behavior and treatment. The patient's relationship to his therapist, both in its administrative and therapeutic aspects, has received the most study. This holds true where the course of treatment is through insight psychotherapy (13, 14), and also where it involves a structuring of the patient's social milieu by prescribing how hospital personnel shall react to him (1, 31, 40). More recently, the influence on the patient of the over-all social structure of the hospital has been investigated (2, 34, 35), as well as the structure of certain types of wards (9, 10), and the social processes at work in the split social field existing between patients and staff (21, 36, 37, 38, 39, 42).

For information on a third social influence, the interpersonal relationships of patients with each other, we must, however, rely largely on patients' autobiographical accounts of their experiences (3, 7, 19, 23, 24, 33). Despite the importance of this area of life in the mental hospital, it has, beyond an occasional astute reference (32), received little systematic attention and no methods have been developed for pursuing such a problem. The problem becomes a particularly crucial one when thought of in terms of the effect on each other of those less disturbed neurotic and psychotic patients who retain intact, and utilize, many of their social personality characteristics and interaction techniques.

Because it is so important a variable, we wished to make a study of this third area of social influence in the lives of patients despite the recognition of the many difficulties which would be encountered in obtaining

* Reprinted from the *American Journal of Orthopsychiatry*, 22 (1952), 314–333.

adequate data. Although we are fully aware of the importance of unconscious determinants of interpersonal behavior, the present study has
concerned itself primarily with a definition of the social reality in which
the patients find themselves. Before field work was begun, an outline was
made of the most pertinent problems to be explored: 1) The interpersonal
relations on the ward between patients and patients, patients and nurses,
and patients and physicians. 2) The social psychological processes involved in becoming a patient after admission, and ceasing to be a patient
as the time of discharge approached. 3) The value and belief systems of
the patient group, and the general attitudes to life in the hospital centering around both administration and therapy. 4) The difficulties experienced by the patients as a group in communicating with the various levels
of the staff hierarchy, and the reflection of these difficulties in the operation of the control and decision-making functions invested in the staff.

Two methods were used in gathering data: Initially, in order to determine some of the social and therapeutic problems of life in a mental
hospital as seen through the eyes of the patients, we decided to have an
observer undergo the experience of being a patient. Known only to two
senior members of the staff, he was admitted to the less disturbed ward of
the hospital and, upon being assigned to one of the psychiatric residents
for therapy, he followed a course of treatment for two months.[1] Secondly,
after a turnover in the patient population, the same observer acted as an
assistant in the activities program for several months. This paper will
present material only from the first set of observations, but the major
points emphasized here were found to hold true for both of the patient
populations.

Neither of the methods used was completely satisfactory. In the first,
the observer, by living on the ward, was in a position to experience the
full round of life and to interact with the patients as people. Coupled with
these advantages there were, however, disadvantages. While to our knowledge no discernible harm was done to the therapeutic progress of any of
the patients, it was recognized that this might have occurred. We were
also mindful of other ethical considerations, of the personal strain on the
observer in undergoing psychotherapy, and of the fact that the observer's
identification with the patients would inevitably result in some degree of
subjectivity in the data. A partial check on such biasing was provided by
having the observer include in his daily record many of his own emotional
reactions to the events of hospital life. As the observer had going-out
privileges after his first week of treatment, he left the hospital each afternoon for a few hours and used this time to work up his material. Despite
its disadvantages, the first method provided a rich body of data concerning many problems, hitherto only incompletely recognized, which were
faced by the patients as a social group in their life on the ward. The
second method, while allowing the observer to be known, had the disad-

vantages of restricting his participation to specific ward activities which were essentially isolated from the flow of day-to-day life. It might be feasible to work out an alternative procedure whereby a known observer could live on the ward on a twenty-four-hour-a-day basis.[2]

The observations were carried out in a small private mental hospital connected with a psychiatric training center. Treatment of the patients was primarily through dynamically oriented psychotherapy. Each patient was assigned to a psychiatric resident who was under the supervision of a physician-in-charge. The resident assumed direct responsibility for most of the management and for the therapeutic care of his patients. Apart from routine contacts on rounds, a patient usually saw his therapist for one hour a day, five days a week. The remainder of a patient's schedule was worked out very sketchily, as only a limited recreational and activities program was available.

The hospital was divided into three wards. Two of these were locked wards located on the second floor where the more severely disturbed psychotic patients were treated. The third was a less disturbed ward on the first floor which accommodated both male and female patients, most of whom were diagnosed as suffering from various types of severe psychoneuroses. This paper will be concerned only with the patients on this last ward, in which each sex occupied a separate wing containing eight private rooms, a four-bed dormitory and a living room. Men and women intermingled in the two living rooms except at mealtime.

As the average stay in the hospital was over two months, the patient population was quite stable during the period in which the observations were made. All told, there were 12 male and 15 female patients on the ward, most of whom were between twenty and thirty-five years of age. The majority came from upper middle class homes, although there were a few from upper lower, lower middle, and upper class backgrounds. Three were Jewish; two were Catholic; the rest were Protestant. There was one Negro patient.

OBSERVATIONS

FROM the moment the observer left his room on his first day in the hospital and joined the patient group at the evening meal, he felt pressure upon him to act in certain ways.[3] As he took his food tray from the cart, he was told by several patients that they had been unable to eat during their first meal at the hospital. As a consequence, he only toyed with his food. During the meal he mentioned that he should write some letters, and was told, "You can't be very sick if you are going to write letters." He feebly parried this by saying that he probably would not get an answer anyway. After the supper trays had been removed by a nurse, and the therapists had made their evening rounds, the group asked him if he played bridge, and was overjoyed to find that he did. After several rubbers, it seemed expected of him that he would retire to his room, and he did so. At ten o'clock he heard a nurse ask the group to go to their rooms, but two of the patients later returned to the living room and he overheard them discussing their problems for several hours until he fell asleep.

Although he would have been unable to categorize them so neatly at the time, there had been, even in his first day's experience, pressures exerted on the observer by the other patients for adherence to certain attitudes in four areas of life—toward the self, toward other patients, toward therapy and the therapist, and toward nurses and other hospital personnel.

Pressures for attitudes toward the self. On the second day, following a conference with his therapist, the observer expressed resentment over not having going-out privileges to visit the library and work on his book— his compulsive concern over his inability to finish this task being one of the factors leading to his hospitalization. Immediately two patients, Mr. Hill and Mrs. Lewis,[4] who were later to become his closest friends, told him he was being "defensive"; since his doctor did not wish him to do such work, it was probably better "to lay off of it." Mr. Hill went on to say that one of his troubles when he first came to the hospital was thinking of things that he had to do or thought he had to do. He said that now he did not bother about anything. Mrs. Lewis said that at first she had treated the hospital as a sort of hotel and had spent her therapeutic hours "charming" her doctor, but it had been pointed out to her by others that this was a mental hospital and that she should actively work with her doctor if she expected to get well.

The observer later saw such pressure applied time and again to other patients, and he came to realize that the group attempted to push its members toward a middle ground where they would not, as in his case and that of Mrs. Lewis, attempt to deny the reality of the hospital. On the other hand, pressure was also brought to bear on those patients who went to other extremes by engaging in too much immature acting-out behavior, who regressed too far, or who denied the emotional basis of their illness. For example, one day shortly after his arrival, the following incident, thereafter to be repeated almost exactly each day, occurred:

Dr. Johnson came by on evening rounds and Mr. Davis made a great fuss, taking him down the hall and swearing violently at him. After Dr. Johnson had left, Mr. Davis stormed back to the table saying that Dr. Johnson told him that by such actions he was trying to destroy all the patients on the ward. But, Mr. Davis continued, all that he wanted out of life was to be a pants presser; he did not want any of that intellectual stuff. Mr. Brown and Mr. Hill told Mr. Davis that he only created these scenes when his doctor showed up; he did not need to do this as he was all right and quiet at all other times. Mr. Davis admitted this.

Equally, the patients sympathized with Mr. Brown when he periodically took to his bed and requested that he be cared for, but they also told him that he was resisting leaving the hospital and that ultimately he would have to go out and get a job. Also, while Mr. Anderson and Mrs. Smith were positive that their ills were "purely physical," and continually attempted to convince others of this, the patients only smiled and pointed out that the doctors would not allow people to come "just for a rest," and that everyone in the hospital had emotional problems.

The patients felt certain that their doctors had as one of their major aims the requiring of patients to give up their "defenses." As the patients interpreted most of their ordinary social activities as defenses, the problem was phrased by Mr. Hill when he said that his doctor kept telling him he had to give up all his defenses but that he could not see this, as what would he have left?

Pressures for attitudes toward other patients. During his first few days in the hospital the observer was frequently told, "You cannot really refuse anything people ask of you around here," and he saw this belief put into action in many small ways. He was also told many stories of recent dramatic incidents, such as that of a recent suicide and what a swell person the patient had been; and he was introduced to what might be called the folklore of the group concerning stories of bizarre and rather humorous behavior on the part of previous patients, such as that of the patient who had been brought in nude upon a stretcher screaming that she expected a telephone call from a producer in Hollywood, and who later did receive the call. Late one night a patient upstairs created a violent and noisy commotion which awakened a number of patients who congregated in the hall. The observer was told, in the warmest terms, of this patient's personal sexual problems and, at the same time, of what a nice person he really was. It was to be noted that such incidents and stories were often treated humorously, but they were almost never treated negatively. The gossip and backbiting that might be expected to develop in a closely confined group were far overshadowed by an emphasis on the positive qualities of a person and a suspension of the direct expression of judgment in other areas.

The patients felt that many of the ordinary conventions and social gestures of the outer world were made temporarily meaningless by hospital life. On one occasion the observer, who had been asked if he cared to go downtown, said he would like to do so if his friend did not mind waiting until he changed his clothes. The friend laughingly chided him to the effect that he had forgotten where he was, that in the hospital one had all the time in the world. On the other hand, small courtesies and expressions of approval that would be carried out almost unconsciously in the outer world often became conscious problems. If one overheard, and enjoyed, a patient playing the piano, should one applaud the performance, or would such approval call forth a neurotic response? Would others overreact and feel hurt if several patients wished to go to a movie alone and did not freely extend the invitation to the entire group? Such problems as these formed part of the belief that one was not free to release oneself fully in the hospital, and that it was very difficult for an individual to satisfy his need to be alone at times.

Although acquaintances among the patients would be made on the basis of similar backgrounds and interests, and much time was spent in gossiping about the social characteristics of others, these activities lacked the invidious overtones they would have carried in the outer world. Along with this went a muting of outer-world distinctions on the basis of race, ethnic group or social class—it was as if the patients had agreed that such categories had little meaning in a hospital. Such an orientation of one's behavior was made easier by the commonly held belief that since none of the group expected to see the others again, it was not necessary to relate one's outside status to life on the ward.

While there was a suspension of the direct expression of judgment, and a much greater tolerance of wide ranges of behavior than would have been true in social situations on the outside, there were limits to such behavior even in the patient group. For example:

One evening a number of the patients had brought in several kinds of cheese, rye bread, and Coca Cola, which they were sharing with the group. Mr. Davis, whose behavior was characterized by aggressive, adolescent outbursts of ranting toward his therapist, immediately began to grab large amounts of the food in a very ill-mannered way. The three women to whom the food belonged became angry and gave Mr. Davis a severe tongue-lashing, calling him "an ill-bred, emotionally immature kid," etc. However, one of the women shortly brought the group together again by saying, "Well, what the hell, we are all in the same boat in this place, so don't worry about it, it's all right." Unity was re-established, the food was shared, and the group then proceeded to get a great deal of enjoyment out of playing a crossword-puzzle game introduced by Mr. Davis.

It was almost as if whenever, within the hospital setting, a disagreeable episode took place, the unity of the group, and its tolerance, had of necessity to reassert itself. Beyond the suspension of judgment, it was also noted that patients expected others to support and sustain them in their activities and roles even if this meant ignoring some of the rules of the hospital:

Mr. Brown very cleverly made stuffed cloth animals which he sold to the other patients at slightly above cost. There was a rule against patients' selling articles to each other; the nurse in charge had spoken to Mr. Brown about this several times, and the patients knew that in buying the animals they were going against the wishes of the hospital. Nevertheless, they felt that it was more important to support Mr. Brown in a productive activity that gave him pleasure than to obey a rule that they thought had little meaning in this case.

Beyond the simple supporting of others, it quickly became apparent that a type of therapy—characterized by sympathetic listening and the making of suggestions—would be carried out among close acquaintances. For example:

Mr. Davis and Mr. Wright were close friends. When Mr. Wright went out with his wife one night, Mr. Davis sat up until 1 A.M. waiting for him in order to see how he would be feeling. On the other hand, the next day Mr. Davis was stirring up a great storm over trying to get out of the ward because he had received some letters from his wife that made him want to leave. Mr. Wright took Mr. Davis to his room, talked to him, got him a glass of milk, and calmed him down. Such scenes were repeated daily between these two patients; after one particularly bad period, Mr. Davis jokingly said that Mr. Wright was going to send him a bill for consultation services since Mr. Wright had sat up and talked with him all night.

Pressures for attitudes toward therapy and therapists. When, on the morning of his second day, the observer attributed his sick stomach to the colorless, liquid sedative that he had been given the night before, the patients told him that this had been paraldehyde, that it was given to alcoholics and was one of the most powerful sedatives used in the hospital. This led to a discussion of the nature of each other's problems which concluded with the agreement that every case was different and that one could not generalize. Partly because of this attitude, there was a strong feeling that a patient should keep his actual relations with his therapist, and what went on during his conference hours, separate from his life on the ward. However, while the patients often adopted the pose that "the conferences weren't helping very much," they would privately discuss their progress with their closer friends, and felt they had to hold to the belief that one's doctor was competent in his therapeutic capacity; one must cooperate with him in order to make any progress and should not question his authority.[5]

The patients believed that therapy was "somehow psychoanalytical," that one had "to go back into childhood," and that therapy went on "twenty-four hours a day." One evening a group of eleven patients were discussing the lack of activities in the hospital, and they came to the conclusion that it was part of a conscious plan by the staff to increase the intensity of "twenty-four-hour-a-day" therapy. The matter was summed up when one patient said he thought that therapy in the hospital was better than having a psychoanalysis on the outside, because in the latter case your hour of therapy was sandwiched between many other activities, whereas in the hospital you could work on your problems all the time.

Not infrequently, many patients despaired of the seemingly endless one-way talk involved in psychotherapy. They felt that they were repeating the same story over and over again until it lost all emotional feeling and became rote. They felt that their doctors never told them anything in their conferences. They were concerned about the end goal of therapy, feeling that this was kept concealed and that they never seemed to be moving toward whatever it was. Somewhat fatalistically, they felt that the doctors took "a long-range view" and did not think of the financial expense involved.[6] While they had to believe that psychotherapy was helpful, they were disturbed because few patients seemed to get better, or to leave the hospital as "cured." Since the patients all shared in such frustrations and doubts, the group was tolerant of occasional aggressive outbursts about one's doctor in his therapeutic capacity, and sanctioned criticism and caricature of the staff's behavior as this manifested itself in attending to administrative duties, making rounds, or in unexpected meetings outside of the hospital.

The patients generally agreed that while they all shared some similar experiences in their conferences, there were also great differences depending on the individual patient and doctor. The characterizations made by the patients of the doctors' personalities seemed to be a blend of projection by the patient of his problems onto the doctor, and a very astute, intuitive grasp of the doctor's own emotional or social problems. For example:

Mr. Hill and Mr. Davis got into a discussion about the differences in their conferences. Mr. Hill said that Dr. Black worries more than he does. He said that they both sit and frown at each other and look worried. Mr. Hill said that he would say something and then sit and worry about it, and Dr. Black would look at him with a worried expression and say, "What do you think that means?" They would then sit in silence and worry together for a while. Usually about that time the sounds of an explosion would occur in the next office and it would be Mr. Davis screaming and swearing at the top of his lungs at Dr. Johnson. Mr. Hill said that one day Dr. Black had inadvertently laughed at something Mr. Davis was shouting at Dr. Johnson in the next office, and then Dr. Black was confused and embarrassed toward Mr. Hill over the effect his laughter might have had on the conference hour.

Pressures for attitudes toward nurses and other hospital personnel. As the observer was playing bridge on his second day, a nurse came by and said to one of the players, "I bet you are beating them at this game, I'll bet." After she had left, Mr. Davis commented that she had "treated us like seven-year-olds." Shortly, another nurse did essentially the same thing. At another time, the staff, without consulting the patients, decided to give them a Valentine party. Many of the patients did not wish to go, but did so anyway as they felt that they should not hurt the feelings of the student nurses who had organized the party. The games introduced by the nurses were on a very childish level; many of the patients felt silly playing them and were glad when the party was over and they could go back to activities of their own choosing.

The patients knew that the nurses, particularly the students, sat around in the living rooms "in order to get material for their reports," and hence the patients felt that the nurses were fair game for occasional kidding. For example:

A nurse was listening to a conversation between Mrs. Lewis and Mr. Brown. So Mrs. Lewis joked with Mr. Brown by saying, "You didn't come in and say good night to me last night." Then she turned to the nurse and said, "You know, Mr. Brown is in and out of my room all night long." Mr. Brown smiled and said, "Yes, of course, that's true."

While the patients ignored the fact that the nurses overheard many of their conversations, there was a definite feeling in the group that one should not inform on another patient in answer to a direct request for information from the nurse:

During the night, Mr. Sullivan had had an anxiety attack and had been taken care of by Mr. Brown, who wrapped him in a blanket and rubbed his temples until he went to sleep. When Mr. Sullivan awakened again, another patient read to him for several hours. The night nurse, of course, must have observed this behavior. Nevertheless, when a student nurse asked at breakfast the next morning how late Mr. Sullivan had been up, none of the group of male patients would answer her.

Since there was little of what is ordinarily thought of as "nursing" to be done on the first-floor ward, the patients utilized the nurses to a considerable degree for domestic or routine service purposes—the nurses served the meals, called cabs, mailed letters, etc. A number of the nurses said that they preferred to work on the locked wards where they felt that there was more "real" nursing. They were ambivalent about their domestic role on the first floor and communicated this feeling to the patients by occasional casual remarks such as, at mealtime, "Be sure and leave a tip for the waitress."[7]

Life on the ward. One of the observer's strongest impressions during his first day on the ward was the feeling of boredom and ennui existing among the patients, several of whom told him that "tomorrow would be just another day with nothing to do but sit around, or play bridge and ping-pong." Actually, as there were few organized activities or secondary types of therapy available, the patients, for the most part, utilized each other to develop a social life. Bridge was played interminably, endless numbers of crossword puzzles were worked cooperatively, while the daily cryptogram in the newspaper was copied out and the patients avidly competed for the solution.

The staff tended to look upon the games and activities of the patients as "fads," in the sense of a passing fashion or fancy. They were much more than this, as they provided simple settings for realistic role taking and helped to bind the group together. The considerable quantity of food the patients brought in from the outside to share with others served much the same function.[8] Snacks, such as *salami*, cheese, pumpernickel, popcorn and Coca Cola, lent a zest lacking in the crackers and chocolate milk provided by the hospital twice a day as "nourishment." Despite the frequent tacit disapproval of the nurses, the consumption of these snacks was usually made into a social rite which complemented the evening-at-home atmosphere the patients created in the living rooms. The social stimulus value of these evening gatherings was heightened by the interaction of small friendship groups which were supported by the patients because they increased the potential for social participation and conversation in the group. Such activities provided reassurance for the patients that they could still, in some measure, interact on an adult level, and also represented a partly conscious resistance to those aspects of the hospital routine which were unduly "infantilizing."

The patients noted that the lack of activities, and the restraint placed on their freedom of action in many areas of life, both by the hospital and the pressure of the patient group, resulted in a great overemphasis on words, and the talking about rather than carrying out of actions. This symptom was labeled "diarrhea of the mouth." For much the same reasons, new physical objects on the ward assumed an importance all out of proportion to that they would have had in the outer world. A new couch placed in the men's living room became a focus of attention and topic of conversation for over a month; while previously the patients had distributed themselves in both living rooms during the evening, they now all congregated on the men's side.

Given the situation in the hospital, the patient group, if it wished a social life, had no choice but to turn inward and, so far as possible, to develop the potentialities of its members. This is what happened, and the resulting social structure is best seen in terms of the implementation of the values of the patient group through the role and clique system that operated in the life on the ward.

VALUE AND ROLE SYSTEMS

As THE sorts of pressures that have been discussed were felt by the observer, he came gradually to realize that the attitudes held by the patients were formed into a pattern of values, some of which were verbalized, while others might be inferred from the consistency of behavior. This *value system* might, in summary form, be stated as follows: 1) Toward oneself. (a) A patient should not deny the reality of being in the hospital for therapeutic purposes, (b) should give up his "defenses," and (c) should try to bring himself to a middle ground where he neither engaged in extreme regressive behavior nor attempted to carry on life as if the hospital did not exist. 2) Toward other patients. (a) A patient should suspend judgment and attempt to see all sides of a person, (b) sustain and support others, and (c) if requested, try actively to help them with their problems by doing a sort of therapy with them. 3) Toward therapy and the therapist. (a) A patient should try to believe in the ability and competence of his doctor, (b) cooperate in working with him, and (c) feel that treatment on a "twenty-four-a-day" basis in the hospital was better than therapy received in the outer world. 4) Toward nurses and other personnel. (a) A patient should try to be thoughful and pleasant, and (b) cooperate by abiding by the rules of the hospital up to the point where either the demands of the nurses became unreasonable, or the rules conflicted with a more important value toward other patients.

This value system of the patient group was translated into action by ascribing to each new member what may be called the *role of a patient*. This role required that one act in accordance with the complex of values and behavior patterns expected of every patient as described above. In addition, each individual played a *personal role* rooted in his background outside the hospital; that is, he presented himself as a certain kind of person to the patient group. The individual patient, then, had the task of integrating his personal role with the role of a patient; or, at least, seeing to it that the values and behavior characteristic of his personal role did not directly conflict with those of the patient role.[9]

If a patient would accept and play the ascribed role of a patient, especially as it entailed mutual tolerance and responsibility for others, then the group would, in turn, support the patient in his personal role. Particularly this was true if the personal role of the patient served some positive function in the group. For example, Mr. Brown's imitations of the doctors, nurses and other patients were a real source of catharsis for the group; and Mr. Davis's immature explosions toward the staff provided vicarious satisfaction for others,[10] while his expertness at bridge and at solving cryptograms was a source of recreation.

The integration of one's personal role with that of the patient role often required that an individual make a conscious effort to channel his personal abilities and resources into the helping of others. For example, Mrs. Lewis was a fashionably dressed woman who purposely went out of her way to help Miss Wood with her clothes; Miss Wood, in her turn, had considerable competence in massage and provided this service for a number of the women patients.[11] The group went so far as to try to establish a function for a patient's personal role if one did not seem self-evident, and through this process the observer's library work and interest in music were drawn into the orbit of the group by having him obtain books and record albums for others.

It was possible to set up a continuum on the basis of the degree of success achieved by the patients in the integration of their personal roles with the role of a patient. The nature of such an integration had a great deal to do with the place occupied by a patient in the total structure of the group.

One extreme was represented by Mr. Hill, whose personal role coincided almost completely with what was expected of him in the role of a patient. He was a passive, nonthreatening person who was very sensitive to group approval and pressure; he had good social techniques and skills for relating to others, and a nice dry sense of humor which he utilized a great deal but never in such a way as to hurt other patients. He was always willing to sustain any activity of the group and was receptive when others came to him for support or therapy. On the other hand, he frequently sought out other patients to ask their advice. While it would be difficult to speak of "leadership" among the patients because, owing to the nature of their situation in the hospital, there were few goals toward which the group as a whole might have been led, Mr. Hill represented the most highly pivotal person on the ward, with whom all of the patients acknowledged some ties.

The other extreme was represented by Miss Ford, whose personal role conflicted in almost all respects with what was expected of her in the role of a patient. Since she felt a need to belong to the patient group, this conflict of roles was a source of anxiety for her. She said that she thought of the hospital as "just like college" and treated her doctor as a professor who would hand her the answers to her problems. She stated that she wanted nothing to do with anyone else's troubles, and hence she made little effort to support other patients. She openly expressed anti-Semitism, was aggressive and hostile to the Negro patient, and was snobbish and class-conscious. Indeed, while she continually tried to participate socially, most of her conversation was derogatory of others. As a consequence, she incurred the hostility of the group and was rejected and isolated because, although she wished to belong to the patient group, she would not carry out its values and responsibilities. Hers was a very different type of isolation from the occasional self-imposed withdrawal of Mrs. Gray, which was respected by the patients, or from the complete isolation imposed on himself by Mr. Reed. Though physically present on the ward, Mr. Reed never entered the social field of the patients, who held an entirely neutral attitude toward him and scarcely recognized his existence.

Most of the patients interacting in the group fell somewhere between the extremes sketched above. Their personal roles did not completely coincide with the role of a patient, but they did accept the society's values and in turn received support. It cannot be said that the place occupied by a patient in the group structure was entirely what might have been expected from his previous psychodynamic history. Mr. Hill was much more highly rewarded for his type of behavior in the patient group than he would have been in the outer world, where he would have been marked as too passive a person. On the other hand, Miss Ford would probably not have been so rigidly censored for her nonsupportive and often hostile behavior by the outer world. This does not mean that she would have exhibited less anxiety, or found life easier, on the outside as the hospital still served as a refuge. It is indicated, however, that the nature of a patient's social integration into the group will affect his therapeutic progress, and both Mr. Hill and Miss Ford, for opposite reasons, experienced more than ordinary difficulty in ultimately leaving the protection of the hospital environment—the former because of his overdependence on the group, the latter because she received too little support.

A further aspect of the social structure of the patient group lay in its encouragement of various types of cliques, one of which was the boy-and-girl team. For example, Mr. Brown and Miss Gaynor spent a great deal of their time together and often joked about the amusing incidents that happened in town when clerks would mistake them for man and wife; they formed a unit in the "evenings at home" held by the group in the living rooms, where Mr. Brown would work on his cloth animals and Miss Gaynor would knit. Once, when Mr. Brown and Miss Gaynor gave a popcorn party for the group, Mrs. Gray jokingly said that all they needed were "His" and "Her" aprons. Such romantic attachments were approved so long as they remained flirtatious and casual because they served to increase social interaction, which was one of the main sociological functions of the clique. If, however, such attachments went beyond this point, they were frowned upon because any behavior which might lead to serious social consequences was felt as threatening by the group.[12] In general, if a clique, for whatever reasons, became so interested in itself that it drew away from the group, this was felt as a social loss and pressure was applied to bring it again into the wider social field.

A second function of the clique, examples of which have already been given, was to act as a mutual therapy group; a third was to provide opportunities to let off steam and thus act as a safety valve since it was not always easy for a patient to maintain a constant attitude of tolerance and support toward all other patients; while a fourth function became operative when a patient felt disturbed and wished to draw away from the group, but did not want to isolate himself completely. The last two functions of the clique can be seen in the following example:

The clique of Mr. Hill, Mr. Porter and Mrs. Lewis frequently joked with each other in an aggressive manner they never used toward other patients. Mrs. Lewis felt free to call Mr. Hill a "fathead"; Mr. Porter kidded Mr. Hill about torturing himself; and Mrs. Hill told Mr. Porter that he seemed to work endlessly on his book, and should just give up academic life. At another time, when the three of them were alone, Mr. Hill told how he disliked Miss Ford, and Mrs. Lewis spoke of how Mrs. Jones hounded and tagged after her. Mr. Hill said that this place stifled him; the boredom got on his nerves. He expressed resentment about the four-bed ward in which he slept, saying that Mr. Sullivan kept the radio on all the time, Mr. Owens was always doing push-ups, and Mr. Miller's only topic of conversation was his "dear old mother." Mr. Hill went on to say that he felt guilty because he had made himself scarce from Mr. Davis today, but that being around Mr. Davis every other day was enough.

Another type of clique, restricted to a predominately social function, was formed, especially among the women, on the basis of similarity in background outside the hospital. There was a clique of young adolescent girls; a second composed of those women who like to sew, cook, and follow other domestic pursuits; while a third consisted of those women with interests in literature, music, art and fashion. There was occasional friction between these cliques as, for example, when Miss Ford was attempting to move into one of the women's groups:

Supper being over, Mrs. Lewis came back to the men's side quite furious and angry. It seemed that there was a "plot" instigated by Miss Ford to break up the group of women who usually ate together at the larger table in the women's living room. Before the meal was served, Miss Ford and Miss Gaynor had spread their knitting paraphernalia over half of the larger table and had said those places were reserved. Miss Ford commented rather pointedly to Mrs. Gray, Mrs. Peterson and Mrs. Lewis about "you intellectuals who play Sark and do crossword puzzles while we sit around and do knitting." Mrs. Lewis said that Mrs. Gray and Mrs. Peterson were really working themselves up to "jumping down Miss Ford's throat" if she continued behavior of this kind.

In general, the women remained separated in small cliques, whereas the men formed a single, loosely integrated group that functioned with little discord. Many patients remarked on the fact that the women's side seemed to be in a state of constant minor turmoil in contrast to the relative peace reigning among the men.

From the patients' point of view, the purpose of the group structure just described was, first of all, to develop among themselves the opportunities for social activities otherwise lacking in the hospital environment by maximizing the number of interpersonal relationships and roles available to an individual, while at the same time trying to keep any serious social consequences of these relationships at a minimum; and, secondly, to provide the members of the group with as supportive and ego-sustaining a milieu as was possible without coming into conflict with the staff or the routine of the hospital.[13] Nevertheless, conflicts did arise because the staff, both doctors and nurses, seemed unacquainted with many aspects of life in the patient group, and dealt with each individual as a separate entity in administrative details as well as in therapeutic matters. In part, this was due to the fact that there was no channel provided by which the patients, as a group, could voice their desires to the staff. If a group of patients wished to make a request, this could be done only by each patient's taking the matter up, as an individual, with his therapist. For example:

A number of the patients had been trying to arrange suitable facilities for listening to music. Their general request was that the hospital either repair the broken phonograph in the living room, or allow another machine—kept in the occupational therapy shop and available only during the time that other patients were using the jig saw, etc.—to be brought on the ward, where it would be more accessible and the surroundings were more conducive to listening. The occupational therapist, however, refused the latter part of this request. Since there was no channel whereby the group could express their desires, the patients who were most interested in music approached their therapists and the nurses on an individual basis. This they did for several weeks. At about this point, the patients' therapists began to use the conference hours to inquire as to the personal meaning music had for the individual patients. Six weeks after the patients made their initial requests, the phonograph in the living room was repaired. The patients were pleased, bought record albums, and formed a music clique. On the afternoon the phonograph was returned, a group of six patients were listening to music at the time the therapists made their rounds, but none of the doctors made a social remark about the pleasure of having the machine in working order.

As a result of this situation, the emphasis placed by the staff upon those aspects of the patients' day-to-day behavior that were brought to their attention was almost solely upon the meaning of this behavior in terms of the patients' individual psychodynamic histories, and seldom was any attention focused on factors inherent in the immediate group situation. When, for example, their doctors attempted to separate the boy-and-girl team of Mr. Brown and Miss Gaynor for therapeutic reasons, they did not fully realize that they were also modifying the place occupied by these two patients in the social group, and hence indirectly affecting the lives of all the patients. Further, since in this case administrative as well as therapeutic control was in the hands of the same doctor, Mr. Brown and Miss Gaynor would be denied permission by their therapists to attend a movie outside the hospital with other patients on one evening, and the next morning would be placed in the position of having to discuss the psychodynamic implications of their desires with the same therapists.

The lack of a channel of communication, and an insufficient separation between administration and therapy, increased the mutual isolation of patients and staff. Both patients and staff structured their actions in accordance with a set of values and beliefs, but because the values and beliefs of each group were only incompletely known or understood by the other, the two groups viewed one another in terms of stereotypes which impeded an accurate evaluation of social reality. Such a situation, when coupled with alternating periods of permissive and restrictive administrative control, probably helps to account for the mood swings in the patient group. One week a general air of depression would prevail, at other times the ward had the atmosphere of a hotel, while again a feeling of rebellion would come over the entire group.

DISCUSSION

THIS paper has emphasized the point that psychoneurotic patients on a less disturbed ward of a mental hospital should not be thought of as an aggregate of individuals, but as a group which tries to meet many of its problems by developing a shared set of values and beliefs translated into action through a system of social roles and cliques. Some of the problems faced by the patient group in ordering the interaction of its members would seem to have been due directly to the factor of emotional illness. Since all of the members were emotionally disturbed, they had all experienced a high level of anxiety during their life in the outer world over their inability to play certain required social roles without introducing extraneous behavior stemming from neurotic conflicts.[14] The particular patient group reported on here recognized this problem and provided for it by its values of suspension of judgment and support. In so doing, the patients were acting in ways very similar to those noted by Rowland (34) for the patients on the less disturbed wards of another mental hospital where interaction was characterized by "small, closed friendship groups," having "a maximum of insight and sympathetic interpenetration," with a "rigid control of affect in terms of group standards."

The patient group also sensed that because of hospitalization, an individual was not only relieved from playing roles in those areas of life where he experienced particular difficulty, but was also cut off from playing those roles in other areas of life which furnished him with some measure of self-esteem. Since few substitutes for these latter roles, in the form of short-range realistic goals and activities, were provided in the hospital, the patient group attempted to meet this problem by increasing opportunities for role taking through utilizing the personal attributes of the patients.

Many other problems of the patient group arose, however, because the patients and staff lived, as Rowland (35) has expressed it, "in two entirely separate social worlds, yet . . . in the closest proximity." While the staff exercised control over the patients, they did not give recognition to the patient world as a social group, but rather, they interpreted the behavior of the patients almost solely in individual dynamic-historical terms. The patient group, thus lacking an adequate channel of communication to the staff, protected itself by turning inward, and by developing a social structure which was insulated as much as possible from friction with the hospital routine. Nevertheless, such friction did occur, and the subsequent frustration led to behavior on the part of the patients which, although it overtly resembled neurotic behavior arising from personal emotional conflicts, was, in fact, to a considerable extent due to factors in the immediate situation.[15] Such phenomena are similar to the "increased agitation and dissociative behavior" observed by Stanton and Schwartz (39) when two staff members with power over a patient disagree as to how the case should be handled. Stanton and Schwartz conclude:

> If our hypothesis is correct that the patient's dissociation is a reflection of, and a mode of participation in, a social field which itself is seriously split, it accounts for the sudden cessation of excitement following any resolution of this split. . . . In other words, the phenomena are not completely "autistic" in the sense that they are not derived entirely from the patient's past history or from an unconscious which is isolated from reality.

Some aspects of the above situation seem almost inevitable in the nature of the hierarchical hospital structure. It is necessary to exercise some degree of control over patients; they will be cut off from the positive as well as the negative aspects of their outside life by hospitalization, and some frustration due to close living will occur in any institutional setting which must, by its nature, restrict the personal liberty of its members. If this is true, then some of the behavior of the patients is due to the nature of the situation rather than to their condition of emotional illness, and such behavior should be shared by groups living in other settings which have some *structural* similarities in common with mental hospitals. Sullivan asks this question in his discussion of the Stanton and Schwartz (37) material when he says: "Is this a pattern which is a function of the particular larger group setting, or is it one that has relatively wide validity? . . . Is it to be seen in essential rudiments among the complements of a naval vessel, among the population of a penitentiary, in any hospital which has a relatively chronic patient population, [or] on the wards of most mental hospitals only . . . ?"

A review of the work done on behavior in such settings would seem, at least tentatively, to answer this question in the affirmative. A group of less disturbed patients in a mental hospital would seem to represent one point on a continuum of types of groups all of which share some structural characteristics—e.g., membership in these groups is transitional, positive goals for the members other than their successful removal from the group are mostly lacking, and control is largely authoritarian. Despite other great differences, such as voluntary or involuntary entrance and helping or punishing aims, these characteristics tend to be shared by groups in mental hospitals (8), tuberculosis sanitariums (30, 43), orphanages (16), displaced persons camps (6, 12), wartime posts relatively free from danger (15, 18), and under various conditions of imprisonment (4, 5, 17,

22, 44). In general, the accounts of behavior in these types of settings all stress the phenomena, so many of which are noted in hospitalized mental patients, of apathy and depersonalization, regression, denial of reality, attempts to maintain threatened self-esteem, increased wish-level and fantasy, and the formation of stereotypes concerning those who control the authority and power.

For example, the previously emotionally mature, female political prisoners observed by Jacobson (22) exhibited, as did many of the patients discussed in this paper, initial feelings of depersonalization and denial of reality; a seeming regression to adolescence with its heightened affect lability; an increased, but unstable, sensitivity to aesthetic and intellectual stimulation; and a strong upsurgence of oral cravings. Also, Jacobson's prisoners and the patients showed, as a sort of group reaction formation, increased morality and superego severity, great concern over the welfare of other members, and a constant effort to control irritability.

Such similarities in behavior as are sketched above for the various types of settings would seem to be in line with the experimental results and theoretical conceptualizations of Lewin, Lippitt, White and others (11, 25, 28, 29) as to the direct effect on behavior of differences in social climate.

Beyond this the patient group seemed to develop certain types of behavior shared with all human groups whether they be, as Homans (20) has pointed out, a bank wiring room in an industrial plant, a street-corner society, or a Polynesian community. Since social life is never wholly utilitarian, the patients were acting like any human group when they tended to overelaborate their interaction beyond the point required by the purely practical problems of the environment in which they found themselves. This tendency, noted by Linton (26) and detailed by Homans (20), accounts, in part, for the fact that the bank wiring employees restricted their output in accordance with their own norms and helped each other on piecework even though this was forbidden by management; similarly, the patients supported the activities of others even if this meant going against a rule of the hospital.

Research stemming from the observations discussed here might lead to an investigation of the following problems: 1) Further studies of the value systems of patient groups, and of the roles by which these values are implemented. 2) An exploration of the somewhat separate value systems of the various communication- and mobility-blocked strata of the hospital staff hierarchy. 3) A detailed analysis of interaction processes between the groups making up the hierarchy in light of the differences in values that might be found to exist. 4) Related to the foregoing problems, a study of what happens to reports on patient behavior, in terms of distortions, omissions and additions, as these reports are channeled upward through the hospital strata to the point where decisions are made, and then down again.

A review would also seem to be indicated of the important question of whether neurotic patients who are still able to function in some areas of life should be admitted to a hospital beyond the need for diagnostic studies. It is quite possible that a great many neurotic patients now admitted to our hospitals would fare better in ambulatory treatment than in a hospital setting. At the same time, many neurotic patients must temporarily be removed from the anxiety-provoking setting of the home in order to facilitate therapeutic progress. This dilemma raises many theoretical and practical problems, and would seem to call for research on other types of environmental settings that might be more conducive to the successful psychotherapeutic treatment of such patients.

There are many questions of ward management to which this study has drawn attention. Our main emphasis, however, has been on a theoretical investigation of basic problems of social structure and interaction processes. Much further study is needed before well-founded, practical applications can be made.

NOTES TO CHAPTER 36

1. Upon admission to the hospital, the observer told his therapist that he had recently been compulsively trying to finish the writing of a scholarly book, but felt that he was not getting ahead; worry over his work drove him to alcoholic episodes ending in fights; he was withdrawn and depressed, and had quarreled with his wife who had then separated from him. Beyond these fictions, the observer gave a somewhat distorted version of his own life in which he consciously attempted to suppress his own solutions to certain problems and to add a pattern of neurotic defenses.

2. The methodological aspects of the study will be reported later in detail.

3. The observer also, of course, felt pressure upon him in his first contacts with nurses, his therapist, and other members of the staff. These are not discussed here, however, because the major focus of this paper is upon the relationships developed by patients with each other.

4. All names appearing here are pseudonyms.

5. From the patient's viewpoint, the therapist was a benign, omnipotent authority beyond whom the patient could not look. Actually, in most instances, the therapist was a psychiatric resident who had to discuss his cases with a supervisor before coming to any major decisions. The patient, however, was not aware of this, and was puzzled by what often appeared to be indecision, arbitrariness and withholding of information, on the part of the therapist. This is one aspect of the whole problem, which cannot be discussed here, of the blocking of the free flow of communication between the various sharply defined strata of the hospital hierarchy due, in part, to the highly formalized nature of interpersonal relationships across these strata.

6. In the opinion of some senior staff members there was a lack of awareness of the patients' economic problems and definite resistance on the part of the residents to recognize these.

7. The role of the psychiatric nurse on a ward of neurotic patients is vaguely

defined and includes many varied services of which traditional medical nursing is probably the least important. The patients sense the vagueness of the nurse's role and act out toward her more than toward the physician. When, in addition to her other duties, the nurse has to assume a policing function, and may be denied at times a humane maternal role, the relationship between nurse and patient may easily become difficult and antitherapeutic. We became increasingly aware of this problem in the course of the study, but more detailed observations will have to be carried out before theoretical conclusions or practical recommendations can be made.

8. This social function of food must be distinguished from the need gratification obtained by a particular patient in the giving of food. Both Mrs. Jones and Mr. Anderson constantly proffered food to other patients and this technique of social participation, which was the only one they had, was intimately related to their personality dynamics. The patients were more or less aware of this personal meaning of food for Mrs. Jones and Mr. Anderson, but they took the food and utilized it for the purpose of increasing group social interaction.

9. These ideas on the social dynamics of the role system in the patient group owe much to Linton's discussion (26, 27) of ascribed and achieved statuses and roles. (Linton has verbally indicated he now prefers the term "acquired" rather than "achieved.")

10. In psychoanalytic terms, much of what would be considered primitive instinctual "antisocial" behavior in the outer world became "social" behavior in the hospital because of the wider range of tolerance and suspension of judgment among the patients. Seen in this way, a mental hospital ward is not only, in the traditional sense, a place where the patient should be free, if need be, to regress with some degree of comfort; but it is also a place where primitive instinctual forces are themselves enmeshed and utilized in the subculture and role system of the patient group. Thus, psychotherapy carried out in the hospital must not only contend with such forces due to regression, but also, with such forces supported by a social system.

11. While such behavior forms a large part of the patients' lives in the hospital, it receives, owing to its undramatic nature, less emphasis in the nurses' reports and the therapists' conversations than do the more dramatic instances of aggressive and destructive neurotic behavior, or that behavior which is precipitated more by frustration inherent in the hospital situation.

12. We realize, of course, that sexual behavior, as well as other behavior, is not only influenced by forces in the social field, but also by powerful genetic and dynamic variables.

13. The role and clique structure of the patient group not only functioned, in a general sense, to provide a social life and personal support for its members, but also helped individuals to meet a number of special situations by making a sympathetic and understanding audience to which a patient could bring his doubts and problems concerning: 1) the visits of friends and relatives, 2) the finding of part-time temporary employment while still in the hospital, 3) the awkward incidents that sometimes occurred during excursions downtown, and 4) the final task of preparing oneself to leave the hospital for good.

14. This is, of course, part of the problem of parataxic distortion discussed by Sullivan (41).

15. The occurrence of such phenomena would seem to make it essential that a systematic understanding be gained of that behavior by patients on the ward which is attributable more to factors in the immediate social situation, and of that behavior which is attributable more to factors in their psychodynamic histories. Once such understanding is gained it would then be possible to investigate a second and very complex problem. This second problem concerns the effect of the patient group on the course of individual behavior that has its main inception in repetitive neurotic patterns. In the hospital the individual is protected from any of the realistic consequences that would follow his actions in the outer world, and he encounters a somewhat different system of rewarding and punishing responses from his fellow patients than he would from persons in ordinary life. Thus, while the patient's action is initially rooted in a repetitive conflict, the behavior flowing from this conflict is carried out in a different social reality than has heretofore been the case, and this may significantly influence the dynamic course of the behavior. The question is how the patient's behavior, set within the context of group interaction, should be met by the staff, given the knowledge that such behavior is both psychodynamically determined and affected by, and itself affects, the immediate social structure of the entire patient group on the ward.

BIBLIOGRAPHY

1. Adams, E. C. *Problems in Attitude Therapy in a Mental Hospital.* Am. J. Psychiatry, 105: 456-461, 1948.

2. Bateman, J. R., and H. W. Dunham. *The State Mental Hospital as a Specialized Community Experience.* Ibid., pp. 445-448.

3. Beers, C. W. *A Mind That Found Itself* (5th ed.). Longmans Green, New York, 1921.

4. Bettelheim, B. *Individual and Mass Behavior in Extreme Situations.* J. Abnorm, Soc. Psychol., 38: 417-452, 1943.

5. Bluhm, H. O. *How Did They Survive? Mechanisms of Defense in Nazi Concentration Camps.* Am. J. Psychotherapy, 2: 3-32, 1948.

6. Boder, D. P. *I Did Not Interview the Dead.* Univ. of Illinois Press, Urbana, 1949.

7. Boison, A. *The Exploration of the Inner World.* Willett Clark, New York, 1936.

8. Dembo, T., and E. Haufmann. *The Patient's Psychological Situation upon Admission to a Mental Hospital.* Am. J. Psychol., 47: 381-408, 1935.

9. Devereux, G. *The Social Structure of a Schizophrenic Ward and Its Therapeutic Fitness.* J. Clin. Psychopathol., 6: 231-265, 1944.

10. ———. *The Social Structure of the Hospital as a Factor in Total Therapy.* Am. J. Orthopsychiatry, 19: 492-500, 1949.

11. French, T. M. *An Analysis of the Goal Concept Based upon Study of Reactions to Frustration.* Psa. Review, 28: 61-71, 1941.

12. Friedman, P. *Some Aspects of Concentration Camp Psychology.* Am. J. Psychiatry, 105: 601-605, 1949.
13. Fromm-Reichmann, F. *Problems of Therapeutic Management in a Psychoanalytic Hospital.* Psa. Quart., 16: 325-356, 1947.
14. ———. *Principles of Intensive Psychotherapy.* Univ. of Chicago Press, Chicago, 1950.
15. Greenson, R. R. *Psychology of Apathy.* Psa. Quart., 18: 290-302, 1949.
16. Goldfarb, W. *The Effects of Early Institutional Care on Adolescent Personality.* J. Experimental Educ., 12: 106-129, 1943.
17. Haynor, N. S., and E. Ash. *The Prisoner Community as a Social Group.* Am. Sociol. Review, 4: 362-369, 1939.
18. Heggen, T. *Mister Roberts.* Houghton Mifflin, Boston, 1946.
19. Hillyer, J. *Reluctantly Told.* Macmillan, New York, 1926.
20. Homans, G. C. *The Human Group.* Harcourt Brace, New York, 1950.
21. Hyde, R. W., and H. C. Solomon. *Patient Government: A New Form of Group Therapy.* Dig. Neurol. and Psychiatry, 18: 207-218, 1950.
22. Jacobson, E. "Observations on the Psychological Effect of Imprisonment on Female Political Prisoners," in *Searchlights on Delinquency* (K. R. Eissler, Ed.). Internat. Univ. Press, New York, 1949.
23. Kindwall, J. A., and E. F. Kinder. *Postscript on a Benign Psychosis.* Psychiatry, 3: 527-534, 1940.
24. King, M. *The Recovery of Myself.* Yale Univ. Press, New Haven, 1931.
25. Lewin, K. *Psychoanalysis and Topological Psychology.* Bull. Menninger Clinic, 1: 202-211, 1937.
26. Linton, R. *The Study of Man.* D. Appleton-Century, New York, 1936.
27. ———. "Problems of Status Personality," in *Culture and Personality* (S. S. Sargent and M. W. Smith, Eds.). Viking Fund, New York, 1949.
28. Lippitt, R. *Field Theory and Experiment in Social Psychology: Autocratic and Democratic Group Atmospheres.* Am. J. Sociol., 45: 26-49, 1939.
29. Lippitt, R., and R. K. White. "An Experimental Study of Leadership and Group Life," in *Readings in Social Psychology* (T. M. Newcomb and E. L. Hartley, Eds.). Holt, New York, 1947.
30. Mann, T. *The Magic Mountain.* Knopf, New York, 1939.
31. Menninger, W. C. *Psychoanalytic Principles Applied to the Treatment of Hospitalized Patients.* Bull. Menninger Clinic, 1: 35-43, 1937.
32. Noble, D. *Some Factors in the Treatment of Schizophrenia.* Psychiatry, 4: 25-30, 1941.
33. Peters, F. *The World Next Door.* Farrar Straus, New York, 1949.
34. Rowland, H. *Interaction Processes in a State Mental Hospital.* Psychiatry, 1:323-337, 1938.
35. ———. *Friendship Patterns in a State Mental Hospital.* Ibid., 2: 363-373, 1939.
36. Schwartz, M. S., and A. F. Stanton. *A Social Psychological Study of Incontinence.* Psychiatry, 13: 399-416, 1950.
37. Stanton, A. F., and M. S. Schwartz. *The Management of a Type of Institutional Participation in Mental Illness.* Ibid., 12: 13-26, 1949.
38. ———. *Medical Opinion and the Social Context in the Mental Hospital.* Ibid., pp. 243-249.

39. ———. *Observations on Dissociation as Social Participation.* Ibid., pp. 339-354.
40. Sullivan, H. S. *Socio-Psychiatric Research: Its Implications for the Schizophrenia Problem and for Mental Hygiene.* Am. J. Psychiatry, 10: 977-991, 1931.
41. ———. *Conceptions of Modern Psychiatry* (3rd printing). William Alanson White Psychiatric Foundation, Washington, D.C., 1947.
42. Szurek, S. A. *Dynamics of Staff Interaction in Hospital Psychiatric Treatment of Children.* Am. J. Orthopsychiatry, 17: 652-664, 1947.
43. Todd, G. S., and E. Wittkower. *The Psychological Aspects of Sanitarium Management.* Lancet, 254: 49-53, 1948.
44. Weinberg, S. K. *Aspects of the Prison's Social Structure.* Am. J. Sociol., 47: 717-726, 1942.

Latency

ぞ☙

CHAPTER 37　A Therapeutic Milieu[*]

BRUNO BETTELHEIM AND EMMY SYLVESTER

THIS paper describes the treatment of emotionally disturbed children in an institutional setting. The clinical material on which this discussion is based concerns a syndrome developed in non-therapeutic institutions which may be called "psychological institutionalism." For the purpose of showing how these children are rehabilitated at the Orthogenic School, two cases will be presented in full.

Psychological institutionalism may be regarded as a deficiency disease in the emotional sense. Absence of meaningful continuous interpersonal relationships leads to impoverishment of the personality. The results of this process are observed in children who have lived in institutional settings for prolonged periods of time, but it is not limited to them. It also occurs in children who are exposed to a succession of foster homes or to disorganized family settings.

Non-institutional living *per se* will therefore not cure or avoid institutionalism. Neither can psychotherapeutic measures be effective which neglect the core of the disturbance. Only measures arising from benign interpersonal relationships among adults and children can combat the impoverishment of the personalities of children who suffer from emotional institutionalism. Since behavior disorders in the common sense do not necessarily form part of the clinical picture, the factors which cause impoverishment of personality are only rarely subjected to psychiatric study. Understanding these factors furnishes leads to the construction of a therapeutic milieu.

A frame of reference that consists of depersonalized rules and regulations may lead the child to become an automaton in his passive adjustment to the institution. There is no need for independent decisions because the child's physical existence is well protected and his activities

* Reprinted from the *American Journal of Orthopsychiatry*, 18 (1948), 191–206. Copyright, the American Orthopsychiatric Association, Inc. Reproduced by permission.

arranged for him. Compliance with stereotyped rules rather than assertive action constitutes adequate adjustment, but does not allow for spontaneity. Reality testing is not extended to variegated life conditions. Complete determination by external rules prevents the development of inner controls. Emotional conflicts cannot be utilized toward personality growth because they are not intrapsychic conflicts, but only occasional clashes between instinctual tendencies and impersonal external rules. The cause of these serious deviations in personality development—the absence of interpersonal relationships—is also responsible for their remaining unrecognized. The child lives in emotional isolation and physical distance from the adult. Even in instances where the child lives in proximity of touch and experience with adults, such closeness does not serve the purpose of personality growth if the significant characteristics of the normal child-adult relationship are not maintained. Frequent change in the personalities and absence of proper and consistent dosage of the adult's distance from and closeness to the child, turn into shadowy acquaintance what should be intimate relationships. This "not knowing" the adult deprives the child of images of integration.

In a therapeutic milieu, on the contrary, the child's development toward increasing mastery must be facilitated. Training in skills and achievements, specialized programs and activities, are of peripheral importance only. They are therapeutically justified solely if they originate from the central issue of the therapeutic milieu. A therapeutic milieu is characterized by its inner cohesiveness which alone permits the child to develop a consistent frame of reference. This cohesiveness is experienced by the child as he becomes part of a well defined hierarchy of meaningful interpersonal relationships. Emphasis on spontaneity and flexibility—not to be misconstrued as license or chaos—makes questions of schedule or routine subservient to the relevance of highly individualized and spontaneous interpersonal relationships. Such conditions permit the emergence and development of the psychological instances, the internalization of controls, and the eventual integration of the child's personality. It may be assumed that these milieu factors which determine the children's rehabilitation in the therapeutic milieu, have validity for the institutional care of children in general.

The personality defects which result from the absence of these factors in an institutional setting are clearly demonstrated by a control group of six to eight year old children who were not considered disturbed by their environment. The reason for the psychiatric study was a "purely administrative one"—they had reached the age limit of the residential institution in which they had spent the greater part of their lives. They arrived at the clinic in groups and presented themselves as physically well developed, neat and well-groomed youngsters. Their behavior in the waiting room was rather striking: they seemed to have an unusual amount of group spirit and had completely accepted their respective positions in the group as leaders, followers, protectors, or proteges.

This apparent social maturity was in marked contrast to their behavior in the individual contact with the psychiatrist, in whose office many were excessively shy whereas others became aggressively demanding. These forms of behavior were fixed. Lack of the flexible adaptability which even disturbed children show during the course of a psychiatric interview, characterized these children. The shy ones remained shy throughout the interview. Others were unable to modify their demands which appeared in two different and mutually exclusive varieties. They took the form of "toy hunger" in the children who had interest in toy material only, and of "touch hunger" in those whose need was exclusively for physical contact. The children who were not overwhelmed by rigid shyness entered conversation readily, and it was possible to get a picture of their subjective world.

In spite of psychometrically good intelligence, all conception of coherence of time, space, and person was lacking. Their lives were oriented to washing, dressing, eating, and resting, experienced as pleasurable and unpleasurable purely in terms of their own bodies, and only loosely connected with the adults responsible for their care. Hardly any of the children referred to the staff by name. Some were able to distinguish individual staff members according to the functions of physical routine they supervised. For many children, there existed one exception in this nameless world: the nurse in charge of the sickroom. This seems significant, since she was the only person who, temporarily at least, was in full charge of all the needs of the child.

The automaton-like rigidity of these children, their egocentric preoccupation with functions of their own body, their inability to master a one-to-one contact with an adult, are indications of a serious lag in personality integration.

The deviation in personality development shown by these children allows important conclusions. It demonstrates the dangers of rearing in a setting where a number of adults take care of isolated functions of the child rather than of the whole child, and stresses the necessity of giving each child the opportunity for a continuous central relationship to one adult in the institution.

Upon admission to the School, the children, whose personality development in the therapeutic milieu will be presented, showed striking similarities to this control group. While the severe psychopathology of the patients will become obvious in the description of their gradual rehabilitation, it should be kept in mind that none of the children in the control group were considered in any way abnormal by those who managed the institutional environment in which they lived.

The following case material demonstrates the slow and gradual emergence of personality structure in two children who showed all the characteristics of emotional institutionalism when they were admitted to the School. Here, the simple activities such as eating, bathing, and going to bed, which had also been provided in the non-therapeutic institution, are carried out within meaningful interpersonal relationships. Thus they become essential therapeutic tools for personality rehabilitation.

Case 1:[1] A ten year old boy of superior intelligence had lived in various institutions since his birth. His adjustment demanded psychiatric attention only when self-destructive tendencies of long standing culminated in a suicidal attempt. His life had been characterized by scarcity and tenuousness of personal ties. During the process of rehabilitation, it became obvious that his self-destructive act was more a desperate than a pathological effort to break through his isolation. This he revealed in a situation which was characteristic for him in the beginning of treatment at the School. An explosion of rage had followed his awkward and ineffectual attempt to get close to other children by provoking their aggression. It was then that he said, "I went up on the Empire State Building and jumped off. After that everybody was my friend."

Although he had always lived in proximity to others, he had never experienced the structured hierarchy which differentiates children from adults and thus permits their interaction. He neither knew how to react to adults nor how to get along with children. For him, adults were those who were bigger than he, individuals who by virtue of greater strength and size enforced rules, inflicted punishment and prevented children from "bothering them."

One counselor devoted herself particularly to him. Though he was for a long time unable to reciprocate the offered relationship, he immediately utilized the additional comfort which the contacts with the counselor offered. Toward the end of the first month, he expressed his first appreciation of her devotion when he snuggled against her and said, "I am a laughing hyena." He could express happiness only by coloring his incorporative tendencies with primitive feeling tones of joy. It took another month before he was able to ask any personal questions of her, the person whom he knew best. Once, when he had assured himself of his hold on his special counselor who had let him cling to her arm, he asked her where she lived. Although it was clear to all other children that the counselor's room was three doors from their dormitory, his deep isolation had to lift before he could envisage her as a living, personal entity.

This breaking through of his isolation was apparently meaningful to him and he feared its return because his ability to maintain contact was still very tenuous. The arrival of a new boy in the dormitory became an immediate threat to him. However, he found means of reassuring himself; he asked his counselor to come over to his bed and asked to kiss her good night for the first time. He then told her a story which he called a "joke": Two people had started to go somewhere but soon found themselves back in the same place from which they had started. His insecurity and fear that the newcomer would set him back with his counselor to where he had started showed that he still lacked faith in the reliability of human ties which he had just learned to appreciate.

He became more aloof for several days, but then realized that his fears of abandonment were not justified. This gave him the courage to display regressive behavior for the first time. Though prompted by the threat of a newcomer, this regression was actually progress, since he experimented actively with his ability to cope with vicissitudes in human contacts. Only with his counselor did he begin to act like a small child. In baby talk he called her his mother, saying, "My mamma washes my hands for me. She gets me clean socks." He asked her to help him dress and to spoon-feed him. He was permitted to experience this primitive child-adult relationship. Two months later, baby talk and desire for spoon-feeding were given up spontaneously and new aspects appeared in his relationship with his favorite counselor. Formerly he could maintain contact with her only as his expectations of immediate and tangible gratification were fulfilled. Now the relationship to her became time-structured. His helplessness, the primitivity and urgency of his needs made him desire the permanency of her support. While walking close to her he said, "I am going to hang on to your arm for the rest of my life." It took a whole year for him to develop a feeling of closeness to two adults, his counselor and his teacher. With the rest of the staff, he got along without conflict since he recognized that they served useful functions.

The relative freedom in the therapeutic milieu remained unacceptable to this boy so long as he lacked inner control and the ability for self-regulation. For many months after entering, he complained that the School was not strict enough. Everyone, including himself, was being too spoiled. He praised the disciplinarian spirit of the orphanage from which he had come. In this way, he expressed the fear of his own as yet unintegrated impulses which at the School were no longer controlled completely by outside rules.

In his eating habits, he experimented with gratification and control of primitive impulses. In addition, through these eating habits he tested the attitudes of the significant figures of his new environment toward his needs.

The boy, who had been well fed and of normal weight upon admission to the Orthogenic School, began to overeat, to suck his thumb, and complain that the staff tried to starve him. Gratification of primitive needs alone gave him a sense of security and means of emotional expression. In eating he also found compensation for the barrenness of his existence, which had to remain limited so long as he could not avail himself of the opportunities for satisfaction offered in the therapeutic milieu. He either insisted that the adults force him to eat, or he ate incessantly. Awareness of his lack of inner control and judgment made it necessary for him to have his devouring tendencies constantly permitted and regulated by others.

He had to check up on the food supplies in kitchen and store rooms to make sure that he could expect continued gratification. This evidence had to be tangible. When he noticed once that the milk supply was lower than usual, his doubts could not be dispelled by verbal assurance; he had to wait around until the milk was delivered.

After he had overcome his starvation fear, he became secure enough to regress once more, and actually recapitulated to the feeding of an infant. He had the courage to discover a baby bottle with nipple which had been on the kitchen shelf since his arrival, and said, "What about that bottle?" When asked, "What about it?" he answered, "I thought I might put some milk in it." He was not prevented from doing it; he used the nipple, then discarded it, but persisted for several days in drinking out of the bottle. Then he began to suck milk out of bottles through straws and for a long time carried a milk bottle around in school and on the playground.

For nearly a year his incorporative needs had been met unconditionally in quantity and form of gratification, before he showed spontaneous attempts to control his gluttony. He began to show some discrimination with regard to food, then he refused second servings, often of dishes he liked best. With self-imposed limitations, his wish for adult control of his eating disappeared. He had begun to have mastery over his primitive desires.

Certainty of unconditional gratification by others and his trust in his ability to master his impulses had to be firmly established before he showed awareness of the needs of others, which is essential in establishing any true interpersonal relationship. Such awareness first centered around eating, the function of such great importance to him. He began to arrange tea parties in which he himself prepared and served all the food. He showed great concern that everybody should have enough to eat. These parties were at first limited to his favorite counselor, the person who for a long time had satisfied all his desires. Then he stopped grabbing food from the plates of the other children and gradually included them in his parties.

Since there had never been any pressure on his table manners, the spontaneous changes in this area are significant indications of his inner changes. His greed, his noisy smacking and sucking, gave way to the eating habits of a normal child. Thumb sucking was relinquished for the socially more acceptable chewing of gum. Personality changes paralleled this process of arriving at mastery of primitive needs through their unconditional gratification. While initially his time was spent mostly in daydreaming, he gradually began to participate in active sports, learned to swim and play baseball and showed pleasure in these achievements.

After two months at the School, his artistic ability spontaneously came to light. His first artistic productions had a bizarre quality and were mainly elaborations of death and cemeteries. While he had up to then continuously disturbed the classroom by hyperactivity, noisiness, and frequent temper tantrums, he now began to isolate himself in painting when the pressure became too great. This temporary and self-chosen isolation was permitted. It made his classroom experience more accept-able to him and to the others. The topic of his drawings changed; while he still needed occasional retreat from the classroom situation, he no longer drew cemeteries but maintained some contact with the class by elaborating on the topics of the moment by painting farmers in the field, Indians, and animals in an aquarium.

His painting lost none of its imaginative and creative qualities. He derived much personal prestige when the principal asked him for one of his paintings for his office; and on the next day he offered paintings to others, indicating that he had accepted the status they were ready to give him. He began to show interest in his clothes and accepted his counselor's suggestion to select them personally. In the store, he showed fear of this personal responsibility which had been delegated to him, but imme-diately utilized the experience of being respected as an individual. During this shopping expedition he talked about his fears for the first time and told his counselor that he often asked her to sit on his bed at night because he worried about death at that time.

Gratification of primitive needs had made possible the emergence of sublimation. He was permitted to use his artistic talent to master the classroom situation. He received prestige and praise for his painting. These freed his intellectual abilities, and in ten months he made academic progress equivalent to fourteen months.

The inability to connect present action, past experience, and future expectation led to many instances of confused and explosive behavior be-cause regular repetition of routine at the orphanage had made the boy's life an "empty" continuum. In the absence of meaningful experiences, his existence had not been structured into past, present, and future.

Maturation as a historical process can proceed only if the child's life experience is structured in the dimension of time. Although in the thera-peutic milieu children are not overwhelmed with too many activities, still the boy complained that there was too much to do. Holidays are made enjoyable in a casual way, to avoid over-excitement. Instead, small everyday activities are made carriers of interpersonal relationships. Al-though he did not yet know what made one day different from another and was still unable to react to the events that structure everyday life, he responded to the major event of Easter. He accepted the present and took part in the egg hunt. He was cautious and not too enthusiastic, but for the first time expressed concern about a future event: he wondered about Christmas and asked whether it would be possible for him to participate in its celebration and what it would be like. He could already envisage an event in the future but was able to tolerate it only on the assumption that it would be similar to the experience in the present which he could accept. He wanted to be sure it would not necessitate new adjustments.

Hallowe'en he enjoyed tremendously. He now took the sources of pleasure in his present existence for granted. On Thanksgiving Day he complained that while living in the orphanage, he had had no fun on holidays. He was now able to appraise his present life in terms of his past, and said "This is my first real Thanksgiving." He went on to complain that at the orphanage the children "never did anything." They just had a meal like any other day. Then he reminisced about Hallowe'en. His story was rather jumbled but he had begun to see his life in the therapeutic milieu as a sequence of meaningful and variegated events which he had the courage to face. He looked forward to Christmas as a new "different" holiday. Structuralization of his existence into present, future, and past was taking shape.

In the service of mastery of the new situation, all mechanisms that had proven their adequacy were activated. New clothes had begun to give him security through prestige. Accordingly, on Christmas morning, he was the only boy who took great care to dress in his best outfit. His tolerance at seeing others receive gratification and the ability to postpone his own gratifications, were recent acquisitions. His behavior was in line with them. He went to the fireplace where the stockings were hanging, and instead of grabbing his presents, he insisted on telling the other children about what he found in his stocking and admiring what they found in theirs. Then he very slowly repacked all the presents in his stocking. It seemed to the adults that he had not noticed a sled and some other presents and they pointed these out to him. He replied harshly and ran out of the room, muttering to himself, "This is enough. I cannot stand more of this." Later, in the afternoon, he unpacked some of his toys and started to play with them.

In a previous step of his rehabilitation, unconditional gratification of his seemingly boundless needs had been therapeutically indicated. This permitted recapitulation and gratification of infantile expectations and established the basis for personality growth. Once he had learned that food is always made available and that presents do not disappear, he could make a further step. His new capacity to permit himself gratification was a new achievement. It represented ego growth even if guilt about receiving it may have prompted him to postpone gratification.

Therapeutic response from the adult had to be in line with the status of his ego development. Because he was not forced to deal with his gifts according to conventional adult expectations of gratitude, he was really able to enjoy the gifts—in his own time. Thus the adults' respect for the patient's self-set limitations again represented unconditional recognition of his autonomous tendencies. Through such attitudes of the adult, the boy derived a sense of personal integrity from incidents in his everyday life. This modified his conception of himself and established self-esteem. He became able to face the "bad" past and also developed trust in a benign and manageable future, while he took his present existence for granted.[2] Two successive dreams which he spontaneously related to his counselor illustrate this.

In the first dream, he was king of the universe, Superman. He had a million dollars and ruled everyone. In the second dream, he went to visit the orphanage. He was in the pool (where the older children had thrown him into the water and never given him a chance to learn to swim). He showed them how well he was able to swim and dive. All the children sat around the pool and admired him and liked him very much.

The first dream shows how he attempted to compensate for his lack of personal status in the orphanage by ideas of omnipotence. In the second dream, his recently acquired real achievements, swimming and diving, give him prestige among those with whom he used to have none. Thus the new strength permitted him a more assuring perspective on past and future. While the past had been bad, a similar situation would not again find him helpless.

He learned to see his past in a light which no longer overwhelmed him. Trust in his ability to master situations which once had overpowered him made his outlook of the future realistic and therefore more optimistic. A similar change occurred in his daydreams: instead of being a great dictator and Superman, he now daydreamed about becoming a street car conductor after having lived in a nice foster home for quite a while.

During the year of his stay at the School, the boy made significant steps in personality growth. Environmental attitudes which made such development possible were to him personified in the first counselor who had gratified his dependent needs, permitted him defensive activity, and mediated between him and the outside world whenever he needed such help. As he experienced the implications of interpersonal relationships in his contacts with her, his total human environment began to take on shape and structure.

When he came to the School, all he knew about people was that there are small children, and big children who tell the small ones what to do. Human interaction was a matter of domination through strength or material possessions. For a long time, contact with other children consisted in forceful attempts to take their toys. This behavior was dented when, on St. Valentine's Day, he unexpectedly received valentines from some of the other children. He was happy that he should have made friends. Gradually, he became able to share his toys occasionally, and there was a lessening of the inner struggle which first arose with such performance.

He was surprised that he had found a new *modus vivendi* with other children and searched for an explanation of their kindness. He came to the conclusion that "the children here act right because the grownups treat them right." This was his first recognition of a benign hierarchy of human interrelations. Such awareness was possible only because he had experienced it explicitly in his contacts with the counselor.

Since he was no longer isolated, the slowness and blocking disappeared which had been equivalents for depressive reactions. The desire and ability to communicate gave new meaning to his artistic creations; he discovered spontaneously that personal ties were the source of his new strength. He told the psychiatrist that he had much more energy now and explained, "Before, I thought that I could get energy and strength from food only; now I know that I get energy from other children, counselors, baseball, swimming, and drawing, that is, if I make a picture for somebody."

In a later interview, about one year after admission to the School, he expressed his contentment in a fictitious telephone conversation. As the chairman of the board of directors, he called the School's principal to check up and offer help. He asked, "What do you need for your children? Candy, paper, paint, crayons, nothing? They know you have all they need? That is good. Good bye."

He became eager to understand the relationship of grownups to one another, since he now knew what adults have to offer children and what children may mean to each other. Their relationships were no longer empty or overwhelming and threatening, and he could therefore accept them. He stated with great pride that he now knew what grownups were —they "act like ladies and gentlemen. They go to college, they care for children, they like children. I will be a grownup too someday, but not for a long time." He had acquired a well defined reference frame and can be expected to proceed further in growth.

Case 2:[3] This case, like the first, is also characterized by a child's desperate effort to cope with an unbearable reality. The outward signs of this struggle for mastery were hyperactivity, destructiveness and stealing, severe inhibition of intellectual functioning, and extreme suspiciousness. These symptoms appeared first when Mary was six years old. She had been transferred to a foster home from the nursery where she had lived after her parents had deserted her at the age of three. While at the nursery, she had not presented any manifest problems, but in the foster homes her behavior became progressively more difficult and led to many changes in homes until she came to the Orthogenic School at the age of nine. Her disturbed actions were only the surface ripples of her megalomaniac fantasies, evidence of the unavoidable clashes between external demands which she could not fulfill, and her magic world to which she could no longer successfully retreat.

Psychiatric study before admission to the School showed that she was quite detached from the many adults and children with whom she had lived. She was utterly confused about their identity. Physiological activities like eating and sleeping were not gratifying experiences, but duties imposed by rules or the wishes of others. She hardly knew what playing meant. She said, "Where I live, there is a doll buggy, but I must not touch it." She explained, "Once I was a baby, but I was never wheeled in a buggy."

When asked where she lived, she answered, "In a place where you get clean clothes after playing. Then you take a nap and eat sometimes." She was unable to name any of the children or adults in the orphanage. When asked whether she had a friend, she said, "They tell me that John is my friend." When asked who took care of her, she replied, "A nurse, that is a lady, any lady."

A large segment of her life was spent in autistic fantasy. She said that she was a good girl because she did not bother anybody. Nothing bothered her either since she, and everything around her, was magic. She only had to open her window, say goodbye to the children, then she could fly to God who was nice always.

A few days after admission Mary said she liked the School. "It is like in the nursery before, but it is better, because it is all in one. The school is just here and not five blocks away." Through simplification in denial of any difference, distance, or discrepancy between the constituents of her outside world, she reduced her new environment to manageable proportion. In the foster homes she had had to protect herself from being overwhelmed by the multitude of external events, since the empty existence of her early years had not equipped her to deal with them adequately. But the autistic mechanisms which she applied did not help her to master the persistent demands of reality; when she attempted to withdraw more deeply, her inadequacy only increased and anxiety resulted. Her confusion which led to constant misinterpretations and contaminations seemed to reduce her intellectual functioning to a near feebleminded level.

In the School her need to avoid anxiety determined the nature of her initial adjustment. This need was met as her spontaneous methods of mastery remained unchallenged by external pressure. At that stage, the existence of actual sources of satisfaction and stimulation in the therapeutic milieu was of value for her only because she was not forced to combat external pressure. Still, the presence of such factors was essential from the beginning for her rehabilitation. They had to be available when she was ready to take advantage of them. Opportunity for stimulation and gratification distinguished the therapeutic milieu from the barrenness of nursery life which had led to impoverishment of her personality, while freedom from the pressure which had made her foster home experiences so deleterious, precluded necessity for further confusion and withdrawal.

Since she could not, *a priori*, expect conditions in the external world to be different from her past experiences, she had to apply her old mechanisms of mastery in the new environment. Her courage to explore reality had first been severely curtailed by lack of stimulation in the orphanage, and later by her experiences in foster homes. Protective withdrawal into a world of all-powerful magic was therefore maintained at the School until she developed sufficient confidence in herself and trust in others gradually to modify her defenses.

Mary had not learned to live without magic protection, and now met benign, relatively powerful figures. In proportion to the abject degree of her helplessness, she needed protective figures of such strength as could only be furnished by endowing them with magic powers. Under the aegis of these figures, she could venture forth to test reality with greater comfort and security. Thus, in a way, she tried to establish magic contact with what seemed to her the most important figures in her new environment, the principal and the psychiatrist. In order to be able to retain them as "magic" figures, all realistic contact with them had to be avoided, and they had to be both depersonalized and unified. To do so was also in line with her past efforts to organize her world by recognizing persons only as carriers of useful or dangerous functions. This tendency she demonstrated by depriving the two figures, the principal and the psychiatrist, of the only personal characteristics of which she was aware, their names. She contaminated them into "Dr. Bettelster." Whenever she used this contamination, it designated both of them in the magic and protective functions she assigned to them. She refused to recognize them as persons and avoided personal contact. Because she rebuffed their efforts, contact was discontinued.

She began to approach the principal about one of his functions with which she had become familiar—his role as mediator. She established a routine of complaining to him, remaining aloof at the same time. She did this in line with her magic expectations, and not in terms of a realistic interpretation of his function. She invariably expected him to take her side, protect her, and punish the others. The fact that she received protection only when she needed it, and that other children were not reprimanded just because she complained about them, did not change her conviction of his role as her special protector. When other children expressed fear about events which were beyond control, she reassured them with the statement, "It cannot happen here because of Dr. Bettelster." Gradually, after she had established personalized contacts with her favorite counselor, she separated the psychiatrist from the principal, still adhering to the conviction of their inherent identity: she then called the one Dr. Bester and the other Dr. Vester. Much later, after she had finally found true security in the relationship to her counselor, it became possible for her to divest them of some of their presumed magic characteristics, to accept them tentatively as real, and recognize them as two different persons with different names.

Under the magic protection of the most powerful figures that she had created for herself, she was able to explore segments of reality and to approach a relationship with her counselor. In the meantime, the other children had to remain anonymous and unreal because to acknowledge their presence would have interfered with her need to claim her counselor for herself.

Gratification of her most urgent needs became the basis for her human contacts. For many months she over-ate, staying in the dining room after the others had left and scavenging for food in spite of the large helpings she had already eaten. After every meal, she wrapped food in a napkin to take with her for fear she might be hungry before the next meal. Whenever a course was put on the table, she jumped up excitedly and looked at her counselor for reassurance that she would get more food. Frequently she ate directly from the plate without utensils in order to finish in time for a third and fourth helping. No limitations were put on her needs. After a month she required fewer helpings of food. Now her eating habits did not reflect greed but became distinctly babyish. She sucked her food and occasionally spat it out. Then she started to carry a small jar with her in which she kept a ration of candy. Her eating habits changed only after she had formed individualized relations to her counselor and to some of the children.

She did not tolerate any closeness and had to be permitted to "float around" in the School for some time. Out of the confused anonymity of her existence, familiarity with carriers of useful functions emerged slowly.

Children remained anonymous to her much longer than adults. A friend was a child who was "bigger and can beat you up; you go to her bed." But she was hardly able to distinguish one child from another. To her, they were nameless and existed only if tangibly present. She spoke of them as "that girl," and the only way she called to them was "Hey, you."

On a walk with a counselor, two of the other children ran ahead and were out of sight for a few minutes. When the rest of the group caught up with them, she said without any sign of being perturbed, "Oh there they are. I thought they were dead."

When she began to individualize the children, it was in terms of their attitudes toward the counselor to whom she had become very attached. She consistently expressed her dislike for some children who called this counselor names. In her first attempts to make friends, she adopted toward other children those attitudes which she expected from her counselor in fantasy, and had to be restrained from giving away all of her possessions. Her tendency to concede to any demand made by other children was inappropriate and had to be modified.

Confusion had been the outcome of her attempts to orient herself toward people around her. Similar disorientation showed her helplessness in other areas. Since she had lived in many parts of the city without sufficient awareness of reality ever to find her way about, she was utterly lost in the neighborhood of the School. She showed pseudologic attitudes when she claimed to know every person and every building, in attempting to compensate for her overwhelming ignorance by such confabulation about persons and places. She claimed to recognize old acquaintances and insisted that she had lived on that or the other street. Isolated actual recollections appeared later and then in connection with functions and activities she had begun to master at the School.

Conventional concepts of time meant nothing to her and she manipulated time purely in terms of her own needs and tensions. On July 10th, she recalled that her birthday had been on "June two and three" (June 23rd). This meant to her that her next birthday would be "in two or three days." Whenever she acquired any valid and usable knowledge, she used it compulsively to orient herself. When she was already sufficiently settled at the School to wish to remain, reassurance that she could stay as long as she wanted was insufficient. She had to orient herself by applying the terms of the seasons she had just learned about in class, and asked repeatedly: "Will I be here in the summer? Will I be here in the winter?" repeating the seasons many times. In this way, she sifted her new knowledge in terms of its value for the reassurance she needed. Facts were accepted and retained only after she had tested their usefulness for her immediate needs.

When she first began to experience activities and events in the external world as more gratifying than complete immersion in fantasy, she could not stand the tension of any delay in the succession of external occurrences. If she wanted to buy something, she could not accept the fact that stores were closed in the evening. She could not stand any moment without activity and continuously asked: "What are we going to do now?" Before an answer could be given, she had already wandered to some other subject and she was unable to comprehend what was said to her.

The same pressure appeared in her manner of talking. While she had been quiet and uncommunicative when she first came to the School, with turning to reality, her speech became rapid and explosive. She deleted syllables and ran words together, so that her talk was difficult to understand. Of this, she was initially unaware. Then she became frustrated about her inability to express herself. Her sentences became even less comprehensible as she now interspersed them with recurring exclamations of disgust. She finally realized this when she stopped herself in the middle of a sentence, looked apologetically at the counselor and said, "I can't even speak the English language. I can never say what I want to."

A process of gradual organization started in and around her daily contacts with her special counselor. At first her counselor was a nameless one of many. Her appreciation was unspecific as to source and form of gratification. She said, "I like them, they are good to you." A few weeks later, she dimly recalled her counselor's name; but she still could describe her life at the School only in a stereotyped enumeration of activities which were related solely to herself, such as eating, bathing, going to bed. She mentioned other children only in terms of their interference or non-interference with these activities.

After about a month, contacts with the counselor centered around such simple activities as Mary initiated herself. She demanded to be carried, to be cuddled and fed. When she saw the counselor after a short absence, she shouted, "I love you," hugged her and playfully bit her. Her attitude then did not yet express the interpersonal relationship of a nine-year-old, but was the possessive clinging of an infant.

After about six months, her haunted, sober expression occasionally gave way to real smiling at her counselor. In these moments, she seemed to be in contact, her voice was natural, she finished her sentences and could be reached by the counselor's reply.

It was then, in her contacts with the counselor that she energetically and actively went about the task of getting order into her immediate world. Temporarily her activities assumed a compulsive character. She was first concerned with the order of things around her and started her new activity around eating situations. She cleaned her candy box repeatedly, stacked candy bars according to color and size, counted them and said spontaneously, "This is fun." Then she cleaned her shelves vigorously, arranged and rearranged her toys and wanted her clothes laid out exactly and neatly for the next morning. Her bed had to be perfect and she liked to sweep the floor around it and even underneath. It was as if orderliness in objects related to her had to precede inner order.

Her counselor made some comment about the amount of cleaning she did and she replied that she liked to clean, and added, "Then when I grow up," and stopped. When asked to go on, she said, "Well, it was silly and I know it is not true, but I thought that I would have all my cleaning-up done by the time I grow up." Thus she experimented with her ability to comprehend and master the objects around her in their relation to each other and to herself. In this experimentation with external order, she achieved mastery over one sector of the outside world. As she became able to internalize this achievement, she made her first steps in integration.

It should be kept in mind that her activity emerged spontaneously within the setting of her contacts with the counselor in which, within a reference frame of predictable and maintained interest, she had already experienced not only order, but also unconditional gratification.

Conclusions. The aim of any psychotherapeutic procedure is to help the patient toward adequate mastery over inner and outer forces.

The importance which milieu factors have for causing emotional disturbances in childhood is well established. It is also realized that manipulation of milieu factors can be used toward the rehabilitation of emotionally disturbed children.

In direct psychotherapy of children, recognition is given to the fact that shaping the individual's biological needs in the earliest years is of decisive importance for later personality structure as well as for prognostic considerations. When distorted growth processes can be recapitulated within the benign setting of the psychotherapeutic relationship, symptoms become unnecessary, personality structure changes, growth phenomena appear, and psychotherapy can be considered successful.

Similarly, emotionally disturbed children can be helped through living in a milieu which is aware of the factors that promote restoration of function growth, and new integration. The two children described improved in the particular therapeutic milieu because there insight was translated into uninterrupted action extending over twenty-four hours a day. The children showed improvement because they lived in an environment which, from the start, provided them with a stable frame of reference. While the adults maintained the interpersonal hierarchy in all their dealings with the children, their actions always remained spontaneous within the indications set by the psychological reality of the individual child. This was the spirit in which every child received such gratification as his instinctual and defensive needs dictated at any given moment.

The use of the continuously maintained one-to-one relationship within a therapeutic milieu as one of the many aspects of milieu-psychotherapy is stressed.

NOTES TO CHAPTER 37

1. Credit for most of the direct work in the rehabilitation of this boy is due to Miss Gayle Shulenberger and Mrs. Marianne Wasson.
2. It should be mentioned that in children whose past experiences have been less malignant, the same process leads to the emergence in memory of the positive factors in their past lives.
3. Credit for most of the direct work in rehabilitating this girl is due to Miss Marjorie Jewell and Miss Joan Little.

CHAPTER 38   Resocialization within Walls[*]

LLOYD W. McCORKLE AND RICHARD KORN

A s the concept "socialization" implies group membership, so the
derivative concept, "resocialization," implies changes in group
memberships. Many findings in the social origins of individual behavior
suggest that the problem of reshaping the antisocial attitudes and values
of offenders is related to the possibility of altering the patterns of group
membership which they bring with them into the prison. The question
therefore arises, To what extent does the prison community provide
opportunities for altering the group memberships and reversing the
socialization process which contributed to the criminal behavior of those
incarcerated in it? A necessary starting point for this inquiry would appear
to be an examination of the prison community as a functional social unit.

A prison is a physical structure in a geographical location where a
number of people, living under highly specialized conditions, utilize the
resources and adjust to the alternatives presented to them by a unique
kind of social environment. The people creating and enmeshed in this
environment include administrative, custodial, and professional employees, habitual petty thieves, one-time offenders, gangsters, professional
racketeers, psychotics, prepsychotics, neurotics, and psychopaths, all living under extreme conditions of physical and psychological compression.
The formal administrative structure of the prison may be comprehended
in a brief glance at its table of organization. This table reveals a series of
bureaucratically arranged positions with the warden at the top, and
formal flow of power downward from his position. A more penetrating
glance at the social structure of the prison reveals an ongoing complex of
processes that can neither be described nor anticipated by a static
enumeration of formal powers and functions. For interacting with this
formal administrative structure—and in many ways independent of it—
is another social structure, the inmate social system, which has evolved a

* Reprinted from the *Annals of the American Academy of Political and Social
Science*, 293 (1959), 88–98, by permission of the authors and the *Annals*.

complex of adaptational processes with which inmates attempt to cope with the major problems of institutional living.

THE INMATE SOCIAL SYSTEM

OBSERVATION suggests that the major problems with which the inmate social system attempts to cope center about the theme of social rejection. In many ways, the inmate social system may be viewed as providing a way of life which enables the inmate to avoid the devastating psychological effects of internalizing and converting social rejection into self-rejection. In effect, it permits the inmate to reject his rejectors rather than himself. If it is valid to assume that the major adjustive function of the inmate social system is to protect its members from the effects of internalizing social rejection, then it would seem to follow that the usages of this system are most beneficial to those who have most experienced the consequences of, and developed defenses around, social rejection. It would also follow that the system would find its strongest supporters among those who have, in the process, become most independent of the larger society's values in their definitions and evaluations of themselves. We might also expect to find that those individuals whose self-evaluations are still relatively dependent on the values of the larger, noncriminal society and whose supportive human relationships are still largely with its members would have the most difficulty in adjusting to a social system whose major values are based on the rejection of that larger society.

If these inferences are correct, we may only conclude that the inmate social system is most supportive and protective to those inmates who are most criminally acculturated—and conversely, most threatening and disruptive to those whose loyalties and personal identifications are still with the noncriminal world. Observation supports this conclusion. The non-acculturated offender is rejected not only by the society which defines him as a person, but he suffers the double jeopardy of rejection from the subsociety in which he is now forced to live. In effect, he is denied membership in both. The adaptive inmate, on the other hand, is not only protected from loss of the group membership which defined him as a person, but he is placed in an environment where that membership is assured and his personal adjustment consequently powerfully bolstered. Continued group acceptance of these individuals is based upon their adherence to inmate codes and values.

CHARACTERISTICS OF THE SYSTEM

THE first and most obvious characteristic of the inmate social system is the absence of escape routes from it. The offender is not only incarcerated in a physical prison without exit; he is enmeshed in a human environment and a pattern of usages from which the only escape is psychological withdrawal. Another aspect of the inmate social system is its rigidly hierarchical character, in which vertical mobility, while possible, is highly difficult. The causes of this immobilizing rigidity are various.

The numbers of roles an individual may play are severely limited and, once assigned, are maintained—particularly at the lower status levels—with enormous group pressure. The degree to which the individual can partake in the selection of his role is similarly limited and conditional. From the moment the new inmate arrives from the court or the county jail, he is exposed to a series of very direct defining experiences. It is of interest to note that those inmates who participate in and administer these experiences are frequently those who recognize that the inmate is somewhat near their level, a perception which stimulates anxiety in them. For example, an obviously tough professional hoodlum will create no special problem to the majority of the lower-status inmates who, responding to minimal clues, will either avoid him or immediately acknowledge his higher status. The arrival of this inmate, however, will pose a threat to the wing's chief "bad man," who will be expected to challenge the newcomer to a battle of mutual definitions.

There is an additional aspect of this defining process which sheds light on another characteristic of the social structure, namely, its extreme authoritarianism. The role-defining conflicts carried on by inmates on or near the same status level point up the fact that any situation of equality is a situation of threat which must be resolved into a relationship of superordinance and subordinance. However vehemently inmates in groups demand equal treatment and condemn favoritism, inmates as individuals continuously press for special personal advantages. Where demands for increased permissiveness have been granted by authorities, the results have almost invariably been that the rigid authoritarian patterns have not been destroyed but merely transferred to a new and less stable center of gravity. The history of inmate self-government reveals that the yielding up of powers by the external ordering authority usually generates patterns of internal group coercion more punitive, more rigid, and incomparably more discriminatory than those which they supplanted. This authoritarian character of inmate relationships suggests that members of the system afford no exception to the general psychological observation that the victims of power tend to regard its possession as the highest personal value.

POSSESSION OF POWER

THE dominating value of the inmate social system seems to be the possession and exercise of coercive power. There are probably no relationship functions which have escaped the influence of this factor. Even usages of mutual aid have been contaminated and made subservient to it. To illustrate: one way to proclaim possessive rights over another inmate is to help him in some way, usually by material aid. New inmates, unaware of the subversive motivations behind these services, are quickly apprised of their coercive character. Once an inmate has accepted any material symbol of service it is understood that the donor of these gifts has thereby established personal rights over the receiver. The extreme degree to which these mutual aid usages have been made dependent to power struggles is illustrated by the custom of forcing other inmates to accept cigarettes, a frequent prison invitation to submission. Aggressive inmates will go to extraordinary lengths to place gifts in the cells of inmates they have selected for personal domination. These intended victims, in order to escape the threatened bondage, must find the owner and insist that the gifts be taken back. Should the donor refuse to take them back, the receiver may be forced to fight him then and there.

One measure of the inherent cohesive strength of any social system is the degree to which behavior controls have been individually internalized, thereby obviating all but a minimal degree of interpersonal coercion. Since the basic values of the inmate social system, personal power and exploitation, are inherently inimical to co-operative group living, enormous pressures are required to prevent the inherently centrifugal forces from disintegrating the system. These pressures are supplied in part by the external control and punitive threats of the official world. In the absence of these external unifying forces, order can be maintained only by the most tyrannical inmate rule.

EVASION OF RULES

Like every other social organization, the inmate system provides not only rules and sanctions for their violation but also methods for evading those rules and escaping the sanctions. The disruptive forces inherent in the basic personal value (personal domination through the exertion of coercive power) have generated techniques for the violation of the most fundamental ordinances in support of group unity. The power of these disruptive forces is indicated by the fact that even the most sacred rule of the inmate code, the law against squealing, is daily violated and evaded with impunity. Contrary to the propaganda generated by the more solemn of the inmate clergy in defense of their code, informers and betrayers require little or no seduction by prison officials. Actually the main administrative problem presented by informers is not gaining them but avoiding them, since they come as volunteers from all levels of the inmate hierarchy.

In face of these weaknesses and internal contradictions the question arises, How does the system avoid breaking down and why have prison officials generally failed in exploiting its weaknesses? A part of the answer may lie in the fact that prison officials have generally tended to use the

inmate power structure as an aid in prison administration and the maintenance of good order—not realizing that in this attempt to manipulate
the structure they themselves are more used than using. Far from systematically attempting to undermine the inmate hierarchy, the institution
generally gives it covert support and recognition by assigning better jobs
and quarters to its high-status members providing they are "good inmates." In this and in other ways the institution buys peace with the system by avoiding battle with it.

THE WORK SITUATION

THE freedom from the necessity of earning a living in prison introduces a
striking difference between the requirements of material success within
and without the walls. A significantly different configuration of traits and
aptitudes acquires value, some of which represent direct reversals of those
developed outside. In prison the direct relationship between work done
and material value received has largely broken down. The relationship
between individual productivity and personal status is even more markedly broken down. From a sophisticated inmate's point of view this relationship seems to become a negative one. Strategic placement and effective informal connections rather than individual productivity are the crucial methods for the attainment of material goods.

As a consumer-producer, the inmate lives and trades in two economic
worlds: he is a barterer in the informal and illicit inmate market and a
wage earner in the prison work system. The contrast between his behavior in these two worlds is most revealing. As a trader in the informal
inmate barter system, he is resourceful, ingenious, and usually co-operative: there is a kind of "Better Business Bureau" tradition which is generally effective in encouraging the liquidation of debts. As a wage earner
in the prison labor system he is, by contrast, encouraged to be non-
productive, dilatory, and contentious, articulating his work relations with
the institution in terms of declarations of rights and grievances. In many
modern institutions, the "workers' rights" of inmates go beyond the most
extreme of those advanced by organized labor on the outside.

INMATES' ATTITUDES

THE following is a summary of the sophisticated inmate's view of his economic rights—those attitudes and values concerning work most frequently
articulated to institutional officials by leading spirits of the inmate social
system:

The fundamental authority in defining the inmate's job obligations is *tradition.* Inmates are to be required to work only so much as the tradition concerning given jobs requires. Any departure from these traditions—especially those

departures in the direction of increased work for the same pay—are violations of the inmates' work rights and justify obstructionism. (In a certain penal institution, for instance, "tradition" had established that one inmate lay out all the salt cellars on the mess tables while a different inmate was required to lay out the pepper.)

Increases in the amount of time or output may only be required under extraordinary circumstances and merit increased pay or special benefits, since these added efforts are "favors" extended by the inmates. The inmates have a right to resent and take reprisals against any of their number who "show the rest up" by doing more than the traditional amount of work. These hostile attitudes toward more energetic inmates effectively condemn them to the deteriorating work patterns enforced by the group. Any inmate who performs more than the usual expectation must prove that he has received a special reward—usually food or informal permission to evade some institutional rule.

The providing of jobs is a duty of prison officials and a right, rather than a privilege, of inmates. Once assigned to a job, there are only a limited number of legitimate reasons for which an inmate may be "fired." None of these legitimate reasons includes adherence to the accepted job tradition. Thus an inmate rarely feels that he may rightfully be dismissed for laziness, if he performs only the usual amount of work traditionally required, despite an increase in institutional needs, since the tradition protects him from any definition of himself as lazy. Inmates generally feel that the fact that they are paid less than comparable civilian workers entitles them to produce less.

The total result of the prevalence of these attitudes has been to reduce "imprisonment at hard labor" to a euphemism existing chiefly in the rhetoric of sentencing judges and in the minds of the uninformed public. The inmate social system not only has succeeded in neutralizing the laboriousness of prison labor in fact, but also has more or less succeeded in convincing prison authorities of the futility of expecting any improvement in output. Responding to a multitude of pressures within and without the prison, most institutional work supervisors have adopted patterns of expectations which are largely supportive of the inmate position.

SUPERVISORS' ATTITUDES

THE following summarizes what the writers have found to be the prevalent attitudes of work supervisors toward convict labor:

Convicts are inherently unindustrious, unintelligent, unresourceful, and uninterested in honest work. They are, generally speaking, a worthless lot of men who have never learned, and can never learn, good work habits. In the face of these facts, the supervisory staff cannot be held in any way responsible for the low output of prison labor. Any attempts to force increases in output of prison labor are dangerous and must be resisted by realistic administrators in order to protect what little work can be secured from inmates.

But there is another reason for the low labor standards of inmates. Convicts may not justifiably be expected to do as much work as their civilian working counterparts because their pay is so much less. It is basically unjust to demand that a man work as much as he would have to work on the outside for as little as he earns on the inside.

One is reluctantly forced to the conclusion that, in adopting a set of expectations which support inmates' attitudes, prison work supervisors have surrendered to the realities of inmate pressure rather than to the realities of the work situation. This surrender has implications that extend far beyond prison walls, since it encourages inmates to fixate work habits which severely cripple their ability to make realistic work adjustments upon release. Since the inmate's ability to make an effective noncriminal adjustment on the outside is directly dependent on his ability to hold a job, the conclusion is inevitable that the fostering of deteriorated work patterns in prison represents a considerable contribution to recidivism. It is probable that the much decried "prison idleness" in its brutal honesty represents far less of a contribution.

There is another far-reaching evil in this surrender to the inmate social system. In manipulating supervisory authorities into support of his position, the adaptive inmate destroys a major therapeutic objective of the prison experience, namely, that of learning compliance to duly constituted authority. By learning that he can successfully deceive, connive, and evade, the inmate is re-encouraged in the hope that, by using the social skills perfected in prison, he may avoid the unfortunate "errors" that first trapped him and sent him there.

THE CUSTODIAN

PROBABLY the most important and strategically placed individuals involved in the problem of reconstruction of attitudes are the cell-block officers and shop instructors—those representatives of the external community who come in direct, face-to-face daily contact with the inmate. How these individuals relate to the inmate determines, in the long run, not only the care and treatment policy of the institution, but that of the larger society as well. Consequently, any attempt to evaluate reconstruction within walls must make a careful and exhaustive analysis of these highly significant relationships.

The responsibility of those who man the locks is as confining, in many ways, as is the imprisonment of those confined by them. The keeper of the keys is a prisoner too. By the time he retires, the custodian will have spent from eight to fifteen years totally within the prison walls. During this time he will have been personally and singly responsible for the custody and discipline of many thousands of inmates. During most of the time he has spent inside the walls he will have been continually outnumbered and continually under the threat of being outwitted by inmates whose obedience to him is protected only by his status as a symbol of power. His duties are as manifold as those of a commander of troops and as hazardous as those of the commander whose forces may at any time cross the brink of rebellion. One of the hazards of his situation paradoxically is the ease with which he can be lulled into forgetfulness of its hazards.

In order to preserve his status as a symbol of authority, the custodian must surround himself with a social distance which prevents the realities of his weaknesses from becoming apparent to the inmates. The realities of his situation are most unfavorable. He is dependent in part on inmate personnel for the physical mechanics of operating his wing. He is also continuously exposed to numerous techniques of deception. However, these tangible weaknesses do not form the main hazards threatening his effective functioning. These are more intangible and, as such, difficult to detect and even more difficult to control.

The inmate social system has developed techniques to exploit the custodian's psychological as well as his physical vulnerability. These techniques are aimed at a reduction of the social distance protecting his role as guard, outflanking it with a personal relationship, and exploiting that relationship for the inmates' own purposes. Once the relationship between keeper and inmate is on a man-to-man basis, the dependency and vulnerability of the custodian become apparent. "Obeying orders" becomes transformed into "doing the guard a favor." When obedience undergoes this transformation, reciprocity becomes operative, "One favor deserves another." Should a keeper now refuse to return the favor, the inmate feels it within his right to become hostile because of the keeper's "ingratitude." Once the Pandora's box of special favoritism is open it cannot be shut again without a painful and dangerous demonstration of how fickle are the personal relations between those improbable "friends"—the keeper and his prisoner. Neither can be loyal without violating the principles and risking the rejection of the groups which define their roles and set the limits of mutual accommodation. Once these limits are passed, and it is usually the inmate who attempts to pass them, one or the other must balk. This is interpreted as a "betrayal" which terminates the relationship and transforms the friends into enemies. In the process, both become discredited by their own groups—which have now victoriously redemonstrated the insurmountability of the mutual antagonism.

It thus becomes apparent that a breakdown of the social distance between the inmate and his keeper must, sooner or later, result in the exploitation of one by the other and the ultimate degradation of one or both. It is at this point that the most hazardous consequences of this breakdown emerge. Having lost, through a personal relationship, a large measure of the control which had previously been protected by his formal, impersonal role, the keeper is far less able to cope with the powerful and

eventually antagonistic emotions which that personal relationship un-
leashed. A violent resolution of the conflict now becomes increasingly
probable, unless harmony can be re-established by a new capitulation or
coerced by a convincing show of force.

THE PROFESSIONAL STAFF MEMBER

WHEN the activities of the various categories of prison personnel—administrative, custodial, maintenance, and professional workers—are compared in terms of a *clear definition of function,* a curious result of the
comparison emerges. Of all the personnel at work at the prison, the professional workers are charged with the most far-reaching and socially
urgent responsibilities. These are, however, the very persons who are
assigned roles and functions which are defined in the most ambiguous
and uncertain terms. The new custodial officer, for instance, comes into a
defined situation, with his expectations concerning his role reinforced by
tradition. Almost anyone he meets has a more or less clear expectation of
what his behavior ought to be in practically every situation, and these
expectations set distinct limits to individual deviation. In well-run institutions, the very uniform he wears functions as a kind of insulation against
personal failings; it is understood that security and discipline require
that the official community organize its responses around the role rather
than the man. Consequently, it is universally acknowledged that the institution will support the uniform, within limits, whatever the personal
characteristics of the individual who wears it. A comparable situation
exists in the cases of the administrative and maintenance personnel. Here,
too, objectives are limited, well defined, and matched with reasonably
effective powers for their realization.

But what of the psychiatrists, the psychologists, the social workers, the
counselors, and classification specialists—those to whom the larger society
has assigned the mission of resocialization within walls? What are the
work aspirations and expectations which are to guide their operations?
What are the traditions which will unify the expectations related to their
work and set standards for their behavior and the behavior of the personnel interacting with them? They do not exist; they never existed.

The professional entered penal treatment through the breach in the
wall forced by the zeal and indignation of the nineteenth-century religious
reformers. His forebears, the humanitarian reformers, moved by a profound faith in the direct educability of human nature, sincerely believed
that the problem of crime could be solved by a combination of decently
treating and religiously exhorting confined criminals.

It is the tragedy of modern correction that the impulse to help has
become confused with treatment and seems to require defense as treatment. One of the more ironic difficulties with this position is that, when

one makes "rehabilitation" the main justification for humane handling of prisoners, one has maneuvered oneself into a position potentially dangerous to the humanitarian viewpoint. What if humane treatment fails to rehabilitate—shall it then be abandoned? The isolated survivals of flogging and other "tough" techniques which still disgrace American penology remain to remind us that this is no mere academic question.

The bleak fact is that, just as the monstrous punishments of the eighteenth century failed to curb crime, so the more humane handling of the twentieth century has equally failed to do so. Professional workers in penology have an overriding obligation to acknowledge this failure and to seek for its causes. In their inquiry they ought not to exempt their own concepts and methods from scrutiny.

We shall now attempt to examine a process by which the professional services, by defining themselves as the rescuers and helpers rather than the rehabilitators of convicts, helped to maneuver themselves into exploitation by the inmate social system and collaborated in their own neutralization.

"TREATMENT BY HELPING" NEUTRALIZED

IN THE first part of this paper the observation was made that the inmate social system appears to function as an adaptation to social rejection and punishment, enabling the offender to avoid the pathological effects of converting the hostility of society into hatred of himself. Rather than internalizing this hostility, as does the typical neurotic, the adaptive inmate appears to be able to turn it back upon society, using the misery of prison life as his reasonable pretext. If this interpretation is correct, it may help explain the failure of any attempt to rehabilitate which is based on easing the harshness of prison life.

In order to externalize hostility, individuals must find external objects or conditions against which to express that hostility. The harshness of prison life has been suggested—and is, in fact, suggested by inmates—as the external condition which satisfies this requirement. The question now arises: given the need to externalize hostility, would the effect of improving specific conditions be to reduce the hostility *or would it require the inmate to find new outlets for it?* Putting the question in a different from: does acceding to the demands of the aggressive adaptive inmates result in a decrease in their protests or does it give rise to new demands around which the hostility generates new protests? Observation and experiences with the results of acceding to inmate pressure strongly suggest the latter.

Much as he protests bad prison conditions, the adaptive inmate *requires them,* because his system of adaptation creates in him a *need to protest.* By finding reasonable pretexts for aggressive protest, he is able to accomplish at least three essential psychological objectives:[1]

1. The cathecting of hostilities originally generated by his failures in human relations generally and his resentment at confinement in particular.

2. Reinforcement of his self-picture in the role of a martyred victim of superior force, with attendant justifications of his "heroic counterattack."

3. Absolution of any personal sense of guilt or responsibility for his offense against society by emphasizing and concentrating on society's real or fancied offenses against him.

The implications of this widespread psychological orientation for any treatment based chiefly on permissiveness and helping will become painfully obvious for any professional staff member who enters the prison with a missionary zeal and a determination to undo, by open-handed giving, the "evils of generations of prison corruption." The inmate social system has an infinite reserve of grievances and injustices with which to capture his sympathies and divert his efforts. The new professional can walk through the corridors of the cell block reserved for the most notorious prison "bad men," and hear the noble principles of the Declaration of Principles of 1870 mouthed by the most cynical and deteriorated of inmates—men who a moment before and a moment after they speak with him will be ridiculing his naïveté to the very "brutal hacks" they complained about to his face. All too frequently the lingo and point of view of the professional becomes the property of the articulate champions of the most aggressive and corrupting inmate forces in prison. Like some strange human hothouse, the prison has a way of developing a species of flowery "bleeding hearts" which put forth especially sticky and luxurious blossoms to ensnare the new professional. It is almost as if the inmate social system recognizes the special value of these articulate inmates and puts them forth as a kind of burnt offering with which the professional can make penitential sacrifices on his personal altar of social conscience. The inmate social system throws a diversionary human screen of institutional "problem cases" around the professional staff member, eating up his time and misdirecting his efforts away from his proper target, the system itself.

LACK OF TREATMENT RATIONALE

Mention has been made of the lack of any systematic theory of correctional treatment. This situation is closely related to the absence of any comprehensive and tested theory of crime causation. Since the majority of professional personnel working on the treatment of offenders have been trained in the field of psychological therapies, it would be of interest to determine to what extent their methods of correctional treatment are in harmony with the larger body of theory and practice available in social and psychological pathology and treatment.

We are not prepared, in this paper, to enter into the controversies concerning the nature of the malady—personal or social—from which the habitual, acculturated offender suffers. Assuming, for the purposes of discussion, that he is suffering from some form of personality deviation or disturbance, we may raise two questions. First, do contemporary theories of psychotherapy, however diverse, agree on any common core of requirements and procedures? Secondly, if this common core be ascertainable, what inference may be drawn from it for some general statement of a treatment rationale for offenders? Our survey of contemporary theories and methods of psychotherapy persuades us that such a common core exists, or is at least implicit in contemporary practice. The following summarizes our understanding of the principles of any form of psychological treatment. These are principles common to all methods, from the most superficial brief counseling to the most intensive and extended depth therapy.

1. The person must somehow be brought to an awareness that his difficulties are related to motives and patterns of perception within himself. His attempts to account for these difficulties by blaming a hostile or unfavorable human environment must be analyzed as deriving at least in part from a natural human tendency to avoid guilt and self-rejection. He must be assisted in the gaining of an awareness and a motivation for the taking of present initiative toward change or growth within himself, and he must be shown the fruitlessness of evading this responsibility by futile attempts to change merely his environment.

2. This assistance toward understanding comes about through some relationship with the therapist (or therapeutic situation) in which the individual actually attempts to make his faulty modes of perception and behavior work. Repeated demonstrations of this failure may be necessary before he is able to abandon them. It is important that these failures be not interpreted by him as indicating that he is a worthless or helpless person.

3. Finally, the individual must be provided with opportunities for the learning, testing, and fixating of newer, more effective modes of perceiving and relating to his human environment. As these new patterns emerge and are found rewarding in terms of increased success in relations with the self and others, they tend to become more and more established in the individual's total pattern of adjustment.

Therapeutic changes based on the processes just cited are critically dependent on the individual's taking the first step of locating the source of his difficulty somewhere within himself. But it is against this first and all-important acknowledgment that the inmate social system mobilizes all its forces and values. This mobilization takes the form of defining all situations in terms of grievances and demands justified by those grievances. On the basis of this orientation, the inmate social system divides the whole world of people with whom it relates in terms of a simple dichotomy: there are people who persecute inmates and people whom inmates may exploit. When the professional staff member defined himself as the friend and helper of the inmate he was automatically redefined by the values of the inmate social system as one to be exploited as a champion of inmates in their grievances against society in general and the custodian in particular. Any deviation from this assigned role—especially in the direction of co-operation with measures of custodial control—were then viewed, quite logically, as a betrayal by the professional of his mission to help the inmate. Treatment—defined as help—at this point becomes the enemy of control.

But it is only through strict and careful measures of control that the inmate may be brought face to face with the inadequacy of his faulty technique of adjustment, as he tries to carry out the same pattern of violation and evasion of rules within the institution that required his institutionalization in the first place. By defining himself as one who only aids and eases the inmate in his prison adjustment, the correctional therapist implicitly contributes to the frustration of the all-important objective of demonstrating to the inmate that his pattern is ineffective. Treatment, viewed in this way, now becomes an obstacle to therapy.

CONCLUSIONS

THE total result of the interacting trends and processes described has been to isolate the confined offender from socially beneficial contact with individuals outside the inmate social world and to prevent the formation of relationship bonds which might redefine him as an acceptable member of the noncriminal community. This is the major dilemma of penology.

The writers see little possibility of a resolution of this dilemma within the universally prevailing context of a large institutional approach. Large institutions (walled and unwalled) are dependent on the development of a bureaucratic apparatus based on formal structuring of human relationships. This formal structuring, which is required for the efficient and secure operation of the large institution, is in turn dependent on the maintenance of a social distance which sets crippling limits on contact with members of the official community—the only available representatives of the larger society. Where these limits have been redefined—as in the case of the professional worker—the results, to date, have largely been supportive to the inmate social system and have contributed to the weakening of measures of control.

Effective measures of control are viewed as essential to any therapeutic program which would attempt to demonstrate the ineffectiveness of the coercive or conniving or evasive personal and social adjustment which the adaptive offender brings with him into prison. Only after this demonstration is made will it be possible to create the relationships and set up

the learning situations required for the fixations of new patterns of behavior. In order to participate effectively in this two-phase therapeutic
process—the breaking down of old and the building up of new behavior
patterns—the professional and the custodian alike must work to heal the
breach which traditionally divided treatment and custody and which
ultimately weakened both. The custodian's definition of the therapist as
an enemy of discipline and the therapist's conception of the custodian as
an obstructor of treatment must be replaced by new definitions which
view both as united collaborators in a unitary therapeutic program.

NOTE TO CHAPTER 38

1. None of the remarks above justifies complacency about vile prison conditions. One of the worse consequences of these conditions is that they supply
   reasonable pretexts for the externalization of hostilities which could be utilized more therapeutically in internal disruption of the inmate social system.

౭৯

CHAPTER 39   Ideology, Personality, and
Instructional Policy in the Mental Hospital[*]

DORIS C. GILBERT AND DANIEL J. LEVINSON[1]

THIS inquiry concerns the ideologies of mental hospital members regarding the nature and causes of mental illness and regarding hospital aims and policies in treating the mentally ill. We are interested in the
nature of these ideologies as well as their institutional and intrapersonal
roots. Mental hospitals are going through a period of ideological ferment
and organizational change. The newly emerging viewpoints involve much
more than the application of new treatment techniques. What gives them
their fundamental quality is their conception of the hospital as a community of citizens rather than a rigidly codified institutional mold, and
their conception of the hospital members as persons rather than as mere
objects and agents of treatment (2, 8, 9, 14). In this respect as in many
others, the ongoing developments in the mental hospital parallel those in
other "correctional" institutions such as schools and prisons, and in larger
bureaucratic structures such as industry and government (10, 12, 15).
Because of their wider relevance, research in the mental hospital can
make use of, and contribute materially to, the main body of sociopsychological theory and knowledge.

The primary aims of this study are the following:

1. To formulate the main characteristics of the old and the newly
   emerging viewpoints regarding mental illness, and to construct an
   ideology scale that will crudely measure the degree of an individual's
   preference for one or the other viewpoint.
2. To investigate the personality contexts within which these orientations most readily develop.
3. To investigate the relationships of individual ideology and person-

* Reprinted from the *Journal of Abnormal and Social Psychology,* 53 (1956), 263–
271, by permission of the authors and the *Journal.*

ality to membership in particular types of hospital systems and occupational statuses.

4. To investigate the ways in which the hospital's over-all policy is related to the modal (most common) ideology and the modal personality of its members.

CUSTODIALISM AND HUMANISM AS IDEOLOGICAL
ORIENTATIONS IN THE MENTAL HOSPITAL

WE HAVE found it most fruitful, in our attempts at ideological analysis, to begin by asking: What are the major "problems" or issues of institutional life for which some kind of adaptive rationale is needed? The mental hospital presents at least the following issues with which every individual member must deal. The *patient:* what is he like, how did he get that way, how much can he be helped and in what ways? *Patient-staff relations:* what should be the role of hospital personnel vis-à-vis the patient; how much interaction should there be, with what emotional qualities and therapeutic aims? *Staff-staff relations:* how should specific functions and responsibilities be distributed; how much communication and status distinction should there be? *General hospital practices:* what formal treatment methods are best; how should ward life be organized; in what ways should patients be encouraged, left alone, controlled, punished?

The traditional and the newly developing viewpoints offer two contrasting sets of answers to the above questions. Each is a mode of thought underlying institutional policy and individual adaptation. A brief, schematic formulation of each ideology is presented below. It is to be emphasized that these are prototypes, probably represented in pure form by few individuals or hospitals. The two types may be thought of as polar extremes of a continuum containing various intermediate positions. We assume that this continuum is *realistic*, in the sense that viewpoints and policies approximating the prototypes will commonly be found, and that the continuum is *significant*, in the sense that adherence to one rather than the other viewpoint will seriously affect the individual's or the hospital's mode of functioning.

We shall use the term "custodialism" to designate the traditional patterns. The model of the custodial orientations is the traditional prison and the "chronic" mental hospital which provide a highly controlled setting concerned mainly with the detention and safekeeping of its inmates. Patients are conceived of in stereotyped terms as categorically different from "normal" people, as totally irrational, insensitive to others, unpredictable, and dangerous. Mental illness is attributed primarily to poor heredity, organic lesion, and the like. In consequence, the staff cannot expect to understand the patients, to engage in meaningful relationships with them, nor in most cases to do them much good. Custodialism is saturated with pessimism, impersonalness, and watchful mistrust. The custodial conception of the hospital is autocratic, involving as it does a rigid status hierarchy, a unilateral downward flow of power, and minimal communication within and across status lines.

The newer orientations will be termed "humanistic" (after Fromm [6]) in view of their concern with the individuality and the human needs of both patients and personnel. These orientations conceive of the hospital as a therapeutic community rather than a custodial institution. They emphasize interpersonal and intrapsychic sources of mental illness, often to the neglect of possible hereditary and somatic sources. They view patients in more psychological and less moralistic terms. They are optimistic, sometimes to an unrealistic degree, about the possibilities of patient recovery in a maximally therapeutic environment. They attempt in varying degrees to democratize the hospital, to maximize the therapeutic functions of nonmedical personnel, to increase patient self-determination individually and collectively, and to open up communication wherever possible. While the humanistic orientations have the above characteristics in common, and even more an opposition to custodialism, they still differ among themselves in important respects. For example, the concrete manifestations of humanism will differ, although the guiding spirit may be the same, in a large, architecturally horrendous, financially limited state hospital, as contrasted with a small, well-subsidized, private hospital that accepts only patients regarded as good therapeutic risks.

This inquiry makes no assumptions about the actual therapeutic effectiveness of the various approaches. Our primary concern here is with the nature and the determinants of custodialism and humanism.

THE CUSTODIAL MENTAL ILLNESS IDEOLOGY SCALE (CMI)

THE initial, field exploration led to the formulation of the "custodialism-humanism" continuum, the polar extremes of which have been described above. The next step was to construct the Custodial Mental Illness Ideology Scale (CMI), an admittedly crude instrument that had two chief functions in the research: (a) To test the hypothesis that a set of seemingly disparate ideas do in fact "go together" to form a relatively coherent orientation in the individual. A derivative function is to determine whether viewpoints approximating our posited prototypes exist with some frequency within various hospital settings. (b) To provide a quantitative and at the same time meaningful measure that facilitates additional study of the nature of these ideas and their relation to other aspects of the individual and his milieu.

The CMI scale consists of 20 statements, broadly diversified to cover numerous facets of the ideological domain: the nature and causes of mental illness, conditions in the hospital, patient-staff relations, and the

TABLE 1.
The Custodial Mental Illness Ideology (CMI) Scale

ITEM	MEAN	DP
1. Only persons with considerable psychiatric training should be allowed to form close relationships with patients.	3.5	2.4
3. It is best to prevent the more disturbed patients from mixing with those who are less sick.	5.0	1.8
5. As soon as a person shows signs of mental disturbance he should be hospitalized.	3.3	4.2
*7. Mental illness is an illness like any other.	2.7	2.7
9. Close association with mentally ill people is liable to make even a normal person break down.	2.0	1.4
11. We can make some improvements, but by and large the conditions of mental hospital wards are about as good as they can be considering the type of disturbed patient living there.	3.0	3.6
15. We should be sympathetic with mental patients, but we cannot expect to understand their odd behavior.	3.2	3.8
17. One of the main causes in mental illness is lack of moral strength.	2.8	3.2
*18. When a patient is discharged from a hospital, he can be expected to carry out his responsibilities as a citizen.	3.0	.5
19. Abnormal people are ruled by their emotions; normal people by their reason.	3.8	4.4
21. A mental patient is in no position to make decisions even everyday living problems.	3.0	3.1
*23. Patients are often kept in the hospital long after they are well enough to get along in the community.	4.2	—.2
25. There is something about mentally ill people that makes it easy to tell them from normal people.	3.0	2.9
27. Few, if any, patients are capable of real friendliness.	2.2	1.7
31. There is hardly a mental patient who isn't liable to attack you unless you take extreme precautions.	2.5	3.0
33. Patients who fail to recover have only themselves to blame; in most cases they have just not tried hard enough.	1.8	1.5
37. "Once a schizophrenic, always a schizophrenic."	2.3	1.3
38. Patients need the same kind of control and discipline as an untrained child.	3.3	2.4
39. With few exceptions most patients haven't the ability to tell right from wrong.	2.4	2.3
40. In experimenting with new methods of ward treatment, hospitals must consider, first and foremost, the safety of patients and personnel.	5.3	2.3

* Items expressing a "humanistic" position; all others are "custodial."

NOTE.—The item means and *DP*s are those obtained by a sample of 196 mental hospital personnel in Hospitals C, T, and H. Similar *DP*s have been obtained in other samples of personnel, patients, and visitors. Items are numbered as they appear in the questionnaire, which contained other scales and questions.

like. The items were derived from interviews, conversations, and observations of conferences and everyday hospital life. The scale is presented in Table 1. A more extensive description of the field work and derivation of the CMI scale can be found in Gilbert (7).

Scoring procedure. The subjects were instructed to indicate the degree of their agreement or disagreement with each item on a scale ranging from +3 (strong agreement) to −3 (strong disagreement). The responses were converted into scores by means of an a priori, 7-point scoring scheme. It was intended that a high score represent strong adherence to "custodial" ideology as here conceived, and that a low score represent opposition to this viewpoint. Of the 20 scale items, 17 were regarded as custodial, 3 as humanistic. For the "custodial" items, seven points were given for the +3 response, one point for −3. For the "humanistic" items the scoring was reversed. For convenience in comparing scores from scales differing in length, we shall use the mean per item, multiplied by 10. The possible range is thus 10-70 points.

The CMI scale was initially developed on a sample of 335 staff members (aides, student nurses, nurses, and psychiatrists) in three Massachusetts mental hospitals: Hospital C, a large (1,800 bed) institution dealing largely with "chronic" patients; Hospital T, a Veterans Administration hospital of about the same size, and Hospital H, a small (120 bed) state institution providing short-term active treatment. The range for this sample was 15-52, the mean being 31.3 and the *SD*, 9.5. Comparative data for various subgroupings are presented below (Table 2). The reliability (split-half correlation, corrected by Spearman-Brown formula) was .85, and test-retest correlations on several small groups were of similar magnitude. Table 1 presents the means and discriminatory powers (*DP*) of the individual items.[2] The *DPs* of all items except numbers 18 and 23 reach the .05 level of statistical significance, and most of them are beyond the .01 level.

The above data indicate that the initial form of the CMI scale has adequate reliability and internal consistency, and they provide a basis for further improvement. They suggest, moreover, that a person's stand on any single issue represented in the scale is part of a broader, fairly coherent (though seldom fully integrated) ideology that embraces numerous issues of hospital life.

Data were obtained on two "validation groups" to determine whether the CMI score adequately gauges an enduring ideological conviction. One group, containing 10 administrators at Hospital H who are known for their advocacy of humanistic policies, earned a CMI mean of 18.8, with an *SD* of 6.1. The second group comprised the professional staff at the Social Rehabilitation Unit, Belmont Hospital, England, (9) and would also be expected to have a low CMI mean. The obtained mean was 22.9, the *SD*, 6.7. These findings offer additional evidence of scale validity.[3]

TABLE 2.

CMI Mean, F Mean, and Index of Status-Custodialism

HOSPITAL-STATUS UNIT	N	INDEX OF STATUS-CUSTODIALISM	CMI SCALE			F SCALE			rCMIᶠ
			MEAN	RANK	SD	MEAN	RANK	SD	
Attendants at Hospital:									
C	29	12	38.0	12	10.2	46.1	12	13.0	.91
T	51	11	37.3	11	10.3	41.4	11	11.7	.82
H	48	10	32.1	8	9.7	32.5	9	13.0	.77
Student Nurses at Hospital:									
C	66	9	33.4	10	7.7	29.0	8	10.9	.44
T	38	8	33.3	9	6.8	28.9	7	8.9	.25
H	16	7	31.3	6	5.7	28.8	6	9.2	.59
Nurses at Hospital:									
C	14	6	31.3	7	9.9	37.3	10	14.5	.90
T	18	5	22.4	2	5.2	26.7	5	8.7	.53
H	21	4	26.9	5	7.7	25.8	3	14.5	.73
Doctors at Hospital:									
C	6	3	25.8	4	7.0	18.1	1	6.2	.75
T	4	2	21.6	1	4.8	26.6	4	12.8	.80
H	24	1	22.7	2	4.5	19.1	2	8.5	.50
Total Status:									
Attendants	128	4	35.3	4	10.4	39.1	4	13.7	.82
Student Nurses	120	3	33.1	3	7.3	28.9	3	10.2	.41
Nurses	53	2	26.5	2	8.3	27.9	2	12.8	.76
Doctors	34	1	23.1	1	5.3	19.7	1	9.1	.46
Total Hospital:									
C	115	3	33.7	3	8.9	33.8	2	14.5	.67
T	111	2	32.9	2	10.2	34.2	3	12.4	.69
H	109	1	29.0	1	8.7	27.7	1	13.1	.76
Total Sample	335		31.3	1	9.5	31.9		13.7	.71

PSYCHOLOGICAL BASES OF CUSTODIALISM AND HUMANISM

WITH the CMI scale developed, it was possible to test the hypothesis that *the custodial orientation is one facet of an authoritarian personality, the humanistic orientation a facet of an equalitarian personality.* Several lines of theory and observation led to this expectation. Custodialism is strongly autocratic in its conception of the hospital and ethnocentric in its conception of patients as an inferior and threatening outgroup entitled to few if any of the rights of "normal" people. Humanism, on the other hand, seeks a more democratic hospital structure and regards patients as individuals to be understood and treated rather than as an outgroup to be pitied or condemned. There is considerable evidence that autocratic viewpoints tend to exist within authoritarian personality structures (1, 5, 6). We accordingly predicted that the CMI scale would correlate significantly with the F scale (1), a relatively nonideological measure of authoritarianism, and with the Traditional Family Ideology (TFI) Scale (11), a measure of autocratic ideology regarding issues such as husband-wife and parent-child relations.[4]

The obtained interscale correlations are as follows: CMI and F correlate .67, .69, and .76 in Hospitals C, T, and H, respectively. The comparable correlations between CMI and TFI are .50, .56, and .77. The respective Ns in the three hospitals were 115, 111, and 109. The scale means and SDs are presented in Table 2. The findings lend support to the hypothesis that an individual's views regarding mental illness and the hospital are imbedded within a broader ideological and psychodynamic matrix.

It may be argued that the F scale is made of the same stuff as CMI, that it taps relatively superficial ideas or values rather than more central aspects of personality. If this be true, then the foregoing inferences concerning the psychodynamic bases of ideology are unjustified. It is certainly possible that a person may accept many of the ideas represented in the F scale without being an "authoritarian personality." However, we propose on both theoretical and empirical grounds that such persons are rather the exception than the rule. The F items taken as a whole do not comprise an organized body of doctrine. The obtained consistency of response to these items is, we believe, determined for the most part by an enduring pattern of intrapersonal dispositions. Empirical support for this view is given by Adorno, *et al.* (1) and others; for a critical summary, see Christie (3). Significant relationships between CMI scores and nonscale measures of authoritarianism have been obtained by Gilbert (7) and Pine (13). These studies utilized content analysis of interviews, TATs, open-ended questions, and the like in assessing authoritarianism. The F scale would seem to provide a relatively valid though by no means infallible estimate of personal authoritarianism.

Custodial ideology has important psychic functions for authoritarian hospital members. The idea that patient behavior is simply irrational and not understandable has great value in reducing inner strain and maintaining self-esteem for personnel who have difficulty at the outset in taking an intraceptive, psychological approach. Again, for the person who has a great defensive need to displace and project aggressive wishes concerning authority figures to those who can be regarded as immoral, custodial ideology has special equilibrium-maintaining value through its justification of punitive, suppressive measures.

Humanistic ideology has corresponding functions for its adherents. By supporting a critical attitude toward the established order, it permits many equalitarian individuals to express generalized anti-authority hostilities in an ego-syntonic form. The principle of "self-control through self-understanding," applied in the treatment of patients, often serves to maintain and consolidate the intellectualizing defenses of equalitarian personnel. In our view, then, both custodialism and humanism have important nonrational functions for their proponents.

RELATIONSHIPS AMONG IDEOLOGY, PERSONALITY, AND
HOSPITAL POLICY

WE have been concerned thus far with ideology as an aspect of personality. We have suggested that the individual's orientation to mental illness is an intrinsic part of his general approach to life problems and is related to deeper-lying personality dynamics. This, however, is only part of the story. Ideology is also an aspect of the social milieu; we must consider both the psychological and the social soil within which ideologies are formed and modified.

Various social factors operate to induce some degree of ideological uniformity among members of a given occupational status, as well as among members of a total hospital system. Many social scientists, including psychologists, argue or implicitly assume that ideological conformity is ordinarily achieved and that some sort of J curve or concentration of viewpoints approximating the institutional requirements will be found among members of a given institution. One serious limitation of this approach, in our view, is its neglect of the part played by personality. We would expect that the achievement of a policy-congruent modal ideology depends in part on the presence of a corresponding modal personality. Conversely, to the extent that there is variability in ideology-relevant personality characteristics, we would expect ideological variability among members of any system.

Our three domains of inquiry are ideology, personality, and system requirements. Within each domain we have measured individual or system differences along a given continuum: (*a*) The custodial-humanistic continuum of individual ideology, as measured by the CMI scale. (*b*) The authoritarian-equalitarian continuum of personality, as measured by the F scale, (*c*) The third continuum, custodialism-humanism in system requirements, which was assessed as follows. The sample contained 12 subsystems: four occupational statuses (aide, student nurse, nurse, and psychiatrist) in each of three hospitals. Our procedure was to rank the 12 systems in order from relatively most custodial to relatively most humanistic with regard to the demands and pressures each system placed on its members. We ranked the hospitals first, then the statuses, and then combined the two sets into one series of 12 ranks.

The hospitals were ranked in terms of their degree of change away from a predominantly custodial emphasis on protection and bodily care of patients. The large state hospital, C, was assessed as the most custodial in view of its structural emphasis on detention, protection, and custodial care of patients in a highly controlled setting. The pressures it exerted on personnel, and the kinds of experience it offered them, seemed most conducive of a custodial orientation. The large VA hospital, T, was considered intermediate or transitional in that it was in process of fairly rapid change away from custodialism. The third hospital, H, was the most humanistic of the three in its program of ward care, patient government, and general staff-patient relationships.

The four statuses were ranked in degree of custodialism on the basis of educational level and job requirements vis-à-vis the patient. In order from high to low in degree of custodialism, they fall as follows: aide, student nurse, nurse, and psychiatrist.

The three hospitals and the four statuses were then combined into a series of 12 hospital-status units ranked according to degree of pressure toward custodialism. Since occupational status pressures operate over a longer period of time, and more selectively, than do hospital pressures, we made status a primary basis of stratification, and hospital secondary. That is, we assumed that statuses are relatively nonoverlapping in degree of custodialism in their policy requirements and that hospitals make a difference only within a single status grouping. Accordingly the rank 12 was given to the most custodial status in the most custodial hospital, namely, the aide status at Hospital C; this is followed by the aide status at Hospital T, and at H; then come the student nurse statuses at C, T, and H; the nurse statuses at C, T, and H; and lastly the doctor statuses at Hospitals C, T, and H with ranks of 3, 2, and 1 respectively (see Table 2). Ideally a more intensive sociological analysis of the structure and policies of each status in each hospital should be carried out. However, the rankings used here seem adequate for our present purposes.

Having roughly assessed the degree of custodialism in the policy requirements of each hospital-status system, we can now investigate the degree to which these requirements are supported by the ideologies, and are congruent with the personalities, of the system members.

Relations between policy requirements and ideology.   What is the relationship between the degree of custodialism in the policy requirements of a hospital-status system and the degree of custodialism in the modal ideology of its members? The relevant data are given in Table 2. We use the CMI mean as a measure of modal ideology, for in the distribution of CMI scores the mean, by and large, corresponds closely to the mode. The obtained rank-order correlation between degree of custodialism in policy requirements (status ranks) and in modal ideology (CMI mean) is .92. There is, in other words, relatively great congruence between policy demands and modal ideology. At the same time, the CMI means of the 12 status units do not correspond fully in absolute degree to the estimated degree of custodialism in their structural pressures. For example, the aide status at Hospital C was ranked most custodial both in policy requirements and in CMI mean; however, in an absolute sense, the policy requirements are highly custodial whereas the CMI mean is only moderate.

The above findings do not tell us how much ideological variability exists within each system. Data on variability are given in Table 2. It will be noted that the *SD*s of most of the 12 units approximate the *SD* for the total sample. Only in the doctor statuses is there anything approaching uniformity of opinion. Thus although *modal* ideology is fairly closely related to policy requirements, the findings on intrasystem variability suggest that an individual's ideology does not reflect in a simple way the demands of his occupational milieu.

In investigating the relationship between *individual* ideology and policy requirements, we consider system pressures as characteristics of the individual. Every individual in the sample of 335 was assigned an index figure representing the relative degree of custodialism in the policy requirements of his particular hospital-status unit. This index figure is simply the rank of the individual's status within the series of 12. For instance, each doctor at H, the least custodial status, is assigned an index figure of 1, and each aide at C is assigned an index of 12.

The obtained product-moment correlation[5] between CMI score and Index of Status-Custodialism is .47. This finding is evidence of a significant but moderate relationship between individual ideology and system pressures. If system pressures were the most weighty determinants of individual ideology, relative ideological homogeneity within statuses should follow, and thus a high correlation (of the order, .7 to .8) between an individual's CMI score and the degree of policy-custodialism of his work unit. However, the degree of uniformity within any system is not as great as a system-centered mode of thinking would require. An individual's ideology can be predicted with only fair accuracy on the basis of his occupational-hospital membership.

Relations between policy requirements and personality.   If the individual's ideological orientation is thought to be simply and directly a result of pressures from his work milieu, relatively independent of his personality, one would not expect the degree of custodialism in system policy to be significantly related to the degree of authoritarianism in modal personality. Rather, the 12 units might be expected to show similar degrees of authoritarianism, as measured by the F-scale means.

In our view, however, some congruence is to be expected between the policy requirements of a system and the modal personality of its members. Such congruence would be facilitated through recruitment, selective turnover, and possible personality changes in the direction of congruence. We are supported in this hypothesis by the finding of congruence (the correlation of .92) between policy requirements and modal ideology in the 12 status units. We would expect a parallel correspondence between policy requirements and modal personality.

For the 12 status units, the obtained rank-order correlation between Index of Status-Custodialism and F mean is .90 (see Table 2). Thus, there is relatively great congruence between policy demands and modal personality. This congruence is as great as that between policy demands and modal ideology.

The obtained correspondence between modal personality (F) and system requirements is accompanied by appreciable variability on the F scale within most of the statuses (Table 2). The size of the variance on F tends to covary with that on CMI ($r = .61$). This leads us to consider the degree to which system membership and personality are related in the individual. We would expect that the correlation found above between status membership and individual CMI score (.47) will hold as well for index of status membership and F score. The findings bear out this prediction. The correlation between the individual's F score and the Index of Custodialism for his status membership is .46.

Relations between ideology and personality. One of our fundamental postulates is that an individual's ideological orientation is intimately bound up with his deeper-lying personality characteristics. We therefore hypothesize, at the collective level, relative congruence between modal ideology and modal personality. The obtained rank-order correlation between CMI mean (our measure of modal ideology) and F mean (our measure of modal personality) for the 12 units is .81. Thus, the congruence between modal personality and modal ideology in a system is relatively great. As noted earlier, the size of the variance on CMI is also associated with that on F.

With the individual hospital member as the focus of analysis, the CMI-F correlation for the total sample of 335 (regardless of specific status membership) is .71. We can now consider the relationship between ideology and personality when system membership is held constant. The F-CMI correlations for the single status groupings are presented in

Table 2. They average .71, a value identical to the CMI-F correlations for the sample as a whole, and 11 of the 12 correlations are significant at the .05 level or better.

We thus have evidence that the differences in modal ideology among the 12 status units are closely related to differences in modal personality. When we find individual differences in ideology within a single status unit, these differences are closely related to differences in personality characteristics.

The theoretical formulations and results presented here concerning the mental hospital have their parallels in other social settings such as the school, the prison, industry, and the family. In all these institutions a small "administrative" elite has the power and responsibility to set goals and to control the destiny of a massive "membership." This larger population, whether children, patients, or prisoners, is a potential threat to society's values; various measures of education and social control are necessary. One of the major forms of conflict arising in these institutions is that between autocratic and democratic orientations. There is considerable evidence from both the present research and related studies that the autocratic-democratic ideological continuum is one aspect of a broader authoritarian-equalitarian personality continuum. Social ideologies have, to a considerable extent, a psychological basis in the personalities of their adherents. A socio-psychological approach provides, we believe, an important adjunct to historic-sociological approaches in the study of ideology.

SUMMARY AND CONCLUSIONS

THIS inquiry has taken as its starting point the distinction between "custodialism" and "humanism" in the mental hospital. These terms refer to two contrasting ideological orientations and to the corresponding forms of hospital policy. We have investigated ideology both as an individual and as a collective phenomena—or, more accurately, we have used both individual and collective modes of analysis in the study of ideology. With regard to the individual, we have tried to assess ideology by means of a specially devised CMI (custodialism-humanism) scale, and to determine the relationships between ideology and other individual characteristics such as psychodynamics and membership in various groups. With regard to the collective unit (e.g., hospital or occupational status), we have tried to assess the degree of custodialism in its policy requirements and in the modal ideology of its personnel, as well as the degree of authoritarianism in the modal personality of its personnel, and to determine the relationships among these.

In the individual, preference for a custodialistic orientation is part of a broader pattern of personal authoritarianism. Correlations averaging about .70 were found between the Custodialism (CMI) scale and the scales measuring autocratic family ideology (TFI) and general authoritarianism (F). Although various hospital groupings differ significantly in mean CMI score, there are appreciable individual differences within most of the groupings studied. These ideological differences within single hospitals and occupations are quite closely related to differences in personality.

In the collective unit, we found relatively great congruence between prevailing policy, modal ideology, and modal personality. The hospital-status units having the most custodial policy requirements had as well the most custodial modal ideologies and the most authoritarian personalities. At the same time, it should be noted that the correspondence among policy, ideology, and personality is far from complete. Each of these aspects of collective life can vary to some extent independently of the others, and the phenomenon of incongruence is as important as that of congruence.

Although none of our groups can be regarded as ideologically homogeneous, some of them showed relatively small dispersion in CMI scores. These groups had a similar dispersion in F scores, and had low CMI and F means. Our data do not tell how the low diversity and the high ideology-personality congruence came about, but they point up the need for answers to at least the following questions. To what extent do relatively homogeneous systems maintain themselves by recruitment and selective maintenance of individuals whose personalities are receptive to the structurally required ideology? To what extent do systems change the personalities which initially are unreceptive to the prevailing policy? Under what conditions can a system induce most of its members to support the required ideology even when this ideology is personality-incongruent? Under what conditions can the "incongruent" members change the system to a personally more congenial form?

Systems characterized by relatively great ideological diversity were very common in our sample. Moreover, the ideological diversity went hand in hand with diversity in personality, the standard deviations on CMI correlating .61 with those on F. We incline to the belief that significant heterogeneity of opinion and of personality obtains in the majority of institutional settings within modern societies undergoing rapid technological and educational change.

NOTES TO CHAPTER 39

1. This investigation was supported in part by research grants M-687 and M-1000 from the National Institute of Mental Health, of the National Institutes of Health, Public Health Service.
2. *DP* of an item reflects its ability to differentiate between extremely high

scorers and extreme low scorers (the upper and lower 25 per cent) on the total scale. It is computed as the difference between the means of the high-scoring and the low-scoring groups.

3. In a study to be published shortly, we have obtained correlations of .5 and .8 between the CMI scale and a measure of custodialism in role performance, in two samples of hospital aides. Since at least a moderate relation between ideology and action would be expected on theoretical grounds, evidence of such a relation has indirect validational relevance for the CMI scale (4).

4. An abbreviated F scale of 8 items was used; it contained Items 9, 13, 18, 25, 26, 37, and 42 from Form 45, and Item 32 from Form 78 of the original F scale (1). The TFI measure contained Items 2, 3, 5, 6, 7, 9, 11, 12 of the short form presented by Levinson and Huffman (14, p. 268).

5. The use of indices based on rank in a product-moment correlation involves the assumption of equal intervals between ranks. This constitutes a possible source of error, but probably not a great one.

REFERENCES

1. Adorno, T. W., Frenkel-Brunswik, Else, Levinson, D. J., & Sanford, R. N. *The authoritarian personality.* New York: Harper, 1950.
2. Bettelheim, B. *Love is not enough.* Glencoe, Ill.: Free Press, 1950.
3. Christie, R. Authoritarianism re-examined. In R. Christie & Marie Jahoda (Eds.), *Studies in the scope and method of "The authoritarian personality."* Glencoe, Ill.: Free Press, 1954.
4. Cronbach, L. J., & Meehl, P. E. Construct validity in psychological tests. *Psychol. Bull.,* 1955, 52, 281-302.
5. Dicks, H. V. Personality traits and national socialist ideology. *Hum. Relat.,* 1950, 3, 111-154.
6. Fromm, E. *Man for himself.* New York: Rinehart, 1947.
7. Gilbert, Doris C. Ideologies concerning mental illness: A sociopsychological study of mental hospital personnel. Unpublished doctor's dissertation, Radcliffe Coll., 1954.
8. Greenblat, M., York, R., & Brown, Esther L. *From custodial to therapeutic care in mental hospitals.* New York: Russell Sage Foundation, 1955.
9. Jones, M. *The therapeutic community.* New York: Basic Books, 1953.
10. Leighton, A. H. *The governing of men.* Princeton: Princeton Univer. Press, 1944.
11. Levinson, D. J., & Huffman, Phyllis E. Traditional family ideology and its relation to personality. *J. Pers.,* 1955, 23, 251-273.
12. Mayo, E. *Human problems of industrial civilization.* Cambridge, Mass.: Harvard Univer. Press, 1933.
13. Pine, F. Conceptions of the mentally ill and the self: A study of psychiatric aides. Unpublished doctor's dissertation, Harvard Univer., 1955.
14. Stanton, A., & Schwartz, M. *The mental hospital.* New York: Basic Books, 1954.
15. Tannenbaum, F. *Crime and the community.* New York: Columbia Univer. Press, 1951.

CHAPTER 40   Psychiatry in Prison*

HARVEY POWELSON AND REINHARD BENDIX

A PRISON—like other large-scale organizations—reflects in its day-to-day operation many of the unresolved conflicts which exist in the society at large. People in our society are of many minds with regard to the major social problems of our time, of which the treatment of prisoners is one. And the people who work together in the prison and who are charged with the responsibility of guarding and supervising prisoners are not likely to be of one mind simply by virtue of their employment. Thus, controversy continues among those who are concerned with the crime problem, officially or otherwise. Some hold that the convicted criminal must be punished to repay his debt to society. Others believe that he must be rehabilitated and restored as a member of society. The actual treatment of convicted offenders in the prison depends upon the way in which these conflicting views are acted upon by the prison staff; and these actions of the staff become intelligible only if they are viewed in the context of the history of prison reform and with regard to the ideological and psychological involvement of the different professionals who make up the prison staff. The following study examines this involvement primarily with regard to the relation between the staff of the psychiatric ward and that of the custodial division in a state prison.

A criminal's conviction and imprisonment confirm his guilt beyond reasonable doubt in the eyes of most people. Moral condemnation by the public and the authority of government are mutually reinforcing, and in

* This article is the outgrowth of repeated discussions between the authors concerning the interrelations between psychiatric and sociological modes of analysis. When Dr. Powelson served as psychiatrist for three months in the psychiatric ward of a prison, an opportunity presented itself to test our preliminary conclusions by means of case studies. The present article is based on Dr. Powelson's observations, which were corroborated so far as possible by several other psychiatrists who had held the same position, and by Dr. Bendix in a series of interviews with a number of the persons involved.
Reprinted by special permission of The William Alanson White Psychiatric Foundation, Inc., and the authors from *Psychiatry*, 14 (1951), 73–86 (copyright by the Foundation).

the face of such overwhelming censure it is difficult indeed to take a detached view of the convicted criminal. Since the guilt of the criminal is established, many people feel that most forms of punishment are justified, because public morality has been violated and the authority of the law has been challenged. We shall designate this approach to the criminal as punitive, and we do not subscribe to it. But we must acknowledge at the same time the tragic involvement which tends to make any prison into an institution that creates criminal behavior. In 1935-36, a survey of state prisons showed that 55,822 prisoners out of a total prison population of 106,818 were idle. It is hard to see how rehabilitation is possible under these conditions, but it is easy to see that the unwitting punishment of enforced idleness is likely to have a more corrosive effect on the personality of the prisoner than most forms of deliberate punishment. What we say subsequently concerning the actions and ideas of a prison staff is written in full appreciation of the burden which the setting of prison work imposes upon the members of the staff.

It is perhaps necessary to add a caveat. The prison is a world by itself. Yet, in the prison, each person acts as a member both of the larger society and of the prison society. And the conflicting views of crime and the criminal which prevail in the larger society vitally affect, though frequently in imperceptible ways, the interpersonal relations within the prison. On a routine visit to Condemned Row where every one of the condemned men was locked behind steel bars, except one who was cleaning up, we were warned by the guard, "Do you really want to go in there? It's dangerous!" We feel sure that the guard had a genuine concern for our safety as well as a routine apprehension which is probably second nature to him by now. Yet, in analyzing his behavior, we would feel justified in saying that his warning reflects an exaggerated concern with physical aggression, which is anticipated in all cases but erupts in only a few. We must observe that this anticipation is the basis for a punitive approach to the prisoner. But we realize that basic to this anticipation is concrete experience with aggressive prisoners and the deep anxiety, prevalent among the public at large, which prompts people to identify violent crime with an image of the perpetually aggressive criminal.

In a situation as emotionally charged as that of a prison, every factually accurate observation will be regarded as an attack. A guard who treats an inmate in a punitive way will regard a statement to this effect as a criticism of his action. We have attempted to analyze the perspectives of different members of the prison staff as accurately as we can, but we have no doubt that our observations will be adjudged as partisan by the participants. It is in the nature of conflict situations that any attempt at objective analysis contributes fuel to the fire, and of course no one is entirely free of bias. The analyst is, moreover, not in the role of umpire, since he has usually not been invited to observe.

THE PRISON ORGANIZATION

THE Official Training Manual for Correctional Employees issued by the state government contains an historical sketch which is highly instructive. It would appear from this survey that the penal and correctional system of the state has progressed over the last sixty years through the addition of new correctional methods, all of which are designed to strengthen the work of rehabilitation and diminish the merely punitive aspects of the penal system. The following excerpts from this historical account illustrate this point:

1893   Parole as a release procedure was adopted. This was an important step away from the classical theory of punishment.

1911   State reformatory is authority. This allowed segregation of younger offenders to prevent further corruption.

1917   The indeterminate sentence became law. The arbitrary sentencing power of the judge was removed and the State Board of Prison Directors were authorized to set sentences within minimum and maximum period as prescribed by law.

1931   Board of Prison Terms and Paroles was created. This Board had the following duties: (1) Fixing of prison terms to be served; (2) Granting of paroles; (3) Restoration of civil rights.

1941   The State Institution for Men was established. It provided a minimum security institution with vocational training and education for younger offenders. This was a major step in the rehabilitation program.

1945   Medical Facility authorized. The primary purpose of this institution is to be care and treatment of males who are: mentally ill or defective, epileptic, narcotic addicts, psychopaths and sex offenders.

Under the State Department of Correction and the Chief Warden of the Prison, the following divisions are operating: (1) Guidance Center; (2) Medical Services; (3) Care and Treatment; (4) Business Management and Correctional Industries; (5) Custody. Each of these divisions is staffed with people whose training predisposes them to look at the problems of the prisoners under their care from different points of view. The Official Training Manual for Correctional Employees, in characterizing the functions of these divisions, seems to endorse this professional specialization. A brief review of these divisions may help one to obtain an initial impression of the problems of prison organization.

The Guidance Center is set up so that a "clinical study may be made of each prisoner" which will serve as the basis for "his care, training and employment." The stated objective of the Guidance Center is to reform the prisoner and protect society. The Official Manual, from which this description is taken, also specifies that the work of the center involves the professional services of psychiatrists, physicians, sociologists, psychologists, guidance and vocational counselors.

During his stay in the Guidance Center, the inmate is assigned to work projects and educational programs. This procedure acclimates the new prisoner to institutional living and provides the necessary time for thorough study of the inmate and the planning of his prison program.

It is apparent from these statements of the Official Manual that the professional specialists in the Guidance Center will look at the prisoner from a social welfare point of view. The prisoner is likely to be viewed as a social deviant whose violation of the law is to be attributed to social and psychological causes—such as broken homes, poverty, harmful recreational facilities, difficulties in school, confusion in moral values, and what not. A page and a half of these causes is enumerated in the Manual.

The reform of the prisoner is sought through the care, training, and employment which he receives. The underlying philosophy of the Guidance Center is that a proper diagnosis of the factors which led to the crime will enable the experts to devise a program of activities for each prisoner which will facilitate his rehabilitation. Specifically, his work in the prison will help to reform him and will give him those skills which will enable him, after his release, to find his place in society. In this way he will lose his criminal tendencies.

The Medical Services in the prison are designed to preserve the health of the prisoner. Specific cases of illness are diagnosed and treated. The sanitation and diet of the prison are supervised, and prisoners are given, when necessary, individual psychiatric treatment. These are the official objectives. They reflect the professional objectives of medicine, which consist in the maintenance of the health of the individual person. Health is the supreme value of the doctor, and that means the health of each person under all circumstances. The supremacy of this value is perhaps indicated by the fact that a prisoner who has been condemned to death and who is at the point of death as the result of a suicide attempt will be restored to health only to be executed. The prison doctor can, therefore, be expected to be concerned with the prisoner as a person whose health is of paramount importance and whose other attributes are consequently of secondary importance.

The Division of Care and Treatment is officially designated as being principally concerned with the prisoner's rehabilitation. Organizationally, this division should execute what the Guidance Center has previously established as in the best interests of the prisoner and of society. Its activities range from education and recreation to the organization of the prison library, religious services, and the preparole program. The principal philosophy of this division is that of the educator. Care and Treatment is concerned with implementing the recommendations of the Guidance Center. The prisoner is taught useful skills on the presumption that this will prompt in him the desire to do useful work. It is also done in the belief that his deviant behavior in the past is due in part to the absence of such desires or of such skills. Moreover, the inmate is taught to distinguish between good and bad actions, as these are conventionally conceived. The expectation is that men who know this distinction will act "appropriately," since some of the criminal's behavior is thought to be due to an atrophy of his moral faculties. "A man who knows good will not do wrong."[1]

Another division is that of Business Management, which is responsible for the operation and maintenance of the physical plant and for the whole range of industrial operations in which the inmates are employed. Unlike the other divisions which have an ostensibly clear purpose, Business Management faces an inherent contradiction. Businessmen and legislators accept the view that prison industries must not compete with outside industries, but they also accept the view that there is no excuse for an insolvent business operation.

The last division which we consider here is that of Custody. This is the largest division of the prison, in terms of personnel. Its program is officially stated to consist of ". . . the custody and security of the inmates committed to the institutions, and . . . the effective application of rehabilitative measures." If one interpreted this literally, he would expect that the Division of Custody would be independently concerned with all problems affecting security, but that it would follow the direction of the other divisions insofar as the rehabilitation of the inmates is concerned. At any rate, so it would appear from the Official Manual, since the personnel who are expert on problems of rehabilitation are employed in the Guidance Center, the Medical Division, and the Division of Care and Treatment. The historical sketch given earlier would also make it appear that the emphasis on the punitive aspects of the penal system had been left behind. With each addition of services, the correctional features of the prison seem to have gained in importance.

Are these impressions in accord with the facts? The personnel of the Custodial Division is the largest numerically. It comprises some three hundred persons, which is equal to the number of employees in all the other divisions taken together. Although the importance of the different divisions in the prison is not indicated simply by the size of their respective staffs, it would appear that the Custodial Division dominates the operation of all the other divisions. A few illustrations will make this clear. In the Guidance Center extensive records are prepared which give in detail the case history of the inmate and the results of a series of tests which are run by the staff psychologist. The Center's recommendation on the prisoner's program of rehabilitation is based on all these assembled data. However, the personnel of the Guidance Center has no authority over the prisoner once he has passed through these screening procedures. He is then under the authority of Custody. Since his program in the prison is directly determined by Custody, the Guidance Center is only effective in determining the program insofar as Custody is guided by its recommendations. Apparently Custody is not so guided to any appreciable extent. Our impression is that Custody has a separate and independent system of classifying prisoners which has little, if anything, to do with the recommendations made by the Guidance Center. Each prisoner, who has been classified in the Center on the basis of his case record and a battery of tests, is now reclassified in accordance with Custody's estimate of the prisoner as a security risk. The three degrees of security risk—minimum, medium, and maximum—are only remotely related to these earlier findings. They also have little to do with any objective standard which might enable one to distinguish between prisoners of different degrees of security risk. The custodial classification seems to be based rather on the conventional middle-class evaluation of different crimes. Crimes involving violence, sexual or other, are rated as maximum security risks, despite the fact that murderers and sex offenders have the best parole records. Similarly, former escapees from reform schools never get less than a medium security classification, presumably on the ground that once an escapee, always an escapee. Yet, the individual case might well warrant less severe treatment.

To classify prisoners as Custody does, involves a theory of criminality for which there is no evidence. The theory holds that those who have committed crimes most severely punished in our society are most likely to repeat them and are, therefore, least likely to benefit from the program of the Care and Treatment Division. The facts point to the opposite conclusion, though our knowledge is very limited in this field. Murderers and sex offenders are rarely professionally so, while confidence men, robbers, holdup men, and others are frequently professional criminals and as a consequence are frequent repeaters. While repeated criminal activity does not necessarily mean that the inmate cannot benefit from rehabilitative measures, his chances of benefiting are certainly not better than those of the nonrepeaters. And similarly, the seriousness of a person's crime or the length of his sentence is not a measure of his chances of rehabilitation. This chance can only be judged on the basis of a careful examination of the individual case. The custodial classification, in terms of security risk, is therefore unrelated to the program of correction. It is solely dictated by the consideration that those who have received the highest sentences must be the "most dangerous" to society and the most incorrigible—a view which coincides with that of the sensationalist press. They must be the most severely punished, therefore, not only in terms of the longer duration of their sentences, but also by the more severe treatment while they are in prison.

Finally, there is the consideration of convenience. Custody supervises the activities of the prisoners and is interested in "smooth operation," regardless of the effect on the individual prisoner. Educational privileges may be extended to inmates as rewards or withdrawn from them as a form of punishment by the custodial personnel. Inmates are assigned to work details under the jurisdiction of Business Management from the point of view of security or convenience. For example, a prisoner who was working as a saw-filer had applied for an assignment in vocational drafting. At the simple request of the custody officer to the Classification Board, the prisoner was kept at saw-filing "because saw-filers are hard to find." The work record may be held for or against the individual inmate and his need or desire for rehabilitation is not considered.[2]

THE CUSTODIAL ORIENTATION

THE only professional group which comes into the prison for positive reasons is that of the custodial employees. They enter the prison with the clear objective of punishing convicted offenders and protecting society. Perhaps members of the other professions (doctors, psychologists, teachers, vocational counsellors, and many others) enter the prison for equally clear reasons, for instance, to promote the rehabilitation and the health of prisoners. Yet, they cannot, in fact, pursue this goal. If, in spite of this, they continue to stay in the prison, it is probable that a number of selective factors enter in which make their continued activity on the prison staff tolerable to them.

There are two principal methods by which the conflict of ostensible goals among the various professional groups on the prison staff could be resolved.[3] The first of these methods, and the one which is in closest correspondence with the formal organization of the prison, would be *compromise for the sake of teamwork*. This would mean, for instance, that the health of the individual prisoner is considered paramount whenever this does not conflict with the security of his retention. An example will indicate that such compromises are not made—that, instead, the constant tension that exists between Custody and the Medical Division breaks out into pitched battles on occasion. At one of the psychiatric staff conferences, a number of staff members complained that whenever the inmates applied for psychiatric treatment, the guards addressed them as "ding" or "queer." Representation against this practice to the Associate Warden, who headed the custodial staff, drew only the reply that this allegation would have to be proved, that none of the guards ever did such a thing, the implication being that the psychiatrists were simply the dupes of malingering prisoners. What is characteristic in this incident is the avoidance of the usual bureaucratic evasion. It would have been easy for the Associate Warden to have stated that this complaint of the Psychiatric Staff would be communicated to the Custodial Staff, although no particular instance of this sort had previously come to his attention. This, of course, would have meant no action, just as the real reply did, but it would have preserved the pretense of cooperation. Instead, the representation of the Psychiatric Staff is rejected as unworthy of attention unless it be proved. In that case, the accused guards would have to testify against themselves since the testimony of the inmates is immediately rejected by Custody. It is apparent that the Warden, in charge of Custody, did not consider it necessary to reach an understanding which would be required for effective teamwork. Compromise, then, is not the method usually resorted to in relations between Custody and the staffs of the other divisions.

The formal organization chart indicates the coordinate position of all divisions. Nevertheless, there is hardly any give-and-take between these divisions. In practice, all activities are subordinate to the decisions of Custody, although not directly. Conflicts between the divisions are most frequently resolved by the effective power of Custody over each prisoner. This makes it possible, incidentally, to preserve in many instances the appearance of cooperation even if there is no cooperation in fact. Custody expresses its attitude toward the activities of the other divisions in terms of its actions concerning the prisoner. The other divisions have power over the inmate only when and as long as Custody permits this.

The *authoritarian solution* to the conflicts between the different divisions makes it necessary to characterize their relationship from the vantage point of each. The custodial view of prison organization is in practice that the activities of all other divisions are subordinate to the security regulations and the disciplinary measures of Custody. Custody regards the prisoner, at least unofficially, as a special form of humanity, as a person who must be guilty unless he can prove his innocence. If questioned, most guards are likely to defend this view as proved by the conviction itself. If the inmate were innocent, then he would not be in prison; since he is in prison, he must demonstrate his "reform" by proving his innocence. Hence Custody looks at the activities of the other divisions as evidence of misguided humanitarianism. It will tolerate them only after it is satisfied that every conceivable breach of security and discipline has been guarded against. The guards suspect the other divisions of being "soft." They take pride in their intimate knowledge of the prisoners' depravity as they see it.[4]

Hence the guards will act on the premise that each prisoner is a cunning malingerer and that each staff member who is not a guard falls an easy prey to the chicanery of the criminal mind. It is as an outgrowth of this orientation that an inmate must convince a guard that he is sick before he can obtain medical or psychiatric attention. But the guard will assume that the inmate is malingering. It is as an outgrowth of the same orientation that Custody acts on purely medical matters in a manner completely unrelated to medicine. The following three examples may show how medical aid to the prisoner is subordinated to the aims of punishment or detection, or is withheld because of the sheer inertia of the Custodial Division.

An inmate who has an ulcer often must first convince a guard that he requires medical help. Once medical tests are positive and the appropriate diets are prescribed, the ulcer patient is put under double lock on order of the medical officer. This means that the prisoner is placed in a regular cell under solitary confinement. Usually he is placed on the most severe diet which can be prescribed for ulcer patients—namely, milk every other hour. However, the patient usually gets milk only three times a day, since the attendants who are responsible for the care of the patient are inmates and are negligent because of ill will towards the patient, or for some other reason. The guards look the other way because they suspect the patient of malingering anyhow. Of course, after a few days of this the patient is so starved that he will do anything to get back into his regular cell although his ulcer is worse as a result of this experience.

A prisoner who had been severely stabbed was bleeding from several deep knife wounds when the doctor arrived. To begin with, the doctor was only asked whether the prisoner was dying; his answer was negative. The prisoner was completely surrounded by guards who questioned him in detail and took photographs of his wounds from various angles. Despite the fact that the prisoner was bleeding acutely, the doctor was allowed to treat the wounds of the patient only after about thirty minutes. The ostensible purpose of this procedure was the detection and punishment of the attacker. It seems then that the doctor was asked whether the patient was dying—not because his death mattered but merely because the guards wanted to question him. At any rate, it is not apparent why the same questioning could not have been done equally well after the wounds had been dressed.

During off-hours, drugs are not handled by the attendants and registered nurses, but by the guards. The guards are completely unacquainted with the drugs. Some guards carry the drugs all mixed up in a small box and pick out a pill at random when medication is needed. In one case, a patient, who was suffering from excruciating pain, needed a morphine injection. The guard, who brought the patient to the doctor, went to get the morphine capsule. He came back with the capsule in his bare hand, violating the most elementary precautions against infection. The morphine, so obtained, had then to be injected into the arm of the patient. "We have always done it that way" was the only answer the doctor could obtain from the guard.

These illustrations may suffice to indicate the orientation of the Custodial Division. They give a picture of the setting in which the Medical and Psychiatric Division has to do its work.

THE RELATION OF THE PSYCHIATRIC AND
THE CUSTODIAL ORIENTATIONS

THERE is a striking contrast between the custodial and the psychiatric view of the prisoner. Psychiatry, like medicine, is concerned primarily with health. Both are also concerned with the individual and his mental and physical welfare, but here the psychiatric emphasis is the more individualistic of the two. Medicine considers health largely in terms of the community and, in the prison, this is reflected in the medical supervision of sanitation and nutrition for the prison as a whole. Psychiatry, on the other hand, deals only with the mental health of the individual.

Regardless of the current fashion of mental hygiene for whole groups or even nations, the hard fact remains that the whole history of psychiatry and of its therapeutic techniques points to the cure of the individual. This aim of therapy necessitates a thorough-going, though not an absolute, ethical relativism. Behavior and emotional disposition are good insofar as they are good for the health of the individual. Psychiatrists are vague enough on what this end-state of mental health is, but they are quite definite in rejecting most of the conventional ethical values as they apply to the individual's attempts at emotional recovery. The prison code regards aggressive behavior as an offense, subject to punishment; yet the psychiatrist will often regard the same behavior as essential for the individual's emotional rehabilitation.

Finally, psychiatrists come into the prison with the belief that the inmate's present action is an outgrowth of his personal history. To the psychiatrist, actions and rationalizations are only the symptoms of underlying causes; hence he will interpret them in this context. To the custodial officer, the inmate's present behavior is the conclusive index of his depravity or of his progressing rehabilitation. How much these views differ is, perhaps, best indicated by the conflict between the custodial and the psychiatric appraisal of the inmate's motivation. Custody thinks of each prisoner as desiring, above all else, to get out of prison by fair means or foul, and so to escape the just punishment of society. Prisoners often present to the psychiatrist a picture of having adjusted to the human jungle of the prison and of fearing the insecurities of the outside world and of their own position in it. Harsh though prison is, it is a knowable world which forces the inmate into an established routine of activities. During the last four weeks before being released on parole, for example, prisoners become tense and are likely to spoil their records. During the period of observation, an inmate was told to clean his cell for the last time within a few hours of his release from the prison. In cleaning his heavy mattress, the inmate dropped it from the height of the fifth tier, seriously injuring another prisoner. After his sentence had been extended by another six years, the inmate showed a notable decrease in tension.

The psychiatrist emphasizes the mental health of the person, the need to consider his present actions as determined by his personal and emotional history, and the need to suspend judgment of the inmate's actions for the sake of therapeutic success. It will be apparent that the prison psychiatrist must come into conflict with the custodial treatment of prisoners if he follows the precepts of his profession. In view of this contradiction, and since there is little effort to minimize it through compromises, it remains for us to show how the subordination of psychiatric to custodial treatment actually transforms psychiatric practice and those who engage in it.

It is apparent that the health of the prisoner, both physical and mental, has become a subordinate consideration under the influence of Custody. Prisoners are well aware that every instance of sickness will be recorded. "Too many" applications for medical or psychiatric aid will be held against them, since it will be interpreted as malingering by the custody officer. The medical officer in the prison, therefore, has to deal with patients who have been discouraged from seeking his help. The same subordination of the prisoner's health is in evidence in the procedure of the sick line which forms daily before the prison clinic at a stipulated hour. Those in line have previously persuaded the guard of the validity of their needs, and they presumably consider their complaints serious, since they are likely to have weighed the disadvantage of another sickness notification on their records. Usually they file by the pharmacist who sits behind a small open window prescribing and dealing out drugs as each prisoner states his complaint. There is also a psychiatric sick line, in which patients are seen only for a few minutes at a time. In the clinic a patient may receive a 'complete' neurological and psychiatric work-up in thirty minutes. One psychiatrist has openly boasted to the members of the staff that he can hold 50 'therapy' interviews during the day, and the fact is that he can. Again, when inmates are selected for group therapy, the custodial officer in charge will give the order that all violators of Section 288 of the Penal Code[5] who are between the ages of 20 and 40 and are nonveterans are to appear for group therapy at a given hour. Thus the physical conditions and the mental climate surrounding medical and psychiatric aid are such as to make ordinary standards of medical and psychiatric practice completely inapplicable.

How can the psychiatric staff do its professional work under these conditions? It seems to us that these are the possibilities:

1. The psychiatrist can become a custody officer and cease all pretense of doing psychiatric work. This is a frequent case in other organizations, as in the case of the professor who has become a university administrator or the medical officer in the army whose duties are administrative and who no longer practices medicine.

2. The psychiatrist may be conscious of a strong antagonism towards Custody; but, in his actual psychiatric work, he adopts Custody's punitive attitude toward the prisoner.

3. The psychiatrist may have a cynical or embittered attitude towards Custody; but, in his actual work, he goes through a routine performance of the job without apparent awareness that his work is

futile from the psychiatric viewpoint, given the conditions under which it must be done.

4. The psychiatrist may become aware of the irreconcilable conflict between Custody and Psychiatry, and, as a result, leave the prison for practice elsewhere.

The subordination of the particular problems of health and personality to the punitive treatment of the inmate is the condition which Custody imposes on psychiatric practice in prison. The responses of the psychiatrist to this condition reveal much about the interrelation between personality and institutional position.

We wish to comment primarily on the second and third types. The psychiatrists whom we have observed in this situation have in fact abandoned their belief in ethical relativism and psychological determinism. They accept a condition of employment in which concern with the health of the individual inmate can at best be perfunctory. Although they accept Custody's view of the prisoner, they feel constantly challenged by Custody and show a strong antagonism toward it. To illustrate, here is a verbatim record of an interview with a 20-year-old Mexican inmate. The patient is a paranoid schizophrenic who received a one-hundred-percent disability discharge from the Navy and who has been sent to prison with the explicit instruction that he be given psychiatric treatment. The following are some questions put to the prisoner:

"You didn't do well in the Navy, did you? . . . You were mostly unsuccessful all your life! . . . Maybe your illness was caused by taking the money [pension for mental illness]."

(*Then with reference to illness in childhood:*) "Were you able to get out of work when you had an earache?" (*With reference to sibling rivalry:*) "Maybe your brother has tried harder?" (*With reference to a choice the patient had made:*) "You took the easy route again."

(*In response to a blocking of the patient's speech:*) "Go ahead, we can take it." [Whereupon the patient replied: "Yes, you can, but can I?"]

The interview clearly shows that the psychiatrist has abandoned that degree of ethical relativism which is the *sine qua non* of his discipline. The questions put to the prisoner assume that he suffers from moral weakness and that if only he had made up his mind, he would not be where he is now. This is in fact Custody's view. It rests on the idea that the prisoner is a criminal by choice or, perhaps, by virtue of his failure to choose the right way. It is instructive to hear this view expressed in psychiatric jargon. The following quotation is taken from the instructions which have been prepared for all new members of the psychiatric staff:

The purpose of the Psychiatric Department is first and foremost to safeguard the total, and, especially, the mental health of the individual, to improve the mental hygiene of each and every individual with whom we have contact, be he a civilian employee or be he an inmate. We, therefore, are interested in helping each individual obtain a better understanding of his own thoughts, motives, feelings, and actions, and then help him to help himself to work out a healthy way of living in which he recognizes his basic needs, wishes, and desires, and work out the ways and means by which he can get the most out of life for himself and for his fellow human beings, so that he can earn his livelihood; get his share of love and affection, his share of friends and learn to work out his own problems a little bit better each day.

It is our desire and purpose and aim to help each man to organize and balance his personality so that he will have a reasonable goal or ambition in life with short term and long term goals in keeping with his assets and capacities, handicaps and opportunities. We want each man to use his intelligence and his judgment to plan ahead with imagination and vision and, at the same time, temper his plans and his imagination and his prayers with reality. It is our aim to help each person develop a true appreciation of the value of time and plan and ration it accordingly; to develop in each individual a skill, or trade, or vocation by which to serve his fellow human beings better—to use sufficient initiative to even develop an avocation or a craft or a spare time interest or hobby. . . .

We hope to help those with whom we work to develop a balance between present pleasure and future needs; to develop good habits—physically, mentally, and emotionally; to use drugs and alcohol only with judgment and understanding. We bend our efforts to fully develop, in ourselves and others, reliability and dependability and responsibility; to develop understanding of emotions and emotional instability and controls of these emotions and their variations; to develop an appreciation of the value of personal and social contacts and so train ourselves to be good friends as well as to deserve good friends—to learn not only the cause of our emotional swings but that we all have moods and that a certain amount of control needs to be exercised in or over our moods.

We all need self satisfaction points of rest and recreation, of play, hobbies, new experiences.

We all have sex needs and we should realize that the ultimate goal of sex needs is the formation of the family. We endeavor to train ourselves to understand our psychosexual development and, when compromises are made, that they be recognized as such. We all need to learn to solve our problems without too much tension, evasion or frustration, and we all need to develop a personal philosophy of life; to learn to Live and Let Live—not to get too upset when things go wrong or too self-sympathetic when things don't turn out as we plan. . . .

Let us, therefore, point every effort to not only understanding ourselves better and training ourselves to develop a healthy way of living; to train ourselves to daily live a healthy personal religion based on the understanding and gaining for ourselves and other fellow human beings the most life has to offer, legitimately.

Let us continue our search for the truth that sets us free in mind and body and help our fellow human beings by giving them a little more of the light that we have been fortunate enough to get ourselves.

The view here expressed might be taken from an after-dinner speech on mental health to any fraternal organization. It endorses the custodial view that the depraved prisoner must be rehabilitated by being confronted with a model of the "clean life." The prisoner must be taught to cherish the values of the family and of "the good deed." He must also be taught never to want more out of life than he can get. In this context, the prisoner, far from being told of the virtues of striving, shall be advised by the psychiatrist that above all he should exercise moderation and self-restraint. The values stated in the Instruction Manual are such that no prisoner could live up to them, if for no other reason than that he is in prison. Witness, for instance, the statement that "the ultimate goal of sex needs is the formation of the family." A prisoner's failure to "adjust" and to "reform" is evidence of his moral inferiority. In the light of the views expressed in the Manual, it is hardly surprising that psychiatry in the prison consists primarily in therapeutic practices which can have punitive or disciplinary implications: electric shock, insulin shock, fever treatment, hydrotherapy, amytal and pentothal interviews, cisternals and spinals, and so on—that is, everything except psychotherapy.

Under the conditions extant in the prison, this conventional and punitive approach to the prisoner will eventually determine the practice and personnel of the ward. This approach to the prisoner requires of the psychiatrist a rigidly prescribed range of behavior. The personality attributes which would permit a person to function effectively under these conditions have been well summarized by A. H. Maslow, who lists the traits which are characteristic of an authoritarian personality. He is a person who looks at the world as a jungle "in which [each] man's hand is necessarily against every other man's, in which the whole world is conceived of as dangerous, threatening, or at least challenging, and in which human beings are conceived of as primarily selfish, or evil or stupid."[6] Such a person has a tendency to view others as superior and therefore to be feared; or as inferior and therefore to be scorned. He tends to have a strong drive for power and for external prestige. Kindness is identified with weakness, and hardness with strength. The sadistic component of his personality is likely to be prominent in his relations to the prisoners, while the sado-masochistic component appears in the relation among staff members. He achieves a superficial feeling of security through compulsive routines, order, discipline, and rigidity. It is a fair guess that these same character traits would be a liability rather than an asset in any extended period of contact between patient and therapist, and as a result very considerable anxiety would be generated in both participants. Moreover, such a doctor might find it very anxiety-provoking to associate with other psychiatrists. Hence, he would experience great insecurity outside the prison; but inside the prison the situation is different. We stated earlier that the custody officers come to their work in the prison for positive reasons. We should now amend this by stating that a psychiatrist of the type we have described would take on a prison job, such as we have described it, for equally positive reasons. The very personality characteristics which are liabilities in outside practice turn into assets in a prison of this kind.

A person of this type is best able to function simultaneously on these five levels: (1) He is antagonistic toward Custody and its encroachments. (2) As opposed to Custody, he gives lip service to the importance of psychiatric treatment. (3) In his psychiatric practice he shows the same attitude toward the prisoner as the guards do. (4) He is only conscious of doing expert psychiatric work and indeed prides himself in being part of a model department. (5) He is conscious of custodial interference but unconscious that he, basically, agrees with the attitude towards the prisoners which lies back of this interference.

It is apparent that a psychiatrist of such disposition is able to tolerate the wide gulf between the stated aims and the actual practice of psychiatry in the prison. Psychologically, this is most tolerable because he has actually adopted the custodial view, although he would, of course, deny this vehemently. He is unconsciously at peace, as it were, though at the conscious level he fights a running battle with the other divisions. And he is able to do this effectively because he can perform each of his incompatible roles in isolation from the other or reconcile them by projecting his internal conflicts on others.[7]

Psychiatrists of less compulsive and sadistic disposition cannot make this adjustment. They will either keep their antagonism toward Custody and their routine psychiatric practice in separate compartments—though the custodial environment makes that practice well-nigh meaningless, or they will become so intensely conscious of the conflict that they will leave the prison because they are unable to tolerate it in any form. The net result will be that the personnel of the psychiatric service will become typed, because, by a gradual process of attrition, those who do not fit in will be eliminated and those who do fit in will stay on. Our period of observation was, of course, too short to see this process in operation, but, on the face of it, it is probable that persons of the personality type we have described will unwittingly help to perpetuate this pattern of character structure and institutional position. In selecting additional personnel, such persons will tend to favor persons like themselves and, in organizing the psychiatric department, they will create conditions sufficiently uncongenial for persons of other types.

CONCLUSIONS

IT MAY be useful to summarize the major conclusions of this study by an explicit statement of the frame of reference on which it is based. We began our observations with the finding that psychiatry, as practiced in the prison, was unlike psychiatric practice in any other context with which we are familiar. This finding pointed to the different views of punishment, rehabilitation, and criminal behavior, as these are institutionalized in the different divisions of the prison. It also pointed to the different historical background of the various professions represented in these divisions. Retention and punishment of convicted criminals is one of the major problems of modern society. The prison brings to sharp focus all of the conflicting views concerning this problem. These conflicts are resolved, after a fashion, in the institutionalized interplay of the professions which represent these views on the outside.

The history of institutional changes. In this field as in others, the history of institutional changes is frequently presented in the form of dated events. In 1893, parole as a release procedure was adopted; in 1911, younger offenders were segregated from older offenders, and so on. Those who espouse the cause of penal reform are likely to take more solace than they should from the apparent progress which has been made. Their concern with legal reform is certainly legitimate, but they tend to overlook that even explicit adoption of these reforms in penal institutions is not an indication of their effect on practical application. The history of dated events is a surface phenomenon.

Formal organization as an ideology. It is odd that the reformer is aided and abetted in this deception by those who stand against reform. We have tried to show how the general trend toward penal reform *is* reflected in the formal organization of the prison. But we have also pointed out that the formal endorsement of correctional, rather than punitive, penology is not acted upon. Formally, each of the divisions has its assigned role in effecting the rehabilitation of the inmate, and rehabilitation is clearly the stated aim of the prison. In fact, Custody prevails, and, with it, the punitive approach to the prisoner. The challenges to this approach have been enacted into law and the letter of the law has been followed; but the effect has been to create a prison in which the inmate is subjected to punitive practices which are represented as designed for his rehabilitation. We are observers, not judges, of this system and we lack the experience required for remedial proposals.[8] But at least it is an open question whether an admittedly punitive treatment of the prisoner might not be preferable to a punitive treatment under the pretense of rehabilitation. This is not an argument for punishment, but, rather, an argument against the false representation of whatever treatment is adopted. The criminal, as a human being, is likely to benefit from a clear statement of purpose corresponding to practice, whether that purpose is punishment or rehabilitation.

Obstacles to institutional change. Institutional changes cannot be effected by gradual accretions. The addition of guidance centers and psychiatric services is necessary but hardly sufficient. These additions will be largely futile so long as the Custodial Division is not completely reorganized, both in the training program for correctional employees and, above all, in the supervisory practices on the job. Yet, a better supervision of guards on the job would encounter a seemingly insurmountable obstacle. This is, perhaps, responsible for the tremendous difficulties which stand in the way of reform. The guards are the disciplinarians of the inmates. They have the responsibility for security as well as for the adherence to prison regulations. If the guards were supervised, the inmate would become aware of the fact that their authority over him is not final. Of course, this is, in principle, true of all strictly authoritarian organizations, though in most of them, including the prison, there are some provisions for complaint; but in the prison the guard's authority is represented to himself and to the inmate as the symbol of just punishment. The guard must be obeyed because the conviction has subjected the morally delinquent inmate to his authority. The moral rightness of authority is called into question when a supervisor can correct a guard's decision. The moral depravity of the prisoner becomes, therefore, an assumption which is necessary for the self-esteem of the guard, because it implies that his authority is symbolic of justice, regardless of how he exercises it. It is apparent that supervision of the guards would jeopardize this system of interlocking assumptions, since a check on the guard's authority over the prisoner seems to challenge the justice of the punishment itself.

It seems to us that vague feelings of this kind lie behind the behavior of custodial employees. In observing the conflicting ideas about prisoners and punishment which are embodied in the divisions of the prison, it is essential to view the activities of each of these as seen by the personnel themselves. This enables the observer to assess the momentum which lies behind the patent discrepancy between formal role and the actual behavior of the individual employees within the organization. To understand how each group looks at its own performance, it is helpful to consider the history and ideology of the profession which it represents. But it is also necessary to consider the situational pressures within the organization. In this instance, these pressures result from the moral gulf which is conventionally assumed to exist between the criminal and the guard. Nothing a prisoner does is ever unequivocally right. His rehabilitation, however, would require many actions which would have to be considered right. Hence, rehabilitation tends to threaten the view that the inmate is a depraved individual whose every action confirms this depravity. On the other hand, there are few actions of the guard which are unequivocally wrong, unless it is a violation of the law which cannot be overlooked. To think that a guard's action might be wrong is to challenge the justice of the punishment and of those who administer it.

The rehabilitation of the prisoner is not likely to succeed so long as these views prevail. Rehabilitation would seem to depend on the willingness of the guards to see their exercise of authority criticized. And this willingness depends, in turn, on the belief that criminal tendencies exist in all men, including one's self.[9]

Personality and institutional position. The prison as an institution does not have an organizational purpose other than the purpose enacted into law. The prison is staffed by a variety of personnel. Each person, as well as each group of persons, performs his duties in terms of formally articulated goals. These are not the same as a person's motive in taking the job. Rather, each will seek to rationalize his activities within the organization in terms of "what is good for the institution" as his professional training and personal disposition prompt him to see it. In doing that, he will encounter the competing rationalizations of others. He will come to terms with the discrepancies between what he does, what he claims to do, and what his profession stands for ideologically. In some measure, this is true of any of the different departments in any organization. It is highlighted in this institution by the striking incompatibilities between psychiatric practice and practice on the psychiatric ward. It illustrates a very frequent source of tension in modern society in which a large number of people work in large-scale organizations and are, thereby, exposed to similar strains. But the prison we have examined is striking in that the internal pressures of prison organization make for a closer fit between personality type and institutional position than is likely to be true of less extreme instances. These internal pressures will help to make psychiatrists of a different bent ineffective or to eliminate them. On the other hand, psychiatrists who have authoritarian tendencies will show an "elective affinity"[10] for work which turns these tendencies into personal and institutional assets.

NOTES TO CHAPTER 40

1. Quotations not otherwise identified are verbatim statements by members of the prison staff.
2. We should add that Custody operates in fact on the basis of three criteria: security, convenience, and discipline. What stands for rehabilitative measures in Custody is, in fact, the insistence on conformity and the punishment for breaches of discipline. (It should be emphasized in this context that the number of prisoners is twice the number provided for by the physical plant of the prison; hence the exaggerated concern with security and discipline has an important factual basis.) The maintenance of discipline involves a symbiotic relationship of prisoners and guards which seems primarily based on a system of frames and counterframes. Since guards and prisoners live in close proximity, they become able to obtain favors and inflict harm on each other by means of concealment and denunciation. An obvious example is that guards and prisoners alike prefer some jobs and seek to avoid others.

Prisoners compete for jobs by compacts and denunciations. They seek to revenge themselves for ill-treatment and to escape the detection of illicit activities. Guards, on the other hand, depend for the performance of work and for the maintenance of discipline on the prisoners themselves. (The disproportion in the number of guards—*circa* three hundred, as against the number of prisoners, fifty-five hundred—is significant in this respect, since it necessitates a considerable delegation of authority to the latter.) For these and other reasons, the inmates and guards are each vitally interested in knowing what goes on in the other group. The inmates are interested because they may be able to use such knowledge to ease prison life; the guards because their obsessive concern with security makes them suspect the worst of the prisoners and they naturally wish to have the feeling of knowing what the prisoners may be about. But of course the concern of the guards with the prisoners is not only punitive, since the latter can frequently render them services. Inside dope is therefore used by both groups as a means of haggling for position.

Temporary participant observation, on which this paper is based, cannot afford more than a glimpse of this system. That it exists became apparent when a sadistic inmate, who would beat up the patients of the psychiatric ward whom he supervised, could not be removed by the head psychiatrist because the Associate Warden was "unable" to effect his transfer.

3. From this point on, our examples will be chosen exclusively from a three months' observation of the medical and psychiatric division.

4. We should add, perhaps, that it is quite possible that the expectation of depravity helps to create it. From informal conversation with inmates, one gathers that the obsessive concern of the guards with security makes the prisoners vie with one another in their ability to evade custodial supervision and to do what is forbidden. Obviously, the prisoners evade supervision in order to ease their life in prison, but we would not dismiss the possibility that elements of play—and of playing with danger—enter in. The prison is a dull place to live in; it is overcrowded and time hangs heavy on the hands of many inmates. It is quite possible that the evasion of supervision is also a form of entertainment.

5. Provision of the Penal Code providing for the prosecution of "lewd and lascivious conduct."

6. A. H. Maslow, "The Authoritarian Character Structure," *J. Social Psychol.* (1943) 18:402.

7. It should be added that psychiatrists also function in a custodial capacity. They sit on the Disciplinary Committee and they do medical examinations, which serve detective functions, at the request of Custody.

8. As an example of possible solutions, we might mention one which has passed the stage of advocacy and is in the process of becoming fact: that for psychiatric disorders prisoners be placed in a prison where the warden is a psychiatrist.

9. In this connection it would be worth while to make a systematic study of the social and psychological characteristics of the attendants, orderlies, or guards who have the most frequent contact with the patients or inmates in mental and correctional institutions.

10. Max Weber has used this term in his psychological analysis of religion. See *From Max Weber: Essays in Sociology;* translated, edited, and with an introduction by H. H. Gerth and C. Wright Mills; New York, Oxford Univ. Press, 1946; pp. 284-288. Cf. also the illuminating comments by the editors in their introduction, pp. 62-63.

Section V

DYNAMICS OF CHANGE

IN RESIDENTIAL SYSTEMS

INTRODUCTION

THE basic task for residential treatment institutions is comparable to what Max Weber called the "routinization of charisma"[1]—to achieve the stability and efficiency which results from bureaucratic organization without sacrificing the qualities of human relations required to bring about change in clients.

Long before recent efforts to see treatment as a scientific endeavor, there were practitioners with personal qualities and skills, not unlike the *mystique* of the charismatic leader, who related to their charges in such a way that rehabilitation was achieved. However, when treatment settings expanded beyond the limits of face-to-face primary group contacts, it has proven difficult to prevent practices from developing which maximize administrative convenience at the expense of helping inmates to learn behavior acceptable in the larger society.

Some aspects of the problem are peculiar to residential treatment institutions. For example, although a certain degree of impersonality is functional for bureaucratic effectiveness, the symptoms of inmates frequently evoke the deepest feelings of those who care for them. Staff members who are subjected to the aggression of delinquent or psychotic inmates need considerable emotional support from their superiors to keep them from retaliating in kind. Rehabilitation requires an atmosphere of emotional warmth, and the ways in which staff members are expected to carry out their responsibilities to each other and to inmates has a profound influence on the emotional atmosphere.

The problem of delegating authority, common in all bureaucratic organizations, encounters special pitfalls in residential treatment. Weber mentions power dispersion as a natural consequence of efforts to routinize charisma in a rationally structured organization, and it is now generally recognized that democratic processes are conducive to attainment of psychological maturity.[2] But, however desirable it may be for inmates to take

[1] Max Weber. *The Theory of Social and Economic Organization*, New York: Free Press, 1964, p. 363.
[2] Jean Piaget. *The Moral Judgment of the Child*. Glencoe, Ill.: Free Press, 1948, pp. 412-413.

part in democratic decision-making, an important reason for their confinement to institutions is impaired social judgment, so that granting any autonomy to institutional inmates is especially frightening to administrators. Similarly, lower echelon staff are often insufficiently trained to be given the burden of responsible decision-making. The fear that dispersion of power will have dire consequences frequently makes administrators reluctant to give any authority to subordinates, but this reluctance also inhibits the goals of rehabilitation.

It is our contention that therapeutic change can be effected only when the social system makes provision for incorporating therapeutic principles at the outset. These principles serve to guide the creation of positions and to clarify administrative expectations of incumbents in these positions. In particular, positions may include specialists who encourage behavior that is therapeutically desirable but may rock the organizational boat, as well as specialists in maintaining order; in consequence, interstitial positions may also be necessary to resolve conflicts. Where responsibility for carrying out multiple functions devolves on subordinate staff and inmates, a therapeutically-oriented social system will provide means of communicating the hierarchy of expectations and clarifying misunderstandings.

Since there can be no rehabilitation without opportunities for inmates to take some decision-making responsibility, and responsibility must consequently also be delegated to subordinate staff members, the structure should make provision for decisions which have proven wrong to be reevaluated, and for this reevaluation to serve as a constructive learning experience. The institution must expect to allocate some of its resources to make restitution for damages resulting from wrong decisions.

Persistence of the therapeutic component in institutional structure, once established, requires an ongoing training program for inducting new staff and a system of rewarding those whose performance achieves therapeutic success. With the criteria of successful rehabilitation constantly in mind, opportunities for experimentation and evaluation must be provided within the structure. The results of these operations should then be fed back to the administrative change agent to use as the basis for making further modifications in the system.

RESISTANCE TO CHANGE

ANYONE who contemplates changing an existing system into a therapeutic community must be alert to sources of system inertia. Kissinger and Pearlin both deal with such problems in their papers. In Kissinger's description of an attempt to institute a therapeutic community within a larger hospital system, strained relations between the therapeutic community unit and the larger hospital system were responsible for its failure. These strains were located primarily at higher levels of administration. The article by Pearlin, on the other hand, locates greater resistance to change among lower echelon staff. Taking Pearlin's paper together with that of Scheff (in Section III above), which indicates how subordinate staff members exercise power over their superiors, one can explain the failure of attempts to change ward practices which have not included adequate methods for overcoming the resistance of lower-ranking staff.

UNPLANNED CHANGE PROCESSES

NEXT are two papers detailing change processes which, though unintended, bear on the therapeutic aims of institutions. Reformatory inmates studied by Wheeler showed increasing prisonization—acceptance of inmate attitudes harmful to rehabilitation—when he compared men in the first six months of their sentences with those in the middle phase, but in the final phase there appears a resocialization effect: prisoners who were to be released within six months scored nearly as high in conformity to staff expectations as the recently admitted group. In the second of these articles Rapoport, who studied Maxwell Jones's therapeutic community at Belmont Hospital, describes oscillations in degree of tension among the patient group. There is, he believes, a level which is optimal for therapeutic purposes; staff can err either by taking steps to relieve tension too quickly, or by letting it get out of hand. In both Wheeler's and Rapoport's studies, awareness of the natural course of change can suggest how timing of therapeutic intervention should be done for best results.

PLANNED REHABILITATION

PROGRAMMATIC proposals are represented by the next four papers. Cressey applies the group dynamics maxim—that it is easier to change individuals in groups than one at a time—to the problem of resocializing criminals, but he reformulates it in terms of Sutherland's theory of differential association. If, as Sutherland said, criminality results when an individual has associated primarily with others who accept crime as a way of life, then rehabilitation occurs by exposing the individual to others who are law-abiding. Cressey mentions group conditions, such as cohesiveness and common purpose, under which change is maximized.

While Polsky also recognizes the importance of group process in changing individuals, he points out the further contribution that awareness of intrapsychic processes can make for planned group change. The effect of individual therapy on value change is often nullified by the force of a delinquent peer group. However, a group worker who is cognizant of each boy's personality dynamics as well as his role in the peer group can make use of these related facts in restructuring the group along more positive lines.

George Devereux sees another way in which psychology can influence structuring of social environment to bring about change. Whereas Polsky shows the bearing of intrapsychic processes on internal differentiation of the group, Devereux relates them to the structuring of ward atmosphere. As an anthropologist sensitive to the impact of culture on personality, he suggests applying ethnographic knowledge to the design of therapeutic environments for particular disorders. If anthropologists can tell us the conditions of social life under which certain psychiatric disorders do not occur, would such conditions, recreated on wards for patients suffering from these disorders, contribute to their recovery? If this environmental manipulation works, return to the community would be accomplished by moving the patients, when they could tolerate it, through a series of wards increasingly like the society to which they will return.

Polsky and Claster have designed a model of group goal attainment for fostering resident autonomy in the institutional setting. The guidance of the counselor attached to the residents' living unit is central. He must work toward a balance between insuring the attainment of successful and gratifying group goals, and training residents to master the components of group process. As a result of such skilled guidance by counselors, the resident group can become a more autonomous force in the institution.

Following these programmatic outlines are four descriptions of actual treatment systems. Elaine Cumming, a sociologist, collaborated with two psychiatrists, I. L. W. Clancey and John Cumming, in a classic example of applying organizational sociology to a mental hospital. Through redefining lines of authority, creating new positions, and delegating decision-making to lower echelons, they were able to build a structure to bring about and maintain those therapeutic attitudes which their predecessors had tried to promote, but which had not persisted. There is no better testimony than this report for the argument that change, to persist, must be accomplished through modification of the social structure.

Ohlin describes the results of structural reorganization in a training school for girls. A major problem, under the old system, arose when demands for control, imposed on houseparents by residential supervisors, conflicted with social workers' recommendations for therapeutic care. The reorganization consisted of giving authority for both disciplinary and treatment matters to the social workers. Placing both horns of the houseparents' dilemma in the social workers' laps took it out of the realm of interpersonal conflict; it forced the social workers to a resolution that was successful because it was based on realistic appraisal of both custody and treatment requirements.

The paper by Sivadon discusses the sociotherapeutic techniques used in various phases of the mental patient's stay at a French psychiatric hospital. At the initial stage of admission, instead of the process common in other institutions, by which inmates are stripped of individuality by taking away their clothes, etc.,[3] the patient is greeted by a hostess and given per-

[3] Erving Goffman, *Asylums,* New York: Doubleday, 1961.

sonal items for use in the hospital. These include visiting cards imprinted with his name to indicate that he is regarded as an individual. Techniques of resocialization vary with the level of regression; for severely withdrawn patients they begin with the most primitive forms of interaction and progress to group activity as patients begin to respond. Most striking, in contrast to institutions which devote a large part of their efforts to enforcing conformity to institutional expectations, is Sivadon's practice of encouraging opposition to the environment as a basis for establishing group solidarity and for learning to cope constructively with frustration.

Last of the programs described is Synanon, a method of rehabilitating drug addicts patterned after Alcoholics Anonymous. There is no professional staff in the usual sense; rather, the essential process in rehabilitation is what Cressey calls "retroflexive reformation": the effort to help others like himself reinforces the addict's own motivation to stay free of drugs.[4] Yablonsky analyzes the principal forces underlying this approach to rehabilitation.

In the last article Raush, Dittman, and Taylor demonstrate, through direct observation over time, that interpersonal behavior shows quantitative changes in the desired direction as a result of residential treatment. Evaluative studies like this one can help clarify relationships between social system treatment methods and the specific changes in behavior that result. The trend toward such studies is a mark of increasing demands that claims for the effectiveness of residential treatment methods be justified by rigorous scientific evidence.

[4] The psychological theory of cognitive dissonance explains how advocating action results in the advocate himself embracing more strongly the conduct advocated. See Leon Festinger, *A Theory of Cognitive Dissonance*. Evanston, Ill.: Row Peterson, 1957.

Resistance to Change

ॐ

C H A P T E R 4 1   The Untherapeutic Community:

A Team Approach That Failed*

R. DAVID KISSINGER

THIS paper will attempt to describe in objective terms the initiation and development of a "therapeutic community." Unlike many such attempts that have been described in the psychiatric literature, this attempt "failed." The intent is to clarify and make explicit those forces which went into this "failure" in order that similar programs might benefit from the attempt which will be described here.

The program was attempted in a typically large 3,000 bed state mental institution. One ward, consisting of 25 beds, was set aside in the Admission building to house the project. Administration of the ward was delegated to co-administrators: a psychologist and a psychiatrist. It was understood at the outset that these individuals would design and execute whatever changes would be necessary to rehabilitate and return to the community the patients included in the project. Overall supervision for the project would be in the hands of the Chief of the Male Admission Service.

THE EXISTING SITUATION

THE ward contained 12 male patients who were all moving toward clinical remission. They were all on privilege or parole status. They ranged in age and diagnosis from a 17-year-old mental defective to a 52-year-old brain damaged, depressed alcoholic. Their care was handled, for the most part, by an attendant who had been in the employ of the hospital for 25 years. Three other psychiatric aides were on duty at intermittent times so that, for the most part, if an aide was needed, one could be reached. Very often, however, one aide would be in care of several wards so that constant su-

* Paper read at Eastern Psychological Association Meetings, 1963. Reprinted by permission of the author.

pervision or contact could not be maintained. At night, one aide handled two wards and the admitting room (in another part of the building) so that contact was quite minimal during the evening hours.

All patients were assigned to psychiatrists (residents in training) who supervised their care. Five of these patients had recently entered individual psychotherapy, either with the personnel of the Psychology Department or with the psychiatric staff.

This writer's first contact with the ward typified the apparent feelings and attitudes of the personnel and the patients. The dayroom was stripped of furniture. The pool table was covered with canvas and the TV and radio were locked in the closet. There was a sign on the door explaining that none of these facilities could be used during the current week in order to give the fresh coat of wax on the floor a chance to dry. Of the 12 patients on the ward only three were to be seen. The aide was concerned with "rounding up" several men to help carry back the furniture into the dayroom. The content of this writer's first meeting with this psychiatric aide was devoted to his discussion of how difficult it was to obtain help on the ward and how men would "slip away" from the jobs assigned to them. Contact with the other aide revealed the same kind of problem. He was concerned with getting help in curtailing the activities of an acting-out adolescent. Help was defined as transfer to another ward. In the main, his focus was upon the patients' lack of responsibility toward work on the ward.

Therapeutic efforts consisted of the administration of tranquilizing drugs, haphazard attendance at occupational therapy, privilege cards and weekends at home. Rounds by the psychiatric staff were held once a week and patients were locked on the ward at that time so that they might be seen. The entire ward was seen for approximately twenty minutes at that time.

THE PLAN OF ACTION

THE term "Therapeutic Community" has been used to describe a wide variety of programs. Broadly defined, it represents an attempt to marshall all the treatment resources together and integrate and coordinate them so that the desocialization and chronicity which seem inherent in institutional settings is inhibited. Every possible action, relationship and administrative decision is defined as having potentially a beneficial and constructive effect on patients. This is an exciting concept and represents an immediate challenge. The question put before this writer, once this assumption was granted was in effect: what changes in attitudes, structure or administration had to be effected to convert the existing situation, as described above, into a program where growth could take place?

The most basic change and perhaps the most difficult change to take place, was to modify the employee attitudes toward the patients to be treated. The direction of this change could be briefly characterized by the formula: from "good patients" to "useful citizens."

The first step toward this goal was to indicate that the administrators were sympathetic to personnel needs and felt that all personnel had important functions in the program. Through a constant emphasis on their therapeutic efforts and a de-emphasis of their custodial functions, it was hoped that the "climate" of the ward would improve. Informal conferences with the night as well as day aides were encouraged. These meetings were ostensibly held to increase the administrator's information about the patients being treated but they also served the purpose of establishing a regular channel for the ventilation of feelings and attitudes which were aroused by the changes taking place on the ward.

Another conference was established including the psychotherapists of the patients on the ward. This conference was intended to facilitate the flow of information and to coordinate administrative efforts so that therapy and administration could work harmoniously and not against each other.

A consciencious effort was made to increase administrator-patient contact. Rounds were made every day and "office hours" were posted so that patients could increase contact on their own initiative. These hours were made open to anyone on the ward—including personnel.

All of these steps were to provide for a climate in which patients could be allowed to grow and take responsibility and inhibit regression and dependency. Once this climate had been established it was the administrator's responsibility to stimulate this growth.

Recognizing that self-initiative and the assumption of responsibility toward the self and others cannot be ordered or directed, the plan was to gently and gradually introduce and suggest possible activities, rather than present and dictate behavior. It was felt that the administrators could not determine in advance the needs and the desires of the group, even though they would have some control over the selection of patients to be included in the project. Ultimately the particular activities would have to emerge from the group itself and not be handed down by administrative fiat. Initially however, we had to combat the feelings of helplessness and dependency which are engendered by custodial care.

First in our program was to help form a group feeling on the ward. One way of fostering this feeling was to present the group with common tasks, i.e., the common responsibilities that living together on the ward entailed. Group therapy was initiated with every member of the ward, with the implication that dealing with the reasons for their current hospitalization and their current psychological difficulties would be part of the group's goals and responsibilities. In essence, providing a climate for growth and the formation of a group were the primary tasks before the administrators. Once this had been achieved we felt sure that the group would begin to express their needs and to strive for some measure of autonomy. Although this was necessarily slow in coming about, exactly this began to occur.

To give the reader an idea of the kinds of activities which were initiated by the group, the following is a partial listing of some of the activities actually accomplished. A rules committee was organized and they produced a set of rules for acceptable behavior on the ward. A patient government was formed which not only distributed the responsibilities of the ward to individual members, but also planned activities, handled disputes, and acted as official liaison between the hospital and the patients of this ward. An activities committee was formed and organized dances (female patients were invited onto the ward for the first time) without any help whatsoever except for the approval of the administrators. The group selected mental health movies and these were shown and discussed as a way of increasing self understanding. Competitions were organized not as "time killing devices," but as a way to involve the whole ward in group activity.

Other plans which did not come to fruition due to the demise of the project were: an integration of the patient's family into the ward, either socially or therapeutically, the introduction of college volunteers, inauguration of a "buddy" system whereby patients would formally take responsibility for other patients, an emphasis on social pressure instead of transfer as a way of curtailing acting out, integration of the ward into the community by housing patients only "part time," and finally some arrangement for aftercare—perhaps in the form of an alumni group.

It must be understood that the above plans only represent the thoughts of this writer and generally reflect the current notions of modern psychiatric and psychological treatment. What might have emerged from the group itself, unfortunately will never be known.

THE PATIENTS TO BE TREATED

AFTER some consultation with the chief of male service, all patients currently living on the ward, save one, would represent the core patients for the program.

It was generally agreed that these individuals represented "treatment failures." These people had gone through the regular treatment regime of the hospital and had not responded positively enough so that they could be discharged. Nor had they regressed sufficiently to demand transfer to a continuous treatment service. Most of these patients were diagnosed as chronic schizophrenics with many having a history of repeated hospitalizations. It was felt by the administrators of this project that an appropriate goal for our patients would be social rehabilitation rather than the attainment of insight into their problems. Group experiences were felt to be instrumental in attaining this goal.

CRISES

WHEN concentrated effort and care is given and this is designated treatment, a number of crises emerge as a process of the changes which occur.
The resolution of these critical incidents give a good index of the growth
or decline of a treatment procedure. It is this writer's purpose to highlight
the development of the project by outlining the crises which developed
within it.

The first such crisis developed when one of our project patients became
verbally abusive to a female attendant on another ward. The attendant
complained to the acting chief of male service (chief of male service was
off during that day) who, after hearing this complaint transferred the
patient to a closed ward. After this decision had been made, the administrators of the project were called in and informed of this move. It was
clear that neither administrator had any voice in the matter. Feeling some
responsibility toward the patient, they attempted to interpret the transfer
to the patient and to the ward. When the administrators arrived on the
ward, they found the patient packing his things, exclaiming loudly that he
had no use for the ward, personnel, nor anyone in the world. At this point
it was impossible to aid the patient in increasing his understanding of
either himself or the situation. Subsequent staff discussion of this matter
revealed that there was agreement that this had been a regrettable situation. Assurances were made that it would not be repeated. This transfer
proved to be, however, an irreversable administrative decision and the
patient remained on the closed ward and was not re-instated in the ward
program.

The second crisis concerned the actions of several patients who had
apparently been holding "clandestine" meetings at night to discuss suicide.
Approximately one week after these "suicide club" meetings and after
they had come to the attention of the administrators, one of the patients
brought in to the hospital a bottle of 500 aspirins. The attendant apparently was informed of this and consequently brought it to the attention
of the collaborating psychiatrist. The patient's night stand was searched
and the aspirins were found. The psychiatrist told the attendant to immediately transfer this patient to a closed ward as soon as the patient
returned from his daily activity. Without explanation the patient was
transferred to a closed ward and within 24 hours broke into a medicine
cabinet and swallowed an overdose of tranquilizing drugs and was shifted
to a medical ward. Another patient involved in the "suicide club" was
shifted to a closed ward, upon the order of the chief of the male service,
and subsequently transferred to a chronic service.

While these events were taking place, another patient, apparently responding to increasing pressure in group therapy, and to his own feelings

of hopelessness, escaped from the hospital. He was returned to the hospital placed on a closed service and then transferred to a chronic building.

The proceeding series of events triggered off some lengthy discussions of the decision making process. It became clear, although not explicit, that the real administrative power resided with the chief of male service and that he was making unilateral decisions which were, for the most part, irreversible. An attempt was made by the administrators to include the chief of male service in our weekly conferences for the dual purpose of helping him to develop some trust in the administrators and to help him delegate some of his power. He joined the meetings for approximately two weeks when the "pressure" of other duties and responsibilities caused him to miss the meetings.

The third crisis was the introduction into the treatment team of a social worker. It became immediately clear that there were profound differences in orientation and considerable conflict concerning the role of each member of the treatment team. Initially, the social worker's perception kept her aloof and seemingly subordinate to the other members of the team. She seemed unsure of her role as well as the roles of the other members. Conflict arose between the psychologist and the social worker and manifested itself in extended discussions of differences in attitudes toward hospitalization, treatment goals and counter-transference arguments about patients' potential. After an initial phase of these rather heated discussions, it became somewhat clear what the purpose of the project was, where the lines of authority lay, and what expectations each member had of one another. These expectations began to come closer to reality and we began to be less concerned with roles.

The fourth crisis emerged when the treatment team began to discharge patients. The group slowly was dwindling in size. Difficulties began to arise in replacing patients who had moved through the program. The administrators began to put pressure on the chief of male service to transfer patients into the program. This pressure brought about a re-evaluation of the criteria for admittance to the project. After some discussion of this, it was decided to include all those male patients who appeared not able to respond in the usual three months' period of hospitalization. In addition, the patients admitted could not have a history of aggressive acting-out. After an initial "flood" of three patients, the admittance pace began to slow down again.

The fifth crisis revolved around the sudden transfer of the collaborating psychiatrist to a continuous treatment building. This decision was reached after discussion between the clinical director and the collaborating psychiatrist. This took place on Sunday (the psychologist's day off) and the actual shift in assignment took place the next day. Due to shortages in staff, it was stated, the psychiatrist could not be replaced and it was understood that the psychologist would function as administrator directly under the chief of male service who would then assume the collaborating psychiatrist's patient load. It soon became clear that other matters were more pressing for the chief of male service. Although the chief of male service would retain the right to make all decisions, the psychologist would continue to function as therapist and liaison between the "team" (now reduced to two members), the patients, and the psychiatric administrator. Communication was becoming increasingly more difficult between professional persons and meetings involving the whole staff on this ward were only called to handle emergencies. The psychologist was given the tacit understanding, however, that the psychiatrist administrator would support most, if not all, of the treatment plans which the "team" would recommend.

The final crisis actually consisted of a number of small events. The first of these was the transfer of the chief of male service to other duties in another part of the hospital. He was replaced by another senior psychiatrist who was to act as administrator. During this time, when communication was most difficult and administratively things had come to a stand-still, this writer went to the clinical director and indicated his desire to incorporate female patients into the group therapy program on the ward. This was, in part, motivated by the shortage of patients on the ward and the difficulty experienced in obtaining patients for the program. Over and above these considerations, however, this therapeutic procedure was congruent with the spirit and direction which the project was taking. Since our primary goal was to help our patients become more socially competent individuals, anything that could be done inside the hospital to help them face the problems which they would encounter in the outside world, was considered to be beneficial. Even though the hospital world is segregated by sex, the community into which the patient might be entering would not be.

Although the clinical director did not recommend any female patients for the project from the admission service, she indicated that more chronic female patients might be available. The psychologist went to this source and approximately one week later began to have integrated group sessions on the ward.

One week after this, the chief of male service returned to his regular duties and informed the psychologist that some difficulties had arisen with the nursing staff concerning the inclusion of female patients in the group therapy sessions. Sensing that there was more in this communication than what was being overtly expressed, the psychologist had a lengthy meeting to discover the possible reasons for difficulty and to achieve some resolution. It became immediately clear that the chief of male service was unwilling to assume the responsibility of having female patients on the male ward. Although he felt that this integration had great therapeutic or rehabilitative potential, he felt that he could not take the administrative risk which it would entail. The psychologist attempted a compromise solution by offering to hold the group therapy meetings off the ward in a more neutral site. The chief of male service agreed fully with this plan. The following day, the psychologist received a telephone call from the clinical director informing him that although there would be a room available for the mixed group, that she felt that the chief of male service had some objections to this kind of therapeutic approach. The psychologist assured the clinical director that this had been resolved in the meeting the previous day.

At approximately the same time, the chief of male service indicated to the psychologist that there was an active TB patient living on the ward and that he would be transferred to a local Veterans Administration Hospital for further diagnostic tests and treatment. In an attempt to clarify this situation, the psychologist called a special meeting of the "team" to discuss when and how this transfer would take place. The psychologist's interest was to help facilitate this move and help prepare the patient for this transfer. After some lengthy discussion in which the chief of male service alluded vaguely to "administrative difficulties" it was decided that the patient would be transferred in approximately two weeks.

At this time the chief of male service asked the psychologist to write monthly progress notes on all patients on the ward. This was done and the psychologist soon discovered that his notes were incorporated in the chart over the chief of male service's signature. At the psychiatrist's next request for progress notes, the psychologist indicated that his professional ethics could not allow this practice and that the psychologist would have to take responsibility for his own notes. However, the psychologist indicated his desire to discuss these patients with the psychiatrist to facilitate the note writing if the psychologist could not enter them as his own. The chief of male service indicated that it was against "hospital policy" for a psychologist to sign notes put in the chart and that only physicians could do this. The chief of male service accepted the psychologist's offer to discuss these patients but did not carry through.

THE DEMISE OF THE PROJECT

THE preceding incidents occurred almost simultaneously. Shortly after their apparent resolution, the chief of male service distributed a memo to the clinical director, the chief of psychology service, the assistant chief of male service and to the nursing supervisor of the building to the effect that the psychologist had been "relieved of his duties on the ward as of that date." In the memo were some references to "personality difficulties" of the psychologist and lack of "leadership qualities." Charge of program was given to the assistant chief of male service who held one group therapy meeting and subsequently disbanded the ward program. The ward now resembles the ward described in the first section of this paper.

DIRECT AND INDIRECT BENEFITS

IN the six months of operation, this project served a total of 36 patients. Twenty-four of these patients were discharged to the community and approximately half of these have returned to the hospital at the time of this writing (a six-month period). Nine patients were transferred off the ward to the continuous treatment buildings. All of these patients, save one, are still in the hospital. A formal evaluation of the project is not possible since provisions were not made at its inception for either a control group or precise measurements.

It is almost a platitude to state that modification of any element within a field will effect the total field. But it was obvious that as we were helping patients to change, positive changes were occurring in the staff. The ongoing experiences of the collaborating psychiatrist, psychologist, and social worker increased their understanding of their respective roles and resulted in feelings of respect for each other. In particular, a greater understanding and appreciation of the role of the social worker in the discharge planning of patients was attained. Industrial therapy as part of a treatment program, which was formally introduced on this ward, maintained a firm "foothold" in the Admissions building, even following the program's demise. In addition, a fuller recognition of the potential therapeutic value of week-end privileges was realized.

In general, the therapeutic usefulness of administrative decisions and a fuller awareness of the value of careful deliberations concerning these matters seemed to have permeated the psychiatric staff as a whole. Last, but by no means least in importance, was the lifting of morale both in patients and staff. Demonstration of the fact that multiple admission cases and "unresponsive" patients could work cooperatively, could plan, could show organized social interests to an extent that had not been seen before, had an immeasurable positive effect on the entire staff. In summarizing the major effects of the program, it focussed attention upon the impact which administrative decisions had on patients. It removed some of the "magic" which is often ascribed to other professional disciplines and it demonstrated to the entire staff that cooperation and communication among staff members could be effective therapeutic tools in themselves.

It is at this point where many accounts of the "therapeutic community" stop. In this instance, however, our program "failed" and it is this writer's task to attempt to find some explanation as to why it did fail. It would be easy to blame a particular member of the "treatment team" and to assume that this person's "personality problems" was the primary factor in bringing about the program's end. In fact, this is precisely what was done in the memo which announced the formal termination of the program. It is the writer's view, however, that there were more important contributing factors than the personality characteristics of those most immediately involved.

AN ANALYSIS OF THE PROGRAM

IN order to highlight those contributing factors, an attempt will be made to enumerate what courses of action might have enhanced the chances of the program's success and compare it to our experiences.

1. One of the glaring weaknesses of the project was that it did not include either in the planning or in the execution those individuals who maintained the greatest influence and power in the hospital. The false assumption had been made that the distribution of power was delegated along the usual lines of authority. When problems did arise, however, the chief of male service was no more able to make independent decisions than were the collaborating psychiatrist and psychologist. His apparent inability to maintain a steady flow of new admissions to the project, his inability to take the therapeutic risks necessary for the assumption of responsibility by our patients, the transfer of vital personnel and the inclusion of the clinical director near the terminal stage of the program are all testimonial to the fact that he was responding to considerable external pressure. It was an erroneous assumption that the program had certain circumscribed boundaries and therefore problems engendered within this setting could be dealt with locally through the cooperation of just the "team" members. A new treatment procedure, or more broadly, any change, involves the whole hospital and produces infinite and often entirely unexpected ramifications throughout the entire institution. The inclusion of all figures who have influence or power in bringing about this change is absolutely essential. In order to insure this inclusion of vital persons, an accurate assessment must first be made of the power structure of the hospital. Power may be distributed to anyone from the business manager or clinical director to a psychiatric aide or nurse. It is this writer's conclusion from his experience gained from this project, that errors of inclusion are considerably better than errors of omission.

2. Related to the last enumerated point, relative autonomy and delegation of specific responsibilities must be granted by those individuals who are in control. Mere lip service is not enough, but a clear specification of which responsibilities are being delegated and which are not must be made explicit. In the program described in this

paper, it had been decided that administrative decisions would be made by the "team." As it was clearly shown in the first episode, however, this appraisal of the decision making process was far from realistic. Once authority and responsibility is delegated, relative autonomy is gained. How far this autonomy goes or the limits which are established must be "spelled out" in detail.

3. Although it has been emphasized time and time again how important clear cut lines of communication are in the coordinated treatment of patients, this writer must also consider failures in communication as a determinant in the termination of this program. Special provisions were made to facilitate the flow of communications and to keep the channels open, but it was obvious, at times, that messages were not getting through. Communication problems are never just "communication problems" per se, they are diagnostic of difficulties in the working relationships of those who are sending messages. Members of the team must be *dedicated* to the principles of free and open communications and willing to deal immediately with blocked or distorted communications. Team members must be highly sensitive to changes which occur in the lines of communication since they are the first sign of "trouble ahead."

4. In forming the team, due allowance must be made to the differences in definition of roles, functions, and experiences which each member of the team brings with him to the relationship. Professional mental health workers, like most people, carry with them both negatively and positively stereotyped sets of prejudices. It is only through contact and interaction that misconceptions can be corrected so that a realistic appraisal of the skills, talents and the special contributions of the team members can take place. It must be made apparent to all, and worked through by all, what the goals, responsibilities, and requirements are of having an effective team. Each member must become aware of his own prejudices and be willing to modify his own orientation for the effective functioning of the team. An essential aspect of this point is an "iron-clad" agreement that unilateral decisions are not to be permitted. Even in emergencies, no decision should be irreversible. Although the process is slow, the full participation of all members must be brought to bear on problems. By all members meeting a common problem an opportunity is raised to work through communication, interprofessional, as well as the clinical problems on hand. Not only does this method facilitate effective team functioning but usually has the effect of raising the quality of the administrative or clinical decision.

Finally, one must be aware that surface problems have deeper ramifications. There are levels of agreement and disagreement. The resolution of surface issues does not always lead to effective nor even constructive team functioning. It was evident in the project described here that many issues reached solution, at least on a superficial level. What did not reach true resolution was the issue of who was taking responsibility and who was making the decisions. Since these issues were not resolved nor even seriously considered, the eventual and inevitable demise of the program took place.

CHAPTER 42   Sources of Resistance to
Change in a Mental Hospital*

LEONARD I. PEARLIN

CHANGE is an ever present part of the scene of any human organization. It is a natural process that can gain impetus from many
quarters: the organization's network of ties to the broader community and
society; the constant realignments that take place between the various
social and personality components of the organization; the conflicts and
adjustments between formal and informal structures; and shifts in organizational functions and goals. Changes can occur very subtly. They can
also be brought about purposefully and dramatically. It is planned,
intended change, initiated through the establishment of new and explicit
policy that will be the concern of this paper. Specifically, we shall deal
with the anticipatory acceptance or resistance to such change among the
members of the nursing force of a large mental hospital.

The initiation of change through conscious decision and its subsequent
course are matters of interest to students of most types of human
organization.[1] It is certainly an issue of crucial relevance to mental institutions. With a pace that has gained momentum over the past decade
mental hospitals have been reappraising their performance and reassign-
ing priorities of their various functions.[2] But the attainment of a goal does
not automatically follow from its high priority, its clarity, or its wisdom.
Not uncommonly, hospitals defer the introduction of new patient care
policies and programs because widespread support for them is lacking.
There are also instances where initiated changes fall short of the goals for
which they were intended because of the opposition they encounter after
they are introduced. Both the initiation of change and the achievement
of its intended effects are determined in part by attitudes toward the

* Reprinted from the *American Journal of Sociology*, 68 (1962), 325–334, by permission of The University of Chicago Press. Copyright © 1962, 1963 by The University of Chicago. All rights reserved.

change. The sources of resistance to change, therefore, represent a matter of great concern to mental institutions, as well as to other human organizations.

Two general points of view used to speculate about resistance to change in the mental hospital can be identified. One of these is psychological and emphasizes resistance as a characteristic response to any modification of the environment by individuals with certain kinds of personality structures.[3] The second view takes as its point of departure the bureaucratic nature of the institution. It also stresses indiscriminate opposition to change but as it is rooted to an organizational structure that engenders and perpetuates ritualized routine.[4]

Both points of view suffer from an overstatement of their cases. While it is probably true that characteristics of individuals prompt their resistance to change, this relationship can apparently be attenuated or enhanced under different organizational conditions. At the same time, while the hospital is bureaucratically organized, within its generic structure there are situational variations that can create greater or lesser resistance.

SETTING AND METHOD OF STUDY

THE subjects of the study are all members of the nursing service below the supervisory level at Saint Elizabeths Hospital.[5] This is a federal institution that draws most of its patients from the District of Columbia. The hospital has about 7,500 inpatients and is organized into 12 services and 156 wards.

Two data-collection instruments were used. One was a self-administered questionnaire addressed to 1,315 individuals, of whom 1,138 returned usable questionnaires; the other was a form that asked for demographic characteristics of ward patient populations, the distribution of certain psychiatric characteristics, and the employment of various ward programs and policies and was filled out by the persons in charge of each of the 156 wards. These two instruments enabled us to examine both the characteristics of individual hospital workers and the characteristics of the wards to which they are assigned.

Three ranks are represented in this study; each differs in responsibilities, authority, and rewards. In the lowest rank are nursing assistants; next are charge attendants who, on the basis of experience and demonstrated ability, are given charge of wards in the absence of a registered nurse; third, and smallest in number, is the group of registered nurses who have authority over the preceding ranks and are usually responsible for running the wards. These three groups are collectively referred to as nursing personnel: 40 per cent are males and 60 per cent are females.

Resistance was assessed through five items proposing diverse changes. While these changes appear to be unrelated, reactions to them form a

Guttman scale, indicating unidimensionality and suggesting the presence of a general attitude toward change rather than series of specific feelings about discrete innovations. For each of the five items that make up the scale, respondents were asked whether the proposed policy "should definitely be done," if they "wouldn't mind seeing it tried out," or if they "would be against it." The items, all dichotomized between the second and third response categories, are presented below in scale order:[6]

1. Pay patients for the work they do.
2. Open the locked wards.
3. Put the most disturbed and least disturbed patients together on the same wards.
4. Let patient groups decide when patients should be discharged.
5. Have males and females on the same wards.

The suggested policies, it might be noted, are not untried or chimerical. They are in effect in some hospitals in various parts of the country, and some are in practice in limited areas of the hospital under study. Nevertheless, the nursing personnel who accepted all items represent vanguard advocates of change toward the creation of what they hope is a therapeutic hospital milieu. The dimension on which the scale rests is a willingness to move from tradition in patient care. It is to be noted that the above scale aims only at patient-care policy. Despite this, there are, we think, processes involved that operate with other types of change as well.

POSITION AND PRECEPT

MOST sources of resistance that are examined in this paper can be understood only by taking into account the positions of personnel in the nursing order. Position is central to resistance in two distinct ways. On one hand, resistance increases markedly from the higher to the lower ranks. On the other hand what constitutes a significant source of resistance for one echelon can be quite irrelevant for another. Thus, the ranks differ both in the proportions of individuals who strongly resist change and in the factors revelant to such resistance. Because of its centrality to the acceptance of, or opposition to, change, position will be taken into consideration throughout the following discussions.

In an examination of the variations in resistance to change that occur between the nursing ranks, it is seen that, of the three ranks represented, resistance is greatest among nursing assistants, the lowest rank, and is least likely to be found among registered nurses (see Table 1). A number of factors undoubtedly contribute to these positional differences, including the level of general educational attainment and the duration and intensity of occupational training.

Another factor that we wish to examine is the influence of professionalization inasmuch as the nursing profession, largely through the

TABLE 1.

*Resistance to Change, Position in Nursing Force, and
Membership in Nursing Organizations*

	NO.	RESISTANCE TO CHANGE (PER CENT)		
		STRONG	MODERATE	LOW
Position in nursing force:†				
Registered nurse	157	46	27	27
Charge attendant	173	59	24	17
Nursing assistant	736	67	23	10
Membership in professional nursing organizations:‡				
None	93	54	28	18
1	26	31	38	31
2 or more	27	33	22	45

* This table, as well as those that follow, does not include "No answers," resulting in slight variation in totals from table to table.

† $\chi^2 = 36.2$; 4 degrees of freedom; $P < .001$.

‡ $\chi^2 = 10.6$; 4 degrees of freedom; $P < .05$.

various organizations it has established, is an important source of values regarding the treatment of patients. The norms and values supported by nursing organizations emphasize practices that stand in marked contrast to custodialism and, generally, are compatible with the directions embodied by our measure of resistance. One probable reason that registered nurses offer relatively little resistance to change, therefore, is because of their exposure to values that are in sympathy with changes of this sort.

If this is so, then we should expect that the more fully a nurse participates in professional organizations the more likely she will accept change. Table 1 compares nurses on the basis of their affiliations with such organizations and shows that nurses having no affiliation are quite similar to charge attendants; resistance decreases, however, among affiliated nurses. It can also be noted that nurses graduating from a university with a Bachelor of Science degree are less resistant than those having only a nursing diploma. Nurses who are most professionally active and who carry the most professional credentials, therefore, take over the current treatment values that prevail in nursing and the psychiatric community. These values constitute the standards by which a favorable evaluation of the changes is produced. It is this process, apparently, that accounts for much of the difference between the positions in resistance to change. There may be some filtering down of the treatment values to charge attendants, but the values do not appear to touch the nursing assistants. Consequently, the lowest group does not possess the same standards by which change is favorably assessed. In the absence of such standards, many hospital changes appear whimsical to them and are therefore resisted.

Exposure to and internalization of advanced treatment values are only part of the story. We would also assume that higher and lower personnel vary in the proportions who resist change because of differences in more specific precepts they hold regarding patients. In this connection, beliefs about the social distance that should properly be maintained with patients is especially pertinent, for this aspect of relations with patients is closely bound to changes of the kinds with which we are dealing. As will be shown, it can be difficult to enlarge the autonomy and decision-making powers of patients while desiring great distance from them.

Two conceptions are considered, both of which entail the social distance which staff members psychologically put between themselves and patients, with each concept in a separate dimension. The first—personal distance —refers to the extent that personnel regards patients impersonally and without affective attachment. The second—status distance—refers to the case in which one sets himself apart from patients by elevating himself above them along an inferior-superior dimension.[7] As expected, we find that (1) resistance tends to increase with both personal and status distance, and (2) nursing assistants on each dimension are more distant than the higher nursing groups. These facts would lead us to believe that the greater opposition to change of assistants may be due to their greater desire to maintain distance between themselves and patients. But what is actually found is that distance is related to opposition only among charge attendants and registered nurses and not among assistants. While these somewhat surprising findings preclude personal and status distance as factors contributing to positional differences in resistance, it will be seen that they nevertheless help to explain the sources of resistance to change.

Let us look at personal distance in detail. Table 2 shows that personal distance has a pronounced association with resistance among those in the higher ranks while there is almost no relationship at all with the assistant group. Considering for the moment only the higher groups, we should recall the nature of the proposed changes in order to understand this association. As do most efforts to make the hospital a "therapeutic milieu," these changes stress the personal qualities of patients as persons. In contrast, highly distant personnel regard patients with little affect and with marked impersonality. The changes, therefore, are sharply inconsistent with an impersonal view of patients. As a result of the dissonance that exists between the precept and the change, the change is rejected.[8]

The same sort of finding emerges with reference to status distance (see Table 2). Although assistants are again more inclined to be high on this measure, status distance bears no relationship to their attitudes toward change. Among the charge attendants and registered nurses an association is once again found. For these groups conceptions of patients built around status difference are not supported by the kinds of changes in patient care that are at issue. The changes constitute a challenge and threaten their belief that patients are status inferiors; consequently, the changes are likely to be resisted. It would appear that, where the meaning attached to these changes is dissonant with the feelings and beliefs held by individuals, resistance is more readily aroused. But this is true only under certain conditions. For although distance from patients is more prevalent among the assistants, it plays no appreciable part in their feelings toward change.

Dissonance between the precept and the change will not produce resistance, we believe, unless the precept is relevant to the work roles and occupational self-images of personnel. Matters of proper distance from patients, along with broader issues of staff-patient relations, are much more likely to be imbedded in the thinking and work of those in the higher positions. Following from the widely held view that functional psychoses represent a maladjustment to painful interpersonal experiences, there is a corresponding stress placed on staff-patient relations as powerful conditions for social relearning. The training of many nurses, their literature, and their reference groups all contribute to an acute awareness of their relations with patients and the possible therapeutic consequences of these relations. Because relations with patients tend to be important problematic issues of work to the higher personnel, their beliefs as to what forms these relations should properly take can result in resistance when these beliefs are dissonant with the change.

By contrast, it is apparent from Table 2 that such aspects of relations with patients are not influential factors in assistants' reactions to change because they are tangential to the central work performed by this group. Assistants' beliefs about the distance they should properly maintain with patients cannot be considered as either consonant or dissonant with the proposed changes; instead, they are irrelevant to these changes.[9] Before dissonance will produce resistance to change, there must be some investment in the precepts involved. Investment, in turn, is created when the precepts are meaningfully tied to the tasks that confront personnel. For assistants, meaningful ties between their work and properly gauged distance in dealing with patients evidently do not exist.

The precepts of assistants that do bear on their resistance to change, therefore, must be of a different order. Just as notions of proper distance are relevant to the resistance of the higher groups, because such precepts are bound to central elements of their work roles, so it is that precepts among assistants derive their relevance from being linked to tasks demanding a major part of their attention. Given the nature of the daily tasks for which they are responsible, it could be expected that certain problems of patient and ward management would be salient elements of

TABLE 2.

Positions of Personnel, Their Personal and Status Distance from Patients, and Resistance to Change

	NO.	RESISTANCE TO CHANGE (PER CENT)		
		STRONG	MODERATE	LOW
		Personal Distance		
Charge attendants and nurses: [*]				
0-1 (high)	33	64	30	6
2	69	64	19	17
3	113	53	26	21
4-5 (low)	113	43	28	29
Nursing assistants: [†]				
0-1 (high)	104	70	19	11
2	206	69	23	8
3	223	69	20	11
4-5 (low)	201	61	26	13
		Status Distance		
Charge attendants and nurses: [‡]				
4-6 (high)	112	64	22	14
2-3	128	48	29	23
0-1 (low)	86	45	26	29
Nursing assistants: [†]				
4-6 (high)	154	65	23	12
2-3	239	68	21	11
0-1 (low)	341	67	23	10

[*] $\chi^2 = 13.7$; 6 degrees of freedom; $P < .05$.
[†] Not significant.
[‡] $\chi^2 = 10.5$; 4 degrees of freedom; $P < .05$.

their work roles and that resistance would depend on whether the proposed changes were seen as potentially interfering with the discharge of these tasks. This line of inquiry can be followed by examining answers to a question in which respondents were asked to rank the types of patients they prefer to work with. Four such types are relevant here: "a patient who does a lot to help with the work on the ward," "a patient who is neat and clean," "a patient who doesn't cause much fuss or trouble," and "a patient with good manners."[10] When one of these types of patients is given top ranking, it indicates that the respondent views patients in terms of how they facilitate or, at least, do not hamper the execution of tasks relating to patient and ward management.

In Table 3 respondents are categorized according to whether they ranked facilitating patients first or second or whether they give these ranks

TABLE 3.
Positions of Personnel, Rank Order of Preferences for Patients Who
Facilitate Ward Management, and Resistance to Change

POSITION AND RANKING	NO.	RESISTANCE TO CHANGE (PER CENT)		
		STRONG	MODERATE	LOW
Charge attendants and nurses:*				
First	8	50	25	25
Second	25	56	16	28
Other	296	51	27	22
Nursing assistants:†				
First	22	86	5	9
Second	83	71	23	6
Other	600	66	23	11

* Not significant.
† $\chi^2 = 13.7$; 4 degrees of freedom; $P < .01$.

to other types of patients. The manner in which the rankings bear on resistance to change for different positions is a complete reversal from those revealed in Table 2. Here a relationship is found between preferences for facilitative patients and resistance, although such preferences make no difference to the feelings of the higher groups. The assistants giving the high priorities see in the changes an altered role for patients that clashes with their present conceptions, for these are patient-centered rather than task-centered changes. But it is essential to note that by itself a high priority attached to facilitative patients is not sufficient to produce resistance; it is also necessary that there be an investment in those conceptions which, in the present instance, stems from the realities and demands of work roles. Ward maintenance duties are of greater relevance to assistants than to charge attendants and registered nurses. The same considerations unequally influence feelings toward change among personnel, for they are not of equal relevance to members of different ranks. Relevance, then, is a condition for dissonance and the subsequent rejection of change.

EXISTING PATIENT-CARE POLICY

IT was just seen that the things with which people are actually occupied in their work determine the relevance of their precepts to proposed change. This directs our attention to broader conditions of work and suggests that the situations in which personnel are located and the experiences allowed by these situations can themselves constitute sources of resistance to change. Indeed, from our examination of some situational factors, it appears that from the working environment stem events that can exert a powerful influence on these attitudes. Policies and programs of patient care, to the extent that they set the structure of the situation and thus create conditions out of which experience flows, have important consequences for attitudes toward change.

We shall consider three policies here: (1) the existence of patient government on the ward; (2) whether the ward doors are open or locked; and (3) the occurrence of regular staff-patient meetings. Although not coextensive with our scale of resistance to change, these policies rest on the same continuum and, in the case of open-locked doors, overlap it. On one hand, the policies are indicators of conditions of patient freedom, autonomy, and decision-making actually extant on wards; on the other hand, the scale asks staff members how far they are willing to go in accepting changes along these lines. Therefore, we are asking, essentially,

TABLE 4.
Positions of Personnel, Ward Patient-Care Policies, and Resistance to Change

POSITION AND POLICY ON WARD	NO.	RESISTANCE TO CHANGE (PER CENT)		
		STRONG	MODERATE	LOW
Charge attendants and nurses:*				
Patient government	73	45	29	26
No patient government	112	66	21	13
Nursing assistants:†				
Patient government	149	56	32	12
No patient government	279	70	21	9
Charge attendants and nurses:‡				
Open wards	21	43	38	19
Closed wards	163	60	22	18
Nursing assistants:§				
Open wards	39	48	31	21
Closed wards	386	67	23	10
Charge attendants and nurses:‖				
Regular staff-patient meetings	78	46	28	26
No meetings	107	66	21	13
Nursing assistants:#				
Regular staff-patient meetings	155	56	32	12
No meetings	273	71	20	9

* $\chi^2 = 8.4$; 2 degrees of freedom; $P < .02$.
† $\chi^2 = 10.1$; 2 degrees of freedom; $P < .01$.
‡ $\chi^2 = 3.0$; 2 degrees of freedom; $P < .30$.
§ $\chi^2 = 6.8$; 2 degrees of freedom; $P < .05$.
‖ $\chi^2 = 8.1$; 2 degrees of freedom; $P < .02$.
$\chi^2 = 9.6$; 2 degrees of freedom; $P < .01$.

whether personnel working under the conditions set by the three policies accept change more readily than those working under other conditions.

Table 4 reveals that this is the case.[11] The table shows that personnel of all ranks are most likely to resist change strongly when they are assigned to wards where these procedures are not followed. This is true in all six combinations, five of which are statistically significant. While we are suggesting that these relationships signify that the absence of the policies produces the resistance, the reverse could be argued; that is, resistance precludes the employment of such patient-care policies. It can be pointed out in this regard, however, that the personnel included in this survey do not make decisive policy. While some, particularly the registered nurses, might exercise influence in establishing programs, it is typically the nursing supervisor or ward psychiatrist who institutes such policies. It is evident, then, that the de facto state of affairs constitutes a foundation for attitudes toward change and not the other way around.[12] When existing conditions are such that there is a discernible continuity between one's present experiences and the changes he anticipates, relatively little opposition is likely. But when conditions provide no bridge to future expectations, resistance becomes more probable.

The above findings bring into question the typical views of change in our society. From both moral conviction and practical considerations, it is usually felt that desired changes should be preceded by favorable attitudes among the people to be affected by the change. Our evidence suggests, however, that a condition for the breakdown of resistance to change is through change itself. This conclusion is consistent with that of Clark, drawn from his review of desegregation through 1953: "the use of necessary power and authority to change the structure of the situation results initially in behavioral changes. These behavioral changes then compel compatible attitudinal accommodations which are required to preserve the assumption of personal rationality and adjustment."[13] It will be seen in the case of the institution under study, however, that the structure of the situation most effectively brings about attitudes favorable to change only where there is a supporting leadership.

OPINION LEADERSHIP

It would appear from the foregoing tables that the work situation has a direct impact in shaping the attitudes of personnel toward change and that this impact is exercised independently of position. There is evidence, however, that the influence of the situation can be intensified or vitiated by the opinions of people in positions of leadership. In this connection we refer specifically to the leadership of the registered nurses over their nursing assistants. As previously noted, registered nurses, on wards on which they are found, are usually responsible for the care given to patients by their staffs. By virtue of these responsibilities, they have a good deal to do with setting the pace and tone of their wards. Also, because of their authority and relatively high status, their behavior and attitudes can be taken as a model on which those working under them pattern themselves.

One question we should ask is whether the nurse has a role in imparting to subordinates her own resistance to or acceptance of change. For this purpose the nurses' attitudes are simply compared to those of the nursing assistants assigned to the same wards. Table 5 would suggest that the assistants do tend to take over the attitudes of their nurses.[14] Thus, assistants working on wards with nurses who strongly resist change are themselves likely to express the same stand; they are far less likely to be strong resistors if the nurses for whom they work are low in resistance. It is apparent that there is a close association between the opinions of nurses and their assistants.[15]

TABLE 5.
Attitudes toward Change of Nurses and Their Assistants

	NO.	ASSISTANTS' RESISTANCE TO CHANGE (PER CENT)		
		STRONG	MODERATE	LOW
Registered nurses who are:*				
Strongly resistant	54	70	17	13
Moderately resistant	39	67	23	10
Low in resistance	36	33	53	12
Assistant's attitudes toward regular staff-patient meetings on wards having:†				
Favorable policy and favorable nurses	37	27	54	19
Favorable policy but unfavorable nurses	26	69	23	8
No favorable policy but favorable nurses	23	78	22	—
No favorable policy and unfavorable nurses	43	70	14	16

* $\chi^2 = 16.2$; 4 degrees of freedom; $P < .01$.
† The first combination is significantly different from the remaining three, in each case beyond the .001 level. There are no significant differences between the remaining three combinations.

The opinions of nurses must also be considered in conjunction with existing ward policies known to create a favorable disposition toward change. By examining these two factors simultaneously we can assess the interplay between conditions of the work situation and opinion leadership as they effect the resistance of assistants. The practice of regular staff-patient meetings is taken for this purpose, since it affords the best distribution of cases. The results of these comparisons are also presented in Table 5. It is apparent that the influence of the existing condition in breaking down resistance to change among assistants is exercised only where it is reinforced through the favorable opinions of the nurse: it has no effect by itself. On the other hand, when the nurse is favorably disposed toward change, this will have no influence on her assistants in the absence of the disposing situational condition. From these findings it would appear that, where existing policies are influential in reducing opposition, the opinions of key personnel are the vehicles through which the influence is exercised. But when these personnel are located in situations whose realities do not support their opinions, the effects of their opinion on the attitudes of assistants are lost.

SUMMARY AND IMPLICATIONS

THERE is little doubt of growing unwillingness to let change take its own time and directions. Although attempts are increasingly being made to initiate and guide change along a purposeful course it is readily apparent that wanting particular changes and achieving them can be quite unrelated. Antagonisms emerge and become barriers to desired ends, or desired changes are held in abeyance out of fear of arousing hostile opposition. This paper attempted to trace some sources of resistance to rather extreme but realistic changes in patient care policies.

Attitudes toward change were found to be related to the values and precepts of personnel and to their positions in the nursing force. Registered nurses, having access to a body of treatment values sympathetic to the orders of changes dealt with here, are least resistant to change. The influence of these values is pointed up by the fact that nurses who, as a result of active professional identification, are likely to adopt and espouse advanced views of patient care are also most inclined to accept change. The specific precepts found to be related to resistance did not hold across the different ranks. Among those in higher positions, conceptions of social distance that should properly be maintained between themselves and patients were associated with their attitudes toward change. What matters to the resistance of assistants, however, is the extent to which they want patients to serve as instruments of ward maintenance functions. Precepts and desiderata, therefore, will have a bearing on resistance only under conditions of relevance. What appears to determine the relevance of these precepts is their centrality to what personnel actually do in their jobs and to the issues they deal with in meeting the demands of their work.

Certain patient-care policies were taken for a more detailed examination of the conditions under which personnel work. These policies, each reflecting the degree of autonomy accorded patients, are consonant with the proposed changes and were found to have an attenuating effect on resistance. But this effect apparently does not come about directly with all personnel. It reaches the assistants through the mechanism of opinion leadership of the head nurse for whom they work. Thus, the resistance of assistants remains high unless the policy is backed by a disposition favorable to change on the part of the nurse.

The data contain a number of implications for strategies of planned change. These begin with the scale devised for the measurement of resistance, which provides a guide to the rank order of acceptability; it indicates empirically the sequence by which changes can be introduced with a minimum of resistance arousal. There is also evidence indicating that the introduction of the most acceptable change might reduce opposition to the changes that originally were less acceptable. Resistance to change can be overcome through change itself, particularly when supported through the feelings of key personnel. The findings further indicate that any effective attempt to alter attitudes toward change through persuasion must take into account what is meaningful and relevant to different personnel. In the case of the mental hospital, it might be effective to stress the somewhat abstract aspects of staff-patient relations when appealing to the higher placed staff. It would be our prediction, however, that the lower groups would be more responsive to appeals that discuss change in terms of everyday ward maintenance.

Finally, the fact that those lowest in position are also most resistant represents a barrier to change. These individuals are most remote, both in position and identification, from the professional goal-setters of the institution. At the same time, a great deal of reliance is placed on them for the achievement of the institution's goals. The organizational separation of goal-setters and goal-getters cannot work effectively, however, as long as they are oriented to different ends. In order to overcome opposition, an institution must recognize and deal with such elements of its structure, either by having the lower groups participate more actively in plans for change or by having the goal-setters participate more actively in the implementation of their goals.

NOTES TO CHAPTER 42

1. The processes and consequences of planned change might be quite different under the direction of an outside expert than when it receives its impetus and guidance exclusively by members of the organization. For studies and discussions of planned change see Ronald Lippitt, Jeanne Watson, and Bruce Westley, *The Dynamics of Planned Change* (New York: Harcourt, Brace & Co., 1958); Cyril Sofer, *The Organization from Within* (London: Tavistock Publications, 1961); F. L. W. Richardson, *Talk, Work, and Action*

(Monograph 3 [Ithaca, N.Y.: Society for Applied Anthropology, Cornell University, 1961]), and a symposium in *Human Organization,* Vol. XVII (Spring, 1959).

2. For examples of work reflecting this reappraisal see Maxwell Jones, *The Therapeutic Community* (New York: Basic Books, 1953); Milton Greenblatt, Richard H. York, and Esther Lucille Brown, *From Custodial to Therapeutic Patient Care in Mental Hospitals* (New York: Russell Sage Foundation, 1955); and Milton Greenblatt, Daniel J. Levinson, and Richard H. Williams (eds.), *The Patient and the Mental Hospital* (Glencoe, Ill.: Free Press, 1957), pp. 20-35, 197-230.

3. This point of view is no stranger to the mental hospital with its psychiatric perspectives. There is a tendency in such a setting to look exclusively "inside" the participants for explanations of behavior. Alfred H. Stanton and Morris S. Schwartz discuss this proclivity and the use of *ad hominem* arguments by psychiatric staffs (*The Mental Hospital* [New York: Basic Books, 1954], pp. 247-48).

4. Peter M. Blau's studies of public bureaucracies tend to refute this view; he discusses the structural features of bureaucracies that make it a type of organization that can easily accept and accommodate to change ("Bureaucracy and Social Change," in *The Dynamics of Bureaucracy* [Chicago: University of Chicago Press, 1955], pp. 182-200).

5. The author wishes to express his gratitude to Dr. Winfred Overholser, superintendent of Saint Elizabeths Hospital, and Miss Lavonne Frey, director of nurses, for their help and support of this study. Responsibility for the data and their interpretation are the author's alone.

6. The reproducibility of this scale is .92; its scalability is .72. In the tables presented, respondents scoring 0 or 1 are categorized as showing "strong" resistance; 2 to 3 "moderate" resistance; and those scoring 4 or 5 are "low."

7. Each dimension of distance is measured by a Guttman scale. The items making up the scale of personal distance are: (1) I often find pleasure in talking about myself to patients, (2) I often become quite personally attached to patients on my ward, and in a way am sorry to see them leave the ward, (3) Whenever possible, it is fun to sit down with a patient and just pass the time of day talking, (4) One patient is more or less the same as any other, and (5) When I get to know a patient well, I find I talk to him just as I would anyone else. Status distance is measured by the following items: (1) If you get too friendly with patients, they often lose respect for you, (2) It's a bad idea to get too friendly with patients, (3) You have to keep your distance from mental patients, otherwise they are liable to forget you are a nurse or nursing assistant, (4) It's hard to be friendly with patients without it becoming too personal, (5) One of the problems in getting friendly with patients is that patients don't know where to draw the line, and (6) It's all right to get friendly with patients but not too friendly. A detailed description of the construction and uses of these scales is found in Leonard I. Pearlin and Morris Rosenberg, "Nurse-Patient Social Distance and the Structural Context of a Mental Hospital," *American Sociological Review,* XXVII (February, 1962), 56-65.

8. Many of our interpretations are based on the theoretical, and empirical

treatment of dissonance and its role in attitude change by Leon Festinger, *A Theory of Cognitive Dissonance* (Evanston, Ill.: Row, Peterson & Co., 1957).

9. Festinger notes that by no means are all cognitive elements related; he refers to such cases as "irrelevant relations." We are dealing with a situation where two elements are irrelevant for one group but quite relevant for others (*ibid.*, pp. 11-12).

10. There are four additional types on the list: "a patient who really needs and wants your help," a patient who appreciates what you do for him," "a patient who has a pleasant personality," and "a patient who means well underneath." These are distinguished from the types enumerated above by their emphasis on personality qualities of patients.

11. The tables have a total N considerably less than the 1,138 included in the survey. The reason for this is that over 40 per cent of the nursing personnel are regularly assigned to more than one ward. In cases of staff having multiple asignments, it would not be possible to use a given ward policy in accounting for resistance. Only personnel with single assignments, therefore, figure in tables using ward information. Their total number is 647.

12. It is possible that psychiatrists seek out the most receptive wards on which to introduce programs or, upon meeting resistance, they might arrange to have the recalcitrants transferred to other wards and replaced by more accepting personnel. Either of these selective actions would contribute to the observed relationships; if such actions do occur, however, they probably contribute quite minimally to the variance.

13. Kenneth Clark, "Desegregation: An Appraisal of the Evidence," *Journal of Social Issues*, IX, No. 2 (1953), 74.

14. The small N of the first part of this table results from the limited number of registered nurses with single ward assignments who have assistants exclusively assigned to their wards.

15. The association in the second part of Table 5 probably derives from opinion leadership rather than from exposure of both groups to a shared environment; for when the attitudes of charge attendants toward change are compared with those of the assistants working under them, no relationship appears, despite the fact that these two groups are in a common environment.

Unplanned Change Processes

ஜ்

C H A P T E R   4 3   Socialization in
Correctional Communities*

STANTON WHEELER

THIS paper grows out of a tradition of sociological investigation established some twenty years ago by Donald Clemmer.[1] One of the
most important of the many contributions in Clemmer's *The Prison Community* was his analysis of the changes inmates undergo during periods of
confinement—changes Clemmer signified by use of the concept of *prisonization*. The present paper reviews the processes Clemmer described,
provides an empirical test of some of his propositions, and attempts to
relate the analysis of socialization processes to other features of correctional communities.

PRISONIZATION

CLEMMER employed the concept of prisonization to describe the central
impact of the prison on its inmates—the impact of an inmate society
whose code, norms, dogma, and myth sustained a view of the prison and
the outside world distinctly harmful to rehabilitation. The core of this
view was indicated in an inmate code or system of norms requiring
loyalty to other inmates and opposition to the prison staff, who served as
representatives of a rejecting society beyond the walls. The consequences
of exposure to the inmate society were summed up by the concept of
prisonization, which Clemmer defined as "the taking on, in greater or
lesser degree, of the folkways, mores, customs and general culture of the
penitentiary."[2] Clemmer saw prisonization as a specific illustration of

* Expanded and revised version of a paper read at the meetings of the American
Sociological Association, Chicago, 1959. The author is greatly indebted to Dr. Clarence
C. Schrag, University of Washington, for aid and criticism in the formulation of the
research, to the inmates and staff of Western State Reformatory for their cooperation.
Reprinted from the *American Sociological Review*, 26 (1961), 697–712, by permis-
sion of the author and the American Sociological Association.

more general processes of assimilation occurring wherever persons are introduced to an unfamiliar culture. The net result of the process was the internalization of a criminal outlook, leaving the "prisonized" individual relatively immune to the influence of a conventional value system. Both Clemmer and the inmates who served as his principal informants felt that the degree of prisonization was the most important factor affecting adjustment after release from the institution.[3]

Clemmer noted that no inmate could remain completely unprisonized. Merely being an incarcerated offender exposed one to certain "universal features" of imprisonment. These included acceptance of an inferior role and recognition that nothing is owed the environment for the supplying of basic needs. Beyond these features were other conditions that he felt influenced both the speed and degree of prisonization. Thus prisonization would be lowest for those inmates who have had "positive" and "socialized" relationships during pre-penal life, those who continue their positive relationships with persons outside the walls, those whose short sentences subject them to only brief exposure to the universal features of imprisonment, those who refuse or are unable to affiliate with inmate primary groups, and those who by chance are placed with other inmates not integrated into the inmate community. Clemmer felt that the most crucial of these factors was the degree of primary group affiliation.[4]

Though some twenty years have passed since Clemmer's work was first published, his account remains the most thorough and detailed description of the socialization process in prisons. The viewpoint expressed by Clemmer is based on a direct social learning theory highly similar to Sutherland's theory of differential association. The variables affecting degree of prisonization reflect the same influences Sutherland noted—the frequency, duration, priority, and intensity of contact with criminal patterns.[5] When the concept of prisonization has been discussed by sociologists, the comments are similar to a chief criticism of Sutherland's theory. Thus Cohen finds the theory of differential association incomplete because it fails to illuminate the conditions determining the presence of the delinquent culture.[6] Sykes and Messinger find the theory of prisonization incomplete because it fails to account for the presence of the inmate culture.[7] The theory is found wanting because it accounts only for the process of cultural transmission and does not explain why the culture is "there" to be transmitted. It is criticized for being incomplete rather than false. But in addition to this omission and the need for more evidence concerning the process, there is a further problem in employing the concept of prisonization that requires clarification before Clemmer's propositions can be adequately tested. It concerns the temporal frame of reference within which socialization effects are studied.

The usual way of treating the time variable in studies of assimilation is to classify persons according to their length of exposure to the new social setting. This conception is usually employed in studies of prison adjustment, and was explicitly stated by Clemmer, who directed his attention to "the manner in which the attitudes of prisoners are modified as the men spend month after month in the penal milieu."[8] Throughout his work Clemmer concentrated on the process of induction into the community. He had little to say about changes that might occur as inmates neared the time for release. His proposition that prisonization is the most important determinant of parole adjustment is based on the assumption that processes observed during the early and middle phases of incarceration continue until the inmate is paroled.

It is easy to understand how this emphasis on the process of induction developed, for it grew out of the awareness that the prison is a community with its own norms and structure. The task of accounting for processes of assimilation into the community developed as a natural concern. In addition there were no well-developed notions of what Merton has called "anticipatory socialization," the preparatory responses that frequently precede an actual change in group membership, such as the movement from prison to the broader community. The result is that we know much more about processes of socialization into the community than we do about re-adaptation to the outside world. There is evidence, however, that from the inmate's perspective the length of time *remaining* to be served may be the most crucial temporal aspect. Many inmates can repeat the precise number of months, weeks, and days until their parole date arrives, whereas few are equally accurate in reporting the length of time they have served. The inmate language system contains terms such as being "short" and having "short-time-itis" that suggest the importance of the last few weeks in the institution, just as the term "fish" denotes the new inmate's status.

These observations merely illustrate that at any given point in time the temporal frame of reference of different types of inmates may have various psychological and social meanings. So long as we restrict our analysis to the length of time since entrance into the prison, we may miss important features of the inmate's response to the institution.[9]

In order to clarify the different temporal aspects of socialization in the prison, the data reported below are divided into two sections. The first uses a definition of time similar to that implied by Clemmer, and allows for the test of his hypotheses. The second classifies inmates according to phases of their institutional career, thus enabling us to observe changes that may occur as inmates are preparing for release from the institution.

RESEARCH SETTING AND METHOD

THE research was conducted in a western state reformatory, one of two adult penal institutions in the state. It is a walled, close custody institu-

tion receiving inmates from 16 to 30 years of age. The only felony offenders excluded by statute from sentence to the reformatory are those
convicted of capital crimes. The physical plant is roughly typical of many
northern state institutions designed to handle young adult offenders.

Samples of inmates were drawn from each of the housing units of the
institution, using stratified random sampling procedures with a variable
sampling rate designed to increase the number of inmates in the sample
who were in the early and late stages of their incarceration. Of 259 men
originally assigned to the sample, 95 per cent completed questionnaires
and 92 per cent of the questionnaires were usable for research purposes.
The only inmates excluded from the sample design were those screened
by the clinical psychologist as psychotic or near psychotic, or too low in
intelligence to understand and respond meaningfully to the questionnaire. The sample n is 237 from an inmate population of approximately 750.[10]

Hypothetical conflict situations were used to develop an index of conformity to staff role-expectations. Several conflict situations were employed in the research. The ones selected for the index were those that
(a) gave evidence of normative consensus on the part of custody and
treatment staff members, and (b) showed variation in inmate response.
Five items adequately met these criteria. The items, arranged in de-
creasing order of "conformity to staff" response, were as follows:

1. An inmate, Owens, is assigned to a work crew. Some other inmates criticize him because he does more work than anybody else on the crew. He works
as hard as he can.
2. Inmate Martin goes before a committee that makes job assignments. He is
given a choice between two jobs. One job would call for hard work, but it would
give Martin training that might be useful to him on the outside. The other job
would allow Martin to do easier time in the institution. But it provides no training for a job on the outside. Martin decides to take the easier job.
3. An inmate, without thinking, commits a minor rule infraction. He is given
a "write-up" by a correctional officer who saw the violation. Later three other
inmates are talking to each other about it. Two of them criticize the officer. The
third inmate, Sykes, defends the officer, saying the officer was only doing his
duty.
4. Inmates Smith and Long are very good friends. Smith has a five-dollar bill
that was smuggled into the institution by a visitor. Smith tells Long he thinks
the officers are suspicious, and asks Long to hide the money for him for a few
days. Long takes the money and carefully hides it.
5. Inmates Brown and Henry are planning an escape. They threaten inmate
Smith with a beating unless he steals a crowbar for them from the tool shop
where he works. He thinks they mean business. While he is trying to smuggle
the crowbar into the cell house, he is caught by an officer, and Smith is charged
with planning to escape. If he doesn't describe the whole situation, he may lose
up to a year of good time. He can avoid it by blaming Brown and Henry.

Responses to the first four items were on a four category approve-disapprove continuum. Response categories for the fifth item were:

What should inmate Smith do?
He should clear himself by telling about the escape plans of Brown and Henry.
He should keep quiet and take the punishment himself.

On each of the items at least 75 per cent of the custody and treatment staff members were in the modal response category: They approve the inmate's conduct in items one and three, disapprove on two and four, and feel that inmate Smith "should clear himself. . . ." Sixty-seven per cent of the staff were in agreement on all five items, and 93 per cent were in agreement on at least four items. Thus for these items there is a relatively high degree of normative consensus among staff as to proper inmate behavior. Inmates are classified into three categories, according to the number of situations in which the inmate response is the same as that of the modal staff response. The high conformity group includes inmates whose own response agreed with the staff in at least four of the five situations, the medium conformists those who agreed in two or three situations and the low conformists those who agreed in none or in one situation. The relatively small number in the extreme nonconformity group has led to their inclusion with the medium conformists at several points in the analysis.[11]

This index of conformity to staff expectations obviously taps only a part of the phenomena referred to as prisonization by Clemmer and others. It does seem to get at a central core: the acceptance or rejection of norms and role definitions applied to inmates by the prison staff. As a crude check on the possibility that the index serves also as a more general reflection of the inmate's support for law abiding values, an additional item was included that refers to behavior in civilian roles. The item was adapted from the studies by Stouffer and Toby designed to measure universalism-particularism and reads as follows:[12]

Barker is riding in a car driven by his close friend, Davis, and Davis hits a person crossing the street. Barker knows that his friend was going at least 40 miles an hour in a 25-mile-an-hour speed zone. There are no other witnesses. Davis's lawyer says that if Barker testifies under oath that the speed was only 25 miles an hour, it may save Davis from serious consequences.

What do you think Barker should do?

He should testify that Davis was going 25 miles an hour.
He should not testify that Davis was going 25 miles an hour.

When this item is used as a criterion in place of the conformity index, the direction of all the relationships reported below still holds, although the degree of relationship is somewhat reduced. Thus there is some evidence that the index used here, although limited in reference to the prison situation, may serve as a more general measure of the inmate's values.

The conflict situations were presented in a questionnaire that also contained a brief self-conception inventory, background items, and items relating to participation in various institution activities. Inmates responded to the questionnaire in groups of ten to twenty, and under conditions of anonymity. Every precaution was taken to insure free, private responses. Although no formal validity checks could be made, there is indirect evidence of validity in the fact that the rank order of proportion high conformity response is what would be expected from knowledge of the administrative process by which inmates are assigned to housing units. Thus the smallest percentage of high conformity response is found in the segregation unit (14%), followed by the close custody unit (21%), medium custody unit (34%), honor farm and reception unit (44% and 47%), and the protection unit (83%), where inmates are held for their own protection from other inmates, chiefly because they are defined as "rats" who have violated inmate norms regarding informing on other inmates.

Our interest is in tracing changes over time in response to the correctional community, from data gathered at one point in time. Several conditions could invalidate the assumption that the observed differences are due to the time variable. These include change in characteristics of inmates, changes in characteristics of the institution, and selective parole procedures. There is no evidence that the first two conditions could have operated in any significant degree. There had been only slight changes in the characteristics of incoming inmates for several years preceding the study, and no major administrative changes in program had been introduced over the previous three year period. The major potential bias concerns selective parole policies. Presumably, inmates who have served longer sentences are more serious offenders who may have been more opposed to the staff at time of entrance into the institution. The average length of sentence in this institution is slightly over three years. The typical inmate serves two thirds of this sentence, and almost all inmates serve at least 18 months. Selective factors may be operating beyond the two year period but are unlikely to be present in significant degree prior to that time. Yet evidence reported below shows changes over time that operate before selective factors are introduced. Thus while panel data are obviously needed to verify the relationships reported here, there is reason to believe that valid inferences may be made about temporal shifts.[13]

The statistical significance of the relationships is assessed by chi square, employed as a one tailed test when Clemmer's hypotheses are being tested, and in the normal manner when inmates are classified into phases of their institutional career.[14] The gamma coefficient described by Goodman and Kruskal is used as a measure of degree of relationship throughout the paper.[15] The small number of cases in some of the tables suggests that the results can best be evaluated in terms of size and consistency of relationships rather than the degree of statistical significance obtained in any one table.

TABLE 1.

Length of Time Served and Conformity to Staff Role Expectations

LENGTH OF TIME SERVED	PER CENT HIGH CONFORMITY	PER CENT MEDIUM CONFORMITY	PER CENT LOW CONFORMITY	TOTAL	N
Less than 6 months	47	44	09	100	77
6 months-2 years	32	54	14	100	99
Over 2 years	16	61	24	100	38
Total	—	—	—		214

$$\chi^2 (4df) = 12.00 \; p < .01$$
$$\gamma = -.35$$

RESULTS: LENGTH OF TIME SERVED AND CONFORMITY TO STAFF EXPECTATIONS

WHEN the usual method of treating the time variable is employed, the results give strong support to Clemmer's propositions regarding prisonization. Table 1 shows the relationship between length of time served and conformity to staff norms. As expressed in this table, the effect of increased length of exposure is to reduce the proportion of men who conform to the staff's expectations. Furthermore, when analysis is made separately for first termers and recidivists, there is evidence of a relearning process among the recidivists. Although recidivists are more likely to be non-conformists than are the first termers, the effect of time served on their non-conformity is about the same. Instead of entering the prison already prisonized, a re-prisonization process appears to occur.

If the process of prisonization is operating effectively we should be able to observe its effects over shorter time periods. And we would expect the effect to be present particularly for offenders serving their first term in an adult penal institution. In Table 3, inmates are classified into as refined time categories as can be justified with a small number of cases. The results are presented for a period up to one year, for which period we can be almost positive that selective factors are not operating. The results again confirm Clemmer's observations, and suggest the importance of the first few months in the socialization process.[10]

A central theme in Clemmer's analysis is that the degree of prisonization will vary according to the degree of involvement in the informal life

TABLE 2.

*Length of Time Served and Conformity to Staff Role Expectations,
for Offenders Differing in Prior Penal Commitments*

PER CENT HIGH CONFORMITY

LENGTH OF TIME SERVED	NO PRIOR ADULT COMMITMENT	N	PRIOR ADULT COMMITMENT	N
Less than 6 months	49	51	40	25
6 months-2 years	31	64	33	33
Over 2 years	19	26	06	12
Total	—	141	—	70

$$x^2 \ (2df) = 7.56 \ p < .025 \qquad x^2 \ (2df) = 2.50 \ p > .10$$
$$\gamma = -.40 \qquad\qquad\qquad \gamma = -.38$$

of the inmate community. In the present research, two items were used to tap the extent of inmate involvement. One item reflects the extensiveness of involvement in terms of the number of close friendships established with other inmates. A second item reflects the intensity of involvement by ascertaining the degree to which inmates spend their free time with other inmates or by themselves. The relationship of each of these indexes of involvement to conformity to staff expectations is presented in Tables 4 and 5.[17]

The results indicated in both tables lend support to the proposition that both the speed and degree of prisonization are a function of informal inmate involvement. During the first time period there is no significant relation between involvement and conformity to staff opinion. However, the percentage of high conformists drops rapidly for inmates who are highly involved. For those who have little contact with other inmates as assessed by our items, the process of prisonization appears to operate, but

TABLE 3.

*Percentage High Conformity For First-Termers Over the
First 12 Months of Incarceration*

LENGTH OF TIME SERVED	PER CENT HIGH CONFORMITY	N
Less than 3 weeks	56	18
3 to 6 weeks	48	21
6 weeks to 6 months	42	12
6 months to 1 year	28	25
Total	—	76

$$x^2 \ (1df) = 2.05 \ p < .10$$
$$\gamma = -.37$$

TABLE 4.

Length of Time Served and Conformity to Staff Role Expectations,
for Inmates Differing in Extensiveness of Primary Group Contacts

PER CENT HIGH CONFORMITY

LENGTH OF TIME SERVED	HIGH GROUP CONTACTS*	N	LOW GROUP CONTACTS*	N
Less than 6 months	45	31	48	46
6 months-2 years	20	44	42	55
Over 2 years	06	18	30	20
Total	—	93	—	121

$$\chi^2 (2df) = 8.37 \ p < .01 \qquad \chi^2 (2df) = 1.82 \ p > .25$$
$$\gamma = -.62 \qquad \gamma = -.20$$

* See footnote 17 for item wording.

the major impact is delayed until after two years have been served, and even then does not operate to the same degree as for highly involved inmates.

While our data do not enable us to specify clearly the time relationship obtaining between involvement and conformity, it is instructive to examine the relationship as though the reverse time sequence were in operation—as though the sequence were from conformity to involvement. As Table 6 shows, the proportion of high conformists who are also involved in intimate interaction with other inmates decreases through time, while there is an increase in social contacts among the non-conformists.

These results of course raise the question of the interplay between social involvement on the one hand, attitudes and values on the other. Rather than thinking of one of these variables as an effect of the other,

TABLE 5.

Length of Time Served and Conformity to Staff Role Expectations,
for Inmates Differing in Intensity of Inmate Contacts

PER CENT HIGH CONFORMITY

LENGTH OF TIME SERVED	HIGH GROUP INTENSITY*	N	LOW GROUP INTENSITY*	N
Less than 6 months	42	40	51	35
6 months-2 years	21	61	49	39
Over 2 years	00	16	27	22
Total	—	117	—	96

$$\chi^2 (2df) = 9.75 \ p < .005 \qquad \chi^2 (2df) = 3.58 \ p < .10$$
$$\gamma = -.63 \qquad \gamma = -.27$$

* See footnote 17 for item wording.

TABLE 6.

Length of Time Served and Extensiveness of Primary Group Contacts,
for Inmates Differing in Conformity to Staff Expectations

PER CENT HIGH EXTENSIVENESS

LENGTH OF TIME SERVED	HIGH CONFORMISTS	N	LOW CONFORMISTS	N
Less than 6 months	39	36	41	41
6 months-2 years	28	32	52	67
Over 2 years	14	7	55	31
Total	—	75	—	139

$$\chi^2 \text{ (1df)} = 1.33 \text{ p} > .10 \qquad \chi^2 \text{ (1df)} = 1.17 \text{ p} > .10$$
$$\gamma = -.31 \qquad\qquad\qquad \gamma = .17$$

a more appropriate model of their interaction in the prison community might stress the structural incompatability of being both highly involved with inmates and an attitudinal conformist to staff expectations. The dominant normative order among inmates (at least in terms of power and visibility if not numbers) is strongly opposed to that of the staff. The inmate who values friendship among his peers and also desires to conform to the staff's norms faces a vivid and real role conflict. The conflict is not apparent or perhaps is not felt so intensely during the earliest stages of confinement, but with increasing length of time in the prison the strain becomes more acute; inmates move to resolve the strain either by giving up or being excluded from primary ties, or by a shift in attitudes. In either case the result leads to a polarization of non-involved conformists and involved non-conformists. One group of inmates become progressively prisonized, the other progressively isolated. And as the marginal frequencies of Tables 4 and 6 suggest, the dominant tendency is to move in the direction of non-conformity rather than isolation.[18]

This interpretation of changes over time in the prison community awaits panel data for its validation. In addition, three further problems may be noted. First, there is the question of what tips the balance in individual cases of conflict between conformity and involvement. Undoubtedly a number of factors come into play. Some inmates may have a stronger need for group affiliations than others, a need which can be satisfied in the prison only by association with other offenders. Still others may possess traits or occupy positions in the prison community that are important to the inmate leadership, and may thus be under greater pressure to become implicated in the inmate system. Another influence is the degree of attachment to families and friends outside the institution, a factor noted by Clemmer but one which the present research does not adequately measure. Partial evidence on the importance of such ties is revealed in the higher rates of conformity to staff expectations for married men, and for those who report that family members "have confidence" in them.

Second, there is the question of how the processes noted above are linked to the informally defined social types and roles noted in many studies of prison social structure. Although the categories suggested by the dimensions of involvement and conformity are too simple and crude to catch up the subtle aspects of inmate roles, certain parallels are evident. For example, the involved non-conformists are roughly equivalent to the "right-guys" noted in Schrag's typology and to the role of "real man" described by Sykes.[10] Our data suggest that the movement of inmates over time is in the direction of the right guy role, with a much weaker tendency toward the isolated role of "Square John." The data also point to the large number of inmates who are nonconformists to the staff but who remain relatively unaffiliated with inmate primary groups. This group is probably quite heterogeneous, being composed in part of those variously labelled outlaws, toughs, ball-busters, etc., highly egocentric in orientation and free of commitment to either the staff or inmate systems, and in part of less striking figures who are unable to establish strong ties with other inmates, even though desirous of doing so. Many of this latter type may have experienced what Cloward refers to as the pattern of double-failure.[20] The size of this category of unaffiliated nonconformists raises some important questions about the operation of inmate society. On the one hand it suggests limits to the conception that the inmate system generates a high degree of cohesiveness among its members. At the same time it suggests that informal involvement in the system is by no means a necessary condition for the emergence of strong opposition to staff norms.

A third problem posed by the above data, as well as Clemmer's earlier analysis and the descriptions of social types in prisons, concerns the absence of social bonds among the conforming inmates. Neither in our data nor in the language system of the prison is there evidence of a category characterized both by conformity to the staff *and* by strong social bonds with other inmates. What is it about the structure of the correctional community that makes conformity possible, apparently, only at the cost of isolation? The question is too complex to receive detailed treatment here, involving as it does at least in part the question of the origin of the negative inmate culture in prisons. Once established, however, the culture exerts pressure on both the inmates and the staff which operates largely to suppress the formation of solidary ties among the conformists. Evidence from other parts of this study suggests that inmates perceive the opinions of others to be more opposed to the staff than they actually are.[21] The resulting pattern of pluralistic ignorance operates to restrain even the initial seeking out of like-minded individuals. The same pressures lead to the frequent warnings from staff members to stay out of involvements with other inmates, and "do your own time." Thus the conforming inmate

646 *Dynamics of Change in Residential Systems*

may be restrained from establishing supportive ties with others by both the official and the inmate systems. If the withdrawal pattern characteristic of those who conform to the staff is not offset by strong ties to persons outside the institution, the effects of social isolation may be quite severe. For these inmates, the modern institution may accomplish by social and psychological pressure what the Pennsylvania system accomplished by its physical design, and perhaps with some of the same consequences.[22]

RESULTS: INSTITUTIONAL CAREER PHASE AND
CONFORMITY TO STAFF EXPECTATIONS

IN THE following analysis inmates are classified into three categories: a) those who have served less than six months in the correctional community and are thus in an *early phase* of their commitment; b) those who have less than six months remaining to serve—the *late phase* inmates; and c) those who have served more than six months and have more than six months left to serve—the *middle phase* inmates. This procedure enables us to examine changes in response that may occur as inmates are preparing for return to the broader community.

TABLE 7.

Phase of Institutional Career and Conformity to Staff Role Expectations

INSTITUTIONAL CAREER PHASE	PER CENT HIGH	PER CENT MEDIUM	PER CENT LOW	TOTAL	N
Early phase	47	44	09	100	77
Middle phase	21	65	14	100	94
Late phase	43	33	25	100	40
Total	—	—	—		211

$$\chi^2 (4df) = 20.48 \; p < .001$$
$$\gamma = -.21$$

The relationship between phase of institutional career and conformity to staff expectations is presented in Table 7. Two trends are apparent. First there is a steady increase in the proportion of low conformity responses. Second, there is a U-shaped distribution of high conformity responses. The trends suggest that two processes may be in operation. One process is that of prisonization. A progressive opposition to staff norms is observed when inmates are classified either by length of time served or by institutional career phase.

The second process appears to be one of differential attachment to the values of the broader society. The U-shaped distribution of high-conformity responses suggests that inmates who recently have been in the broader community and inmates who are soon to return to that community are more frequently oriented in terms of conventional values.

Inmates conform least to conventional standards during the middle phase of their institutional career. These inmates appear to shed the prison culture before they leave it, such that there are almost as many conforming inmates at time of release as at time of entrance into the system.[23]

Empirical verification of these two processes will require panel studies. If future research supports the findings reported here, other important questions would be raised. What types of inmates follow the pattern of prisonization vs. the pattern of reattachment to the extra-institutional world? Where are these types located within the prison social structure? What events or conditions lead to one process rather than the other? Can institutional authorities exert control over the processes by policy decisions?

TABLE 8.

Phase of Institutional Career and Conformity to Staff Role Expectations, for Inmates Differing in Extensiveness of Primary Group Contacts

| | PER CENT HIGH CONFORMITY | | | |
INSTITUTIONAL CAREER PHASE	HIGH GROUP CONTACTS	N	LOW GROUP CONTACTS	N
Early phase	45	31	48	46
Middle phase	12	50	30	47
Late phase	33	12	48	27
Total	—	93	—	120

$$x^2 \,(2df) = 11.38 \; p < .01 \qquad x^2 \,(2df) = 4.06 \; p > .10$$
$$\gamma = -.38 \qquad\qquad\qquad \gamma = -.07$$

The resocialization effect is apparent among inmates who have established close friendships in the institution, as well as among those who have not. Table 8 shows that inmates who stay out of close friendship ties exhibit as great an attachment to law-abiding standards during the late phase as during the early phase. The process of resocialization is evident among highly involved inmates, but not to the same degree.[24] And as the marginal distributions indicate, the rate of group involvement is highest during the middle phase. When the rate of involvement is examined separately for high and low conformists, the high conformists show a decline at each stage and the low conformists a sharp rise during the middle phase with a decline as time for release approaches.

Further evidence regarding the process of resocialization appears when recidivists are compared with first offenders. As presented in Table 9, the pattern for recidivists is similar to that for first termers. Both groups show the decline in conformity during the middle phase with a rise in conformity in the late phase. The recidivists begin at a lower point and end at a lower point, but the adaptive response pattern is still evident.

TABLE 9.

Phase of Institutional Career and Conformity to Staff Role Expectations,
for Offenders Differing in Prior Penal Commitments

	PER CENT HIGH CONFORMITY			
INSTITUTIONAL CAREER PHASE	NO PRIOR ADULT COMMITMENT	N	PRIOR ADULT COMMITMENT	N
Early phase	49	51	40	25
Middle phase	21	63	22	32
Late phase	44	27	33	12
Total	—	141	—	69

$$\chi^2 \text{ (2df)} = 11.1 \text{ p} < .01 \qquad \chi^2 \text{ (2df)} = 1.44 \text{ p} > .30$$
$$\gamma = -.19 \qquad\qquad\qquad \gamma = -.19$$

The findings concerning career phase for first termers and recidivists suggest some revision of our thinking regarding the impact of time. Instead of viewing successive institutional careers as the development of an increasingly negative pattern, the results would suggest that a cyclical pattern of adjustment may hold for a sizable number of inmates—a cycle which has its lowest point during the middle of a period of institutional confinement, and may have its high point at some period on parole. If observations could be made on parolees it is possible that we could locate other points in the cycle. The results suggest a complex process of socialization and resocialization as offenders move into and out of the correctional community. The model is that of a cycle with a negative trend rather than a monotonically increasing commitment to a criminal value system.[25]

DISCUSSION

The prisonization theory is strongly supported when inmates are classified according to the length of time they have served. When they are classified into phases of their institutional career, however, the prisonization theory is inadequate as a description of changes over time. While it accounts for the increase in extreme non-conformity, it fails to account for the U-shaped distribution of high conformity responses. Recent attempts to develop a theory accounting for the content of the inmate culture provide some understanding of the possible bases for these two types of change.

The Inmate Culture. Two explanations have been offered to account for the content of the inmate culture, one focusing on the process of "negative selection," the other on problem-solving processes. The *negative selection* approach begins with the obvious fact that the single trait held in common by all inmates is participation in criminal activity. Their criminal acts indicate in varying degrees an opposition to conventional norms. It follows that the inmate culture should give expression to the values of those who are most committed to a criminal value system—the long termers, those who have followed systematic criminal careers, etc. And if the culture is viewed as an outgrowth of the criminogenic character of inmates, it is reasonable to expect a reinforcement process operating throughout the duration of confinement. This is consistent with the image of correctional institutions as "crime schools" and with a theory that accounts for changes in response to the prison largely in terms of prisonization.

The alternative view stresses the problem-solving nature of sub-cultures, and interprets the content of the inmate culture as a response to the adjustment problems posed by imprisonment, with all its accompanying frustrations and deprivations. In his analysis of social types in a state penitentiary, Schrag noted the way in which these types are focused around the problems of loyalty relations, of "doing time," of sexual outlet, etc.—problems which are not a direct carry-over from the outside world.[26] In a more recent functional analysis of the inmate social system, Sykes and Messinger note five major deprivations or attacks on the inmate's self-conception, including the rejected status of being an inmate, the material and sexual deprivations of imprisonment, the constant social control exercised by the custodians, and the presence of other offenders. They conclude:[27]

"In short, imprisonment 'punishes' the offender in a variety of ways extending far beyond the simple fact of incarceration. However just or necessary such punishments may be, their importance for our present analysis lies in the fact that they form a set of harsh social conditions to which the population of prisoners must respond or *adapt itself*. The inmate feels that the deprivations and frustrations of prison life, with all their implications for the destruction of his self-esteem, somehow must be alleviated. It is, we suggest, as an answer to this need that the functional significance of the inmate code or system of values exhibited so frequently by men in prison can best be understood."

Elsewhere they note:[28]

"The maxims of the inmate code do not simply reflect the individual values of imprisoned criminals; rather, they represent a system of group norms that are directly related to mitigating the pains of imprisonment under a custodial regime having nearly total power."

If this interpretation is valid we might expect that the culture would exert its major impact on inmates during the *middle* of their stay, at the point in time when they are farthest removed from the outside world. We might also expect that as time for release approaches, the problems deriving from imprisonment recede relative to prospective adjustment problems on parole. Such a shift in reference should give rise to a resocialization process beginning prior to release. And if the culture has this problem-solving character, then recidivists as well as first termers should exhibit the U-shaped pattern of response.[29]

These observations merely indicate that the two trends suggested by the data are consistent with two different interpretations of the inmate culture. On both theoretical and empirical grounds, the adaptive pattern would seem to deserve more attention than it has received in discussions of socialization in the prison. But whether either or both of these types of response are dominant patterns of adjustment in the prison cannot be assessed with the cross-sectional design used in the present study. A panel study in which inmates were interviewed in the early, middle, and late phases of incarceration, and scored as conformist $(+)$ or deviant $(-)$ in their orientation to the staff and the outside world, would yield eight possible response patterns describing the inmate's movement through his institutional career. In addition to the prisonization and adaptation patterns $(+--$ and $+-+)$ there are patterns of stable conformity and stable deviance $(+++$ and $---)$, a delayed prisonization pattern $(++-)$, patterns of rehabilitation or delayed rehabilitation $(-++$ and $--+)$, and a counter-adaptive pattern $(-+-)$ in which the inmate appears to move toward a conventional orientation during the middle of his stay only to return to the deviant response as he approaches parole. Anecdotal evidence and informal observation suggest that all of these patterns might be found, though the prisonization and adaptation patterns may be the most frequent of those in which change occurs. One suggestion emerging from our analysis of the adaptive pattern is that while changes from early to middle phase may reflect events within the institution, changes near release are largely a response to the external world. As correctional programs develop their emphases on liberal visiting, family counseling and pre-release programs they may be able to strengthen tendencies toward a positive change in attitude during the late phases of imprisonment. In turn, current sociological accounts of the inmate culture and adjustment processes may have to be revised to deal more systematically with these external influences.

Conditions affecting type of response. When Clemmer wrote *The Prison Community* it was perhaps reasonable to note under "conditions affecting degree of prisonization" only the personal characteristics of offenders. Prisons were pretty much alike, classification between institutions was weak, and the processes Clemmer noted could be assumed to be relatively constant across a range of institutions. Current correctional systems increasingly depart from this image, and it is likely that both type of clientele and institutional program exert an effect on socialization processes. For example, the fate of those who enter prison with an initially conformist orientation probably depends in large part on the balance between initial conformists and deviants: as the proportion of initial deviants increases, there is greater pressure on the conformists to move away from the pattern of stable conformity. This relationship in turn probably depends on the average age of offenders in the institution. Thus adult maximum security prisons tend to get a very large proportion of inmates who are deviant at time of entrance, but the advanced age of initial conformists may mean that they are less susceptible to influence from the inmate culture. Juvenile institutions are likely to receive a larger number of offenders whose frames of reference are not solidified, and who may thus be more susceptible to peer-group influence. A less "negative" inmate culture may still produce the prisonization response. These features of the inmate population probably interact with staff programs (including the attempts in some institutions to neutralize the inmate culture) to create further modifications in the socialization process in different institutions. The growing differentiation of correctional institutions reinforces the need for comparative analyses and serves as a reminder of the limits of generalization from studies of the type reported in this paper.

Prison and Parole Adjustment. The suggestion that the inmate's response to the prison is adaptive—that he becomes deprisonized as well as prisonized—raises the question of the impact of incarceration on parole conduct. Failure on parole is frequently viewed as the result of internalization of a criminal value system while in prison. But evidence of a cyclical type of adjustment suggests that the process is more complex than is implied in the prisonization scheme. The value system learned in prison may serve as a set of rationalizations activated only when the parolee faces what he defines as barriers to success on parole. Even though the inmate sheds the culture of the prison it will have provided him with justifications for criminal behavior that may be invoked in the event of post-release adjustment difficulties. The prisonization effect may still be operating, though not in the simple and direct fashion implied by the "crime school" image. Its effect is probably modified in important ways by different types of parole settings.

There is a danger, however, of pressing the concept of prisonization too far as an explanation of the prison's impact on parole behavior. Another feature of imprisonment would appear to have an extremely potent influence. This is the impact on the offender's self-conception rather than upon his attitudes toward the outside world. Almost all accounts of correctional processes note what Ohlin has referred to as the "self defining character of the experiences to which the offender is exposed by correctional agencies."[30] In many instances, these effects appear to be highly related to the prisonization process. The offender learns to reject society and in doing so comes to accept a conception of himself as a criminal, with an elaborate set of supporting justifications. But much of the impact of imprisonment appears to lie along another dimension of self-image—the tendency for the offender to internalize the social rejection implicit in his status and suffer the pains of a lowered self-esteem and self rejection. In the work of McCorkle and Korn and more recently in Sykes and Messinger, these potential attacks on the offender's self-image are taken as a crucial condition giving rise to the inmate value system. Self esteem is restored by participation in a system that enables the offender to "reject his rejectors, rather than himself."[31] But if the inmate culture has the problem solving function stressed in these accounts, and if many men show an adaptive response, it follows that the salience of the culture is reduced as men prepare to leave it. This reduction is probably "functional" in the sense that many of the problems of imprisonment do in fact decrease as the inmate nears release. This would seem to be true of most of the threats to self noted by Sykes and Messinger, including the extensive social control of the custodians, the constant presence of other inmates, and the material and sexual deprivations. However, the sense of rejection and degradation implicit in the offender's status does not necessarily decline with release, for the ex-con label still applies. The inmate who sheds the negative outlook required by the inmate system may inherit in its place the rejecting feelings the culture served largely to deny. In this sense the function of the inmate culture may be to *delay* the facing of problems imposed by a degraded social status, rather than to solve them.

This interpretation may help account for the profound states of anxiety and lack of confidence in themselves which even seemingly "tough" inmates frequently display prior to release.[32] As the inmate turns his attention from the inside to the free community, as he makes contacts with employers and relatives, the definition of his status provided by the inmate code loses much of its significance. But it is precisely at this point when the meaning of being an inmate, *as it is viewed by the outside world,* is most likely to have its impact. Some inmates find an atmosphere of acceptance and encouragement. Many others may find that certain jobs are not open to them, that there is some question as to how welcome they are in the community, that they are generally defined as "risks" and not accorded full status. They may return to associations with other ex-offenders not so much to continue a criminal career as to find a more supportive social setting, though further crimes may well grow out of such contacts.

If this interpretation is correct, many of the psychological pains of imprisonment are revealed most clearly at time of release rather than entry. It suggests a basis for a cyclical fluctuation of attitudes as the offender sheds the culture of the prison, experiences social rejection, finds support among other former inmates, returns to crime and to prison, reincorporates prison values, and so on. If true, it points to another possible reason for the organization of therapeutic efforts around the time of release, as well as to the limitations of such efforts unless they can bring about a change in the response to the offender on the part of those in his parole environment. And it suggests that sociological research should be as concerned with the process of re-entry into the community as it has been historically with the problem of assimilation in prison.[33]

One final problem may be noted. Prisons along with other types of "total institutions" are usually assumed to have deep and long-lasting effects on the values of their members. The assumption is natural, deriving as it does largely from the potential effect of 24 hour living establishments that allow only psychological means of escape. The view is supported by a tendency to study the processes of *induction* into such institutions, where the initial effects stand out very clearly.[34] But in most such institutions, membership is temporary. Inmates leave as well as enter. If the institutions tend to develop sub-cultures specific to the problems imposed by their rather unique character, their members may be insulated from lasting socialization effects. In the case of prisons, this insulation provides a less negative picture of the effects of the institution than emerges from analysis of the inmate culture. In therapeutically oriented total institutions, the positive effects may be suppressed. We might expect this suppression of lasting effects to occur particularly in institutions where membership is involuntary. Another relevant condition may be a known and relatively brief duration of confinement.[35] Both of these conditions are present in reformatories.

NOTES TO CHAPTER 43

1. Donald Clemmer, *The Prison Community*, New York: Rinehart and Co., 1958. (Reissue of Original 1940 edition.)
2. *Ibid.*, p. 299.
3. *Ibid.*, pp. 300-302; 312.
4. *Ibid.*, p. 312. Clemmer noted two other conditions that affect degree of prisonization: degree of "blind acceptance" of the dogmas and codes of the inmate population, and degree of participation in gambling and abnormal sex activity. Since these variables seem so closely tied to the concept of prisonization, they might be thought of as indicators of that concept rather than as conditions that affect it.
5. Edwin H. Sutherland and Donald R. Cressey, *Principles of Criminology,* revised edition, New York: J. B. Lippincott Co., 1955, pp. 78-79.
6. Albert K. Cohen, *Delinquent Boys,* Glencoe: Free Press, 1955, pp. 18-19.
7. Gresham M Sykes and Sheldon L. Messinger, "The Inmate Social System," in Richard A. Cloward, Donald R. Cressey, George H. Grosser, Richard McCleery, Lloyd E. Ohlin, Gresham M. Sykes, and Sheldon Messinger, *Theoretical Studies in Social Organization of the Prison,* New York: Social Science Research Council, 1960, pp. 11-13.

8. Clemmer, *op. cit.*, p. 294.

9. In addition to possible differences in response depending on whether the inmate has a time orientation to the past, the present or the future, (or perhaps an orientation which encompasses all these by stressing the total expected duration of confinement) there is of course the important variable of indefiniteness of knowledge about the date of release. Cf. Maurice L. Farber, "Suffering and Time Perspective of the Prisoner," *University of Iowa Studies in Child Welfare*, 20 (1944), pp. 153-227. The indefiniteness is probably more important in other types of total institutions, especially concentration camps, tuberculosis sanitoria, and mental hospitals. In correctional institutions the sentence and release authorities tend to develop routinized forms of administering the indeterminate sentence laws, so that most offenders know quite early in their stay about how long they will have to serve.

10. The analysis below excludes from the protection and segregation units fourteen inmates for whom data were lacking on the time variable. Another eight inmates were excluded because of non-response to one of the five items in the conformity index. The resulting n is 214. Wherever the reported n's fall below that figure it is due to lack of complete information on one of the independent variables. Results from each sampling unit have been combined in the analysis but have not been weighted for differences in sampling rates. Such differences could affect the results only if r_{ab} in sampling unit x differs from r_{ab} in sampling unit y. Snedecor's test for heterogeneity showed no significant differences for ten of the most important relationships in the study. Therefore the simplification achieved by unweighted combining would seem to be justifiable.

11. Staff responses were based on samples of 81 of 111 custody staff members, and 18 of 21 treatment staff members. For a fuller discussion of the methodology employed, see Stanton Wheeler, *Social Organization in a Correctional Community*, unpublished Ph.D. dissertation, University of Washington, 1958. More recent analysis of the index suggests that the items form a Guttman scale with reproducibility = .92, only moderately high for five items. Results reported below are based, however, on the Likert scoring system used earlier. Differences are very slight and do not affect the conclusions.

12. Samuel A. Stouffer and Jackson Toby, "Role Conflict and Personality," in Talcott Parsons and Edward A. Shils, editors, *Toward a General Theory of Action*, Cambridge: Harvard University Press, 1951, p. 483.

13. It is not at all certain that those who have served longer are necessarily the more criminally mature inmates. Many who receive long sentences are first offenders who have committed what the law judges to be the more serious offenses. This judgment bears no necessary relationship to the inmate's orientation to staff or to other inmates. For evidence on the complex relationship between length of time served and adjustment after release, see Donald L. Garrity, *The Effects of Length of Incarceration Upon Parole Adjustment and Estimation of Optimum Sentence: Washington State Correctional Institutions*. Unpublished Ph.D. dissertation, University of Washington, 1956.

14. The one-tailed chi square test may be ambiguous in tables with df greater than 1. Inspection of the tables presented below suggests that the one-tailed test in these cases is justified. Cf. the discussion between Grusky and Shaw, *American Journal of Sociology*, 65 (November, 1959), pp. 301-302.

15. Leo A. Goodman and William H. Kruskal, "Measures of Association for Cross-Classifications," *Journal of the American Statistical Association*, 49 (December, 1954), pp. 747-754. The "gamma" measure reflects the probability of like vs. unlike orders in the classification. It is a useful measure when one deals with ordered classes, and it avoids some of the problems of chi-square based measures. However, it has one property in common with most other measures of association for cross-classifications in that its value depends in part on the marginal distributions. This effect is relatively minor when the measure is used for comparisons within a given set of data provided the marginals on the independent variables are roughly similar across the tables. The effect of differing marginals should probably be controlled, however, in any comparison with data from a different sample. See the discussion on pages 745-747 of the Goodman and Kruskal paper.

16. Richard Cloward reports a similar finding based on research in a military prison. See Helen Witmer and Ruth Kotinsky, editors, *New Perspectives for Research on Juvenile Delinquency*, Washington, D.C.: U.S. Department of Health, Education and Welfare, Children's Bureau, 1956, pp. 80-91.

17. The items used to measure extensiveness and intensity were:
    Have you developed any close friendships with other inmates since you have been in the reformatory?
    _____ Yes, several, (more than 5)
    _____ Yes, a few, (3 to 5)
    _____ Yes, one or two
    _____ No
    Think back over the past month in the reformatory. How would you say you spent most of your free time?
    _____ Mostly with a group of inmates who are together quite a lot
    _____ With one or two inmates
    _____ With several different inmates, but not in any one group
    _____ Mostly by myself
    In Tables 4 and 5, the top two categories are combined for high involvement, the bottom two for low involvement.

18. The strain may be similar to that noted in small group research, between the expressive and instrumental roles. Persons who initially play both the best-ideas and best-liked roles tend to drop the former role for the latter as interaction continues. Talcott Parsons, Robert F. Bales and Edward A. Shils, *Working Papers in the Theory of Action*, Glencoe: The Free Press, 1953, pp. 150-161.

19. Gresham M. Sykes, *The Society of Captives*, Princeton: Princeton University Press, 1958, pp. 84-108. Clarence C. Schrag, *Social Types in a Prison Community*, unpublished Master's thesis, University of Washington, 1944.

20. Richard A. Cloward, "Illegitimate Means, Anomie, and Deviant Behavior," *American Sociological Review*, 24 (April, 1959), p. 175.

21. "Role Conflict in Correctional Communities," in Donald R. Cressey, editor,

The Prison: Studies in Institutional Organization and Change, New York: Holt-Rinehart-Winston Co., 1961.

22. The suggestion that prisonization and social isolation are alternative forms of response to the prison, each posing different problems of adjustment upon release, does not preclude the possibility that inmates may adopt both forms of response at different stages in their incarceration. Again, panel studies are required to trace the interactions between these forms of response. For some suggestions of possible linkages between the two patterns, see Lloyd E. Ohlin, *Sociology and the Field of Corrections,* New York: Russell Sage Foundation, 1956, pp. 37-40.

23. Another potential bias required analysis at this point. Inmates receiving the longest sentences are more likely to be included in the middle phase, while inmates receiving short sentences are over-represented in the late phase. The differences between middle and late phase inmates could thus be due to selective factors.

   The best available check on the existence of such a bias is to consider the responses of middle and late phase inmates separately in terms of total expected time to be served. If the result is due to selection, the differences between middle and late phases should disappear.

   This procedure yielded the following results: For low total time inmates, the percentage high conformity was 28 per cent in the middle phase, 44 per cent in the late phase, for low conformity from 11 per cent to 25 per cent. For high total time inmates, the percent high conformity moved from 21 per cent in the middle phase to 38 per cent in the late phase; for low conformity from 15 per cent to 25 per cent. Thus the relationships hold when total length of sentence is controlled. Use of other cutting points for total time served produced roughly similar results, though suggesting that resocialization operates more strongly for inmates with short sentences, much less strongly for inmates with long sentences.

24. One may question the use of gamma as a measure of association for U-shaped distributions such as those indicated in Table 8, for (provided the marginals are balanced) the measure will give a value of zero for a perfectly U-shaped distribution, although obviously there is "a relationship." One might think of the measure in the present case as reflecting the "net effect" of imprisonment, in which case the measure appropriately gives a value of zero if changes between the early and middle phase are offset by changes between the middle and late phase. Table 8 also demonstrates the dependence of gamma on the marginal distribution. If our sample contained equal numbers of inmates in the early, middle and last phases, the gamma for the relationship among the "high contacts" group would drop from −.38 to −.18, and for the "low contacts" group from −.07 to zero.

25. A pattern similar to that found here has been observed in a state penitentiary. See Peter Garabedian, *Western Penitentiary: A Study in Social Organization,* unpublished Ph.D. dissertation, University of Washington, 1959.

26. Clarence C. Schrag, *op. cit.* See also Gresham M. Sykes, *op. cit.,* pp. 84-108.

27. Gresham M. Sykes and Sheldon L. Messinger, *op. cit.,* p. 15.

28. *Ibid.,* p. 19.

29. A third possible interpretation is that the U-shaped distribution would disappear if one could control adequately for a "social desirability" response set which may be more likely during the early and late stages of confinement. The conditions of administration of the research were designed, of course, to reduce this possibility, but further controls are necessary before this interpretation can be ruled out. The increase in extreme non-conformity during the late stage shows that the effect is not a general one. Also, one would expect that if the effect is operating, it would be sustained at least until inmates had received their sentences, (sometimes between the third and sixth month of incarceration). But the evidence from Table 3 suggests that the decline in conformity operates before this major administrative decision is made.

30. Ohlin, *op. cit.*, p. 33.

31. Lloyd W. McCorkle and Richard Korn, "Resocialization Within Walls," *The Annals of the Academy of Political and Social Science*, 293 (May, 1954), pp. 88-98.

32. Robert Lindner, *Stone Walls and Men*, New York: Odyssey Press, Inc., 1946, p. 422.

33. Prison officials have long been aware of the potential changes in offenders as they near release, and in some institutions special programs are devoted to "pre-release" training or therapy. Useful information on changes in adjustment associated with release is being developed by Daniel Glaser in his panel study of inmates in the federal prison system.

34. It appears that studies of mental hospitals as well as prisons have emphasized the induction process. For a perceptive account of induction phenomena in mental hospitals, see Erving Goffman, "The Moral Career of the Mental Patient," *Psychiatry*, 22 (May, 1959), pp. 123-142. For a suggestion that the effects of these processes in mental hospitals and other types of total institutions may well disappear with release, see Goffman, "On the Characteristics of Total Institutions," *Proceedings of the Symposium on Preventive and Social Psychiatry*, Walter Reed Army Institute of Research, Washington, D.C., April, 1957, pp. 35-36.

35. Some of the effects of involuntary membership have been outlined by Festinger, "An Analysis of Compliant Behavior," in Sherif and Wilson, editors, *Groups Relations at the Crossroads*, New York: Harper and Brothers, 1953. See also John W. Thibaut and Harold H. Kelley, *The Social Psychology of Groups*, New York: John Wiley and Sons, Inc., 1959, pp. 168-190. The concept of voluntary membership itself deserves further clarification. Membership in colleges and professional schools is usually regarded as voluntary since the member chooses to apply. Since membership in such institutions is frequently the only means of achieving other desired ends, (such as the legal right to teach, practice medicine, etc.) elements of involuntary membership are present. Membership may be something to be endured rather than enjoyed. Such settings may produce less overall change in values than is usually supposed. Thus Becker and Geer found a U-shaped attitudinal shift in medical students similar in form to our findings for the reformatory. The idealism of entering students was corroded during the middle of their stay, under the pressure to get the training and grades

necessary for graduation, though it emerged again as they neared "release." See "The Fate of Idealism in Medical School," *American Sociological Review*, 23 (February, 1958), pp. 50-56. Newcomb's finding of a steadily increasing commitment to the institution's values at Bennington College may be attributed in part to the relatively earlier age at entrance, the spirit of newness, and the high prestige of the institution and its staff. As such it may not be typical of the pattern of value change to be found in many colleges or universities lacking these qualities. Theodore Newcomb, *Personality and Social Change*, New York: Dryden Press, 1943.

ॐ

CHAPTER 44 Oscillations and Sociotherapy*

ROBERT N. RAPOPORT[1]

THE term "therapeutic community" has come into vogue among those who seek to create a social milieu beneficial to psychiatric treatment. The appeal of the term and the enthusiasm with which it is applied, however, do not betoken a well-defined and validated set of rational procedures. The situation is rather one in which new and inviting perspectives are added to the burgeoning field of psychotherapy.

Pioneer research in the new field has brought to light factors that hinder effective utilization of the social environment for therapy—wasted energies of informal ward interaction (1), disturbing effects of hidden staff disagreements (11), social barriers between patients and staff in the treatment situation (2), personal barriers to liberalizing hospital staff attitudes (6). On the positive side there is less clarity, though a great variety of assertions have been made about the characteristics of the social environment to which one might attribute therapeutic influence (8, 9). For the present they remain largely speculative in nature.

This paper explores some possible therapeutic implications of a social process, that of oscillation. This process is not explicitly formulated as a part of the therapeutic programme. The staff of the psychiatric Unit described, tend, rather, to emphasize other aspects of their community therapy, e.g. the development of a humanistic approach, permissiveness rather than punitiveness toward symptomatic behaviour, levelling of the authority hierarchy, and so on. The argument of this paper runs as follows:

Hospital systems like that of the Belmont Unit, organized according to permissive, humanistic ideology and populated by patients of the "acting-out" type (12) who tend to express their conflicts interpersonally, will be subject to endemic episodes of social disorganization. Indeed, any focus of patterned interpersonal relationships in such a setting can be observed to *oscillate* between states of more harmonious functioning and states of

* Reprinted from the *Journal of Human Relations*, 9 (1956), 357–373, by permission of the author and the *Journal*.

greater discord. The frequency and intensity of these oscillations is determined, hypothetically, by the degree to which the individual patients are
susceptible to disturbance, because of personal instabilities, the degree to
which permissiveness is exercised, and the degree to which the social
structure fosters interpersonal "contagion"—i.e. "feed-back" of communications. Deviant behaviour and the accompanying social disorganization within this framework are attended by intrapersonal and interpersonal tensions. These tension states need not be seen as antitherapeutic
and therefore categorically to be avoided. On the contrary, they may
have therapeutic value. The activities associated with the didactic, beneficial resolution of these tension states may be termed *sociotherapeutic*.
It is, of course, common experience that some interpersonal tensions—
e.g. wars, feuds, duels—may be *reduced* without benefit to the participants. Furthermore, not all *beneficial* tension-reducing activities would
be called sociotherapeutic in the sense intended here. The resolution of a
hidden staff conflict might alleviate a patient's disturbance and thus be
beneficial, but it would only become sociotherapeutic if it were done to
the accompaniment of any analysis of the patterned personal significance
of the development and alleviation of discordant relationships for those
concerned. The criterion of *didactic* accompaniment to tension-reduction
is conceived of as important in enhancing the possibility that persisting
change in capacity to sustain harmonious relations will occur. The intention of this paper is to indicate how sociotherapy has been observed to
function in association with the oscillatory process within one therapeutic community. Some of the shortcomings and pitfalls implicit in the
use of the method will also be delineated.

THE THERAPEUTIC COMMUNITY AT BELMONT (3, 4, 5, 10)

THE Social Rehabilitation Unit at Belmont is a semi-autonomous treatment centre within a larger neurosis centre serving all England under the
National Health Service. The present Unit is an outgrowth of wartime
experimentation with therapeutic and transitional communities (13). Currently it houses 100 patients, and in the course of a year it discharges just
over 250 patients. The treatment is voluntary and the average length of
hospitalization is between three and four months. This average is perhaps
smaller than the average effective treatment period, since a high percentage of cases take their own discharge soon after entry.[2] The Unit sets an
arbitrary limit of one year as the maximum treatment period. The majority of cases are of the personality disorder, "acting-out" type, with a
wide variety of psychoneurotic and early psychotic cases constituting the
balance.[3] Since the treatment consists largely of group discussions, a
minimum level of normal intelligence is required for admission.

The staff of the Unit resemble, formally, the familiar psychiatric "teams" that have grown out of wartime experience.[4] It is not so much in their composition, as in their pattern of role performance, that they differ from conventional treatment teams.

Basing its views on the assumption that its cases are treatable through contemporary social experience and that they are basically amenable to constructive self-conducted group activities, the Unit has developed a set of relatively explicit convictions about the ideal principles according to which a therapeutic community should be organized. These may be abstracted and presented as four interrelated themes. The Unit functions more or less in accordance with these ideals.

1. *"Permissiveness"*: it is considered valuable diagnostically and therapeutically to allow patients to express their feelings in words or actions, without fear of punishment or retaliation.

2. *"Equalitarian-democracy"*: it is considered valuable to blur status differentiation and to "flatten" hierarchical structure so that participation in the policy and treatment affairs may be enjoyed by all. This is seen as enhancing the patients' opportunities for role-rehearsals, through which empathy, a crucial social capacity, may develop.

3. *"Communalism"*: social connectedness and the sense of sharing and belonging are considered to be enhanced through maximum face-to-face interaction and intimate "free" communication.

4. *"Reality-testing"*: it is considered valuable for treatment to confront patients with an accurate picture of themselves as others see them and with an awareness of how their actions affect others. The Unit "mirror" aims at having rehabilitative value by replicating within the Unit as closely as possible the social situations of ordinary life outside.

1. The Unit is *permissive* in that there are relatively few explicitly stated "formal" rules for conduct and the limits of tolerance for behaviour ordinarily punishable in the outside world are extended. Instead of punishment, patients are "pin-pointed" by one another, and the nature, causes, and social ramifications of their "acting out" are analysed. This may be as difficult for the individual patient to accept as punishment would be, but it is conceptualized differently, and efforts are made to keep activities consistent, in spirit at least, with the ideological tenet of permissiveness.

2. *Equalitarianism* is promoted by legitimizing patient participation in all Unit problems, administrative or therapeutic. Many differentiating symbols like uniforms, titles, and the like are dropped. Staff as well as patients are subjected to critical public discussion of their behaviour within the Unit. Everyone, regardless of formal role, is expected to participate in activities conventionally allocated according to special qualifications, and there is a deliberate blurring of status differences, particularly of a hierarchical nature. The fact that these differences exist formally

as inherent in the hospital system of which the Unit is a part is a precondition that the Unit cannot remove in its present circumstances, but that its staff tend to blur as much as possible in order to achieve a quasi-equalitarian mode of functioning.

3. The ideal of *Communalism* is enhanced by the characteristics of the social structure. All patients are assigned to three formally organized subgroups within the Unit—a ward, a doctor's group, and a workshop.[5] Wards are segregated by sex, one female and three male, but all other groups are mixed in membership as between the two sexes and by cross-cutting—i.e. a given patient will have in his workshop members of his ward and of other wards, members of his doctor's group and of other doctors' groups, and similarly for other activities. This means that each patient will have a chance to interact with all the others in the Unit, and that people will be present in any given group to give perceptions of his relationships in other groups. Informally, patients and staff form pairs and cliques of many kinds that cross-cut these formal groups. The communal aspect of Unit life is implemented not only by the interlocking membership in groups and by the continuous nature of meetings, but by the kinds of task in which the groups engage. Workshops, for example, are engaged in tasks of practical use to the community as a whole—tailoring, furniture repair, painting and decorating, gardening, cleaning. The socials bring the total community together for expressive group activity. The community meetings each morning focus attention on problems that affect the community as a whole.

4. *Reality-testing* is similarly implemented by the factory-like workshop activities, by the attitude of fostering "free" communication to provide a "mirror" for each person of how his behaviour impinges on others with whom he interacts, and by the way in which the groups are organized. *Table 1* shows how groups provide for an alternating pattern of staff-patient contact. This pattern provides comprehensive feed-back channels for the utilization of data on social interactions in all the types of situation provided in the Unit. It also provides a variety of groups in which to test for consensus. Staff members have opportunities to stabilize their perceptions of current events by intermittent contact and detachment from involvement with patients.

The actual functioning of the Unit as a social system approximates these ideals and this structuring of activities only partially. The factors that govern the "goodness of fit" between the ideal and real aspects of Unit life are extremely complex and vary through time. They involve personality composition, role differentiation, pressures and limits imposed through the Unit's network of external relations, contradictory elements in the set of ideals itself, and so on. The present paper describes only those factors associated with one social process in the Unit—that of oscillation.

TABLE 1.

TABLE 1.

The Pattern of Group Activities
(usual day's round)

TIME	PATIENTS ONLY	STAFF AND PATIENTS TOGETHER	STAFF ONLY
07:30	Breakfast		Breakfast
08:30		Community Meeting	
09:45	Tea		Tea
10:15		"Doctors' Groups"	
12:00	Lunch		Lunch
12:30		Ward Meeting*	
13:00	Workshops		Staff Meeting
14:00		Workshops and Private Therapeutic Interviews	Nurses' Tutorials
16:00	Tea		Tea
16:30	Free Time	Some Private Interviews, Conferences	
19:00	Supper		Supper
19:30		Unit Social	
20:30	Retire and sleep		Retire and sleep

* Ward Meetings are held once weekly for each ward, Staff Meetings thrice weekly.

OSCILLATIONS IN SOCIAL ORGANIZATION

THE concept of social organization has to do with the interrelatedness of persons representing parts of a social system at any given time. A state of perfect organization, only hypothetical in any social system, would exist when every participant performed his social role in such a way as consistently to fulfil the expectations of all the others. The system would function harmoniously and would efficiently fulfil the goals or values according to which it was organized. Complete disorganization, on the other hand, would mean the termination of the social system through the death of its members, their absorption into other systems, their cessation of motivation, or other defections of behaviour crucial to the survival of the system.

Both poles of the continuum may be conceived of as ideal-typical constructs between which actual social systems oscillate. The degree to which any given system oscillates and the varieties of patterning that characterize its internal alignments in the course of their movements are extremely diverse. An organization like the Unit, with its disruptive type of patient, its permissive ideology, and its interlocking social groups, seems to foster great fluctuations of many kinds.

Visitors to the Unit are impressed with the fact that its "emotional climate" varies very greatly from time to time. On one morning a query about why a patient did not go to his workshop might be taken as an attack and responded to defensively by counter-attack, withdrawal, or an emotional display. On another morning, what would appear to be a far more disturbing topic—e.g. murder or incest—might be discussed calmly and rationally by all who have something to contribute to understanding the problem. It is further apparent that the differences cannot be explained in terms of the disturbance-value of the content, when one notes that similar problems—e.g. the use of a ward kitchen—are differently handled on different occasions. Furthermore, it is noted that there are wide variations in attendance at groups, in quantity and quality of participation in various activities, and so on. Even more striking is the observation that there is a wide range of variation in the ways in which the ideals of the Unit are put into practice. Some situations are handled, by any criteria, more democratically, permissively, communally, and realistically than others.

Just as it proves fruitless to attempt to find a comprehensive explanation for these variations atomistically in terms of any single factor, such as content of the discussion or activity, so it proves fruitless to attempt to demonstrate its association with an all-embracing molar process. Individuals or small groups within the Unit stand in a great variety of kinds of relationship with one another. Different kinds of real and imaginary alignment cross-cut the larger structure, and these relationships change somewhat independently of the other processes in the organization. However, it may serve to clarify some of the implications for therapy of the process itself if it is considered as a global phenomenon recurring within the Unit and having certain common features that can be abstracted from extended observations.[6]

Each oscillation may be contrived as varying around the ideal-typical pattern represented in *Figure I*.

FIGURE 1   *OSCILLATORY PATTERN*

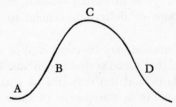

Phase A. This is the point of greatest organization. The system is well integrated, its members performing their social roles most in accord with the expectations of others. Interpersonal tensions and environmental stimulation of intrapersonal tensions are minimal. The Unit is able to function most consistently with staff ideals. Staff find it less anxiety-arousing to be permissive, since deviation is minimal. Group decisions are likely to be taken in the best interests of the Unit as a whole, so that staff need not be apprehensive about having diffused responsibility for Unit affairs through its entire population. Consensus is relatively easy to reach, and the social climate is a relaxed one that fosters trust. Since all these patterns of behaviour in the Unit are taken to be indicative of a good general capacity for social adjustment, there is a tendency to encourage those who have consistently shown socially integrative behaviour to resume their ordinary social roles outside the Unit.

Phase B. As "constructive" patients are discharged and replaced by new patients who bring with them predispositions to disrupt their interpersonal contacts, the potential for disorganization mounts. Patients are permitted to "act out," in keeping with Unit ideals, and interpersonal tensions begin to mount. The new patients are not the only ones who contribute to these tensions. Sometimes older patients who have come through Phase A have interpreted the relative inactivity of the staff as neglect or rejection, and act out in an effort to gain attention. Interpersonal tensions generating around any particular focus, e.g. a ward, tend to ramify into the workshops, socials, and other groups in which its members participate. As personal anxieties mount, the fulfilment of social role-expectations is impaired. Attendance at groups falls off, participation tends to become defective, communications through "official" channels are inhibited through fear and distrust. This last blockage cuts down the flow of spontaneous information on which the staff depend for their own feeling of security in the informal transfer of responsibility for the running of the Unit to the community as a whole. The Unit, indeed, becomes less and less a functioning whole. Cliques form, their members turn inward frightened to trust outsiders with information that might be used against them. Isolates withdraw even further, sometimes leaving the Unit altogether by taking their own discharge. New patients are not as effectively absorbed or welcomed by the old ones, who have become sceptical of the value of Unit treatment and absorbed with their own personal problems. Even some of those patients whose problems do not centre on authority relations tend to resent the staff's failure to act authoritatively to solve the interpersonal problems. Those patients who had been staunch upholders of Unit staff ideology become targets for the aggressiveness of others who feel hostility toward the staff. The patients who symbolize staff members among fellow-patients are less dangerous hate-objects on to whom feelings toward the staff can be displaced. Prestige is gained among the patients through demonstrating "anti-unit" values—defiance, symptomatic acting-out (drinking, taking drugs, fighting, etc.). Patients who communicate openly or take staff-like attitudes in meetings are negatively sanctioned. Staff members are seen as "snoopers," "gestapo," incompetent, exploiting, hypocritical, or insensitive. Adjustment to society is seen as undesirable and those prompting it as loathsome.

Phase C. The crescendo of tension has mounted to such a pitch that a turning-point must be reached if the health of individuals is to be safeguarded and the perpetuation of the institution assured. Several kinds of things characteristically happen to mark the turning-point in the trend.

Complaints from outside may threaten the existence of the Unit—e.g. from local citizens about housebreaking, from the local police about public indecencies, from the larger hospital system about disturbance to other patients or damage to hospital property. Internally the threat of disintegration, personal and social, may reach alarming proportions. A patient may attempt suicide, another may intensify psychotic manifestations imminently threatening uncontrolled behaviour, meetings may become so poorly attended and so unproductive as to cause alarm, disturbances in the wards at night may place severe strain on the night staff.

Several kinds of action serve to bring the situation more under control. Staff may "certify" a patient, sending him to a mental hospital for his own protection (if he is suicidal) or to safeguard others (if he threatens uncontrolled behaviour). The director may insist on the discharge of patients whose behaviour is disturbing the external authorities or the local community. The "pruning" process becomes more than usually active in pressure for the discharge of "dead wood," "untreatables," and others defined as too ill to be helped by Unit methods, too uninterested in receiving treatment really to participate, too disruptive to be tolerated in the interests of the community as a whole or of other patients who might benefit if relieved of pathogenic influences, and so on.

In ordinary circumstances, the staff would seek positive sanctions from the entire Unit before performing such authoritative acts. At points of external threat or internal disintegration it becomes increasingly difficult to count on patients being willing or able to assume overall responsibility for taking the action deemed appropriate by those who are formally responsible, and it becomes increasingly difficult to reach consensus in discussions. When the staff perceive the threats to be intense enough to warrant action regardless of internal sanctions, they act authoritatively. In this sense they evoke their "latent" or "submerged" authority, formally vested in them by the hospital system but more or less obscured informally in the ordinary functioning of the Unit according to its ideals of equalitarian-democracy.

Other kinds of event that can serve to reverse the trend without staff authoritative action may be the unusual displays of leadership by patients who suceed in mustering courage and support even in the face of severe opposition, timely and astute interpretations by staff members or by constructive patients, or more active efforts by staff members to absorb antisocial patients into the larger Unit life through non-authoritative, informal contacts.

Phase D, the reorganizing phase, gains momentum as reparative forces come into play. The fact that disruptive patients have been discharged in itself alleviates some interpersonal tension. Some of those who remain identify with the ones who have been sent to mental hospitals. In favourable circumstances, cases of this kind may redouble their efforts to come into treatment. They may lower their resistances in the face of circumstances that they can recognize as possible extrapolations of their own careers unless they accept help in time. Others, feeling that they have failed in their informal responsibility as therapists or that they have contributed to the precipitation of the disturbances so vividly experienced, seem to feel a strong wish to "repair" the damage in which they have been involved. The staff too, sometimes feel their own departure from behaving consistently with their ideological tenets, though they may have acted in accordance with some other set of commendable principles—e.g. those of medical ethics. In such cases they often make special efforts to regain a more valued mode of operation. Having acted more autocratically and less permissively than they would have wished, having lowered their standards for communality and communications, they renew their efforts to regain, through the alleviation of tensions, a social situation that will once again allow a greater degree of permissiveness, democracy, communality, and reality-testing. They take a more active, didactic role in group discussions. Constructive leaders among the patients now feel secure to speak up. Consensus becomes easier to reach. Patients' attitudes toward one another are more positive and constructive. Participation in the Unit's round of activities improves and becomes more conjunctive. Phase A is once more regained.

The general picture is summarized in *Table 2*.

THERAPEUTIC PROBLEMS

IMPLICIT in the analysis of this process is the assumption of a relationship between intrapersonal and interpersonal tensions. In ordinary extra-hospital settings, particularly in complex urban society, social tensions need not be accompanied by intrapersonal tensions in the participants. Conflict groups like sects, political parties, and so on may generate tensions between members and non-members without necessarily building up correlative intrapersonal tensions. They tend, in fact, to give scope to the expression and alleviation of tensions in socially acceptable channels. When these conflict groups are anti-social, e.g. criminal gangs, society brings to bear negative sanctions. Where the conflict is between an individual and society because of that individual's incapacity to empathize with others, one finds the type of case conceptualized in its extreme form by psychiatrists as the "phychopathic personality." Such individuals tend to set up disturbances with persons around them without feeling the correlative, socially appropriate remorse within themselves. The enlight-

TABLE 2.

Social Functioning and the Oscillatory Process

		PHASE A	PHASE B	PHASE C	PHASE D
Interpersonal Relations	*Role Performance*	Conforming	Deviancy mounts	Deviancy peak	Strain to conformity
	Social organization	Integrated	Disorganization mounts	Disorganization peak	Reorganization
	Mood	Relaxed	Tension mounts	Tension peak	Tension abatement
Ideal-Real Relations	*"Permissiveness"*	Free	Limits strained	Limits set, deviancy repressed	Restoring trust
	"Democracy"	Universal participation	Staff anxiety mounts	Emergence of staff "latent authority"	Staff leadership
	"Communalism"	Community	Cliques form	Fragmentation	Surging together
	"Reality"	Consensus	Disagreement mounts	Dissensus	Eagerness for agreement
Goal Fulfilment	*Treatment*	Success	Symptoms increase, premature self-discharge mounts	"Pruning" failures	Symptoms analysed, energy focused in system, few discharges

ened prescription for such cases is treatment. The problem is what kind of treatment.

The Unit, whose population is made up in good part by people who tend toward the "psychopathic" type, works to forge a more positive relationship between interpersonal and intrapersonal processes. Its tremendous pressures toward communal participation enhance the probability that patients will identify with individuals and groups throughout the total social system. Each person or segment of the Unit is a potential "significant other" for everyone else in the system, to be symbolically invested with emotions derived from earlier relationships in life outside the Unit. Patients tend to reconstitute their effective social environment from among the Unit personnel. To the extent that this occurs, the didactic resolution of interpersonal conflicts among them may be postulated as being accompanied by the resolution of internal conflicts in the individual.

Which aspects of the social environment of a "therapeutic community" most serve to foster this sociotherapeutic blending of individual and social considerations? The speculations that have been conventionally proposed by milieu therapists tends to emphasize one or another of the elements of the present analysis (i.e. role performance, mood, social integration, consistent staff adherence to ideological tenets). Publications in the field announce that such things as the provision of opportunities for ordinary role performance (e.g. in factory-like workshops), the "freeing of communications," the adoption of permissive attitudes, and so on result in therapeutic gains. It seems reasonable to assume that all of these assertions contain elements of validity in that one may note for each of them a certain percentage of improvement for some of the cases who are exposed to the treatment. Some psychiatrists, lacking greater specificity of knowledge in the field, even seek to maximize these gains in an eclectic "shotgun" approach known as the "total-push" method. Even in these approaches, however, one notes failures as well as successes. Attempts at differentiating among the reaction types associated with particular socio-environmental treatment methods are as yet rudimentary.

It is possible to observe, in a place like the Unit, that some persons recover after exposure and conformative participation in most of these types or conditions of treatment, others do not participate conformatively nor do they recover. These reaction types are consistent with the hypothesis implied in the milieu therapists' prescription, viz. participation leads to recovery and non-participation leads to non-recovery. The therapeutic problem in such cases becomes how to get the patient to "swallow the pill" of participation. On the other hand, one also observes theoretically deviant types. The "chameleon-reaction" type, for example, participates in overt behaviour to the hospital programme but does not sustain an enduring change in *capacity* to adjust outside. This type, like the "sleeper-effect" type—the patient who *does not* participate overtly in the prescribed behavioural forms and yet *does* sustain an improvement in capacity to adjust to the outside world following treatment—is covered by postulating *levels* of participation. *True* participation becomes adherence to the prescribed modes at a deep as well as at a superficial level. For therapeutic goals that seek to restore the patient to social roles in ordinary society rather than sheltered artificial roles in hospitals, the covert level is particularly important. The special difficulty it offers both for clinical and for scientific work is its elusiveness to reliable detection and appraisal. On the basis of observations, however, some relationships between intrapersonal and behavioural participation within the framework of the oscillatory process may be hypothetically delineated.

Fundamental to the discussion is the point that the milieu conditions postulated as effective in psychiatric treatment are not found in a stable state of "being," as many descriptions of the methods imply. Permissiveness, equalitarian social relations, free communications, and so on exist in a recurring process of "becoming," partly because they contain implicit within them the scope and stimulus for their own undoing. As patients who habitually "act out" are given free rein to do so, their reactions initially, at least, tend to be socially disruptive. However, the episodes of disorganization or "collective upset" that occur in this connection may be seen as having potential therapeutic value. If understood and managed sociotherapeutically, the process of oscillation in the overall state of social organization may harness energies more effective for some therapeutic problems than would be available by creating and maintaining, if it were possible, a steady facsimile of the idealized (Phase A) set of conditions.

The energies made available by oscillatory tensions, particularly in Phase D, that could implement therapeutic learning-experiences seem to include the following:

Patients sometimes prospectively identify with the casualties of the process. That is, they see others "break down" under the stress of social disorganization and see themselves as potentially in the place of the casualty unless they focus their energies on receiving the timely benefits of treatment. This, in favourable circumstances, enhances identification with the Unit staff.

Patients also feel a sense of responsibility for the casualties of the process since they have been given, within the Unit, a share of the staff's treatment responsibility. Their desire to repair the harm that they feel themselves to have been involved in may be channeled, in favourable circumstances, into constructive sociotherapeutic work.

Staff members, too, may feel in such circumstances a resurgence of their own reparative motives. The departure from their own ideal standards for a therapeutic milieu has been particularly great just prior to Phase D, and this further stimulates reparative behaviour.

Increased staff participation is called for in discussion groups as constructive patient-leaders are discharged (early in the process) or inhibited (later in the process). This may enhance staff leadership and didactic functions. Patients may be stimulated to more active participation by numerous kinds of identifications. Those who identify with the staff may become incipient "constructive" patient-leaders. Those who identify with the casualties who have left the Unit may take a more active interest in preventing this eventuality for themselves. Those who have identified with internal casualties of disturbed interpersonal behaviour or have themselves experienced disturbing interpersonal contacts may participate more actively in bringing the disruptive stimulators to light. In cases where there is consensus in the group that a given patient's acting-out indeed has this harmful interpersonal effect, the stimulator is presented with the "realities" of his problem. The continuous round of discussion groups provides opportunities for confronting him with these data while the situation is "hot"—and attention of all concerned is heightened by being poignantly involved. In cases where consensus indicates the reaction to be much more deviant than the stimulus, it is the reactor rather than the stimulator whose fantasies and perceptions are analysed. In a place like the Unit, where such a large proportion of the population are psychiatric cases, and where all of the population are subjected to stimuli that could bias perceptions, this becomes a very tricky problem. Often there are distortions on both sides of interactions, and the validity of the consensus itself is subject to query.

Feelings that the existence and validity of the Unit methods may be called into more focused criticism, as disturbances ramify into the surrounding society, stimulate further activity that could serve learning. From the staff point of view, the processes that it fosters may be taken under serious reconsideration. From the patients' point of view, the approaches to this region of anxiety may serve to enhance their identification with staff members, who may be seen as people who are taking personal risks in the interests of promoting a treatment method in which they believe.

Some of the problems and pitfalls in this process have already been implied. These same oscillatory tensions may, in unfavourable circumstances, contribute to undesired consequences. Patients whose fears and anxieties rise too high before the oscillatory cycle takes its turn may take their own discharges prematurely. They may be motivated either by an excess of intrapersonal disturbance—as with persons showing symptoms of anxiety states, obsessional neuroses, or schizophrenia—or by an excess of interpersonal disturbance—as with those showing extreme "psychopathic" personality disorders. The first types, for example, might tend to leave more readily in Phase B; the second types more readily in Phase D, having interpreted the staff's authoritative activities as punitive and betrayals of trust. Those whose conditions do not mobilize them to express their tensions maladaptively through self-discharge may "break down" within the Unit and be excluded from the subsequent sociotherapeutic process, e.g. by certification and referral to a mental hospital. These are only extreme cases of reactions that are present to a lesser extent in other patients. If the tensions generated occur in circumstances unfavourable for the development of the kinds of identification mentioned above they may subtly block sociotherapeutic effectiveness, even where there are no extreme reactions. Patients' anxieties about their treatment responsibilities, for example, may lead in some cases to inhibiting worry and detachment rather than to reparative involvement, even though the patients concerned are not severely enough disturbed to take their own discharges or to "break down" emotionally. The determinants of these reactions seem extremely complex and require a great deal of further study. They include factors like timing of staff action, personality of the patient, interpersonal influences operating on him both inside and outside the Unit to create cross-pressures, and so on.

The staff, too, may encounter undesired aspects of the tension mobilization. Being less close to the "breakdown threshold," on the whole, than the patients, they do not show as high an incidence of symptomatic behaviour, though this too is noted in some degree. Being more bound to the local situation by professional contract they do not easily leave the Unit, though occasionally this does occur, and very often it happens in fantasy and conversation. Maladaptive staff concomitants of this process include lowered morale, disjunctive participation, and distortion of perceptions. Where the distortions gain sufficient group support to be carried into action, they may be called collusions. Two types of collusion have been observed in connection with the process described, that of collusive anxiety and that of collusive denial. Their implications may be discussed in connection with *Figure 2*.

In the first cycle presented, the hypothetically optimal pattern is achieved. The staff allow deviation and disorganization to occur and tension to mount until the "optimal tension ceiling" is reached. While there may have been losses through self-discharge and through pruning and unproductive emotional disturbances, the net gain in the direction of didactically utilizing the tensions of the equilibrating phase (D_1) seems great, and consensus can be found that in the circumstances casualties were unavoidable and minimal.

In the second cycle, where collusive anxiety is graphically portrayed, authoritative action is taken by the staff because of an exaggerated perception of danger. The collusion might occur, for example, in the following way. A member of the permanent staff, perceiving possible danger because of a patient's destructive behaviour in the neighbouring community, might feel more alarmed than another, less permanently established, less

FIGURE 2   *PATTERNS OF COLLUSIVE MODIFICATION*
OF THE OPTIMAL OSCILLATORY CYCLE

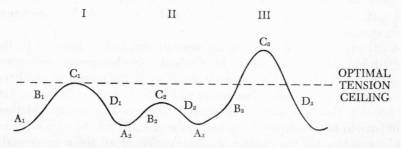

formally responsible member of the staff. A third, however, might share the alarm through identification with the first; another might be easily aroused to it for personality reasons; another might resonate to the sense of danger possibly displaced from another source, e.g. a feeling of being out of touch with his groups—which would usually indicate the kind of inhibition of communications characteristic of Phase C, and so on. If an effective coalition is formed around this sense of alarm, premature action may be taken (C_2), e.g. by asking the patient to leave, without strong patient support for the staff action, before the optimal tension ceiling had been reached. This premature action might hamper the utilization of the tensions implicit in the oscillation. Aside from the unnecessary loss of the patient through staff action, there may be other effects. The maladaptive tensions of patients who remain, e.g. anger and disillusionment at what seems to them to be the unreasonable abandonment of valued ways of operating, would be higher than necessary. Their trust and confidence in the staff's sincerity might be undermined, and communications essential to therapeutic relationships inhibited. Moreover, there is the loss of the tension itself, which might have built up to a more powerful pitch to be harnessed in the ways outlined above.

In the third cycle, collusive denial is pictured. This might, for example, occur if a particularly influential member of the core staff group, for conscious or unconscious reasons, idealizes the state of affairs. He might, for example, assert that everything was quite all right, that the patients were handling things adequately in a communal manner, and that there was nothing to worry about, while in fact the optimal tension ceiling had been reached. The idealization might become collusive if staff consensus is reached for inaction—one person giving silent pseudo-assent through a personal fear of contradicting the idealizer; another remaining silent because of a feeling of newness in the situation; another because of the feeling that his loyalty to the ideals was in question; another because of deference to the social status superiority of the idealizer, etc. If, in such a situation, real dangers were present in the Unit, grave difficulties might go unattended until something of a very serious nature occurred—e.g. a psychotic breakdown or an episode involving extensive destruction to property or disturbance to the neighbouring community. Similar losses in patients, confidence, energy-utilization, and so on would be experienced here as with collusive anxiety.

Further study is called for to differentiate the various types of participation and their consequences in a mixed sociotherapeutic programme like that of the Unit. A better understanding of the nature of oscillatory processes and of the conditions under which tension can enhance the kind of learning that will achieve personality changes is necessary. Methods will have to be developed for reducing the casualty rate of such a process and for enhancing the quality of participation of all those concerned—those giving as well as those receiving the treatment.

SUMMARY

1. SOCIAL psychiatrists emphasizing the influence of socio-environmental factors in mental health have adopted the concept of the "therapeutic community." This concept implies "humanistic" social values and a permissive yet rehabilitative environment within the hospital, but its specific functions relative to the goals of psychiatric treatment are still in a rudimentary stage of exploration.
2. The Belmont Social Rehabilitation Unit is a treatment centre of this kind. Its ideology includes humanistic themes of permissiveness, democracy, communalism, and reality-testing. Its social structure includes social roles for patients that in some degree foster a repetition of their problems in social relationships outside the hospital. These roles are organized in such a way as to foster maximal interaction and feed-back of communications among all members of the community.
3. Given the tendencies of patients toward disturbed interpersonal relations, the permissive ideology of the staff, and the interactive capacity of the social structure, there is a recurring tendency for social disorganization and intrapersonal and interpersonal tensions to be generated in the system. These recurring tendencies and their resolutions set up a pattern of oscillations in social organization.
4. These oscillations are not to be seen as necessarily anti-therapeutic. In fact, it seems that very powerful therapeutic forces are harnessed when the oscillations are optimally managed. The didactic resolution of these interpersonal tension states is called sociotherapy.
5. Sociotherapy is a process that has unique potentials for large-scale intensive psychotherapy. It is also fraught with complexities and pitfalls. Two of the latter, collusive anxiety and collusive denial, are delineated.
6. Further study is needed to lead to greater specification of personality

characteristics, fields of social forces, and other conditions of operation that will enhance the maximal realization of the potentialities of the sociotherapy conception.

NOTES TO CHAPTER 44

1. An early draft of this paper was delivered at Professor Max Gluckman's seminar at the University of Manchester in March 1955. The research from which it is excerpted has been supported by the British Medical Research Council and by the Nuffield Foundation. Thanks are due to them, and to Dr. Maxwell Jones and his staff at Belmont Hospital Social Rehabilitation Unit. Many friends in and out of the Unit have discussed the concepts associated with this research, and for clarification of the ideas presented here I am especially indebted to Dr. Daniel Levinson, Dr. Irving Rosow, Dr. Rhona Sofer, and Eileen Skellern, S.R.N.

2. In 1954, 22 per cent of the patients were discharged within 25 days of admission, a further 12 per cent in their second 25 day period, 11 per cent in their third, and 5 per cent in their fourth, 25 day period. Another mode is noted in the fifth period, when 14 per cent of the patients were discharged, followed by diminishing percentages thereafter.

3. In 1954, about 60 per cent were diagnosed as in the "personality disorder" group (psychopaths, character disorders, etc.), about 20 per cent in the psychoneurotic group, about 10 per cent as psychotics, with the remainder mixed indeterminate or organic cases.

4. The Unit is under the directorship of a psychiatrist, who is assisted medically by three more junior psychiatrists. Four trained nurses and eleven untrained assistant nurses (called "social therapists"), a psychiatric social worker, a clinical psychologist, two disablement resettlement officers assigned from the Ministry of Labour to assist with work placement, four workshop instructors, three domestic workers, and two secretaries complete the Unit staff. Night-nursing, catering, and administrative services are provided by the larger hospital.

5. Other formally constituted sub-groups exist for patients, but they are optional or based on special selection procedures—e.g. membership of committees, special interest groups, etc.

6. The oscillations observed were of varying scope. Minimally they involved a two-person relationship in which patterned expectations were operating. More often they were of larger scope. The ramifications of any given interpersonal disturbance are increased by the sensitivity of the Unit population, their "inward-facing" and "interlocking" group structure. This is illustrated substantively in an episode described in (7).

REFERENCES

1. Caudill, W., Redlich, F. C., Gilmore, H., and Brody, E. "Social Structure and Interaction Processes on a Psychiatric Ward." *Amer. J. Orthopsychiat.*, Vol. 22, pp. 314-34, 1952.

2. Hollingshead, A. B., and Redlich, F. C. "Social Stratification and Psychiatric Disorders." *Amer. sociol. Rev.*, Vol. 18, 1953.

3. Jones, M., *et al. Social Psychiatry*. London: Tavistock Publications, 1952; New York: Basic Books, 1953 (under the title *The Therapeutic Community*).

4. Jones, M. "The Concept of a Therapeutic Community." *Amer. J. Psychiat.*, Vol. 112, No. 8, pp. 647-50, 1956.

5. Jones, M., and Rapoport, R. N. "The Absorption of New Doctors into a Therapeutic Community." In the press.

6. Levinson, D., and Gilmore, D. C. "Ideology, Personality and Institutional Policy in the Mental Hospital." *J. abnorm. soc. Psychol.* In the press.

7. Rapoport, R. N., and Skellern, E. "Some Therapeutic Functions of Administrative Disturbance." *Adm. Sc. Quart.* In the press.

8. Rioch, D. McK., and Stanton, A. "Milieu Therapy." *Psychiatry*, Vol. 16, No. 1, 1953.

9. Schwartz, C. "Rehabilitation of Mental Hospital Patients." U.S. Department of Health, Education and Welfare: Public Health Monograph No. 17, 1953.

10. Skellern, E. "A Therapeutic Community." *Nursing Times*, April 1955.

11. Stanton, A., and Schwartz, M. *The Mental Hospital*. New York: Basic Books, 1954; London: Tavistock Publications, 1955.

12. Weinberg, S. K. *Society and Personality Disorders*. New York: Prentice-Hall, 1952.

13. Wilson, A. T. M., Trist, E. L., and Curle, Adam. "Transitional Communities and Social Reconnection: a Study of the Civil Resettlement of British Prisoners of War." In Swanson, G. E., Newcomb, T. M., and Hartley, E. L. (Eds.), *Readings in Social Psychology*. New York: Henry Holt, 1952.

Planned Rehabilitation

ৡৢ

CHAPTER 45   Changing Criminals: The
Application of the Theory of
Differential Association*

DONALD R. CRESSEY

SOCIOLOGICAL theories and hypotheses have had great influence on
development of general correctional policies, such as probation and
parole, but they have been used only intermittently and haphazardly in
reforming individual criminals. Since sociology is essentially a research
discipline, sociologist-criminologists have devoted most of their time and
energy to understanding and explaining crime, leaving to psychiatrists and
others the problem of reforming criminals. Even the sociologists employed
in correctional work have ordinarily committed themselves to nonsocio-
logical theories and techniques of reformation, leading the authors of one
popular criminology textbook to ask just what correctional sociologists can
accomplish which cannot be accomplished by other professional
workers.[1]

Perhaps the major impediment to the application of sociological theories
lies not in the nature of the theories themselves but, instead, in the futile
attempt to adapt them to clinical use. Strictly speaking, the now popular
policy of "individualized treatment" for delinquents and criminals does
not commit one to any specific theory of criminality or any specific theory
of reformation, but, rather, to the proposition that the conditions considered as causing an individual to behave criminally will be taken into
account in the effort to change him. An attempt is made to diagnose the
cause of the criminality and to base the techniques of reform upon the
diagnosis. Analogy with the *method* of clinical medicine (diagnosis, prescription, and therapy) is obvious. However, by far the most popular

* Reprinted from the *American Journal of Sociology*, 61 (1955), 116–120, by permission of The University of Chicago Press. Copyright © 1954, 1955 by The University of Chicago. All rights reserved.

interpretation of the policy of individualization is that the *theories,* as well as the methods, of clinical medicine must be used in diagnosing and changing criminals. The emphasis on this clinical principle has impeded the application of sociological theories and, it may be conjectured, success in correctional work.

The adherents of the clinical principle consider criminality to be an individual defect or disorder or a symptom of either, and the criminal as one unable to canalize or sublimate his "primitive," antisocial impulses or tendencies,[2] who may be expressing symbolically in criminal behavior some unconscious urge or wish arising from an early traumatic emotional experience,[3] or as a person suffering from some other kind of defective trait or condition.

In all cases the implication is that the individual disorder, like a biological disorder, should be treated on a clinical basis. An extreme position is that criminality actually is a biological disorder, to be treated by modification of the physiology or anatomy of the individual. However, the more popular notion is that criminality is analogous to an infectious disease like syphilis—while group contacts of various kinds are necessary to the disorder, the disorder can be treated in a clinic, without reference to the persons from whom it was acquired.

Sociologists and social psychologists have provided an alternative principle on which to base the diagnosis and treatment of criminals, namely, that the behavior, attitudes, beliefs, and values which a person exhibits are not only the *products* of group contacts but also the *properties* of groups. If the behavior of an individual is an intrinsic part of groups to which he belongs, attempts to change the behavior must be directed at groups.[4] While this principle is generally accepted by sociologists, there has been no consistent or organized effort by sociologist-criminologists to base techniques or principles of treatment on it. Traditionally, we have emphasized that sociologists can make unique contributions to *clinical* diagnoses, and we have advocated the development of a "clinical sociology" which would enable us to improve these diagnoses.[5] But here we reach an impasse: if a case of criminality is attributed to the individual's group relations, there is little that can be done *in the clinic* to modify the diagnosed cause of the criminality. Moreover, extra-clinical work with criminals and delinquents ordinarily has merely extended the clinical principle to the offender's community and has largely ignored the group-relations principle. For example, in the "group work" of correctional agencies the emphasis usually is upon the role of the group merely in satisfying the needs of an individual. Thus the criminal is induced to join an "interest-activity" group, such as a hiking club, on the assumption that membership in the group somehow will enable him to overcome the defects or tendencies considered conducive to his delinquency.[6] Similarly, in correctional group therapy the emphasis is almost always on the use of a group to enable the individual to rid himself of undesirable psychological disorders, not criminality.[7] Even in group-work programs directed at entire groups, such as delinquent gangs, emphasis usually is on new and different formal group activities rather than on new group attitudes and values.

The differential association theory of criminal behavior presents implications for diagnosis and treatment consistent with the group-relations principle for changing behavior and could be advantageously utilized in correctional work. According to it, persons become criminals principally because they have been relatively isolated from groups whose behavior patterns (including attitudes, motives, and rationalizations) are anticriminal, or because their residence, employment, social position, native capacities, or something else has brought them into relatively frequent association with the behavior patterns of criminal groups.[8] A diagnosis of criminality based on this theory would be directed at analysis of the criminal's attitudes, motives, and rationalizations regarding criminality and would recognize that those characteristics depend upon the groups to which the criminal belongs. Then, if criminals are to be changed, either they must become members of anticriminal groups, or their present pro-criminal group relations must be changed.[9]

The following set of interrelated principles, adapted in part from a more general statement by Dorwin Cartwright,[10] is intended as a guide to specific application of the differential association theory to correctional work. It is tentative and directs attention to areas where research and experimentation should prove fruitful. Two underlying assumptions are that small groups existing for the specific purpose of reforming criminals can be set up by correctional workers and that criminals can be induced to join them. The first five principles deal with the use of anticriminal groups as *media* of change, and the last principle emphasizes, further, the possibility of a criminal group's becoming the *target* of change.

1. If criminals are to be changed, they must be assimilated into groups which emphasize values conducive to law-abiding behavior and, concurrently, alienated from groups emphasizing values conducive to criminality. Since our experience has been that the majority of criminals experience great difficulty in securing intimate contacts in ordinary groups, special groups whose major common goal is the reformation of criminals must be created. This general principle, emphasized by Sutherland, has been recognized and used by Gersten, apparently with some success, in connection with a group therapy program in the New York Training School for Boys.[11]

2. The more relevant the common purpose of the group to the reformation of criminals, the greater will be its influence on the criminal members' attitudes and values. Just as a labor union exerts strong influence over its members' attitudes toward management but less influence on their atti-

tudes toward say, Negroes, so a group organized for recreational or welfare purposes will have less success in influencing criminalistic attitudes and values than will one whose explicit purpose is to change criminals. Interesting recreational activities, employment possibilities, and material assistance may serve effectively to attract criminals away from pro-criminal groups temporarily and may give the group some control over the criminals. But merely inducing a criminal to join a group to satisfy his personal needs is not enough. Probably the failure to recognize this, more than anything else, was responsible for the failure of the efforts at rehabilitation of the Cambridge-Somerville Youth Study workers.[12]

3. The more cohesive the group, the greater the members' readiness to influence others and the more relevant the problem of conformity to group norms. The criminals who are to be reformed and the persons expected to effect the change must, then, have a strong sense of belonging to one group: between them there must be a genuine "we" feeling. The reformers, consequently, should not be identifiable as correctional workers, probation or parole officers, or social workers. This principle has been extensively documented by Festinger and his co-workers.[13]

4. Both reformers and those to be reformed must achieve status within the group by exhibition of "pro-reform" or anticriminal values and behavior patterns. As a novitiate, the one to be reformed is likely to assign status according to social position outside the group, and part of the reformation process consists of influencing him both to assign and to achieve status on the basis of behavior patterns relevant to reformation. If he should assign status solely on the basis of social position in the community, he is likely to be influenced only slightly by the group. Even if he becomes better adjusted, socially and psychologically, by association with members having high status in the community, he is a therapeutic parasite and not actually a member until he accepts the group's own system for assigning status.

5. The most effective mechanism for exerting group pressure on members will be found in groups so organized that criminals are induced to join with noncriminals for the purpose of changing other criminals. A group in which criminal A joins with some noncriminals to change criminal B is probably most effective in changing criminal A, not B; in order to change criminal B, criminal A must necessarily share the values of the anticriminal members.

This process may be called "retroflexive reformation"; in attempting to reform others, the criminal almost automatically accepts the relevant common purpose of the group, identifies himself closely with other persons engaging in reformation, and assigns status on the basis of anticriminal behavior. He becomes a genuine member of this group, and at the same time he is alienated from his previous pro-criminal groups. This principle is used successfully by Alcoholics Anonymous to "cure" alcoholism; it has been applied to the treatment of psychotics by McCann and Almada; and its usefulness in criminology has been demonstrated by Konopka.[14] Ex-convicts have been used in the Chicago Area Projects, which, generally, are organized in accordance with this principle, but its effect on the ex-convicts, either in their roles as reformers or as objects of reform, appears not to have been evaluated.

6. When an entire group is the target of change, as in a prison or among delinquent gangs, strong pressure for change can be achieved by convincing the members of the need for a change, thus making the group itself the source of pressure for change. Rather than inducing criminals to become members of pre-established anticriminal groups, the problem here is to change antireform and pro-criminal subcultures, so that group leaders evolve from among those who show the most marked hospitality to anti-criminal values, attitudes, and behavior. Neither mere lectures, sermons, or exhortations by correctional workers nor mere redirection of the activities of a group nor individual psychotherapy, academic education, vocational training, or counseling will necessarily change a group's culture. If the subculture is not changed, the person to be reformed is likely to exhibit two sets of attitudes and behaviors, one characteristic of the agency or person trying to change him, the other of the subculture.[15] Changes in the subculture probably can best be instigated by eliciting the co-operation of the type of criminal who, in prisons, is considered a "right guy."[16] This principle has been demonstrated in a recent experiment with hospitalized drug addicts, whose essentially antireform culture was changed, under the guise of group therapy, to a proreform culture.[17] To some extent, the principle was used in the experimental system of prison administration developed by Gill in the Massachusetts State Prison Colony.[18]

NOTES TO CHAPTER 45

1. Harry Elmer Barnes and Negley K. Teeters, *New Horizons in Criminology* (New York: Prentice-Hall, Inc., 1951), p. 644.
2. Sheldon and Eleanor T. Glueck, *Delinquents in the Making* (New York: Harper & Bros., 1952), pp. 162-63; see also Ruth Jacobs Levy, *Reductions in Recidivism through Therapy* (New York: Seltzer, 1941), pp. 16, 28.
3. Edwin J. Lukas, "Crime Prevention: A Confusion in Goal," in Paul W. Tappan (ed.), *Contemporary Correction* (New York: McGraw-Hill Book Co., 1951), pp. 397-409.
4. Cf. Dorwin Cartwright, "Achieving Change in People: Some Applications of Group Dynamics Theory," *Human Relations*, IV (1951), 381-92.
5. See Louis Wirth, "Clinical Sociology," *American Journal of Sociology*, XXVII (July, 1931), 49-66; and Saul D. Alinsky, "A Sociological Technique in Clinical Criminology," *Proceedings of the American Prison Association*, LXIV (1934), 167-78.

6. See the discussion by Robert G. Hinckley and Lydia Hermann, *Group Treatment in Psychotherapy* (Minneapolis: University of Minnesota Press, 1951), pp. 8-11.

7. See Donald R. Cressey, "Contradictory Theories in Correctional Group Therapy Programs," *Federal Probation*, XVIII (June, 1954), 20-26.

8. Edwin H. Sutherland, *Principles of Criminology* (New York: J. B. Lippincott Co., 1947), pp. 6-9, 595, 616-17.

9. Cf. Donald R. Taft, "The Group and Community Organization Approach to Prison Administration," *Proceedings of the American Prison Association*, LXXII (1942), 275-84; and George B. Vold, "Discussion of *Guided Group Interaction in Correctional Work* by F. Lovell Bixby and Lloyd W. Mc-Corkle," *American Sociological Review*, XVI (August, 1951), 460-61.

10. *Op. cit.*

11. Sutherland, *op. cit.*, p. 451; Charles Gersten, "An Experimental Evaluation of Group Therapy with Juvenile Delinquents," *International Journal of Group Psychotherapy*, I (November, 1951), 311-18.

12. See Margaret G. Reilly and Robert A. Young, "Agency-initiated Treatment of a Potentially Delinquent Boy," *American Journal of Orthopsychiatry*, XVI (October, 1946), 697-706; Edwin Powers, "An Experiment in Prevention of Delinquency," *Annals of the American Academy of Political and Social Science*, CCLXI (January, 1949), 77-88; Edwin Powers and Helen L. Witmer, *An Experiment in Prevention of Delinquency—the Cambridge-Somerville Youth Study* (New York: Columbia University Press, 1951).

13. L. Festinger *et al.*, *Theory and Experiment in Social Communication: Collected Papers* (Ann Arbor: Institute for Social Research, 1951).

14. Freed Bales, "Types of Social Structure as Factors in 'Cures' for Alcohol Addiction," *Applied Anthropology*, I (April-June, 1942), 1-13; Willis H. McCann and Albert A. Almada, "Round-Table Psychotherapy: A Technique in Group Psychotherapy," *Journal of Consulting Psychology*, XIV (December, 1950), 421-35; Gisela Konopka, "The Group Worker's Role in an Institution for Juvenile Delinquents," *Federal Probation*, XV (June, 1951), 15-23.

15. See Edwin A. Fleishman, "A Study in the Leadership Role of the Foreman in an Industrial Situation" (Columbus: Personnel Research Board, Ohio State University, 1951) (mimeographed).

16. See Hans Riemer, "Socialization in the Prison Community," *Proceedings of the American Prison Association*, LXVII (1937), 151-55.

17. James J. Thorpe and Bernard Smith, "Phases in Group Development in Treatment of Drug Addicts," *International Journal of Group Psychotherapy*, III (January, 1953), 66-78.

18. Howard B. Gill, "The Norfolk Prison Colony of Massachusetts," *Journal of Criminal Law and Criminology*, XXII (September, 1937), 389-95; see also Eric K. Clarke, "Group Therapy in Rehabilitation," *Federal Probation*, XVI (December, 1952), 28-32.

$\partial\!\!\!\!\partial$

CHAPTER 46   Changing Delinquent

Sub-Cultures: A Social-Psychological Approach*

HOWARD W. POLSKY

I N increasing numbers, psychologists, anthropologists, and sociologists
are turning their attention to the interpersonal dynamics of juvenile
delinquent groups.[1] One important source for investigation has been the
training schools and residential treatment centers.[2] We have come to
realize after considerable trial and error that it is no easy matter to
intervene effectively in the delinquent subcultures established by aggressive adolescents. This paper is a contribution to an understanding of
delinquent social structures and the bearing this has upon group intervention and individual rehabilitation. Our fundamental source is an
intensive participant-observation analysis over the period of a year in a
cottage containing the oldest, toughest, and most delinquent boys in a
residential treatment center.[3]

The sociologist attempts to find the mainsprings for human behavior
within the matrix of interpersonal relationships in which the individual
functions. He tries to determine the significant people in the delinquent's
life and how they are influencing him. To be sure, the press of the
environment—the external frame of reference—has as its counterpoint
the individual's internal reference structure. We must evaluate the pathology inherent in the psychic structure, lest we overestimate the extent to
which group norms influence individuals. This must be carefully assessed
in any intervention program. Our primary focus in this paper, however, is
to delineate some of the social and cultural forces that shape delinquent
group life and individual "careers" within it.

The theory of delinquency as a subculture has left many gaps in the
analysis of its organizational character. We know little about how delinquent boys interrelate between antisocial outbreaks. What are the norma-

* Reprinted with permission of the National Association of Social Workers, from
Social Work, Vol. 4, No. 4 (October 1959), pp. 3–15.

tive interpersonal relationships in a delinquent subculture which periodically spill over in the form of aggression against society?

An organized delinquent peer group is not merely the sum of hostile
projections of disturbed boys who are externalizing intrapsychic conflicts.
A large variety of diagnostic types can be found to "fit" the alternative
roles the delinquent culture assigns its recruits. An important need today
is a better understanding of the *system of norms and statuses* which
delinquent groups create and the interpersonal soil in which antisocial
acts, values, and personalities are nurtured.[4] "Economic" principles appear
to operate not only in the individual, but in the group as well; delinquents
are able to articulate a highly stylized social and cultural organization to
which all its members must contribute and respond—often at great personal risk and deterioration.

Thus far sociologists have tended to concentrate their fire on the
accommodation patterns by way of which the leaders and activists in the
delinquent gangs gain recognition by adults in the community.[5] But this is
akin to describing American society only by analyzing its international
relations. We need more empirical studies of delinquency as a social
system, emphasizing the sources of strain and anomie generated by "internal" social and cultural normative processes. As long as this approach
is lacking, we shall have a distorted concept of the emergence and
maintenance of delinquent groups as viable organizations.

For example, we analyzed a runaway which culminated in the theft of
an auto in a town near the institution. Two boys, an introverted isolate
and a rebellious scapegoated newcomer, combined forces to escape from
both their peer group and adult authorities. The significant precipitating
cause was the rejection of both boys by the cottage peer group. The
sources of stress within the peer group on this microscopic level can be
multiplied many times.

In our analysis we shall stress the "internal" systemic aspects of delinquency, which means that our focus will be upon the normative interpersonal relationships and processes within the group, and the values
upon which they are based.[6] At a minimum four questions must be posed:
(1) What is a delinquent subculture? (2) To what do we want to change
it? (3) How can we change it? (4) How can we evaluate culture and
individual change?

THE AGGRESSIVE SOCIETY

EVERY social system consists of ideal or expected patterns of action and
statuses and is stratified so that power, prestige, and income are differentially distributed among its members. The recruitment for positions
and their consolidation vary with the character of the group and its stage
of crystallization. The criteria which distinguish the superior and inferior

strata depend upon the core norms of the group. The rigidity of the delinquent social structure is formed by underlying sanctions of brute force and manipulation which are used by the top clique boys and filter down through the entire social order. The boys in Cottage 6 believed that no other boy had a right to enter their cottage, but if they suspected someone else of taking something from their cottage, they felt they had the unqualified right to ransack other cottages.

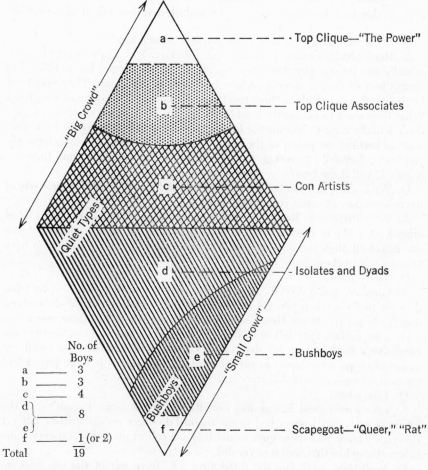

Within the cottages, there are several variants of a stratified social structure based on toughness, "brains," deviant activities, and status-deflating, rigidly controlling interpersonal processes. In some groups the tough boys—the "power," "big men," or "take"—maintain absolute hegemony and assign the "con-artists" subsidiary positions. In other groups, the gamblers and con-artists unite with the tough leaders and maintain a pressing rule over the "punks" or "bushboys"—the weak and less able boys. In any case, muscles, brains, and deviant activities are united in one form or another to insure a flow of psychic and material services upward to the boys in the upper half of the status hierarchy. Brute force maintains the rigid pecking order and is exemplified in violence, manipulation, exploitation, "ranking," and scapegoating. These processes occur not only between delinquent groups, but are the essential dynamic of social control *within* the delinquent group.[7]

The paradigm above was vividly corroborated by a perceptive cottage leader and has been verified by detailed independent observation:

Q: Well, who ran the cottage when you first came into 7?

A: Hank Shade, Frankie Gorman, Spiffy Weiner. You see, a cottage is never actually run by one guy. One guy has brains, the other guy has muscles, but always four or five, or three guys are the power in the group. They might not be the roughest guys, these three together, but they are the power of the group. What they want to do mostly is what the group does, and a lot of smart guys don't actually want to become the leader, they want to be the guy in back, they want to become the *power* of the group. And then the cottage guys clique up, you know, they fall into certain groups where they hang together and they stay together. And these groups, you know, are your power.

Q: Well, when did you become a power in 7? I know you did. It was one of the reasons they changed you. Right?

A: Well, that's true. But I came about power in a different way than a lot of other kids. I like to gamble and I'm good at it, and through the fact that you can win, well, then you have money. That automatically makes the group have to come to you at one point or another.

Q: That's right.

A: Guys are going AWOL, they got to come to you to get money. So what they try to do is when you get money and they're looking out for themselves, they try to get you to like them. And in order to get you to like them, when you make a suggestion they follow it, because there is no reason to antagonize the hand that's feeding you. So that's how I came into power. Guys owed me money, so guys were afraid to get me mad because they'd have to pay. I had my own strong-arm boys that were willing to collect for me. . . .

Q: Like who?

A: Like Foster, and Simon, like myself. You see, I mean I wasn't . . . the whole point is that I never had to use them. I'd collect my own debts, but yet everybody knew that these guys would help me collect my debts if it ever came to something like that, and it never did.

Q: Well then, were you the three guys who were sort of the top guys up there?

A: Yes.[8]

We have found in several cottages a diamond-shaped social system which persists over time as old leaders leave and middle- and low-status boys rise in the hierarchy.[9] Delinquent status positions are useful in predicting the boys' interrelationships in the cottage. This is why we view their behavior as a social system. Every stratum combines a cluster of privileges and duties. The translation of each clique's norms into concrete action is the function of the diverse roles in the cottage.

The top clique is the "power"; within it boys of inferior status were ranked and exploited by the tougher boys; the former attempted to take over the cottage when the toughs left. Below the top clique are the "con-artists," who are not afraid to fight, but more typically employed their manipulative abilities and skill at deviant activities to exploit boys further down in the hierarchy. The "quiet types"—or "regular guys"—have abandoned gross delinquent activities, but are not typed "punks"; several are regarded as mentally or socially retarded by the older boys and have a long history of foster home and institutional placement. The bottom stratum consists of "bushboys" or "punks," the targets of the boys above; they carry out the menial tasks in the cottage, are looked upon as "dirt" or "sneaks," not to be trusted, and are frequently singled out for violence and ranking. At the very bottom are the scapegoats—the "queers"—who are the focal targets for the entire cottage; some break down under the pressure and run from the institution; others compulsively ingratiate themselves with higher-status boys or accept the minimum duties required at this station and, biding their time and using violence and ranking upon boys arriving after them, eventually climb up the status hierarchy.

Social distance between the cliques within a cottage is quite large. The cliques are ranked and each person recognizes to which one he belongs, and its relationship to the others. Clique members share common activities and outlooks. They reinforce each other in opposing "out-cliques" and exert social control throughout the group.

The statuses are unusually "frozen." A new boy coming into the cottage must identify with the lowest stratum. He is put into the "punk bedroom" and undergoes a period of severe manipulation and testing. This includes social ostracism as well as performance of menial duties for older boys. He learns how to take it and if he survives, how to dish it out too. One of the chief ways a boy can change his status is through physically challenging higher-status individuals. This frequently culminates in a fight or "stand-off." The outcomes of these fights are burned into the boys' memories and can drastically change one's status and horizons in the cottage.

The delinquent social system is essentially inequalitarian. Individual boys become alerted, sensitized, and preoccupied with power relationships; it is to each according to his status, from each according to his status. This colors the most incidental interactions. I have observed unbelievable anxiety in the simplest request for milk on the part of a low-status member who was addressing a high-status boy. It is our feeling that this authoritarian type of social structure organizes and controls the major portion of the boys' lives, inculcates delinquent norms, defends them from facing threatening problems—school, girls, jobs, community disgrace—and blocks involvement in constructive activities.

Among the boys hostility is so pervasive that after a while it becomes the automatic response and is displaced readily upon any available target. The stultifying process works as follows: when violence is used against individuals within the group (and they are always around), it creates an intense need on the part of the perpetrators to rationalize their behavior. Thus they condemn those against whom they commit violence by citing the latter's "queerness," "sneakiness," and "grubbiness." This justifies increased violence and manipulation against them, which in turn reinforces stereotypes. The omnipresence of the strong-weak continuum, the followers' identification with power figures, and the lack of *alternative identifications* exaggerate the importance of toughness. The vigilant alertness for potential "pretenders to the throne" leads to projection of hostility in situations in which it does not actually exist.

The analysis of delinquency as a social system enables us to view the developmental phases of the group. With each turnover in the cottage, especially when the leaders leave, a crisis is precipitated. The boys then subject one another to a period of intensified manipulation and testing until each recognizes where he stands in the total system. Out of this interregnum of testing and manipulation new alliances and out-groups are formed. New members become extremely vulnerable because of their function as targets for the other boys to gain prestige. The punk "invites" his oppressors to harass him. The scapegoat's fears are monitored by his tormentors as they stimulate one another to exclude him from their midst. Thus by examining the total social system we have a better understanding of its hierarchical components. All the group members must learn how to orient themselves to one another.

There is another dimension to cottage social control based upon personality factors. Within each clique there are pecking triangles which are miniature reproductions of the larger social organization. Regardless of the extrinsic characteristics of each clique we believe that there are intrinsic personality factors which predispose individual boys to fulfill specific roles. Psychodynamically, a high-placed punk in Clique I has more in common with a punk in Clique IV than he does with a dominant member of his own clique. What specific personality traits huddle together with each role is now being explored. We want to emphasize that the complementary role sets in each clique that fulfill the requirements of the aggressive society can be understood fully only if we are flexible enough to shift from group to personality variables when the analysis demands it.

Several sociologists have asserted that delinquents pursue "malicious, negativistic, and non-utilitarian" goals.[10] However, this appears to be a cultural bias. If one evaluates their culture according to society's value system, their actions appear nonutilitarian. Looking at the delinquent social system from within, however, our perspective changes. The drastic restrictions for achieving status within a delinquent group lead to exaggerated conformity with the group's norms. If one can gain prestige by showing defiance against adults, this is not a negativistic activity from the point of view of the boy who is attempting to gain recognition within his group. Thus before we conclude that a boy trying to swing from one of the trees is trying to kill himself because he cannot control repressed conflicts, we have to analyze such an act in the context of his strivings in his primary group.

Group participation shapes personality organization; the latter partially determines role incumbency. Peer interpersonal patterns are crucial for the development of the boy's attitudes and philosophy of life, his aspirations for the future, the kinds of activities in which he will excel, and the form and content of relationships he will make with adults. In short, we must challenge the delinquent subculture as well as its individual constituents.

CONTROL VERSUS CHANGE

STAFF members who have to deal with these boys on a day-to-day basis learn to accommodate themselves to the delinquents' system of social control. Counselors will assign a bushboy to a "regular guy's" bedroom and thereby help him avoid extreme forms of ranking and violence. Social workers have been known to prod their charges to fight in order to change their social status. The "pro-academic" youngster is removed from an "anti-academic" cottage. Top delinquent leaders are accorded community-wide prestige; one "tough boy," a dictator who exercised rigid control over the other boys in a cottage, inadvertently was given the top award for the most improvement.[11]

In order to maintain a state of equilibrium the cottage parent "strikes a bargain" with the delinquent leadership. The latter "agrees" not to cause disturbances within the institution outside of the cottage. The price that the staff pays is "restricting" the aggression and hostility to the cottage. The unintended consequence of such compromises is reinforcement of the authoritarian social structure. Our observation of the cottage parents in the senior unit indicates that their background, their isolation from the professional staff, and the dense interaction with twenty disturbed delinquents results in a role adaptation which alienates them from the relevant structures of the treatment institution and its philosophy.

Many of the inequalities institutionalized in the peer group are reminiscent of the boys' typical family situations in which we find the incipient cause for delinquent acting-out. Many of these boys are in revolt against highly unstable, controlling, narcissistic mothers and weak, indifferent fathers with whom they are unable to identify. These parents and delinquent gang leaders have served as the chief models for the boys' superegos. The natural inequality between parents and child is further exploited in the peer group so that "the whole relationship is not one of universal goodness but of arbitrary power."[12]

It is important to point out that we not only have to change the stereotyped ideology upon which the boys' social structure is based, but modify their interrelationships as well. The leadership in the delinquent group we analyzed frequently verbalized democratic and laissez-faire principles:

Observer: Did you stay in the same bedroom with Red Leon and Stein?
Steve: No, when I first came, I roomed with two other guys. Then I started buddying around with Red Leon and I finally moved into the end room. It was me, Red Leon, and Wolf. Then it was the big room.
Observer: Then it was the big room? What do you mean by that?
Steve: Well, I mean by the big room is that we were about the only guys in the cottage who were considered big around the campus—me, Red Leon, and Wolf. We were considered the biggest on the campus.
Observer: By biggest, you mean toughest? Because you certainly weren't the tallest or heaviest.
Steve: Well, all the guys considered us the toughest, me and Leon especially. But we never really looked for trouble. The only time we'd fight was when trouble came to us.

This vocabulary has to be challenged in concrete situations. The toughest boys claim that "they never look for trouble." Yet they are the chief controllers and perpetrators of the delinquent orientation. How does this occur? Steve Davis, the undisputed leader in the group, talked about Ricky Kahn as follows:

Well, Rick Kahn, when he first came up, he was a bushboy. I got that slang word from the gang. They call a guy a bushboy when he does another guy's clothes for him, or runs errands for him. Another guy tells him to do that and do that, and he runs and does it. That's what we mean by bushboy. But he used to do a lot of that for me and we got along.

In other words, "getting along" with the top delinquent leader is conforming to his expectations for behaving as a bushboy. In turn, the latter internalizes the delinquent leader's image and practices the same kind of exploitation with new boys who enter the cottage after him. Thus the delinquent cycle is perpetuated.

We have discovered that these very disturbed ("maladaptive") delinquents are able to create a well-organized social structure. Critical questions in an institutional setting concern not only individual pathologies, but the ways in which they are mutually reinforced in the peer group and between it and the staff. Therefore we believe that to maximize the therapeutic influence we must go beyond the concept of accommodation with the intact delinquent social system and think in terms of penetration and change.

WHAT KIND OF CULTURE SHOULD BE PROMOTED?

THE foregoing presentation has stressed the concept of group delinquency in terms of authoritarian interpersonal processes, fascistic values, and deviant activities. We want to change the boys' activities, goals, and interpersonal relationships. Gambling, liquor parties, and "kangaroo courts" are gross activities that we agree should be prohibited: what is less stressed is changing the boys' interrelationships.

Social work is committed to a democratic ideology.[13] We would like to influence delinquent groups toward democratic rather than authoritarian relationships. Each individual has a right to participate in the decision-making process. Might is not right. Activities should fulfill rather than negate human dignity and integrity. The stress upon *democratic* procedures is crucial because we know that the boys can become involved in many nondelinquent activities using authoritarian methods. (This is why spotless cottages in institutions are suspect.) The boys must be enabled to formulate realistic goals and handle frustration constructively. We would emphasize the boys' acceptance of each other even though they may differ about the criteria of acceptability. High evaluation of other human beings should be stressed, apart from their social status. Basic social rights should be so institutionalized that all have an equal chance to gain satisfaction on bases other than authoritarian. The group worker and other adults should strive to promote consensus for *democratic procedures* as the ground rules under which individual interests may be pursued.

We have found that intragroup (and out-group) aggression and manipulation alternate with long periods of apathy, boredom, aimlessness, and depression:

"It's boring around here. We're around all day, then stay up all night shooting the shit, just shooting the shit, and playing with *Oscar*." The guys chimed in agreement: "The trouble is, there isn't anything to do around here all day, it gets boring. In the morning we have a couple of details and work . . . imagine on our vacation [recorded during Christmas]. Spend a little time in the gym in the afternoon and then there's nothing to do until we eat and then we come back and look at television, play a little cards . . . and just sit around shooting the shit."

This is the cottage milieu which is structured by the boys' aggressive tendencies. One of the key tasks of the professional worker responsible for the cottage is motivating the boys toward goals which are realistic in terms of individual and group achievement and which are meaningful *to them*.

THE BASIC INSTITUTIONAL CHANGE

THE boys do become aware of positive values and goals in their individual casework interviews. However, the pressure encountered in the daily cottage living situation can be so overwhelming that it counteracts values which are and could be engendered in the social worker's office. The first step necessary for change is to acknowledge the existence of the delinquent subculture with all its ramifying importance for individual and group rehabilitation.

The next step is to fashion an institutional arrangement whereby we can place at the center of the cottage a professional person who works directly with the boys on a cottage level. This residential worker, together with cottage parents, caseworker, and other adults who come in contact with the boys, must begin thinking creatively about supplanting the aggressive vicious cycles in the cottage with positive relationships, activities, values, and goals. No longer satisfied to react merely to the boys' internal delinquency, we propose that they take the initiative to plan a viable cottage program which unites the group's propensities for health and all the available resources in the institution. Only by constant feedback with a professional (or professionally oriented) residential worker responsible for the boys' collective living situation do we create the possibility of continuous and cumulative development rather than having to start all over with every major turnover of boys. This resident worker is a middleman between the boys and the administration. We assume he will be primarily a social group worker, but with experience and background in working with disturbed individuals.

One way of conceptualizing our approach is by visualizing the delinquent culture as being "invaded" by the culture of the group worker. He will be resisted as he tries to maintain his standards. Increased social tension is inevitable. The boys will try to resolve the situation by making the intervener conform to their values. They may be enraged at the threat to the system that has served them. Thus we have to evaluate carefully the investment of the different strata in the cottage violence, ranking, and manipulative patterns. We must know not only each boy's role but his attitude toward it, and carefully assess his actual behavior vis-à-vis members of his own status and above and below it. The crux of the group worker's problem is focused in emphathizing with the boys' gripes, constantly challenging them to resolve their collective problems, and at the same time retaining adult standards. One cannot underestimate the amount of pressure in the form of testing and seduction to which the worker will be exposed.

We view remotivation as confronting the boys with constructive alternatives to achieve satisfactions articulated with meaningful realizable goals. As long as the conduct routines in the peer group remain unchallenged, the boys will continue to elaborate authoritarian roles via delinquent interpersonal processes. If we present the cottage with other expectations, then we introduce the element of choice and "constructive conflict" which can lead to new self-images.[14]

ASSUMPTIONS UNDERLYING INDIVIDUAL AND CULTURE CHANGE

THERE are two ways of looking at maladjusted adolescents. Above we have emphasized delinquency as a social system. We have to go further. We have to ask ourselves what childhood compulsions force individual boys to behave destructively and reinforce authoritarian group adaptations. We have to pinpoint the specific intrapsychic processes that lead them to fashion this way of life. We believe that an adequate social-psychological formulation must comprehend intrapersonal and interpersonal approaches—with varying degrees of emphasis on each.[15] Thus a boy who is a punk but also a paranoid may need special supports beyond revamping the group's standards and changing his role. Youngsters with severe neurotic pathology benefit substantially from a close relationship with an individual therapist or caseworker. It provides a transference experience on the basis of which neurotic delinquents can acquire insight and new identifications.

The conflicts arising out of changing peer group relationships and between the standards of the boys and the group worker will tend to heighten intrapersonality conflicts. Pressures stemming from interpersonal and intrapsychic stresses increase the possibilities of reactive deviant behavior. For extremely defensive, irrational, emotionally disturbed youngsters the group worker will have to call on his caseworker colleague. An important contribution can be made here by a combined group work and casework attack upon juvenile delinquency in the residential treatment center. Each has a unique contribution to make toward helping the disturbed delinquent; learning about each other's perspective and skills by working together with specific groups and individuals will result, we believe, in more effective treatment.

This leads us to one of the major problems which the group and "island culture" therapists have not as yet posed for themselves. How much real personality change is effected through group participation? Sociologists involved in group treatment claim that delinquents for the most part are normal boys reacting to abnormal situations. Change the culture and individuals will change by assimilating new roles and values. However, the implication here is that *basically* the character structure of these youngsters is sound. Nevertheless, a contradiction remains—when the delinquent boy returns from a physically or psychologically removed therapeutic milieu to a disorganized neighborhood, should he not, according to the theory, after a short period resume his delinquent way of life?

Apparently the sociologists fall into an obsolete "imitation theory" of personality. Psychological processes are oversimplified. The boys are perceived as nuts and bolts which have been pressed into a cultural mold. In order to understand the complex interplay of personality and social and cultural forces, we must incorporate into our thinking dynamic explanations of personality; the impact of the milieu upon the personality must be detailed in light of clinical experience. We shall not be able to do this until we welcome into our interdisciplinary family psychoanalytically oriented practitioners who are trained to diagnose the manifest and latent intrapsychic factors in personality structure. Once this is done we can then seek to explore how the "role expectations of the social system" become the "need dispositions of the personality."[16]

THE TECHNIQUE OF CHANGING DELINQUENT SUBCULTURES

THE theory for changing individuals by changing the group's norms and structure can be summarized briefly:[17]

1. People are influenced to behave antisocially in much the same manner as they are conditioned to behave in socially conforming ways. The basis for change is that the individual will accept new values, perspectives, and modes of conduct if he will accept a new group as an instrument in which to achieve satisfactions. Boys "out of step" with society strongly feel their peculiarity and alienation from socially conforming peers and adults. By affording them an opportunity to express their hostility in a permissive setting, they learn that they are not as "queer" as they imagine people think them to be.

2. It is also assumed that delinquents have, in addition to a great storehouse of negative and distorted values, positive strengths. They will be manifested only if the boys have a feeling that they are not being attacked.[18] Given an opportunity to make constructive choices, they will do so if they are properly guided. Two prerequisites are freedom to make meaningful decisions (this does not mean the absence of limits) and confidence that adults are there to help them *achieve, individually and collectively*—not only to restrict them.

3. It is indispensable to this approach to have attached to the cottage a professional practitioner who would (a) be able to serve as a socially ideal model in his transactions with the boys and (b) be able to use himself as a link to the administration and community to enable boys to release pent-up emotions by affording them constructive outlets for resolving problems which emerge in the institution and which come out of their group interaction.

4. It is assumed that with continued positive interaction and successes

in resolving problems, the group can become a positive instrument which the boys want to utilize in order to achieve further satisfactions and rewards. Prestige is allotted to group members not because of antisocial behavior, but according to the contribution made toward the achievement of collective goals which rise out of the boys' interaction in the group. Prestige is added to a boy's stature as he fashions a role which helps the others achieve recognition and group goals. Conversely, individuals who obstruct the group's goals are pressured to conform. Authority begins to inhere in the consensus of the group, which now has a more positive orbit and is gaining a more constructive self-image.

5. In addition to these social dynamics within the group, its relation to outside groups and individuals is critical. Part of the group worker's job is protecting the boys from delinquent-prone adults. He must help his charges graduate from the group if consistent improvement is demonstrated; a feeling of direction is helpful, and the knowledge that the others have been instrumental in helping him to gain the maturity he needed to strike out on his own.

6. The extremely disturbed youngster in the cottage will need special support at every phase of the group intervention; this can be given only partially by the resident worker in the cottage situation. The one-to-one social worker-client relationship appears to be the ideal setting for the youngster to "explode" or reveal *privatissima* which are disabling him from satisfactory interpersonal relationships. In his special setting the psychiatric caseworker may be able to give the kind of support the extremely disturbed youngster needs in order to survive in the cottage without disrupting the group.

It is important to conceive of the total therapeutic approach to the boys and evaluate its steps in relation to the sum process. The over-all goal is to move the boys to a level of collaboration in which they feel free to (1) raise all kinds of questions—concerning family, sex, peer group, work, school, recreation; (2) become accustomed to having the group, or cliques, including the intervener, discuss these issues constructively; and (3) develop an action program in which they can carry out the decisions they reach as a result of democratic discussion. Only when these criteria are met can the group become a constructive source of authority, new roles develop, and socially acceptable values form the norms of the group's activity.[19]

ONE STEP BACKWARD—TWO STEPS FORWARD

DYNAMICALLY, the attempt to change delinquent subcultures is similar to the process of Western colonialism, which sometimes leads to native movements that rally the most reactionary elements to ward off all change.[20] This is sparked by the invested leadership. Our intentions, materially or spiritually, are not exploitative, but can be so defined by delinquents.

The presentation of new rewards and tasks to the boys is the opening tactic. The first step is to convince the boys that by cooperating they can undertake new activities which they cannot engage in now. If the boys accept new ways of relating on a superficial level as *conditions* to receiving concrete rewards, we may ultimately move toward a point where they will co-operate without such "bribes." If they can be persuaded to conform to new values and conduct on utilitarian terms, we might then explore how these changes can be incorporated permanently into superego structures. We believe that this "superficial" manipulation is an important intermediate step for delinquents from actively *opposing* to *internalizing* new norms of conduct.

Psychodynamically, there are important gains for each member if he can overcome his initial resistance. The aggressive leader rests uneasily with his power because of its tenuous foundation; the manipulator constantly seeks opportunities for exploitation, not only because of satisfactions he gains, but because of his own fear of being a sucker; the bushboy must develop a whole strategy of distasteful ingratiating tactics in order to survive. A permissive peer group environment would free these boys to expend their psychic energy in ego-strengthening pursuits rather than in futile efforts to dispel anxiety through delinquency.

We feel that if the group worker "sticks" to the boys during this rough period of mutual adjustment and active opposition, they will come to realize gradually that he is there not to "do them in" or to assume the role of the unconditional giver, but to help them. We need much more experience in learning how to work through "group transferences," with specification of the important group and individual variables in the process.[21]

MEASURING CULTURE CHANGE

ANY evaluative program for gauging change in a group in a natural setting offers tremendous problems for those who are sticklers for reliability and validity. The fact is, we have little systematic knowledge of successful intervention in a delinquent group as an ongoing social system. Although there have been more than seventy years of experimentation with these strategies, little work has been done to date to validate their therapeutic influence. Empirical experiments are sorely lacking in the field.

The measurement of change from a delinquent social structure to a less delinquent one involves focusing upon the boys' interactions, the group norms and roles, and the extent of involvement in nondeviant activities. Each one of these realms of group process can be defined in operational terms. In our studies we have focused primarily on peer group interactional processes as a basic criterion of change.[22] In any culture, norms, activities, and interactions are all interrelated and the researcher can select one or several key variables to evaluate change as a function of intervention.

The process of intervention is dynamic and dialectical; it includes not only stages of peer group development but, concurrently, stages of acceptance of the adult—the purveyor of socially acceptable norms. Once he is accepted, he must be cautious about the issues he can raise with the group. At first he may take up general issues. Only later when the group begins to crystallize and gains a positive identity will it feel secure enough to explore individual or group problems of a more threatening nature. Regression and rebellion may occur at any stage and will have a different meaning each time.

Methodologically, the next steps in research in group treatment can be summarized as follows:

1. Measurement of group processes so that we can objectively state: *Group X has moved so far from a negative hostile aggressive orbit to a positive one.*[23] We have begun to approach this problem in our utilization of Bales's interaction instrument to determine the extent of delinquent processes in one group of extremely aggressive boys.[24]

2. Measurement of individuals' attitudes toward peers, adults, themselves, school, work, and so on.

3. Measurement of the role performances of group members.[25] (This is revealed by Bales's instrument.)

4. Finally we must try to quantify the highly qualitative dynamic clinical diagnoses of psychiatric practitioners; this must be done before and after group treatment, so that we can determine whether members have changed fundamentally—internalized nondelinquent outlook and conduct—or are merely superficially adapting to a new behavioral setting.

When these four methodological prerequisites have been fulfilled adequately, we shall be in a much better position to shed some light on the effectiveness of group treatment for fundamental personality reorganization, and *how* new role and value assumptions become part of and change group members' basic character structures.

In the foregoing we have tried to conceptualize delinquency as a peer group authoritarian social system with terrifying internal conflicts as well as anticommunity outbreaks. We have outlined the difficulties of introducing a group worker amidst the boys in their daily lives. We have anticipated the boys' resistances and how best to overcome them by *not controlling* but *changing* their culture. This cannot be done by remote control; our best professionals with maximum support of the institution have to learn how to create truly therapeutic day-to-day cottage living situations. Speculation is now momentarily suspended and the larger complexities of experimentation begin. In this way theory and practice never cease building upon each other.

NOTES TO CHAPTER 46

1. This sociological tradition in America goes back at least to 1930-1931 with the publication of Clifford R. Shaw's *The Jack Roller* and *The Natural History of a Delinquent* (Chicago: University of Chicago Press, 1930 and 1931). Recent cross-cultural work in this vein can be found in Herbert Bloch and Arthur Niedenhoffer, *The Gang: A Study in Adolescent Behavior* (New York: Philosophical Library, 1958).

2. See for example Richard D. Trent, *An Exploratory Study of the Inmate Social Organization*, Vol. 5 of Warwick Child Welfare Services Project, 1954-1957, ed. Bettina Warburg (New York: State Board of Social Welfare, 1957). (Mimeographed.)

3. Howard W. Polsky and Martin Kohn, *Progress Report: Analysis of the Peer Group in a Residential Treatment Center* (Hawthorne, N.Y.: Hawthorne Cedar Knolls School, 1957, mimeographed); "Participant-observation in a Delinquent Subculture," *American Journal of Orthopsychiatry*, Vol. 29, No. 4 (October 1959).

4. Albert K. Cohen, "The Study of Social Disorganization and Deviant Behavior" in Robert K. Merton, Leonard Broom, and Leonard S. Cottrell, eds., *Sociology Today* (New York: Basic Books, 1959).

5. For an excellent summary and analysis of new developments in this approach see Richard A. Cloward, "Illegitimate Means, Anomie, and Deviant Behavior," *American Sociological Review*, Vol. 24, No. 2 (April 1959).

6. Our analysis of the social structure of the delinquent group has been observed by others who have described juvenile gangs. See William Poster, "T'was a Dark Night in Brownsville," *Commentary*, Vol. 9, No. 5 (May 1950); Dale Kramer and Madeline Karr, *Teen-age Gangs* (New York: Henry Holt & Co., 1953); Stacy V. Jones, "The Cougars—Life with a Brooklyn Gang," *Harper's Magazine* (November 1954), pp. 35-43; Harrison E. Salisbury, *The Shook-up Generation* (New York: Harper & Brothers, 1958).

7. Delinquent interpersonal processes are discussed in detail in a forthcoming book by the writer, *Cottage 6: A Study of Delinquency as a Social System.*

8. Howard W. Polsky, *A Treatment Center Alumnus' Own Story* (Hawthorne, N.Y.: Hawthorne Cedar Knolls School, 1958). (Mimeographed.)

9. Howard W. Polsky, *Continuity and Change in a Delinquent Sub-culture* (Hawthorne, N.Y.: Hawthorne Cedar Knolls School, 1959). (Mimeographed.)

10. Albert Cohen, *Delinquent Boys: The Culture of the Gang* (Glencoe, Ill.: The Free Press, 1955).

11. We have analyzed the relationship between the cottage culture and the institution in a paper entitled *Why Delinquent Subcultures Persist—The Double Standard "Interaction" Hypothesis* (Hawthorne, N.Y.: Hawthorne Cedar Knolls School, 1959). (Mimeographed.)

12. Eric Homburger Erickson, "Growth and Crises of the Healthy Personality," in Clyde Kluckhohn and Henry A. Murray, eds., *Personality in Nature, Society and Culture* (New York: Alfred A. Knopf, 1956), p. 209.

13. See among numerous writings Herbert Bisno, *The Philosophy of Social Work* (Washington, D.C.: Public Affairs Press, 1952); Gisela Konopka, "The Generic and the Specific in Group Work Practice in the Psychiatric Setting," *Social Work*, Vol. 1, No. 1 (January 1956), p. 72.
14. George H. Grosser, "The Role of Informal Inmate Groups in Change of Values," *Children*, Vol. 5, No. 1 (January-February 1958).
15. Talcott Parsons, "Psychoanalysis and Social Science," in Franz Alexander and Helen Ross, eds., *Twenty Years of Psychoanalysis* (New York: W. W. Norton & Co., 1953), pp. 186-215.
16. Talcott Parsons, *The Social System* (Glencoe, Ill.: The Free Press, 1951).
17. Kurt Lewin, *Resolving Social Conflicts* (New York: Harper & Brothers, 1948), chap. entitled "Conduct, Knowledge and the Acceptance of New Values."
18. Gordon W. Allport, "A Psychological Approach to the Study of Love and Hate," in P. A. Sorokin, ed., *Explorations in Altruistic Love and Behavior* (Boston: Beacon Press, 1950).
19. Lewin, *op. cit.*
20. A. Irving Hallowell, "Sociopsychological Aspects of Acculturation," in Ralph Linton, ed., *The Science of Man in the World Crisis* (New York: Columbia University Press, 1950).
21. Harold Esterson, Martin Kohn, and R. Magnus, *Countertransference in a Clinical Group* (Hawthorne, N.Y.: Hawthorne Cedar Knolls School, 1957). (Mimeographed.)
22. Howard W. Polsky and Martin Kohn, *A Pilot Study of Delinquent Group Processes* (Hawthorne, N.Y.: Hawthorne Cedar Knolls School). Paper read at American Sociological Society Meeting, Seattle, Wash., August 1958. (Mimeographed.)
23. Harold L. Raush, Allen T. Dittman, and Thaddeus J. Taylor, "The Interpersonal Behavior of Children in Residential Treatment," *Journal of Abnormal and Social Psychology*, Vol. 58, No. 1 (January 1959).
24. Robert F. Bales, *Interaction Process Analysis* (Cambridge, Mass.: Addison-Wesley Press, 1950).
25. Norman A. Polansky, Robert B. White, and Stuart C. Miller, "Determinants of the Role-image of the Patient in a Psychiatric Hospital," in Milton Greenblatt, Daniel J. Levinson, and Richard H. Williams, eds., *The Patient and the Mental Hospital* (Glencoe, Ill.: The Free Press, 1957).

ౖ➷

CHAPTER 47   The Social Structure of the

Hospital as a Factor in Total Therapy*

GEORGE DEVEREUX[1]

THE present study is divided into two parts: 1. Since every rational
    system of therapy presupposes some etiological hypotheses, I propose
to offer, first, a tentative theory of the *partial* sociogenesis of mental
disease.

2. The second part of the study outlines some of the therapeutic implications of our etiological hypotheses, which are also susceptible of
serving as a point of departure for the further exploration of the possibilities and limitations of the social therapy of mental diseases. Since the
development as well as the practice of social therapy presupposes a close
cooperation between the psychiatrist and the anthropologist, the section
on social therapy is, at the same time, a description of the services which
the social anthropologist may render to the psychiatrist.

THEORETICAL CONSIDERATIONS

"CULTURE AND PERSONALITY STUDIES" are today a recognized field of psychiatric, psychological, and anthropological inquiry, whose logical foundations have been studied in some detail (9). It is generally conceded that
the characteristic child-training techniques of a given society tend to
affect the personality make-up of the members of that society (22). It
does not matter *in this context,* as regards the personality structure of the
living members of a given society, whether these child-rearing techniques
are, according to Róheim (26), a *product* of the distinctive way of life of a
given society or the *cause* thereof, as claimed by Kardiner (17, 18). Nor is
it important, *from the practical point of view,* to become involved in the
"nature vs. nurture" controversy, since I have shown elsewhere that,

* Reprinted from the *American Journal of Orthopsychiatry,* 19 (1949), 492–500.
Copyright, the American Orthopsychiatric Association, Inc. Reproduced by permission.

methodologically, the "nature vs. nurture" problem can be reduced to the question, "When is it scientifically expedient and economical to cease using the biological frame of reference, and to begin to use the sociological frame of reference" (9)? All we need to remember in this context is that no competent scholar contests today the thesis that culture tends to affect personality make-up.

"Culture and the Abnormal Personality Studies" are a natural extension of the field of culture and personality studies. Dynamic psychiatry, and especially psychoanalysis, assigns to traumata produced by interpersonal (social) relations an important role in the etiology of the neuroses and of the psychoses; witness the emphasis on mother-child relations, the oedipal situation, etc. These relationships and situations are known to be determined by the characteristic way of life of each society. Traditions governing nursing and weaning practices (10, 20), as well as methods of toilet training (12), determine to an appreciable extent the amount and kind of pregenital gratification or frustration of children living in various cultures. Custom and social structure also play a role in sibling rivalry (16). The personnel, as well as the intensity and form of the oedipus situation, is likewise affected by such characteristic features of the social structure as avunculate (24), polyandry, or the instability of the biological family (7). Social attitudes toward early sex play are largely responsible for the occurrence or absence of the latency period, etc. In brief, each society has its characteristic ways of gratifying and traumatizing the child. We suspect, therefore, that social factors are partly responsible for the formation of personalities which eventually succumb to certain neuroses or psychoses.

Social factors are also present in the constellation of forces usually spoken of as "precipitating causes." It is plausible to assume that some potential psychotics may go through life without becoming acutely psychotic, if they are able to avoid certain situations too traumatic for their labile or defective egos. Many of these situations, such as combat, unemployment, etc., are socially determined.

Just as infantile frustrations and gratifications vary from society to society, so adult strains and satisfactions are, to a large extent, socially determined. Marquesans may legitimately fear crop failures (17), but need not worry about technological unemployment. The exploited Japanese peasant (2) and the Hindu farmer (3) may have no hope of breaking into an upper caste, but they do not live on a constantly descending social escalator, since advancement is not the *only* alternative to social degradation. Their social environment frustrates ambition, but gratifies the need for security and stability.

Since different sets of infantile and adult traumata and satisfactions tend to play a role in the formation of various types of prepsychotic personalities, and in the precipitation of acute psychotic breaks, and since these frustrations and gratifications are to some extent socially determined, it is to be expected that the incidence of various syndromes will not be the same in various societies, or within the same society, throughout recorded history. Existing studies tend to confirm this expectation.

Seligman (28) did not find a single case of schizophrenia among relatively untouched primitives; whereas Laubscher (19) has shown that schizophrenia is relatively frequent among the natives of South Africa, where the impact of White society is a particularly traumatic and intense one. Dhunjibhoy (11), an Indian psychiatrist, found that schizophrenia is more frequent among Hindus who have been abroad than among those who have never left India, and that the highly urbanized Parsee have a higher rate of schizophrenia than have rural Indian groups. The fact that Kardiner and Linton (17) make no mention of schizophrenia among the Marquesans, whose oral frustrations are exceptionally early and severe, does not abolish the validity of attempts to connect oral traumata with the etiology of schizophrenia. It merely suggests the possibility that the Marquesan way of life may provide substitute gratifications, and may perhaps be characterized by a lack of other factors which play a role in precipitating acute schizophrenic episodes. I have attempted elsewhere (5) to list a set of social factors which may conceivably play a role in the occurrence of schizophrenia.

Skliar and Starikowa (29) have shown that the relative incidence of various types of psychiatric syndromes varies from tribe to tribe in the Russian Turkestan and in adjacent areas. Carothers (4) provides us with similar data for certain African tribes. Faris and Dunham (13) have demonstrated that whereas some sections of Chicago have an unusually high incidence of schizophrenia, other areas produce more than their quota of manic-depressive states.

As regards changes in the relative incidence of various syndromes in the course of the history of a given society, we know that *la grande hystérie,* so frequent in the time of Charcot, Liébault, and Bernheim, is today a relatively rare neurosis.

Due allowances being made for the fact that comparative studies of this type are few, as well as for changing diagnostic conceptions, and for individual variations in diagnostic tendencies, existing data are sufficiently important to encourage us to formulate a working hypothesis of the *partial* sociogenesis of various psychiatric syndromes. In brief, there are reasons to assume that social and cultural factors which play a role in the formation of the characteristic basic personality of certain ethnic or social types, also promote the formation of a characteristic "predisposition" to certain neuroses and psychoses, and are part of the constellation of forces usually spoken of as "precipitating factors."

Therapeutic Implications: If the above working hypothesis is adopted, the social phases of milieu therapy will have to be analyzed by means of techniques familiar to social anthropologists, in order to ascertain precisely what kind of social life in the hospital will be most beneficial in the total therapy of various syndromes. The above working hypothesis clearly implies that a mode of life which places no pressures on the "sensitive spots" of the hysteric may be quite traumatic for a schizophrenic, and vice versa.

Our greatest difficulty in this connection is our ignorance of the *specific* social factors involved in the sociogenesis and in the precipitation of various syndromes, with the possible exception of schizophrenia (5).

Yet if we knew precisely what features of social life are partly responsible for the occurrence of various "dispositions to psychosis," and in "precipitating" various psychoses, we could perhaps manipulate the social life of various wards in such a manner as to increase rates of recovery.

We must not disregard, in this context, important psychiatric contributions to the solution of this problem, even though these contributions were the result of intuitive psychiatric "know-how," rather than of a systematic inquiry into the pathogenic or therapeutic effects of the social situation. The social factors which appear to play a certain role in the occurrence of schizophrenia (5) were found to be conspicuously absent in the social life of the Schizophrenia Research Ward of Worcester State Hospital (8). Nonetheless, the psychiatrically informed social anthropologist can perhaps be of some use to the psychiatrist in the exploration of this aspect of milieu therapy.

It is not possible to present in detail the social factors involved in the genesis and precipitation of every major psychiatric syndrome, nor would such an undertaking be feasible in the present state of our knowledge. Suffice to say that some initial guidance may be derived from the study of societies in which the incidence of certain syndromes is very low. Speaking both broadly and tentatively, the social therapy of a given syndrome might conceivably consist in providing the patient with an environment approximating the social life of a society in which that syndrome is rare or absent.

Since the entire problem is still relatively unexplored, it would be both presumptuous and inexpedient to labor this point, except to point out that *several types* of societies may show a characteristically low incidence of a given psychiatric syndrome. On the theoretical level, this observation enables us to seek out the basic similarities of these diverse cultures, and to utilize them therapeutically. On the practical level, it gives us a certain range of social structures from which to select the one most compatible with the laws and mores of our own society.

A few words may now be said about the therapeutic implications of Benedict's psychiatric diagnosis of cultures (1). Benedict's thesis has sometimes been misunderstood and distorted to such an extent that some actually seem to believe that every Kwakiutl is an acute case of megalomaniacal paranoia, and every Dobuan an acutely persecutory paranoiac, and that these societies are actually "sick" societies. Such a meaning is entirely alien to Benedict's very temperate formulations, since she never failed to emphasize the realistic satisfactions which these cultures provide for their members, and since these societies are obviously not involved in self-destructive, vicious circles. Only when the incidence of mental diseases becomes very high, and when, simultaneously, the society seems to destroy itself—be it only by inviting aggression from its neighbors—can one speak of a truly "sick" society. This, I think, is implicit in Benedict's valuable scheme.

In brief, we suggest that patients suffering from a certain psychiatric syndrome might benefit by living in a hospital environment which is made to resemble a society in which that particular syndrome happens to be rare or absent. The practical implementation of this suggestion must, however, give due consideration to two important implications of our theoretical scheme:

1. Each society has its gratifications as well as its frustrations, both of which are important in the prevention of certain types of psychic disorders. The implications of this observation will be discussed under the heading of "permissiveness."

2. The therapeutic social environment must be reasonably compatible with the mores of that segment of society in which the patient is ultimately expected to live. This problem will be discussed under the heading of "therapeutic objectives."

Permissiveness: The outstanding characteristic of the modern mental hospital is its selectively permissive atmosphere. Psychiatrists question, however, the value of *total* permissiveness. They point out that one does not do a favor to a patient, who must eventually return to extramural society, by being totally permissive; e.g., as regards wanton aggressiveness, or as regards other severely tabooed modes of behavior. This observation can be profitably discussed in some detail.

a) *Permissiveness and the Superego:* In an overly permissive situation the patient can simply "get away with" certain things which are taboo in society, which is different from a positive exercise of freedom. "Getting away with it" does not weaken the tyranny of the superego, and may even increase guilt feelings. It is known that some religious fanatics react to a permissive atmosphere rather violently, and view the hospital as a den of iniquity. A positive code of freedom, on the other hand, may perhaps lead to the strengthening of a realistic ego ideal, which can sometimes be successfully played off against the tyrannical superego.

b) *Permissiveness and Orientation:* An overly permissive situation resembles somewhat the sociologist's "undefined situation." The patient is compelled to determine for himself the boundaries of tolerance; he must constantly take the initiative, etc.; and he must do all this in an unfamiliar setting, which is half-authoritarian (administrative regulations, etc.) and half-permissive. This calls for a degree of reality testing and for more spontaneity than many a weak and constricted ego can muster. Some patients react to uncertain and undefined permissiveness by a further constriction of their personalities—just to be neurotically "on the safe side."

c) *Permissiveness and Reality:* In many ways hospital life is unlike society at large. It is "unreal"—an "imitation of life," "time out of mind." Hence, hospitalization in a simple protective environment sometimes encourages a further regression and constriction of the personality, i.e., an "institutional cure." Another difficulty is the fact that hospital life corresponds to the *healthy* man's idea of what is a "good society" and what is "good for the patient." This viewpoint ignores the fact that psychotics had to be hospitalized precisely because the healthy man's "good society" was not good *for them.*

Summing up, in the present state of our knowledge, our proposals must be tentative ones. For practical reasons the following outline tends to emphasize possible areas of cooperation between the psychiatrist and the anthropologist in the social therapy of patients.

SOCIAL THERAPY

I. *Special Diagnosis:* The proper planning of social therapy presupposes an initial cooperation between the psychiatrist and the anthropologist in the area of social diagnosis. The social anthropologist can make the following contributions to the social diagnosis of the patient:

1. He can rectify misinterpretations of the patient's social behavior; e.g., he can point out that a "constant changing of jobs" does not suggest psychopathy, but great ingenuity and skill in the management of reality, if the patient happens to be a Negro (30), or if the changing of jobs took place during the depression.

2. He can identify culturally determined reactions which, in an average middle-class White, would be abnormal; e.g., he can point out the cultural determination of a Crow Indian veteran's water phobia (25).

3. He can assist the psychiatrist in assessing a patient's social "allergies," etc.

II. *Social Therapy.* 1. *Acute Wards:* It may be worth while to experiment with wards having a relatively uniform population of patients, i.e., schizophrenia wards, paraphrenia wards, etc. Each of these wards could attempt to approximate, within the limitations imposed by existing mores, the social structure of some society in which the incidence of that particular syndrome is very low. The permissive aspects of that society would tend to relieve tensions of the type most painful to the patient, while the regulations and frustrations of that society would provide ego support.

This "natural" mixture of duties and obligations would tend to decrease the "unreality" of hospital life.

2. *Closed Convalescent Wards:* It may be desirable to experiment with schizophrenia or paraphrenia, etc., wards of graded social complexity, each successive ward through which the patient passes in the course of his convalescence approximating more and more closely the structure of that segment of society in which he will eventually live.

3. *Open Wards:* The last "grade" should be represented perhaps by wards approximating rather closely the real future extramural situation of the patient. In the open wards the various diagnostic categories would no longer be separated, since patients must be taught to get along once more with all kinds of people.

Throughout the treatment period it may be worth while to attempt a systematic, intellectual reorientation of the patient in the real social world. Anthropologists know how little even the average native knows of his own "simple" society and its customs. A systematic social reeducation and reorientation of the patient may be worth our while. I have reported elsewhere (8) the case of a catatonic who, after being made to assist me in my study of the schizophrenia ward, began to understand the world in which he lived, and soon afterward was discharged from the hospital where he had spent a number of years. The emotional reeducation of patients may likewise be attempted. Rowland (27) has pointed out that babies and passive catatonics, who cannot "hit back," are excellent love objects for the timid. The hospital could perhaps provide passive love objects, such as pets, for patients who cannot yet face the risks of adult emotional involvements. I know that William C. Menninger is in sympathy with this proposal. Generally speaking, life in the hospital should provide an opportunity for a risk-free retesting of reality and of the patient's own capacity to love and to receive love.

The anthropologist can be of service in such an over-all therapeutic program by helping the administration to organize various types of wards, by assisting psychiatrists in the preparation of "social therapy prescriptions," which should be at least as individualized as occupational therapy and group therapy prescriptions are, etc. In particular, he can help formulate social settings and plots for psychodrama, a useful method of retesting reality.

III. *Therapeutic Objectives:* In the past, psychiatry aimed simply at a restoration of the *status quo ante.* Frieda Fromm-Reichmann insists, however, that mental disease should be thought of not as a calamity, but as an opportunity for a fresh start toward higher goals, this fresh start being presumably made possible by regression itself (15). She feels that the patient should be primarily restored *to himself* and, regardless of past commitments, should be taught to find his own optimum social milieu and level of adjustment. This viewpoint seems to be a sound one. It is obviously useless to attempt to force a noncompulsive former bookkeeper back into his previous occupation, to compel an independent and enterprising Negro to return to the deep South, etc. It would also be fallacious to consider such forced returns to an uncongenial environment or occupation an adequate means of testing the extent of the patient's "social recovery." A proper formulation of therapeutic objectives would attempt to take full advantage of the great regional and cultural diversity of the United States, which is an invaluable asset to the therapist. The anthropologist can assist the psychiatrist and the specialist in vocational guidance, in their search for a social environment and for an occupation best suited to the needs of a given patient. The United States, with its great regional variations, is still a land of unlimited opportunity for the patient seeking a suitable environment, and with some slight anthropological assistance, the psychiatrist can make the most of this fact (6).

Summing up, social therapy can be made to fit the patient's individual needs as completely as can psychotherapy. Our therapeutic sights can be appreciably raised if we recognize the patient's right to his individuality, and help him seek out an environment suitable for the unfolding of his individuality.

IV. *The Ethics of Social Therapy:* R. M. MacIver (23) has stated that maximum individualization and maximum socialization go hand in hand; just as the individual cannot unfold his potentialities to the utmost without the help of society, so society derives the fullest benefit only from those of its members who are free to be themselves. This statement is not contradicted by Linton's remark that the average social role can be adequately filled by almost anyone (21). On the whole, it is safe to say that the healthiest societies are those which attempt to socialize, and to take advantage of, the *diversity* rather than the *similarity* of their citizens. This point of view is strongly supported by Fromm's distinction between the negative "freedom from" and the positive "freedom to," which encourages constructive individualization (14).

In brief, systematic social therapy is the very opposite of the conscious manipulation of persons, or of the deliberate exploitation of human plasticity for the purpose of making man wholly subservient to society or to the state. The ethics of social therapy are identical in essence with the great tradition of the West, that society and the state were made *for* the individual, and that all men have a dignity inherent in their human status. Social therapy merely extends man's right to be himself also to the mental patient, who, because he was not permitted to be himself, ceased to be himself altogether. The ethics of social therapy are the Magna Charta of the human being, even though he be a deviate. The philosophy of social therapy is the belief that man was not made for the Sabbath, but Sabbath for man. The therapeutic philosophy of Karl Menninger, which calls for "love unsolicited" for the patient, is still another way of affirming the human dignity of the patient's *own* personality. The unconditional acceptance of the patient's personality is the main guiding line of our work at Winter Veterans Administration Hospital, where a systematic exploration of the possibilities of social therapy is now under way.

NOTE TO CHAPTER 47

1. Published with permission of the Chief Medical Director, Department of Medicine and Surgery, Veterans Administration, who assumes no responsibility for the opinions expressed or the conclusions drawn by the author.

BIBLIOGRAPHY

1. Benedict, R. *Patterns of Culture.* Houghton Mifflin, Boston, 1934.
2. ———. *The Chrysanthemum and the Sword.* Houghton Mifflin, Boston, 1946.
3. Bouglé, C. *Essai sur le Régime des Castes.* Felix Alcan, Paris, 1935.
4. Carothers, J. C. *A Study of Mental Derangement in Africans, and An Attempt to Explain Its Peculiarities in Relation to the African Attitude to Life.* J. Mental Science, 93: 548-597, 1947.
5. Devereux, G. *A Sociological Theory of Schizophrenia.* Psa. Review, 26: 315-342, 1939.
6. ———. *Maladjustment and Social Neurosis.* Am. Sociological Review, 4: 844-851, 1939.
7. ———. *The Social and Cultural Implications of Incest Among the Mohave Indians.* Psa. Quarterly, 8: 510-533, 1939.
8. ———. *The Social Structure of a Schizophrenia Ward and Its Therapeutic Fitness.* J. Clin. Psychopathology, 6: 231-265, 1944.
9. ———. *The Logical Foundations of Culture and Personality Studies.* Trans. New York Acad. Sciences, Series II, 7: 110-130, 1945.
10. ———. *Mohave Orality.* Psa. Quarterly, 16: 519-546, 1947.
11. Dhunjibhoy, J. E. *A Brief Résumé of the Types of Insanity Commonly Met with in India, with a Full Description of "Indian Hemp Insanity" Peculiar to the Country.* J. Mental Science, 76: 254-264, 1930.
12. DuBois, C. *The People of Alor.* Univ. of Minnesota Press, Minneapolis, 1944.
13. Faris, R. E. L., and H. W. Dunham. *Mental Disorders in Urban Areas.* Univ. of Chicago Press, Chicago, 1939.
14. Fromm, E. *Escape From Freedom.* Farrar and Rinehart, New York, 1941.
15. Fromm-Reichmann, F. *Remarks on the Philosophy of Mental Disorder.* Psychiatry, 9: 293-308, 1946.
16. Henry, J. and Z. *Doll Play of Pilagá Indian Children.* Res. Monog. 4, Am. Orthopsychiatric Assoc., New York, 1944.
17. Kardiner, A. *The Individual and His Society.* Columbia Univ. Press, New York, 1939.
18. ———. *The Psychological Frontiers of Society.* Columbia Univ. Press, New York, 1945.

19. Laubscher, B. J. F. *Sex, Custom and Psychopathology*. Routledge, London, 1937.
20. Leighton, D., and C. Kluckhohn. *Children of the People*. Harvard Univ. Press, Cambridge, 1947.
21. Linton, R. *The Study of Man*. D. Appleton-Century, New York, 1936.
22. ———. *The Cultural Background of Personality*. D. Appleton-Century, New York, 1945.
23. MacIver, R. M. *Community* (3rd ed.). Macmillan, London, 1936.
24. Malinowski, B. *The Sexual Life of Savages* (3rd ed.). Routledge, London, 1932.
25. McAllester, D. *Water as a Disciplinary Agent Among the Crow and Blackfoot*. Am. Anthropologist, n.s., 43: 593-604, 1941.
26. Róheim, G. *The Origin and Function of Culture*. Nerv. and Ment. Dis. Monogs. 69, New York, 1943.
27. Rowland, H. *Friendship Patterns in a State Mental Hospital*. Psychiatry, 2: 363-373, 1939.
28. Seligman, C. G. *Anthropological Perspective and Psychological Theory*. (Huxley Memorial Lecture.) J. Royal Anthrop. Institute, 62: 193-228, 1932.
29. Skliar, N., and F. Starikowa. *Zur Vergleichenden Psychiatrie*. Archiv für Psychiatrie und Nervenkrankheiten, 88: 554-585, 1929.
30. Stevens, R. B. *Racial Aspects of Emotional Problems of Negro Soldiers*. Am. J. Psychiatry, 103: 493-498, 1947.

ॐ

Chapter 48   Fostering Resident Autonomy
in an Institutional Setting*

HOWARD W. POLSKY AND DANIEL S. CLASTER

AUTONOMY AS A GOAL OF RESIDENTIAL TREATMENT

THE point of departure of our orientation to residential treatment is contained in a World Health Organization report which noted that in order to create a "therapeutic atmosphere," patients must be regarded as "capable of responsibility and initiative and provided with planned purposeful activity."[1]

Residential treatment seeks to change its clients so that they can cope more effectively with their environment during and after their stay in the institution. It is thereby distinguished from custodial care where inmates are forced or allow themselves to be taken care of. When inmates stand in a dependent relationship to authority, as in custodial institutions, routine management tasks can be carried out most conveniently; for example, menus, time schedules, and work assignments can be handled by administrative fiat if no need for residents to direct their own affairs is recognized.

Residential treatment, however, assumes that clients are to be encouraged to exercise and maximize their autonomy in the institution so that they may learn to cope better with the world outside. Thus one of the central problems in residential treatment is to maintain the press toward resident autonomy in the face of powerful countervailing forces for institutional conformity.

There are special problems, moreover, in encouraging autonomy among residents who have been placed in institutions because of antisocial behavior. Such inmates tend to mistrust opportunities for independent action when offered and refuse them; or if accepted, they exploit the opportunities to repeat past delinquent patterns. To help such clients exer-

* Paper read at annual meeting, American Sociological Association, Aug. 28-31, 1967, San Francisco.

cise autonomy in a socially adaptive way involves much more than simply handing over to them more power to control their lives in the institution. It involves sustained relations and intervention by personnel trained in special techniques for introducing residents to new goals and processes of autonomous functioning.

THE FORMAL AND INFORMAL SYSTEMS

IT IS WIDELY accepted that in residential institutions, no less than in other organizations, the organizational behavior and culture of the less powerful sub-system is to the most important extent determined by the more powerful supersystems to which it is accountable. Equally applicable to institutions is the importance of the somewhat independent informal peer culture that emerges among the rank and file or less powerful groups in the organizational hierarchy. What has not been sufficiently attended to, however, is the interrelationships between the informal culture among workers and patients and the administrative and managerial systems that have power over them.

Our previous research[2] focused on this issue. We studied also the interaction between the kind of management exercised by workers in the cottage and the resultant peer culture. The analysis becomes complicated when we consider that cottage counselors are superordinate to the residents in the cottage, but in turn are subordinate to the higher administrative level within the institution.

THE COTTAGE WORKER'S ROLE

OUR past research at the Hawthorne Cedar Knolls School has focused on the cottage as a unit of treatment.[3] We have conceptualized the relationship between the institution and the emergent cottage culture in a way comparable to Homans' concepts of external and internal systems.

The cottages are relatively self-enclosed systems so that workers and residents build up and elaborate separate cottage identities. The institution does not encourage extensive interaction between the cottages (a special pass is required for a resident to leave the cottage), and so the youngsters within each cottage create a distinctive culture.

The cottage counselor is on the border of these two systems. He represents the institution to the youngsters and the youngsters to the institution.

The first requirement of the cottage is to adapt to the rules and regulations of the institution. The worker's other main task traditionally has been managing in the cottage the inevitable deviations stemming from institutional pressures and the residents' general suspicion and hostility to authority.

Often the cottage living units are very restricted in developing their own goals because the counselors are unable to negotiate effectively with the institution. Moreover, the residents have to be stimulated by the workers to develop their own goals and then the worker has to help the youngsters negotiate with each other and the larger system to implement them.[4] The totalistic character of residential institutions leaves little "space" open for counselors and residents to exercise initiative and autonomy in formulating and implementing indigenous goals.

Our previous research indicates that counselors generally emphasize the custodial role. This emphasis upon carrying out rules and regulations can detract from fashioning a therapeutic milieu in the cottage. When counselors define their role *essentially* as maintaining order and overseeing routines, little "local initiative" is expended in enabling the residents to make other spheres of cottage life a more gratifying experience. If youngsters could be stimulated and taught how to develop and implement their own goals, we believe that the custodial sphere would diminish in importance. The counselor's central role should be to enable the residents to assume more self-direction over their life situation. Custodialism becomes less an issue if there are significant activities in the cottage organized by the youngsters for which they are taking responsibility.

We broadened and converged upon the concept of goal-oriented activity as the chief vehicle for promoting resident group autonomy in the cottage living situation. We gradually realized that it would be possible for youngsters to be engaged much more in a self-directed group process in all of the functional spheres of cottage life, provided they could become more skilled and responsible for formulating and implementing group goals that could become their own. This we envisaged as the heart of our treatment approach.

THE PEER GROUP AS A VEHICLE FOR AUTONOMOUS GOAL ACTIVITY

THE main thrust of our present work is to redefine the role of cottage workers. Specifically, we are interested in how they can carry out their responsibilities through resident group activity and shared goals. Group confrontation, we feel, provides a testing ground for common needs and interests, goal-formulation and strategies for reaching goals. For one thing, many of the kinds of problems that residents will be confronted with on discharge from the institution will arise in a group context and call for group solutions. For another, these adolescents tend to be suspicious of adult authority and are prone to express themselves in antisocial activity. The peer group helps to mobilize and sustain their anti-authority posture.

The skill that counselors have to develop, therefore, is mobilizing the strengths of the group toward constructive goals and processes rather than delinquency and yet not being trapped into a repressive authority role.

As a theoretical problem of attitude change, our goal may be seen in terms of Herbert Kelman's theory.[5] Change, in our view, should not rest with external conformity, or compliance, in Kelman's terms. Nor should it be ultimately based on identification with the super-ordinate.

Our concept of autonomy assumes another psychological basis for the residents' performance—internalization. That is, residents may also perform according to the values of the adults in the institution because the adults' values and goals coincide or are complementary with the residents' own value system. The thrust of our project is premised on this social psychological basis. We are concerned with how residents can internalize new values and ways of behaving that are part and parcel of their own developing philosophy and value system.

PHASES AND COMPONENTS OF AUTONOMOUS GROUP FUNCTIONING

IN THINKING about the central problem of how counselors can encourage youngsters to take more initiative over their lives in the cottage and institution, we become concerned with specifying the methods that can be used by counselors and residents in approaching and articulating a problem, interest or need and devising plans to cope effectively with an issue. We sought to distinguish the components of the group process which culminates in goal-attainment. As we did so, it occurred to us that this component-analysis could serve as a device for workers to approach the key problem of fostering resident autonomy in the process of goal-oriented activities. A scheme was devised from the literature and our experimentation in the cottage on group goal processes, ranging from the initial problem encountered to evaluation of the outcome. Below is a description of each of these sub-processes relevant to carrying out group goal-oriented activities.

In order for a group to work on a problem or issue, communication channels have to be established and members convened so that they can talk to one another. This is what we mean by *convening* the members.

We think the following sources of group action can be reworked by the group into a goal perspective. "Needs" refers to individual or group psychological pressures—the internal condition of the group members. "Interests" refers to more objective concerns, for example, leisure time activities that cottage members are attracted to. "Problems" refers to difficulties and frustrations in the living situation.

Needs, interests and problems when shared by a group result in a kind of group *diagnosis,* so that the issue is further clarified and defined in the minds of the initiating members and the rest of the group.

The third step entails converting the need, interest or problem into a shared concrete realizable goal.

This is followed by *developing a plan and formulating strategies* for reaching the goal. A next logical step is defining and *allocating roles and tasks* among the group members to carry out the plan to attain the group goal. Some kind of differentiation of tasks and roles occurs.

Essentially we view goal-attainment as a boundary exchange process. In order for the cottages to formulate and carry out goals of its own, they have to negotiate with the institution to procure necessary resources for implementation that only it can provide. Furthermore, if the cottage is to become more autonomous it will have to secure permission from the institution to broaden the scope of its responsibilities. This too is a matter of negotiation with the institution. Hence we make the distinction between *securing resources* and *negotiating with the external authority structure* to increase the latitude for autonomous goal-functioning.

The phrase *"carrying out goal activities"* means actual implementation of the goal. We can distinguish this phase, actual implementation from the preparatory activities of setting goals and planning strategies.

The next phase or component, evaluation, consists of workers and residents talking about and assessing what they have done. Evaluation may be used also to discuss how the next activity can be more efficiently or effectively implemented.

The components discussed above emphasize the instrumental activities in consummating group goals. We are well aware that working at goals sparks all kinds of feelings and attitudes. Thus we also directed our attention to the *integration* sphere—the informal, expressive dimension of group activity that we divided into three components: solidarity among the members, degree of commitment to the task and goal, and affect expressed during an activity.

THE COTTAGE WORKER'S TASKS IN
FOSTERING PEER GROUP AUTONOMY

OUR research evaluation of autonomous resident goal attainment postulates three main dimensions[6] that can be visualized in their inter-relationships as follows (the mnemonic phrase, *C DIGS ARNIE I* comprises the components in goal-attainment):

FIGURE 1

THREE DIMENSIONS OF AUTONOMOUS GOAL-ATTAINMENT

Dimensions   The Components of Goal-formulation and Implementation

```
  Depth:        C    DI G  S       A R N I  E          I
                O    A  O  T       L E E M  V          N
Degree of       N    G  A  R       L S G P  A          T
autonomy        V    N  L  A       O O O L  L          E
exercised by    E    O     T       C U T E  U          G
peers           N    S  F  E       . R I M  A          R
                I    I  O  G         C A E  T          A
                N    S  R  Y       O E T N  I          T
                G    M             F S I T  O          I
                     U             O   A N             O
                     L             R   N T             N
                     A               O I
                     T             L   O
                     I             E   N
                     O             S
                     N
```

Progression: Degree of extension of an activity (consummation)

Breadth: Degree of cumulative goal-attainment and autonomy with diverse cottage activities.

The system principle of cottage life that underlies our theoretical orientation is the double dynamic pattern in group life formed by two major trends: The trend toward specification, formulation and attainment of group goals, and the involvement of the residents in the process to enhance their individual and group autonomy. These trends divide and sub-divide, and branch out from very general into more specific attitudes and skills toward shared group goals. These tendencies interact with the opportunities and contraventions presented by the institutional environment.

The domain in which the goal attainment sphere of cottage life processes are distributed and arranged has three dimensions. The *dimension of progression* implies a teleological or means-ends organization, each phase being the end for the preceding and the means for the following phase. In studying these sequences, the practitioner (and researcher, for that matter,) has a certain choice to the size of the parts and phases that are to be considered. But the internal articulation of the process is determined by the nature of the goal, the timing and pace in order to attain it, its complexity, etc.

The *dimension of depth* is designed to help us focus specifically on the quality and extent of initiation and participation in the goal-activity by the resident. We call it "depth" because it is a trend that leads from potentiality to actuality and is formed by individual members in their increasingly individualized elaboration of group skills which come to the surface and are expressed by manifest behavior that becomes accessible to direct observation. The arrangement of this vertical or depth structure is a concretization or partial manifestation of responsibility and decision-making, obligation-assumption and feeling of solidarity, etc., that residents are willing to express toward one another, the staff and the institution in becoming integral parts of institutional life.

The *dimension of breadth.* In addition to differentiating activities on a means-ends and consummation continuum and "depth-to-surface" quality of participation by the residents, another basic dimension in the cumulative development of the culture of cottage life is concerned with the build-up of more complex processes and activities upon simpler editions. Perhaps the key principle underlying this dimension is the residents' increased skill to coordinate their various abilities and interests to attain more complex group goals and evolve cottage solidarity.

These dimensions represent principle aspects of the cumulative development of a cottage culture based upon the ways in which the cottage organizes itself to meet individual and group problems, interests and needs. Long range personal and group goals are organized by many diverse activities into a hierarchy of superordinate and subordinate goals and consist of the coordination of cumulative multiple efforts along the progression, depth and breadth dimensions.

THE COTTAGE WORKER'S DILEMMA

THE child care worker, confronting these major foci of our orientation—autonomy and goal attainment—inevitably comes face to face with a dilemma. Shall he emphasize progression along the phases that culminate in attainment of complex goals, *production,* in the language of the marketplace? Or, shall he emphasize the resident group's autonomy in the process? The dilemma may be schematized as shown in Figure 2.

Theoretically, six major types of worker's orientations can be postulated as well as numerous mixed types. Orientations also vary according to developmental phase, pressures exerted upon the cottage, residents' and staff's skills and personalities, etc. 1,1 is an orientation defined by low concerns in both areas—the transitory, uninvolved worker who is in the cottage, not really part of it and wants either a sinecure or cannot wait to

FIGURE 2

THE COTTAGE WORKER'S GRID

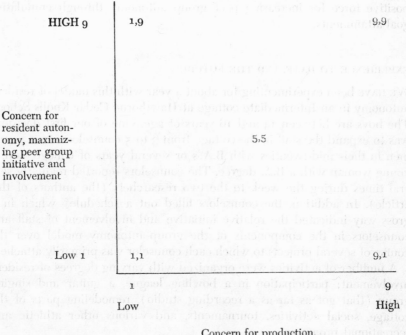

HIGH 9   1,9   9,9

Concern for
resident auton-
omy, maximiz-   5,5
ing peer group
initiative and
involvement

Low 1   1,1   9,1

           1   9

        Low   High

Concern for production,
goal consummation

leave; 9,1 gets things done, often primarily in the custodial sphere, by imposing his authority; 1,9 characterizes the overly permissive, non-directive counselor who believes in "order out of chaos"; 5,5 goes halfway in both concerns, and 9,9, manifests skill in both planning for complex goals and strategies and thinking through imaginatively how to motivate and inspire the residents in the process.

Frequently we have noted "pendulum swings" from 1,9 to 9,9 approaches, alternate periods of crises and calm. Workers often manifest not only a major orientation but a "back-up style" for varying situations.

We have also noted that a 9,9 orientation can be better approximated when the worker has thought through an initiation plan as well as continuity projections of the goal components as the group is mobilized to implement a peer group activity.

We still have much to learn about the inter-relationship of these two concerns and the varying orientations that result from their integration or lack of it. Limited application of the above theoretical orientation has also revealed an intermediate stage of group conflict related to the varying interests, skills, motivation and personality strengths of cottage members.

We have been able to identify "positive," "neutral" and "resistant" (or "negative") factions in the course of a series of goal-activities and have begun to think through strategies for converting stultifying conflict into a positive force for increasing peer group autonomy through cumulative goal-attainments.

EXPERIENCE TO DATE AND THE FUTURE

WE HAVE been experimenting for about a year with this model of resident autonomy in an Intermediate cottage at Hawthorne Cedar Knolls School. The boys are between 14 and 16 years of age. One of our first decisions was to expand the staff in the cottage from 3 to 5 counselors: four young men in their mid-twenties with B.A.'s or several years of college, and, a young woman with a B.A. degree. The counselors reported regularly several times during the week to the two researchers (the authors of this article). In addition, the counselors filled out a schedule* which in a gross way indicated the relative initiative and involvement of staff and counselors in the components of the group-autonomy model over the course of several projects to which each counselor was primarily attached.

A number of activities were organized with varying degrees of resident involvement: participation in a bowling league, a guitar and singing group (that got as far as a recording studio), remodeling parts of the cottage, social activities, tournaments, and various other athletic and recreational programs.

Three substantial obstacles were never overcome: difficulties in the custodial sphere—getting the boys to conform to standard institutional rules and regulations, generation of sustained motivation for the youngsters to persist in an indigenous activity, and lack of resources. We also felt that the counselors were unsuccessful in creating a significantly trustful climate in the cottage. We now believe that much more intensive pre-service and in-service training programs were necessary to train the counselors in group methods and institutional confrontation.

The other major deficiency of the program was lack of basic involvement, cooperation and commitment to the demonstration program by the administration. We mistakenly believed that it would be possible to experiment in one cottage and demonstrate our methods to the administration. Actually we became unduly isolated from the institution. There was a constant lack of resources, conflicting supervision, and distortion of difficulties in the custodial sphere. The institution was not able to create meaningful opportunities which could be exploited by counselors and residents' collective efforts.

It is our feeling that the introduction of an action program for foster-

* See following page for sample rating scale.

ing resident autonomy in an institutional setting demands much more extensive commitment by the administration. It may be possible to introduce change of some kinds in a fragmented manner, but the program that we envisaged required much more commitment by the entire institution. Such involvement could only be won by engaging all staff across hierarchical lines in cooperatively exploring how to design an institution which can afford opportunities for creative group efforts by residents and counselors in the basic living units.

Such thorough-going discussions on the basic purposes and methodology for restructuring the cottage living unit to foster autonomy could perhaps be initiated by methods pioneered by the National Training Laboratory.[7] The philosophy and practical techniques developed by the National Training Labs, in creating a trustful climate and specific procedures for feed-back and promotion of helping relationships between individuals and groups among all strata in the institution, could possibly open up new avenues of institutional living. Top echelon staff especially have to be drawn into redesigning their social system to maximally expand the opportunities for autonomy among personnel at all levels as well as the residents. The combination of NTL sensitivity training programs and our process model of building autonomy through group goal-attainment could very well usher in a new era in milieu therapy.

In summary: we feel that the crucial issue in residential treatment pivots on enabling residents to become more autonomous and self-directive in their total living situation. Our approach addresses itself specifically to the processes of encouraging and developing resident autonomy through group goal-attainment. We believe that this orientation has important implications for work with residents in other kinds of treatment settings. We want to unlock the process whereby groups of patients in a total institution can be provided with the opportunities and taught the skills to become more responsible and autonomous, and to assume more direction over their lives so that they can be better prepared to function with others in the outside community.

NOTES TO CHAPTER 48

1. "World Health Organization Report," 1953, page 17, par. 4.1.1, quoted in Morris Schwartz and Charlotte Green Schwartz, "*Social Approaches to Mental Patient Care,* New York: Columbia University Press, 1964.
2. *Fairline, Hearthstone and Concord, a Social System Analysis of Residential Care in Three Cottages,* now being considered for publication.
3. Howard W. Polsky and Martin Kohn, "Participant Observation in a Delinquent Subculture," *American Journal of Orthopsychiatry,* 29 (1959), pp. 737-751; Howard W. Polsky, Irving Karp and Irwin Berman, "The Triple Bind: Toward a Unified Theory of Individual and Social Deviancy," *Journal of Human Relations,* 11 (1962), pp. 68-87; Howard W. Polsky, "Changing

Sample Rating Scale for Each Component in Goal-Attainment*

a. Overt Behavior

9	8	7	6	5	4	3	2	1

b. Relative Attention

9	8	7	6	5	4	3	2	1
Practically the only process		Major but not only process		Notable but not major process		Occasional attention to this process		Almost none of this process

c. Boys vs. Staff Impetus

9	8	7	6	5	4	3	2	1
Boys impetus alone; no staff help		Mostly boys impetus; little staff direction		Staff and boys equal in impetus		Mostly staff impetus; boys follow directions		Staff impetus alone; boys take little part

d. Success or Failure

9	8	7	6	5	4	3	2	1
Nearly complete success		Mostly successful		Partial success; partial failure		Mostly failed		Nearly complete failure

e. Problems

*See Figure 1 for list of components.

[720]

Delinquent Subcultures: a Social Psychological Approach," *Social Work,* 4 (1959), pp. 3-15. Howard W. Polsky, *Cottage Six: The Social System of Delinquent Boys in Residential Treatment.* New York: Russell Sage Foundation, 1962. Howard W. Polsky and Daniel S. Claster, "The Structure and Functions of Adult-Youth Systems," in Muzafer Sherif, *Problems of Youth: Transition to Adulthood in a Changing World,* Chicago: Aldine, 1965, pp. 189-211; Howard W. Polsky, "A Social System Approach to Residential Treatment," in Henry W. Maier (ed.), *Group Work as Part of Residential Treatment.* New York: National Association of Social Workers, 1965, pp. 116-130.

4. Paul Daniel Sivadon, "Techniques of Sociotherapy," *Psychiatry,* 20 (1957), pp. 205-210.

5. Herbert C. Kelman, "Compliance, Identification, and Internalization: Three Processes of Attitude Change," *Journal of Conflict Resolution,* 2 (1958), pp. 51-60.

6. For an analysis of these three action dimensions—depth, progression and breadth—in the development of individual autonomy see Andras Angyal, "Personality as an Organized Whole," in Angyal *Neurosis and Treatment: a Holistic Theory.* New York: Wiley, 1965, pp. 48-51.

7. See Leland P. Bradford, Jack R. Gibb, and Kenneth D. Beene, *T-Group Theory and Laboratory Method.* New York: Wiley & Sons, Inc., 1964.

CHAPTER 49   Improving Patient Care Through Organizational Changes in the Mental Hospital[*]

ELAINE CUMMING, I. L. W. CLANCEY AND JOHN CUMMING

THIS paper reports substantial changes made in the organizational structure of a 2,000-bed, state-supported mental hospital, mainly through the application of principles developed and tested in the industrial-sociological field.[1] Although our larger goal was the rehabilitation of chronic patients and the treatment of new patients so as to avoid chronicity, we found that our most important single operational approach was to improve the morale and change the basically custodial attitudes of the nursing staff. In a hospital such as this, where the ratio of patients to doctors is high, almost all contact of the hospital staff with patients takes place through the nursing staff. Thus although the whole social structure of the hospital was in some measure changed, this paper is concerned specifically with the mechanics of changing the policy, the structure, and the function of the nursing hierarchy.

The authors of this paper, working as a team, undertook, with the support of the Hospital Superintendent,[2] the general task of designing and carrying out changes which would lead to improved patient care. One member of the team was a sociologist whose role included research and consultation. Another was Clinical Director of the hospital and thus had an executive role, and the third was a senior psychiatrist who had administrative, clinical, and research duties, and whose role on the team was a linking one.

At the beginning of our study, the hospital described in this paper, like many other large, state-supported mental hospitals, constituted a reasonably permanent social system. Its location in a geographically remote place, far from cities, gave it a striking "total community" quality. The

* Reprinted by special permission of The William Alanson White Psychiatric Foundation, Inc., and the author from *Psychiatry*, 19 (1956), 249–261 (copyright by the Foundation).

social structure of its staff was granulated—that is, crosscut horizontally by caste lines, and vertically by the functional autonomy of its parts. The medical staff turnover was high, a few patients were treated with insulin and electric shock, and the patients on the "back wards" were "deteriorated."

On paper, the formal structure of the hospital staff was that of a modern bureaucracy; promotion was based upon specified standards of qualification and performance, jobs were described in terms of specific functions, and authority lines were clear-cut. But much of this was on paper only; informally, the hospital had many of the features of a paternalistic, traditional society, rather than a democratic, rational one. There were cliques of elite who exercised power which went far beyond their legitimate authority; this they could do because some members abrogated their authority through ignorance, error, or a desire to be relieved of it. As traditional ways of doing things were emphasized, once such authority was abrogated, it was difficult to return it to its legitimate holders. Since one group of legitimate authority holders, the doctors, were often not the people with the longest tenure in the hospital, tradition tended to support ways of doing things which resulted in the withholding of power from them. In consequence, informal groupings were very important, a fact expressed in phrases such as, "So-and-so *really* runs the place." No one knew how this had come to be; it was vaguely attributed to "political influence," or nepotism.

With this pattern of traditional ways of doing things, there was a devaluation of new ways, and a compensating ideology that "this is the best hospital in this part of the country." Obviously, innovations were not needed in a society which was already so satisfactory! In the higher reaches of the hierarchy, few regulations were committed to paper; rules, guiding principles, and even the personal records of the nurses[3] and attendants were filed in the memories of the senior staff members. This lore was passed from role-holder to role-holder by word of mouth. Rumors were the lifeblood of the institution because they were often the only way of receiving vital information.

In this hospital, like most institutions of its kind, there was seldom more than one doctor for every two hundred patients. This meant that although the doctor might influence the condition of the patients, he must do it through the nurses. But the doctor was often much less acquainted with the hospital and its lore than were the nurses. Furthermore, there was little interaction across the caste lines.[4] Because of this, and because of traditionalism, it became important to "know the ropes," seniority was valuable, and having "been through the mill" was a virtue. Young doctors attempting to make changes were discouraged by the repeated, "When you've been here as long as I have, Doctor . . . ," which they heard from senior ward staff. Traditional and static, such a mental hospital is hard to change, and especially hard for the doctor to change because he is always outnumbered and usually outmaneuvered.

These were not the only reasons why this mental hospital was hard to change; just as important was the low level of integration at which it operated. There was, in other words, a high level of functional autonomy in the various hospital departments regarding both goals and methods of reaching them. For example, the farm had its traditional patterns of using patient labor in order to reach its goal of food production, while the wards had different goals and patterns of reaching them. The members of these two systems seldom interacted except in the ritualistic handing over of patients in the morning and evening. Thus the policies and procedures throughout the hospital were not closely integrated, and there was little chance of effecting change by reorganizing one part of the greater social system and waiting for the other parts to fall in line, through a necessary adaptive process. If, for example, the occupational therapy department changed its daily routine, all that would happen would be that a few patients affected by the change would stop attending O.T. sessions, and slowly a few would replace them. There would be no corresponding shift in the routines of other departments, no planned adaptive process.

Autonomy was strikingly evident between the "male side" and the "female side." For instance, during the early part of our reorganization, when some fifty female patients from a chronic ward were allowed to go out unaccompanied for the first time, the resulting incidents caused rather dramatic reactions on the part of the townfolk; but the staff on the male side did not know until these incidents had been reported in the press that the female side had even contemplated such a program.

The level of communication between departments was low because there was little need of much communication as long as the hospital functioned mainly custodially. The resulting type of integration was the "mechanical solidarity" of Durkheim;[5] that is, the hospital organization hung together because all were concerned ultimately in the custody of the patients; it was a common task, undertaken for a common goal to earn a living. There was, on the other hand, a low level of the interdependence, or "organic solidarity," which arises from a greater division of labor. Because each person or unit did a more or less complete task—either ran a ward, or administered a portion of the hospital—people were not forced to communicate and to integrate their activities. In our hospital we lacked that specialization which, as Durkheim says, "creates among men an entire system of rights and duties which link them together in a durable way . . . and gives rise to rules which assure pacific and regular concourse of divided functions." Such integration as existed in the hospital was brought about high in the hierarchy; at the ward level no decisions were made which might affect general policy; thus a minimum was done, for nothing could be done without decisions.[6] Therefore changing the hospital entailed raising the level of integration of the system.

In general, our hospital was neither better nor worse than most. Many hospitals such as ours have wrestled with the problem of improving the condition of their chronic wards, lifting the level of their treatment programs, and changing staff attitudes. We propose here to describe some of the techniques which we employed, we believe successfully, in our attempt.

Our goal was to integrate the system so that a new 'therapeutic' policy could be introduced to displace the older 'custodial' one. The meaning we assigned to these terms is a little different from that used by other workers. Briefly, we designated those attitudes as custodial which centered in the conviction that most mental illness, particularly schizophrenia, is incurable. We called those attitudes therapeutic which centered in the assumption that *most mental illness, and particularly schizophrenia, are, like rheumatoid arthritis, chronic, recurrent disorders for which there is no known cure, but which can be so treated as to allow the patients long periods of remission.* Two secondary assumptions we felt necessary for a therapeutic attitude were, first, that mentally ill patients require a high level of interaction with other patients and with staff members in order to improve; and, second, that in almost every case, life in the community is preferable to life in a state mental hospital. The small number of doctors made a goal of personality transformation untenable; our last assumption implied that in our hospital a 'social recovery' would be the goal of choice for most patients.

TWO EARLIER ATTEMPTS AT CHANGE

As WITH most 'reforms,' we stood upon the shoulders of others. Our first step was to examine past attempts at change in the hospital under study. Of these, two were outstanding, although neither had been entirely successful.

THE NURSES' TRAINING PROGRAM

THE first of these attempts at change had been a new nursing training program, which had been introduced seven years before our study. This program was designed to introduce more modern and humane attitudes, and to raise the prestige of the psychiatric nurse. It has been fully described by McKerracher,[7] and, as is evident from his description, it was an excellent program. However, by the time of our study the new training staff had in fact failed to gain access to the wards for teaching purposes, and the most frequent complaint we heard from the training staff was, "We train the new nurses, but after a while the ward culture gets them; the old-line staff ridicule them if they use our ideas, and they are gradually broken down." Thus the training program was, in its effect, encapsulated and academic, and did not seem to have much impact upon the custodial quality of the hospital. It was said, on the other hand, to have raised the standard of physical nursing care, and through its affiliation with the Provincial University, it did raise the prestige of the nursing group.

We tried to find the answer to the vital questions, Why did the program fail to change the ward culture? Why did not the old-line staff learn at least as much from the new trainees as they taught them? We found three main answers. First, the failure to change the ward culture could be attributed to the failure to introduce structural changes in the social system so as to raise the level of integration of the hospital. We know from many sources[8] that values, beliefs, and attitudes—that is, norms— are changed, as they are made, in interaction. This is as true for the work group as for the friendship group or the family group. As Brown says, "The primary group is the instrument of society through which in large measure the individual acquires his attitudes, opinions, goals, and ideals; it is also one of the fundamental sources of discipline and social controls."[9]

If this is true, in a granulated system where the rate of interaction is low, one must either raise the level of integration and hence of interaction of the total system, or else arrange for persistent interaction between members at all parts of the system, thus changing each semiautonomous part separately. Clearly, the latter approach would require a tremendous number of training staff members. The training staff, in fact, interacted only with student nurses, who not only were at the bottom of the nursing hierarchy, but were also unable to support one another on the wards because they were spread out over the hospital. This failure to integrate the granulated social structure acted against the new training course.

The second reason for the failure of the program lay with the failure of its designers to recognize the importance of seniority in the static hospital society.[10] They had by-passed numerous senior ward supervisors by promoting two capable but junior staff members to high-ranking training positions, on the basis of their attitudes and orientation. At the same time they made the training staff independent of the nursing hierarchy and responsible, under a director trained in pedagogy rather than nursing, directly to the Medical Superintendent.

As we have said before, little is written down in a large mental hospital; what is actually expected of a ward supervisor, beyond a minimal list of duties, is never recorded. If the principle of seniority is violated in making promotions, it throws great doubt into the minds of the old-line staff as to their own status. They have no way of knowing whether or not they are performing well enough to be promoted.

Moreover, just as the designers of the training program had not reckoned with the meaning of seniority, so they overlooked the earlier and somewhat less adequate training program, unrecognized by the University, in which the old-line staff had been trained. There was a tendency to refer to "before the training course," and to think of the old-line staff as "untrained." In fact, most employees who had been in the hospital only two or three years were unaware that there had been an "old training course." While the old-line employees were given honorary membership in the new nursing organization, their traditional training was not incorporated into the new program. It was to be new, and it failed by being too new.

A third error lay in the violation of the principle that the most highly chosen people are most likely to be the normbearers.[11] The two men chosen from the nursing ranks to join the training staff were both *deviant by definition,* for they were selected as being the *least custodial* people in a custodial institution. The old-line supervisors had reason to be adamant in the face of this innovation; one of the problems which faces all mental hospitals is the performance of the function of "protection of the public" without slipping into custodialism.[12] Medical men do not like being charged with the duty of "protecting the public," for it runs counter to their perception of themselves as therapists. Yet this function must be performed and the doctor must, by giving certain orders about the patients' daily routines, take his part in performing it. But he is in conflict, and one of his resolutions of this conflict is to exaggerate the "custodialism" of the nursing hierarchy. Many times we have heard a physician complain of "nursing office" attitudes and how they cripple his attempts to give the patients maximum freedom. We believe that our senior nursing staff members had been assigned the mantle of custodialism, and that they had no way of refusing it. Furthermore, the old-line nurse had certain compensations. *In effect* he had made an even trade with the doctors; he had tacitly agreed to wear the mantle of custodialism in return for the power to run the custodial wards himself, in his own way, and with a minimum of interference. In spite of this, when we interviewed senior ward supervisors we found that their reference point for advice and guidance in the care of patients tended to be the medical staff and not the custodially oriented head nursing offices, as had been generally supposed. They had, in short, latent therapeutic attitudes, never called into play.

When all of the foregoing factors are considered, it is not surprising that the efforts of the recently promoted training staff members to teach on the wards were blocked by the old-line people over whose heads they had been promoted. On the other hand, the training program undoubtedly did a good deal of useful work, both in teaching nursing techniques, especially of the concrete, physical sort, and in constantly reminding the students of a more ideal sort of psychiatric nursing care than they were seeing on the wards.

THE "TOTAL-PUSH" WARD

A SECOND and quite different attempt at change had been undertaken four years before by an enterprising and energetic team of two doctors.[13] They had demonstrated on a treatment ward that deteriorated and incontinent schizophrenic patients would show social improvement if they were placed in an improved social environment, *no matter whether they had physical treatment or not.* This demonstration, though strikingly successful, was not followed by any sustained attempt to improve the status of deteriorated patients in the hospital; and indeed it had been intended only as a demonstration. Our assumption is that one cannot create *permanent* changes in attitudes, values, and behavior by such an example, no matter how good, because there seems little doubt that values and beliefs are changed *in interaction,* and only a small proportion of the staff members had a chance to interact in the improved situation. Further, the structure of the organization which had been serving the purposes of the old values was literally unchanged. As soon as the tremendous energy of the two doctors was removed, the old situation reappeared. Thus, some of the staff said cynically, "What is the use of improving the patients' condition, if it is inevitable that they revert to a deteriorated state?" Yet there was an important residue of change in the personal outlook of a few staff members, who hoped that this sort of improvement could some day be made permanent throughout the hospital. This small group of nurses represented a strain in the nursing ranks, for they had a constant latent role conflict. They knew that as nurses they could be doing better, but they did not know how, and their membership in the staff group kept them from voicing this belief very often. But had it not been for them, our task would have been much more difficult. Our predecessors had demonstrated that change was possible, and although they were unable to interact with sufficient people to change the culture of the total group, they had overcome an immense hurdle by convincing a certain number of the old-line staff that something could be done.

Recapitulating, we found that we had before us the task of raising the level of integration of the formal structure, and of providing a high level of interaction with staff members so as to succeed in motivating them to adopt more therapeutic attitudes.

THE STRUCTURAL CHANGE

So FAR, while we have tried to describe the general characteristics of the hospital, we have touched only peripherally on its structure. At this point, a brief but more specific description of the old structure will help evaluate the new one. Our hospital, like many others, had two separate nursing hierarchies, one for the male side and one for the female side, each headed by a chief nursing officer.[14] One of the main characteristics of the nursing structure was a lack of coordination between these two services. In theory, both were responsible to a Superintendent of Nursing, but in practice this post was often empty. Even when it was filled—always by a woman, since the post required general hospital training as well as psychiatric nursing training—there was never an effective coordination of the two nursing services; in actual fact, the role-holder tended to do the job of the chief nursing officer on the female side, while the holder of this role did the job of her deputy.

The two chief nursing officers were responsible directly to the Medical Superintendent, and a system of daily reporting kept a routine communication going between them. Actually the nursing services had been run by their chief offices almost without interference through the years. Since promotion to positions in these offices was based almost exclusively on seniority, the role-holders, on the male side of the hospital especially, were people who had been trained in those custodial principles of mental hospital care which existed when they had first joined the hospital staff.

While the two chief nursing offices were the fulcrum of the medical side of the hospital, beyond this very little was laid down regarding proper lines of communication. Therefore, entrenched informal groupings tended to control the flow of information. These offices often received information directly when it should have come through ward supervisors, and they often withheld information which should have been distributed to the ward staffs. This, of course, greatly enhanced the power of the chief nursing offices, as the control over communication must always do.[15]

Another major characteristic of the old structure was the limited authority of the doctors. The doctors on both sides were responsible to the Clinical Director and hence to the Medical Superintendent, but no one was responsible directly to the doctors. Ward staff had, of course, to obey medical orders from the doctors, but in all other matters their final authority was their chief nursing office. Differences of opinion between doctors and one or the other of these chief nursing offices were resolved by the Medical Superintendent, usually in favor of the nursing hierarchy, for doctors were, by and large, expendable, but the good will of the nursing hierarchy was not. The doctors, themselves, furthermore, did not wish the responsibility for running the wards which authority over the staff would entail.[16]

One of the outstanding aspects of the structure of the nursing service was the small size of the executive echelon, which consisted of the two chief nursing officers, a deputy for each, and three administrative assistants on the male side, and two on the female side. Considering that there are nearly 2,000 patients and a nursing staff of about 350, the nursing executive echelon was large enough for only the most routine daily administrative duties. This, together with an almost total absence of meetings with staff, and the lack of formal job specifications, practically guaranteed that the minimum would be done, and that integration would be low.[17]

All socio-structural changes in our hospital were timed to take place on one day. Just prior to this, meetings were held with various staff groups, and formal announcements were made of the new social structure within which they had to work. We did this not because we felt that they would absorb the information particularly well, but to put the formal intention of the highest hospital authorities before the total staff. This move had a latent purpose, preventing rumors about the change. In a sense it was a rite of passage: the formal announcement of a new status for the hospital.

THE NEW EXECUTIVE ECHELON

Our first move was to expand the executive echelon by creating ten new "coordinating" roles in the nursing hierarchy. Two of these were at the Deputy Nursing Officer level, and the remainder at the Assistant Nursing Officer level. The general purpose was a double one—to increase the efficiency and improve the quality of the nursing service and to integrate ward activities. The number selected was small enough for intensive interaction with the medical doctors in discussions and meetings, yet large enough to meet with the ward staffs sufficiently often to have an appreciable effect upon their attitudes and beliefs—that is, to change their norms. In this way, the new therapeutic approach could be spread out fan-wise through the hospital.

Among their specific duties, these new officers were charged with the job of total hospital planning for the ancillary services, such as recreational and occupational therapies, and of securing the cooperation of the people engaged in these services. Since the development of the special therapeutic departments had been slight, there were no entrenched positions to consider in placing the new Nursing Officers in a coordinating role with respect to them.

Furthermore, the simple matter of getting things and getting things done fell within the scope of these new roles—the kinds of activity necessary in a large bureaucracy for procuring needed equipment and material. Hitherto the nursing hierarchy had been too weakly staffed at the executive level to spend any time on such matters, especially if anything the least bit out of the ordinary was required. For instance, the doctors who had run the total-push ward had experienced great difficulty in getting wood for carpentry activities; since carpentry had not been done on the ward before, obtaining the materials was a major operation.

The new roles, then, in their acting out, were to provide a more efficient, integrated, and therapeutic nursing service, and the medical staff could use the nursing structure to introduce their own attitudes right down to the ward level.

THE NEW FORMAL LINES OF AUTHORITY COMMUNICATION

As a second step, we laid down firm lines of communication and announced that for the time being protocol would in all cases be observed. We did not want people to fall back into their old patterns of informal communication, which would be bound to short-circuit some of the new role-holders, especially as most of these people had only recently been subordinate to the chief nursing offices. Furthermore, although we were prepared to allow some informal channels to develop, we were determined that this should not happen until the proper channels were institutionalized enough so that every time any person used an informal channel he would be perfectly well aware he was doing it. If vital information was withheld or misdirected, formal sanctions could be employed against the act. Sanctions had, in fact, to be used in this regard on several occasions.

THE TRAINING OFFICE

A DRASTIC change was made in the authority position of the Training Office. It had stood outside the nursing hierarchy, and the old-line nurses in the chief nursing offices had had no power to discipline the training staff, who in turn had had no power to force their program upon the nursing hierarchy. The result was an almost inevitable stalemate, and encapsulation. Nursing training was restored to the Nursing Service under a well-qualified Nursing Officer. The creation of a Personnel Department to perform a previous function of the training staff informally allowed some members of the training staff to remain outside the nursing hierarchy, but the training staff—itself long insulated from the nursing service—once again became an integral part of it.

This step not only greatly facilitated the use of ward staff for practical training purposes, but also was designed to break up the granulation of the structure and to bring the training staff, with its therapeutic orientation, into close contact with the ward staffs. At the time of writing, the process of institutionalization is incomplete, and the training staff and personnel staff informally appear to consider themselves unitary.

AUTHORITY OF THE MEDICAL STAFF

A FINAL change in lines of authority gave the doctors authority over the new Nursing Officers in charge of coordinating therapeutic activities. In administrative matters these Nursing Officers were still responsible to the Superintendent of Nursing, and therefore formal regulations regarding communication with the Nursing Office were introduced. It was important not to have overlapping areas in the divided authority;[18] moreover, until the responsibilities of the new officers to the Nursing Office were institutionalized, we felt that they might be tempted to communicate solely with the medical staff, who were, after all, in charge of the more interesting of the activities required by their roles.

INTEGRATION OF THE TWO SIDES

GETTING the hospital to operate as one institution was the biggest single undertaking. After all, it had run along fairly comfortably for years without much contact between the two sides. It is true that some female nurses had been nursing on the male side, but only because of the inability of the hospital to recruit male staff in sufficient numbers, and not because anyone had planned it as a desirable thing.

The first step we took in this direction was to place the two chief nursing offices, together with all the new appointees and the Training Office staff, in new common quarters.[19] Previously, they had been separately housed on their own sides, but now they were in the administration wing of the building together, on neutral ground.

Since the choice of people to fill the new coordinating positions was very important to hospital integration, we will digress here to discuss the selection process. The new appointees had to be able to work with both male and female patients if necessary—not an easy task for some; they must be amenable to the therapeutic approach, although we did not feel that they had to be already enthusiastic about it; and finally, they had to be acceptable to the nurses with whom they would have to work.

With these considerations in mind, we took advantage of the waiting period, while the new posts were being formally approved through bureaucratic channels, to conduct a campaign of anticipation. The following examples of the preliminary work are taken from the male side, because, while that term is fast becoming less meaningful in our hospital, two of us[20] were working closely with the male staff at the time of the reorganization.

A meeting of all the ward supervisors was called; the new jobs, of which six were to be filled by men, were described to them and they were asked to fill out sociometric ballots indicating which male staff members they thought should be promoted to these new positions, as well as to two administrative nursing posts which happened to be vacant. Although the voting did not follow rigid seniority lines, all of the eight men who received *almost all* of the votes were among the fifteen most senior male staff members in the hospital. (Five of the remaining seven men were within a year or two of retirement and had expressed their disinclination for promotion to the new jobs.) Thus only two of the most senior old-line men were considered inappropriate for the new therapeutic positions by their peers.

When we examined this list of highly chosen men, we found it to coincide exactly with our own list of the senior men most able to do a good job. Although we knew that there were some exceptionally good young men of less seniority, we had decided that the following three principles were too important to violate:

(1) Norm-bearers—those who most clearly express the attitudes and beliefs of a group—are highly chosen. New programs, to be accepted, should be introduced by norm-bearers rather than by deviants.

(2) In a stable system, when all else is equal, seniority is the fairest criterion for promotion.

(3) Very few roles in any society should be structured so that only exceptional people can hold them, since most people are unexceptional.[21]

The next step in anticipatory socialization was to assign special tasks to these highly chosen men in order to orient them to the type of problem with which they would be dealing when they were formally appointed. From among the chosen men, several small committees were set up to study ward procedures such as the condemning of old clothing and the requisitioning of new, in order to recommend how these procedures could be changed so as to maximize patient welfare. A committee drafted a plan for the reorganization of a geriatrics ward, and a key man was assigned the task of preparing a weekly bulletin to keep all branches of the hospital informed of any news which might otherwise circulate only by rumor.

These activities proceeded while the men still held their old roles. Although they were never asked to work overtime, they put in many evening hours.[22] Although we asked our staff to work hard at specific jobs for specific purposes during this period, and although we expected them to orient themselves to the welfare of the patient, it was through activity, not through formal teaching of any special attitude, that we hoped that a common sentiment of involvement in therapeutic goals would emerge. These planning committees reported to us, and in these reports we were able to discern a good deal of the 'ward culture.' In this way we knew which of our planned changes would be immediately acceptable, which might be acceptable eventually, and which would be intolerable to this group of men.

During this anticipatory period we made a great many informal contacts among the staff. A lot of our effort was spent in persuading the "old guard" that things *could* be done. A great deal of their skepticism about improving the hospital was founded upon their own experience in attempting minor enterprises of their own. The low level of integration of the structure had convinced them, for example, that it was impossible to get the cooperation of the tinsmith to repair the lockers. Unless they could be fixed, how could the men be expected to care for their clothes? There was a tendency to some defeatist grumbling about past frustrations, even among the new appointees. A certain amount of 'charisma' was needed at this stage, as well as demonstrations that the reorganizing team meant business.

All of the above-mentioned activity took place before the new appointments were made. By the time we made them, we had a fairly good idea of the kind of people we were dealing with and the kind of job we could expect them to do. The restructuring of the nursing hierarchy followed.

Besides the establishment of the new executive positions, two main changes were made in the interests of a closer integration of the two sides. The three top nursing roles, the Superintendent of Nursing—long unfilled, at this time—and the two chief nursing officers were consolidated into two posts, the Superintendent of Nursing, and her Deputy. It was stipulated that if the Superintendent were a woman, the Deputy would be a man, and vice versa, and that one of them must have a general nursing training. These two role-holders were made jointly responsible for nursing services, and charged with the duty of unifying these services across the two sides of the hospital.

At the same time, it was announced that applicants for the Ward Supervisors' posts, made vacant by promotion to the new positions, would be received from both male and female nurses for both sides of the hospital. This broke cleanly with tradition. Men went for the first time into supervisors' posts on the female side of the hospital, because many male staff members had a great deal more seniority than any female members.[23]

Neither the sick rate nor the resignation rate among the women changed in the months following the introduction of this practice. There were undoubtedly certain advantages to the women nurses in working on teams which also included men, for certain work on the wards is more easily done by men because they are stronger, and certain work is more appropriately done by men because of the difference in male and female roles in this society. We predicted that the women would appreciate a division of labor along these male and female role lines, and we have informal evidence that they did; for instance, nurses have commented that they are less exhausted, are less afraid on certain wards, and so on. These compensations appear to offset the dissatisfaction resulting from the women's reduced chances of promotion.

DIVISION OF LABOR BY FUNCTION

As WE have said before, the lack of integration in the hospital was partly a result of the low level of functional specialization. As an example of the increased division of labor at the executive level, we consolidated the booking procedures—that is, the assignment of nurses to wards and shifts—into the hands of one staff member. Previously each side had done its own booking and each had operated on the basis of a different set of principles. Now one person, in consultation with the Deputy Nursing Officer in charge of training and the Superintendent of Nursing, was assigned this task for the whole hospital.

On the same principle, two large male wards were consolidated for the purpose of administration. One supervisor was put in charge of administration and two shared the responsibility for the therapeutic program. This division of labor forced communication and coordination across these two wards, with a rise in efficiency. Such administrative roles seemed an important safety valve for certain senior staff members, whose old, military-like indoctrination into mental hospital procedures made them uncomfortable in the new 'therapeutic' situation.

INTERACTION AND COMMUNICATION

THE importance of changing norms and values through interaction, and of appointing norm-bearers to key positions, which we have mentioned in describing the structural changes, cannot be emphasized too strongly. The impossibility of changing norms in a didactic fashion is aptly illustrated by an unsolicited comment from a Training Office staff member, now attached to the Personnel Office: "All my stereotypes of the old, custodial ward supervisors have gone down the drain." He went on to say, "I see people going around doing all sorts of things that we've been trying to talk them into for years."

An important element in our program was the committee work we have described, which is now being continued in other committees all over the hospital. When a change was considered we tried to ask a committee to find the most therapeutic way of doing it. We did not ask our staff to have good attitudes toward the patients; we assigned them the job of finding out which of several alternatives would most favorably influence the patients. A by-product of this technique was the delegation of the decision-making function to the executive nursing echelon. These people had never in the past had to assume the responsibility for making decisions about changes, and a feeling of increased status and involvement resulted. They became identified through this program of action with the goals of the medical staff, and with the remembered goals of the two doctors who had engineered the total-push ward.

A second by-product of our technique was a high level of communication of vital information where it was needed. Not only did the nursing executive echelon meet together and establish therapeutic norms in interaction, but they also started meeting with groups of ward nurses. Their discussions were focused on the relationship of the new jobs to the starting of therapeutic activities. Thus for the first time, the problems generated on the ward were discussed on the ward, and were passed on for discussion, coordination, and action at the top of the nursing hierarchy.

To coordinate these nursing activities with medical and clinical activities, policy-making committees were formed, composed of the Clinical Director, two Senior Psychiatrists, the Superintendent of Nursing, her Deputy, and, when applicable, the Deputy Nursing Officer in charge of training.

THE DIDACTIC PROGRAM

SINCE many of our older nurses were unfamiliar with the content of modern psychological theory, a series of evening lectures was offered, and morning meetings were held to review papers, discuss problems, and evaluate changes. Didactic material included principles of psycho-dynamic psychiatry, but the emphasis was on social dynamics and inter-action patterns. The social process on the wards was the focus.

In the meantime, one of us[24] started a group therapy training seminar with the new Nursing Officers, and each of these in turn started one group therapy program among the admission ward patients, and one among chronic ward patients. Thus, through the manipulation of the interaction pattern in our hospital, we were able to make the new nursing program very shortly reach the patients.

THE EFFECTS OF THE CHANGES

THE success of the techniques we have described must be measured by the results, as indicated by better staff morale and improved patient care. For both of these there are accepted indices, but since the change is very recent these cannot yet be reported on.[25] Some immediate signs of success are discernible, however. We had expected that there might be a tempo-rary recession in morale as a result of the dislocation of old patterns, but sickness and absenteeism rates, staff resignations, and the frequency of secluding and restraining patients have remained stable. This encourages us to believe that not only have we avoided arousing the antagonism of the old-line staff but have perhaps aroused in them latent thera-peutic attitudes which have in turn provided them sufficient satisfaction to compensate for the dislocation of their accepted ways of doing things.

This impression is strengthened by spontaneous revolt among the male nursing staff against the entrenched practice of using them to relieve shortages in the cleaning and servicing departments. They actively de-manded relief from the non-nursing chores which they had always done, such as carting mattresses to and from the upholsterer. They complained that they were being hampered in their rehabilitative and nursing efforts by routine jobs of cleaning, sanitation, and maintenance which could in no way be considered therapeutic.

Evidence of increased integration of goals has appeared in increased cooperation between departments. For example, the Maintenance Depart-ment, through a spokesman, has suggested that some of their patient-laborers should be placed under the supervision of the nursing staff in order that these patients might have planned therapeutic occupations.

Increased patient activity, both in occupations and in recreation, is evident. We estimate an increase to date of twenty-five percent in the number of chronic patients who are occupied rather than idle. All admis-sion ward patients and many chronic ward patients are in group therapy. The significant point is that this raised level of activity comes from the initiative, planning, and action of the nursing staff. We believe that we have succeeded in some measure in creating a hospital less dependent for its therapeutic activities upon the initiative of the doctors, who are so few and so much less permanent in tenure than the nurses.

There have been some unexpected and negative consequences of the change, which are at present being worked out. On the female wards three of the four new male supervisors were well accepted, but the fourth man was rejected in a curious way. He was cut off from ward activities by the female staff and forced into an inactive role of making out charts in the office. After complaining for some time about it, he "went off sick" and remained so for a long period.

Another problem arose when a small group of men from the old chief nursing office suffered serious loss of status relative to the new members of the executive echelon. Their complaints were of "increased work," although there was no objective reason for this complaint. They had, however, inadvertently been put in the position of working more evening and night shifts than they had done before the reorganization; and not having to do shift work is an important sign of status in any organization which works around the clock.

In many ways, our task is far from completed; for instance, the training staff are only formally attached to the nursing program, and their functional attachment awaits the restatement of training goals and the changes in function which this will imply. There are, moreover, general signs of a tendency to slip back into old patterns; perhaps the most outstanding of these is the occasional automatic response of a nurse to a doctor: "I agree, Doctor, but the ward staff don't have time for that." This is the phrase which for years was used to maintain the *status quo* in the face of the attacks of interfering newcomers; it usually has little to do with time, and expresses mainly desire to resist. On the other hand, we have much evidence that most nurses are more involved in their work than they ever were before, and we have confidence that the hospital can never quite return, under the worst of circumstances, to where it was before.

In general, we worked with our nursing group as we would have with any other staff of workers, assuming that they would do a better job in the interests of our new therapeutic approach if they felt a sense of involvement in our goals and if their statuses were not called into question by the reorganization. Changing the attitudes and values of the staff was accomplished, as such changes are always accomplished, by interacting with norm-bearers in primary groups. We believe that our efforts have resulted in higher morale, in much improved patient care, and in a fundamental change in the basically pessimistic 'custodialism' of the nursing staff.

NOTES TO CHAPTER 49

1. J. A. C. Brown, *The Social Psychology of Industry*, Harmondsworth, Middlesex, Penguin Books, 1954.
2. Dr. Humphry Osmond.

3. The word *nurse* in this paper refers to psychiatric nurses trained in mental hospitals, not to registered nurses.

4. See in this connection: Edwin M. Lemert, *Social Pathology;* New York, McGraw-Hill, 1951; p. 417. Howard Rowland, "Friendship Patterns in the State Mental Hospital," *Psychiatry* (1939) 2:363-373.

5. Emile Durkheim, *The Division of Labor in Society;* Glencoe, The Free Press, 1947; see especially pp. 396-409.

6. See, in this connection, C. I. Barnard, *The Functions of the Executive;* Cambridge, Harvard Univ. Press, 1938.

7. D. G. McKerracher, "A New Program in the Training and Employment of Ward Personnel," *Amer. J. Psychiatry* (1949) 106:259-264.

8. See, for instance, Brown, reference footnote 1. See also: Kurt Lewin, "Group Decision and Social Change"; in *Readings in Social Psychology,* edited by Guy E. Swanson, Theodore M. Newcomb, and Eugene L. Hartley, New York, Henry Holt, 1952. George Homans, *The Human Group;* New York, Harcourt, Brace, 1950.

9. Reference footnote 1, p. 126.

10. Questioning revealed that no old-line supervisor could remember a doctor or training staff member ever asking his opinion on the grounds that his *long tenure alone* made his a valuable opinion.

11. For a discussion of this point, see, for instance, William Foote Whyte, "Corner Boys: A Study of Clique Behavior," *Amer. J. Sociol.* (1941) 46: 647-664.

12. This problem is discussed by Alfred H. Stanton and Morris S. Schwartz in *The Mental Hospital;* New York, Basic Books, 1954.

13. This program has been described by Derek H. Miller and John Clancey in "An Approach to the Social Rehabilitation of Chronic Psychotic Patients," *Psychiatry* (1952) 15:435-443.

14. The chief nursing officer on the male side was called the Chief Attendant, and on the female side the Head Nurse, titles which were dispensed with in our reorganization.

15. Reference footnote 12.

16. This will be discussed further in a forthcoming article in *Psychiatry*.

17. The relationship of the nursing service to the business hierarchy will be discussed in a forthcoming article in *Psychiatry*. We should like to mention here only that the tradesmen who attended to the maintenance of the hospital were on strained terms with the ward staffs. Without going into detail, we can say that this was another evidence of the low level of integration of the hospital structure. The tradesmen thought the nursing staff irrationally demanding; the latter considered the tradesmen to be arbitrary and withholding in their approach to ward needs.

18. This problem has been discussed by Jules Henry in "The Formal Social Structure of a Psychiatric Hospital," *Psychiatry* (1954) 17:139-151.

19. This move was suggested to us by Dr. Robert Hyde, Assistant Superintendent, Boston Psychopathic Hospital.

20. John Cumming and Elaine Cumming.

21. This point is discussed by Ralph Linton in *The Study of Man;* New York, Appleton-Century, 1936; see Chapter 8, "Status and Role."

22. We tried to avoid the pitfall of assuming that nursing is an avocation and that we were justified in asking more than a day's work for a day's pay.

23. This had resulted from the higher turnover among the female staff: approximately three years' seniority had been needed before promotion to the supervisor post on the female side, and fifteen years on the male. However, the trend is toward a greater proportion of women, and while the supervisors' posts will be overweighted with men in the near future, almost all senior posts will eventually belong to women, if this trend continues.

24. John Cumming.

25. Since this paper was written, more specific information has become available. Against a steadily rising admissions rate, there has been a slow but steady decline in hospital population. For 1954, the total admissions were 533, while the hospital population on December 31 of that year was 1,880. For 1955, the total admissions were 683, while the hospital population on December 31 was 1,809. By June 19, 1956, the population had further decreased to 1,790.

    While there have also been dramatic decreases in the use of isolation, restraint, and electroconvulsive therapy to control behavior, clear-cut conclusions are complicated by the fact that the tranquillizing drugs have come into use during the period under study. The use of these drugs does not, however, appear to be a factor in the decrease of hospital population; the initial drop occurred well before the use of any of these drugs, and, so far as we are able to determine, the later discharges of patients have not been attributable to these drugs.

ॐ

CHAPTER 50   The Reduction of Role
Conflict in Institutional Staff[*]

LLOYD E. OHLIN

CORRECTIONAL institutions throughout the United States today are undergoing a process of transformation. They are changing from relatively simple institutions with punishment, custody, and security as objectives to much more complex organizations with such difficult goals as vocational training, education, and personality and value reorganization superimposed on the older custodial expectations.

Such changes require fundamental redefinition of the roles which institution staff members must play, the relationships they maintain with one another and with their charges, and the various activities of their jobs. Basic conflicts are bound to occur in the process. Nowhere is this more clearly apparent than in the dilemma experienced by cottage staff, or houseparents, in juvenile institutions.

Older forms of correctional organization were based on highly authoritarian systems of relationship created to achieve the goals of custody and moral regeneration. The institutions operated through an established set of rules, the violation of which called for predictable forms of punishment. Classification took the form of grading offenders in terms of custodial risk.

In such systems the clarity of the objectives was matched by the clarity with which the role of houseparent was defined. He was expected to treat his charges all alike without regard to favoritism or special considerations arising out of individual need. Only in this way, it was thought, could order be maintained and justice be done. The houseparent who secured the greatest rule conformity by punishing rule violators consistently and impartially was evaluated most highly by the administration.

[*] Based on a paper presented at an advanced seminar in authoritative settings at the New York School of Social Work in December 1956.

Reprinted from *Children* (U.S. Department of Health, Education, and Welfare, Social Security Administration, Children's Bureau), 5 (1958), 65–69, by permission of the author.

SOURCES OF CONFLICT

THE current movement from this type of institution to one in which treatment interests are dominant precipitates a form of role conflict for cottage staff members. Where custodial requirements are minimized and treatment is stressed, they are faced with a dual obligation. On the one hand, they must continue to preserve order and discipline, since this is essential for keeping the institution going and a necessary precondition for effective treatment. On the other hand, they must individualize the handling of their charges according to the unique personality problems of each, so as to aid rather than hinder the therapeutic efforts of the professional staff.

The houseparent in this situation is confronted with a dilemma. The only way he knows of preserving order is to secure conformity to a set of rules which are clearly understood by all members of his cottage. His commitment to democratic values of equality and justice impels him to enforce these rules by punishing violators appropriately. However, he is told that punishment may often make treatment more difficult and that the proper attention to individual needs would make it unnecessary. He is torn between a recognition that an unenforced rule is no rule at all and an interest in abetting treatment efforts.

In most institutions the houseparent in this situation has little training and receives little help from his superiors. Ordinarily his supervisors are persons with greater seniority who have risen from the ranks. Frequently though they have learned to talk about the houseparent's role in terms of its treatment obligations they actually evaluate performance in relation to the houseparent's ability to run a quiet and orderly cottage. Constant referrals of disciplinary problems from a particular cottage mean to the supervisor that the houseparent is not doing a good job, an assumption based on the belief that if the houseparent understood his charges he could prevent disciplinary infractions. The effect of this type of evaluation is to reinforce the houseparent's control-treatment dilemma.

In most training schools too the houseparent receives little help from professional staff members. The latter work from a central office and carry caseloads of individuals scattered throughout the institution. They are not routinely faced with the problem of maintaining group control within a cottage. They tend to become isolated from the disciplinary responsibilities faced by the houseparent and to feel unprepared for and uninterested in intervention in problems of order or security. Interested primarily in therapy, they tend to assess the houseparent's disciplinary action in relation to its effect on the offending individual without regard to its consequences for other members of the cottage. They strongly resist the tendency of administrators and cottage staff supervisors to place primary emphasis on the maintenance of routine, order, and custody.

TRAPPED HOUSEPARENTS

THE inevitable result of these various expectations of the houseparent is to produce considerable conflict between staff units—cottage, supervisory or administrative, and professional. The confusion arising as to the division of authority and responsibility is quickly aggravated and exploited by those juvenile offenders who are most opposed to the institution's goals.

Faced with the necessity of maintaining order and discipline within the cottage without anyone outside knowing of trouble, many houseparents resolve the dilemma by forming friendships with the natural leaders among their charges.[1] Through conferring special privileges and rewards on these persons the houseparent secures their help in controlling the activities of his other charges. This makes him vulnerable to threats of disciplinary violation unless he meets the young people's demands for control over cottage affairs. Thus, the most rebellious and hostile young persons become dominant and exact conformity from their more tractable peers.

The houseparent who is trapped in such a situation is apt to struggle to regain control through occasional inconsistent attempts to enforce his rules to the letter by meting out severe punishments for infractions. There follows a rash of runaways, riots, property destruction, and other rebellious behavior which cannot be hidden. Soon the old order is restored.

A PROBLEM

I HAVE thus far described only a few of the major aspects of role conflict among houseparents in modern institutions for juvenile offenders. Many other pressures and counterpressures operate in this situation, and many variations exist in its form and content. I have, however, delineated the background against which one institution—the New York State Training School for Girls—set about trying to resolve the dilemma in the houseparent's problem of maintaining a quiet, orderly, but treatment-oriented cottage. The following description of this experiment and its effects derives from searching discussions with the superintendent and the members of his staff and from personal observation.

A change of management in this institution in 1953 resulted in a stronger emphasis on professional treatment goals. This transformation was directed by an experienced administrator trained in social work and committed to the values of his profession. He assembled a group of social workers to implement his program. The process of change was facilitated by a high turnover in cottage staff in the first year of the new administration, which made it somewhat easier to set up and enforce new role expectations for both cottage and professional staff.

In the beginning of the new administration the role definition for houseparents at this institution closely paralleled the conflicting expectations described in the preceding general statement. Cottage staff members were supervised by a small group of "seniors," former houseparents carrying supervisory and administrative functions. The seniors made up the institution's "home life department," a referral center for all administrative and disciplinary problems with which the cottage staff felt unable to cope. They provided the houseparents with guidance in carrying out their jobs and evaluated their performance. Though the seniors had acquired an ability to talk in terms of treatment objectives, their evaluations in effect reflected the degree to which the houseparents maintained discipline and order within the cottages and achieved an involvement of the girls in their care into institutional routines.

A houseparent's failure to fulfill these expectations was interpreted as a mark of incompetence and an evidence of inability to adopt a "treatment" orientation toward individual girls. As a result the houseparents felt that their requests to supervisors for support of disciplinary actions were handled in an inconsistent and unpredictable fashion. They could secure little guidance in resolving their basic dilemma—how to maintain a quiet cottage without interfering with individual treatment objectives when confronted with a group of girls largely hostile to the institution's purposes and informally organized for achieving their own ends.

The houseparents also felt unable to get full understanding of the nature of their problem or help in resolving it from the institution's social caseworkers. These formed a separate unit and were assigned their cases on an individual basis after the initial intake examination. Though they made numerous efforts to confer with the houseparents, communication centered about special problems of individuals. The caseworker was not prepared to deal with the houseparent's relationship with an individual girl as a part of the total context of relationships in the cottage. As a consequence the emphasis on solving problems of group discipline through understanding the treatment needs of the individual case only intensified the houseparent's basic conflict and sense of inadequacy.

The organizational arrangement made for division of responsibility and resulting confusion in regard to treatment and disciplinary decisions. It thrust back on the houseparent the basic task of resolving the role dilemma and tended to produce considerable hostility among the three staff units.

The caseworkers were not kept informed of what others were doing to persons in their caseload. They felt that both the seniors and the houseparents failed to work effectively because they were not basically oriented to treatment objectives and were not making an effort to understand and deal with the actions of individuals in relation to their treatment needs.

The houseparents' hostility reflected feelings of being abandoned and left to face their role problem without adequate understanding and support from their superiors. Under the pressure of day-to-day situations they resorted to devious ways of resolving their anxiety on an intuitive basis, but with relatively little success. Some retreated to a fixed and rigid set of rules which they enforced uniformly with whatever disciplinary tools were available to them within the cottage, while others developed cajoling relationships with their charges. In both cases the adjustment indicated an abandonment of treatment goals within the cottage.

The girls generally responded to this state of confusion and divided responsibility by manipulative tactics in which they sought to play various staff members off against one another. The houseparents shopped around for acceptable prescriptions in individual cases of misbehavior by presenting their problems alternately to the seniors and the caseworkers, frequently playing off one against the other. No single unit had access to all information known about an individual girl. Each unit pursued different objectives, collected different types of information about the girls, and arrived at different assessments of what ought to be done. The resulting intrastaff conflicts provided ample reason for the new administration to be concerned about their effect on both the custodial and treatment objectives of the institutions.

AN EXPERIMENT

IN THE face of these conditions the superintendent and his staff of social workers concluded that much more intensive and close supervision of cottage activities by professionally trained persons should be arranged. Consequently, the home life department and the casework service unit were combined into an integrated "cottage service department," with a trained social worker as director. Each social worker was assigned to supervise the activities of the girls and staff in two cottages.

At the present time 12 of the 16 cottages are under the authority of a social-work supervisor. The 4 remaining cottages are supervised by seniors, who also carry general troubleshooting responsibilities on the shifts to which they are assigned. The social workers have line authority over the staffs in the cottages under their direction and are expected to provide them with direct support and guidance in the handling of the girls. They are also required to provide treatment to the girls in these cottages.

This reorganization of the institution's structure firmly locates ultimate responsibility with the supervisors for all administrative, disciplinary, and treatment problems in the cottages. The social-work supervisors are also expected to provide routine evaluations and recordings on the work of the cottage staff. As a matter of practice, though they carry final authority for decisions, they make a conscious effort to share decision making with the cottage staff and to delegate authority to those houseparents who can safely and willingly assume it.

The effort is to present a united front to the girls of the cottage. Where a difficult disciplinary action has to be taken both the houseparent and the supervisor jointly present the decision to the offending girl. The supervisor refrains from openly countermanding inappropriate decisions reached by a houseparent but attempts to use the incident to prepare the houseparent for more adequate handling of similar cases in the future.

RELOCATION OF POWER

THE net effect of this change has been to relocate power in the hands of the supervisors, unify the authority structure, decentralize treatment and disciplinary decision-making to the various supervisory units, provide for professional attention to the total range of cottage problems, and preserve central control and continuity in the handling of individual cases.

The change was met by a considerable amount of initial hostility by houseparents. Some were afraid that they could not measure up to the social workers' expectations of them. Others felt that supervision by treatment-oriented social workers would challenge the disciplinary and treatment measures which they had evolved to maintain order. This hostility gradually turned to enthusiastic acceptance as the houseparents found that they could share the total range of their problems with their new supervisors, that the supervisors were ready to help with the complicated decisions posed by the necessity to carry on control and treatment simultaneously. The houseparents found that the basic role conflict with which they had been struggling was no longer theirs alone but could now be passed on or at least shared with the social-work supervisor.

Though the behavior of the girls improved during the integration experiment, the superintendent and his staff were primarily concerned with a "desire to increase, expand, and refine treatment techniques." In evaluating the results, consideration must be given to the experiment's effects on relationships among the staff, between the staff and the girls, and among the girls themselves.

THE RESULTS

INSUFFICIENT time has elapsed for more than a brief observation of the apparent consequences. Furthermore, resources have not been available to support the independent, objective, and probing type of inquiry which is necessary to assess fully the impact of this staff reorganization at all levels of institutional activity. The following indications, therefore, drawn primarily from staff observations and reactions, should be viewed only as preliminary and suggestive:

1. In the structural change which took place, what has happened to the customary institutional role relationships between social caseworkers and houseparents?

The clear reorganization and clarification of the location of power, authority, and decision making have resulted in a redefinition of the duties of the social worker, making them more nearly coextensive with those of the houseparent. Problems of administration, cottage organization, and discipline have been added to the social worker's traditional concern with individual treatment.

The cottage staff has passed on its role dilemma to the new social-work supervisor. The houseparents are no longer expected to have the competency derived from training, philosophy, or experience to solve the basic conflicts of cottage life. According to the social-work supervisors, as a result of these changed expectations the houseparents are happier, more amenable to suggestions, less rigid in their relationships with the girls, more interested in understanding the girls' treatment needs, more flexible in disciplinary decisions, and more concerned with acquiring a reputation for running a well-adjusted cottage.

This concern with campus reputation indicates an interest on the part of the houseparents in conforming to a developing unified concept of their role. It also shows some willingness to be identified with the girls in the cottage, as well as with the supervisor, in a shared conception of achieving a "good cottage."

In general, a very marked increase in staff harmony has occurred through the minimizing of the basic sources of misunderstanding, competition for control, and factional pursuit of different objectives inherent in the former separation of role obligations.

2. What has happened by virtue of this organizational change to the traditional social-work relationship with the client?

Clearly a stronger authority identification has been built into the new role of the social worker. The social workers have expressed the opinion that the new role offers greater opportunities for treatment than formerly and that there is nothing inconsistent in the various duties or activities of this role from the standpoint of treatment effectiveness. The social-work supervisors have said that the girls do not restrict the information they offer about their problems any more than they did formerly. In fact, the girls seek the social workers out even more frequently and volunteer personal information just as freely.

The social workers report, moreover, that new sources of information drawn from the affairs of cottage life have been opened to them which have enhanced their ability to deal with the individual girl's personal problems. They are now able to relate these problems more successfully to the content of the girl's daily experience in her cottage. This has minimized misrepresentations in the girls' communications to them and has permitted more effective use of the realities of cottage experience as a treatment resource.

The administration places special emphasis on the contribution of the staff reorganization to the staff's ability to present a united front to the girls in the institution. The opportunity for the girls to exploit communication failures between houseparents and social workers has been largely eliminated. The new structural arrangement has greatly facilitated the exchange and sharing of information, thus blocking the girls' ability to manipulate staff and exploit staff misunderstandings as a way of solving or evading personal problems.

3. What has been the effect of the staff integration on the girls' relationships with one another and on their subsequent careers?

An adequate answer to this question would require much more intensive investigation of attitudes and relationships among the girls. While it seems clear that the new system has helped to lessen manipulative and deviant responses on the part of the girls in their relations with staff members, it is not clear how much the decrease in misbehavior is simply due to the greater control potential in the new staff arrangement rather than to greater acceptance and internalization of staff values on the part of the girls.

Possibly the increased centralization of authority among staff has been matched by a greater centralization of relationships among the girls and a heightening of the effectiveness of their informal controls over one another's behavior. The relatively untroubled smoothness with which the new integration has occurred suggests that the basic accommodations which formerly existed between the girls' informal organization and the official system have not been materially altered. The ease with which "acting-up" members are being controlled to preserve a good-cottage reputation suggests the presence of a fairly well-structured arrangement of roles set by the girls themselves. This would mean that the girls' values as opposed to administrative values are still intact, thus blocking effective internalization of official values except by the "squares" who already have them anyway.

OBSERVATION NEEDED

THE foregoing comments on the girls' relationships can only be advanced as a possible hypothesis of the girls' response to staff integration. Currently no evidence is available to provide a clear picture. Observations point to many advantages in the new staff organization from an administrative point of view. It greatly facilitates the management and control of the institutional population. It seems to offer greater opportunities for staff to pool their observations to arrive at more realistic treatment decisions in individual cases. Information is not yet available, however, to determine whether the benefits to the staff in their handling of the girls and in their relations to other staff members are matched by benefits to the girls in their peer experiences and in their subsequent careers.

The results thus far appear to be highly desirable and to point to the general success of the experiment. They also suggest the need for more intensive observations of the girls' responses.

NOTE TO CHAPTER 50

1. Sykes, Gresham: The corruption of authority and rehabilitation. Social Forces, March 1956. (P. 257.)

CHAPTER 51   Techniques of Sociotherapy*

PAUL DANIEL SIVADON

A PSYCHIATRIC hospital, in order to fulfill its role as a therapeutic milieu, ought to be able to do three things: First, to offer to the new patient, whatever the nature of his illness, living conditions suited to his present level of functioning. Second, to obtain for him those circumstances which will permit him to establish satisfactory relationships with his physical and social environments, and to perfect progressively his ways of relating to them. Third, to furnish at all times, to the largest possible number of patients, opportunity for a means of developing toward social behavior more and more approximating the normal.

All of this requires certain conditions which may vary within limits from one hospital to another but which rest upon principles that are undoubtedly quite general. I should like to try now to elucidate these principles, basing my statements upon the experience of my own service at the Hospital of Ville-Evrard in Paris.[1]

THE PROBLEM OF STRUCTURE AND DIMENSIONS

IF THE patient is to benefit from the therapeutic milieu, it is necessary that he should participate in it, and therefore, that this milieu should be structured in such a way that it becomes a "social field." A social field exists if every modification in the behavior of an individual reverberates

---

* Reprinted by special permission of The William Alanson White Psychiatric Foundation, Inc., and the author from *Psychiatry*, 20 (1957), 205–210 (copyright by the Foundation).

This article, written in 1957, is based on the author's experiences while serving at the Hospital of Ville-Evrard in Paris. Since 1958, he has been applying these ideas to the construction of a three-hundred-bed psychiatric hospital (Institut Marcel Rivère, La Verrière, Le Mesnil-Saint-Denis near Paris), where these techniques are being further developed.

upon the whole and if every influence exercised upon this whole is felt by each individual.

In order to realize this goal, the population must be large enough to permit certain diversification of groups and activities and yet small enough to be perceived as a whole by each patient. A population of the order of 250 to 300 patients seems to fulfill these conditions if it is not reconstituted more than once a year—which means 300 admissions per annum. If the mobility of the population is greater than this, the number should be smaller. On the other hand, 500 or 600 patients are not too many if the number of admissions per year is only 100. These numbers are meant, of course, only as a general indication.

It appears to be important that this total population should be divided into groups of about thirty patients and that these groups themselves, in the course of various activities, be divided into subgroups of from 3 to 12 patients.

A pavilion system which allows for living units of 30 patients each, subdivided into smaller units of 5 to 6 cubicles and including small assembly rooms and workrooms, as well as a large common hall, fulfills these needs perfectly.

The architectural whole ought to be sufficiently dispersed to give each pavilion its individuality, but also sufficiently concentrated to preserve the unity of the "field." A circular arrangement or, still better, an oval built around the center of interest—workshops, restaurant, party rooms, and so on—seems to be a desirable one.

Any impairment of the higher nervous functions expresses itself in a difficulty in the integration of space—both physical and social space— and thus the reduction of distances as well as of social groups is one of the primary conditions for the patient's entrance into the "field."

It is desirable also that the population constituting the therapeutic milieu should be well balanced by the right proportions of patients of various categories and ages, and of staff of both sexes. It is in fact important that the patients should be able to find in the midst of the community small unisexual groups and larger bisexual groups in the restaurant, at recreation, and sometimes at work.

Certain particular arrangements do not contradict this general rule: one can provide for a club of adolescents or of elderly patients, but it is detrimental to specialize a whole service, and, above all, a whole hospital, in this way. The same thing holds for epileptics, who are quite well tolerated by other patients if they do not constitute more than 2 or 3 percent of the population, but who become totally unsocial if their proportion is higher.

A good therapeutic community should offer to the patient an opportunity to enter into whatever kind of group suits his condition, whether the group be large or small, homogeneous or heterogeneous. The community should also offer him an opportunity to devote himself to the kind of activity which will promote his need for expression or creation, whether this be in useful work or in play.

TECHNIQUES OF ADMISSION AND WELCOME

ONE of the critical moments in the community treatment is the admission of the new patient. Because of his emotional regression he needs to be accepted, or, still better, to be desired by the new society of which henceforth he will be a part.

In my service I have had for the past ten years a psychologist who functions as a hostess to welcome each new patient. She is the first person with whom the patient comes in contact. Instead of taking away his personal effects, she gives him whatever he needs—toilet articles, cigarettes, writing paper, and so on. She introduces him to fellow patients and to his attendants, nurses, and doctors. She tries immediately to make him feel that he is expected and that he is needed—that his help is needed, perhaps, with a party that is being prepared, with a game, or with some little service which no one else can render, such as repairing a bell or a broken chair. Then she shows him around the grounds and buildings, the workshops, the recreation rooms, the bar, and the hairdressing parlor. Very quickly, often by joining in a game, the patient makes the acquaintance of two or three comrades with whom he will soon work in the shops. The welcome is rounded out by introducing the patient at the weekly meeting of the committee of patients, of which I shall speak later.

Finally, each week there is a friendly gathering at which the medical director and the hostess meet with the patients who have been admitted during the past seven days. The medical director and hostess find out whether they are provided with everything they need and solicit their criticisms and their ideas. Then each patient is given a brochure with his own name printed on it, in which he finds, following some words of welcome, the principal kinds of information which are likely to relieve his anxieties. In particular, he finds there the name of his personal physician and of his social worker. He is also given some visiting cards with which he can introduce himself to his comrades and which he can place at the head of his bed or at the entrance to his cubicle.

Techniques of welcome such as these turn out to be of considerable importance in promoting the rapid participation of the new arrival in the community. In effect, the more one wishes the patient to allow himself to slip quietly into the communal life in a relaxed way, the more important it is to individualize him as much as possible and to make him feel himself to be a person. It is for this reason—namely, to counterbalance

the communitarian atmosphere into which he is plunged—that the patient
is at first seen privately by his personal physician, who gives him an appointment by a written personal invitation.

THE TECHNIQUES OF RESOCIALIZATION

FOR patients at very low levels of regression—catatonic schizophrenics in
particular—methods of progressive re-education are used which permit
development toward modes of social contact compatible with their integration in the communal life. This is often a long-term procedure lasting
two or three years, but sometimes it occurs within weeks or months. The
methods used are essentially psychomotor and expressive techniques. In
psychomotor re-education, ball play is chiefly used. At first the instructor
and the patient squat on the floor very close together in a confined space
and toss a ball back and forth to each other. Then a second patient and a
third are introduced. Finally the play is complicated by modifying the
position and the number of patients, by introducing a second ball, and by
interposing first an obstacle, later a screen, between the patient and the
instructor and so on.

Through this technique it is possible to mobilize more and more complex functional structures by enlarging the space within which the patient
can function adequately and by shifting from direct perception of an
object to its representation. In short, the patient passes from simple, near-
at-hand, immediate relations of the "physical" type to complex, distant,
mediate relations of the "mental" type.

At the same time, the patients are offered expressive activity with the
help of modeling clay or paints. At first they simply knead or mold the
clay directly with their hands, making small, rather unformed objects.
Then the objects become increasingly large and forms begin to appear.
Thus series of objects appear in which a whole symbolism can be found,
recalling that of prehistoric civilizations or mythological allegories, and
which develop finally into objects with a social character, such as vases
and various receptacles. In these, the archaic style is often quite striking.
Only later can the patients make designs which necessitate the use of an
instrument such as a pencil, paintbrush, or paper. The forms, which are
at first undifferentiated, become progressively more differentiated, become more complicated and lead finally to abstract designs. Here too, one
finds at first symbolic, archaic styles and themes before designs of normal
appearance emerge.

From this moment on the patients are ready to participate in the life
of the group, and their development is accelerated. This development,
however, is not necessarily steadily progressive. It is often interrupted by
standstills or even by transitory phases of regression. As a general rule, it

seems that all developmental progress is preceded by an oppositional phase, sometimes accompanied by aggressiveness.

TECHNIQUES OF ACTIVE SOCIOTHERAPY

IT IS precisely this notion of opposition and of aggressiveness which is the basis of the method employed. It is as if the developing energy of the patient, to the extent that it does not meet with an environment favorable to its utilization, is either repressed or externalized in the form of aggressiveness—whence the two types of morbid behavior which one must try to avoid: namely, passivity and inertia on the one hand, and violence and flight on the other. The aim is to promote the freeing and opening-up of latent energy, to avoid its repression, and to permit its investment in adaptive behavior.

Further, it seems that promoting the opposition of a group of patients to their environment facilitates the mobilization of the energy of each one and promotes the cohesion of the group, thus facilitating the resumption of interpersonal relationships. It is well known that in a group of normal but heterogeneous people who are seeking to establish good neighborly relations in an alien environment, the group's first step toward coherence consists in its opposition to its environment. Thus people in a compartment of a railroad car become irritated together against the poor organization of the trains, against the responsible personages in authority, against the government, and so on—whatever may happen in the United States, this is what happens in France.

At the hospital, our service is composed of six pavilions of about 45 patients each. The population of each pavilion meets once each week and is at these times invited—either by certain natural protesters among the patients or by the more or less insidious suggestions of the staff—to take cognizance of the imperfections of the service. Motives are seldom lacking—such and such an apparatus is not functioning; the meals are served too slowly; there is not enough diversion in the evening; and so on. Soon almost the entire group participates in the common protest, and many patients who have up to this point been isolated in their indifference emerge from their mutism. Now human relations have been established. It is only a question of improving upon all the inconveniences of which one is a victim. The premises, the staff, the doctors, the administration, and society in general bear the brunt of the criticism. Immediately the group tends to organize itself. A delegate is elected who is charged with the transmission of the protests to the authorities. Thus six pavilions furnish six delegates who constitute the Committee of Patients. This committee meets once a week with the doctor and the hostess. In the course of long discussions, which turn into real group therapy, the demands are studied, and the whole art of the sociotherapists consists of channeling the aggressive tendencies thus manifested toward useful activities. The first result obtained is that the doctors, attendants, and the nurses, by not seeking to suppress the opposition but by adopting an understanding attitude, find themselves included in the group, and the group is extended henceforth to include the whole of the service. An esprit de corps, the basis for a community atmosphere, is already created; it still remains, however, founded upon common opposition to the environment.

This is a delicate task but one which, by experience, is practically always crowned with success. It promotes the maturation of the protesting attitude into an objective one which is expressed in the need for concrete actualization. For example, there is general agreement about the boredom of the long evenings. The initial attitude is one of protest against the negligence of the administration. But, finally, a decision emerges to organize discussions, lectures, movies, and other diversions.

By this mechanism, the activities which are organized—whether in work or play—the expeditions, or the rules of discipline correspond to the needs of the patients, since they result from their own opposition to their situation. From this it follows that their aggressiveness is invested in an activity which they themselves have decided to undertake and is no longer manifested in the form of violence or the need to escape.

The more passive patients are led to participate in these common activities, which are not imposed upon them by authority but which are linked to the resumption of their social relations. Very frequently the patients experience, first of all, the need for modifying their physical environment. After having torn out the iron fences which formerly surrounded the grounds and planted flower borders, they are happy to repaint and decorate their day rooms. They build new workshops and a miniature golf course, and they organize parties and camping trips. All this is done in friendly collaboration with the staff and with the approval of the doctors. Of course, the ever renascent opposition expresses itself in the need to destroy what has previously been done so that something better may be constructed. It is to the extent that this real metabolism of energy is perpetuated—in opposition, aggressiveness, activity, and creation—that the hospital community remains alive and maintains its active therapeutic character.

Now it does indeed occur, because of the lack of emotional differentiation in the majority of patients, that the situation of being hospitalized is often confused with the state of being sick. To the extent that the patient does not oppose the situation of being hospitalized, he has a tendency to be satisfied with his state of being sick, and his chances of recovery are thus compromised. On the other hand, if he opposes his situation and if this opposition is not utilized therapeutically, it will be expressed by his refusal of treatment or even by escape or violence.

It does not seem to us to be possible to escape from this dilemma except by accepting the opposition—or even by promoting it—and using it as a therapeutic element. It becomes thus not only the foundation of the homogeneity of the group but also the motive power of sociotherapy and the regulator of the collective energy.

Thirty years ago Georges Dumas wrote that mental patients are not capable of social organization. It appears, however, that all they need in order to become capable of it is to have the possibility offered to them.

The criteria of success in this matter are simple: Success is evident when it is possible to leave doors unlocked, and the number of elopements decreases nevertheless; when violent reactions become the exception; when inertia gives way to adaptive activities; and, above all, when the average length of stay in the hospital decreases—when the patients no longer have a tendency to "install themselves" in their sickness and in the hospital. Finally, faced with a situation which is difficult for them, they learn to adopt an objective and pragmatic attitude, to give up their inhibited reactions and to control their aggressive tendencies.

GENERAL CONSIDERATIONS

IN THESE examples I have attempted to show that the therapeutic community, which a psychiatric hospital should be, derives its value from the fact that it is a balanced, living whole. Each patient must find in it an opportunity for adapting himself to a mode of life suited to his capacities, and he must be challenged constantly by other modes of life which will lead him to develop toward perfecting his adaptive capacities. This development is expressed particularly by a progressive integration of time and space, by an increasing capacity for personalization in the midst of larger and more heterogeneous groups, and by a change from infantile, dependent attitudes to adult, autonomous attitudes.

Thus the therapeutic milieu ought to offer the patient multiple possibilities. It seems difficult for the physician to foresee and to organize these. Even if it were possible, such an organization would always be experienced by the patient as coercion, to which he can respond only by passivity or aggression. It seems, then, more sure and more efficacious to allow the community to organize itself according to its needs. In order that this may occur, it is sufficient to keep in one's hands the motive power of the whole; that is to say, to maintain under therapeutic control the social organization of the group. Hospital sociotherapy ought to consist not in organizing activities, but in promoting their spontaneous appearance by mobilizing the energy of the group, channeling it, and balancing it so the entire group may be imbued with it.

No infallible method exists to achieve this, but there are certain conditions, especially of space and of density, which cannot be neglected with impunity.

NOTE TO CHAPTER 51

1. This is a public hospital admitting all mental patients—acute and chronic, certified or voluntary—of the masculine sex from a sector of the Department of the Seine which has a population of 700,000. For this population sector, the medicosocial team operates 6 outpatient clinics: one for children, four for adults, and one specifically for alcoholics. Whenever possible, the patients are treated through consultations in the outpatients clinics; if hospitalization is required, the same medicosocial team supervises the treatment. Upon discharge, the patients are followed up by means of outpatient consultations. The team also operates a club of ex-patients and a post-cure home for discharged patients who can no longer be integrated into their families. The hospital service itself has 250 beds. Their personnel comprises 1 chief doctor; 2 assistants; 8 residents; 1 psychologist; 2 psychiatric social workers; 1 vocational counselor; 120 nurses, of whom 20 are re-education monitors (in sports, work, play, and so on); and 3 secretaries. The staff for outpatient consultations consists of 6 doctors and 7 psychiatric social workers, half of whom belong to the hospital team.

Thanks to the intensive organization of the social life of the hospital, the doors of five out of a total of six pavilions are open. Aggressivity and agitation have practically disappeared. The rate of discharge is 83 per 100 admissions, and the average length of hospitalization for those discharged is about 120 days. The hospital admitted in 1956, 600 patients of all categories.

ॐ

CHAPTER 52   The Anticriminal

Society: Synanon*

LEWIS YABLONSKY

A READER of the *Terminal Island News* of April 12, 1962 would be
somewhat surprised to note an unusual statement called "Breaking
the Invisible Wall" authored by a former criminal and inmate of the
Federal Correctional Institution at Terminal Island, Calif., the U. S.
Public Health Service Hospital at Fort Worth, Texas, the State Prison of
Southern Michigan, and various juvenile reformatories. James Middleton,
the writer of the statement, had served a total of 15 years in these institutions. He has currently been clean of his past lengthy addiction and
criminal history for almost 3 years. Middleton is one of a group of seven
ex-offenders and former prisoners who go to the Terminal Island institution once a week to run group counseling sessions with about 25 addict
inmates. This is the way Middleton described this project in the Terminal
Island News:

As a former using addict and inmate of Terminal Island and other prisons,
having been free from the use of drugs for the past 2½ years by being a resident of Synanon House, I have been aware of the lack of communication between inmates and all those in positions of authority. Perhaps the most difficult
problem to overcome for penologists, prison officials, and others dealing with
the socially rejected group, the criminal, is the problem of establishing an area
of communication, some feeling of rapport. The convict, criminal, or any rebellious delinquent has a defiance of all authority. This he carried to such an extent
that he will refuse to even talk to a person in any position of authority whom he
considers his enemy. He takes the attitudes that "If you are not on my side, you
are against me."
On November 26, 1961, six members of the Synanon Foundation were invited

* Reprinted from *Federal Probation*, 26 (1962), 50–57, by permission of the author
and the journal. This article is derived from *Synanon: The Tunnel Back* (New York:
Macmillan Co., 1965; Baltimore: Penguin Books, 1967).

to the Terminal Island correctional institution by Chief Parole Officer Frank E. Saunders who believed that the Synanon approach might have something to offer the prisoners who had an addiction history.

Of paramount significance perhaps is the effect synanon has had in bridging this gap in communication between prisoner and official. This has been accomplished by the prisoners being encouraged to verbalize their problem, frustration, attitudes, opinions, etc., in the synanon.

Synanon is a form of intense group interaction. In these meetings synanites and inmate addicts, are encouraged to break down this wall and see their problems in a more realistic light. Part of the success of these meetings can be attributed to the fact that an inmate can often lie to the officials and get away with it, however with his fellow inmates, those who know him intimately, and can identify with his problems and his unsatisfactory reaction to them, he can't get away with as much. They see him as he is. Once a person has admitted his failures and inadequacies to others, and as an eventual consequence, to himself, he finds that he can discuss these things with almost anyone.

They are no longer deep, dark secrets which he must hide from others and himself. As Dr. Yablonsky, U.C.L.A. criminologist said, "This is the most significant break-through in the field of criminology in the past 50 years."

It is conceivable to me as an ex-inmate myself that someday Synanon could become an established part of the prison program throughout the United States.

THE BACKGROUND OF SYNANON

THE Synanon organization,[1] of which Middleton is a significant member, has been in operation about 4 years. As a result of exposure to this unique social system approximately 100 persons, most with long criminal and addiction records, no longer find it necessary to use drugs or commit crimes. Some Synanon residents have been clean of these deviant patterns for periods of up to 4 years.

This antiaddiction society originated with Charles E. Dederich, a former business executive, who had worked through an alcoholic problem and was motivated to transmit the forces which had led to his own recovery. A strong personality with characteristics of a charismatic leader, Dederich attracted to his residence by the beach in Ocean Park a coterie of alcoholics and drug addicts who found stimulating and interesting the lengthy philosophical discussions which he led. Many of these persons had no roots and moved into Dederich's "pad." Within a short time a small colony of about 15 addicts moved into the various apartments in the immediate area and emerged as the early core of the Synanon movement. At this point, about 6 months after its inception, there emerged an idealized assumption that no one was using drugs; although this fact was only true for about half the residents at the time.

Two incidents sharply changed the nature of this unusual collectivity and projected the evolution of a clean Synanon community. One was what later became known as the "big cop-out." This involved the open admission of occasional use by several key residents. Shortly after this episode the balance of power shifted over to a community with a majority of *clean addicts*. This new situation gave strength and credence to an anti-addiction, anticriminal ethos. To my knowledge, it was the first time anywhere that a group of nonprisoner ex-addicts could be found in one location.

By the summer of 1959 about 40 to 50 men and women, not using drugs, were living in a Synanon colony in one large building. The Synanon movement had become more established and aroused the interest of many significant professionals. *Time* magazine in its April 7, 1961 issue published an extensive description of the Synanon organization at that time.

S. S. HANG TOUGH

Early in August 1959, homeowners along the stylish Pacific Ocean beaches in Santa Monica, Calif., were dismayed to get a new set of neighbors: a bedraggled platoon of half a hundred men and women, who moved into a run-down, three story, red brick building that once was a National Guard armory. White and black, young and middle-aged, criminals and innocents, artists and loafers, the unlikely assortment shared one trait: they were narcotics addicts determined to kick their habit for good.

Scrounging lumber, paint and old furniture, the group converted the top floor of the armory into a barracks-style men's dormitory. They turned the second floor into offices, kitchen, dining hall and living room, and the main floor into women's sleeping quarters. Over the doors in the living room they hung their emblem: a life preserver with the words "S. S. *Hang Tough*," slang for "don't give up." . . .

Such was the formal dedication of Synanon House a self-run, haphazardly financed experiment in human reclamation whose success has been hailed by Dr. Donald Cressey, University of California at Los Angeles sociologist, as "the most significant attempt to keep addicts off drugs that has ever been made." . . . The technique was patterned roughly after the group-therapy methods of Alcoholics Anonymous. . . . Dr. Cressey describes the psychology: "A group in which Criminal A joins with some noncriminals to change Criminal B is probably most effective in changing Criminal A."

In the often brutally frank personal exchanges, the addicts slowly reveal themselves . . . and through daily contact with similarly beset persons are reinforced in their determination to quit narcotics permanently. Says the founder of Synanon House, 48-year-old Charles E. Dederich . . . , once an alcoholic but never a drug addict: "It is something that works."

The Synanon curriculum is divided into three stages. During the first phase, the emotionally shaken, physically weak addict gradually adjusts to his new surroundings. . . . During the second stage, the ex-addict works at a regular job on the outside, contributes part of his wages to the group, continues to live at the house. . . . In its final stage, Synanon sends its member out into society.

Interestingly, the potential of this type of an anticriminal society for modifying difficult offenders had been forecast by Professor Cressey in an article published in 1955 in *The American Journal of Sociology*.[2] His projection of the need for this treatment approach was based upon Sutherland's causal theory of criminal "differential association." Cressey logically speculated that, "if the behavior of an individual is an intrinsic part of the groups to which he belongs, attempts to change the behavior must be directed at groups."[3]

Cressey utilizing "differential association" theory as a diagnostic base projected the necessity for an anticriminal society to modify deviant behavior.

> The differential association theory of criminal behavior presents implications for diagnosis and treatment consistent with the group-relations principle for changing behavior and could be advantageously utilized in correctional work. According to it, persons become criminals principally because they have been relatively isolated from groups whose behavior patterns (including attitudes, motives, and rationalizations) are anticriminal, or because their residence, employment, social position, native capacities, or something else has brought them into relatively frequent association with the behavior patterns of criminal groups. A diagnosis of criminality based on this theory would be directed at analysis of the criminal's attitudes, motives, and rationalizations regarding criminality and would recognize that those characteristics depend upon the groups to which the criminal belongs. Then if criminals are to be changed, either they must become members of anticriminal groups, or their present pro-criminal group relations must be changed.[4]

Life in the Synanon anticriminal society revolves around a set of educational and apparently group therapeutic procedures developed by Dederich and the group of ex-addict leaders he had personally trained. Synanon by this time had many characteristics of an extended father-dominated family. As Dederich himself described it in an address before The Southern California Parole Officers Association:

> We have here a climate consisting of a family structure similar in some areas to a primitive tribal structure, which seems to affect individuals on a subconscious level. The structure also contains overtones of a 19th century family set-up of the type which produced inner-directed personalities. It is the feeling of the Synanon Foundation that an undetermined percentage of narcotic addicts are potentially inner-directed people as differentiated from tradition-directed people. A more or less autocratic family structure appears to be necessary as a pre-conditioning environment to buy time for the recovering addict.
>
> . . . The autocratic overtone of the family structure demands that the patients or members of the family perform tasks as part of the group. As a member is able to take direction in small tasks such as helping in the preparation of meals, housecleaning and so forth, regardless of his rebellion of being "told what to do," his activity seems to provide exercise of emotions of giving or creating which have lain dormant. As these muscles strengthen, it seems that the resistance to cooperating with the group tends to dissipate.

SYNANON GROUP THERAPY

THE daily program for the Synanon resident includes some type of work, a noon educational seminar, the synanon (a form of leaderless group therapy in which all residents participate three times a week), and daily interaction and communication with hundreds of "squares" (nonaddicts) from all walks of life who visit the building regularly.

The synanon, a form of group interaction vital to the overall approach, tends to be a unique form of aggressive leaderless nonprofessional group psychotherapy, directed by what Dederich has referred to as a Synanist. According to Dederich:

> The Synanist leans heavily on his own insight into his own problems of personality in trying to help others find themselves, and will use the weapons of ridicule, cross-examination, and hostile attack as it becomes necessary. Synanon sessions seem to provide an emotional catharsis and trigger an atmosphere of truth-seeking which is reflected in the social life of the family structure. The Synanist does not try to convey to another that he himself is a stable personality. In fact, it may very well be the destructive drives of the recovered or recovering addictive personality embodied in a Synanist which makes him a good therapeutic tool—fighting fire with fire.

This form of group therapy is ideally suited for the overall Synanon community. The group sessions do not have any official leader. They are autonomous; however, leaders emerge in each session in a natural fashion. The emergent leader tells much about himself in his questioning of another. Because he is intensely involved with the subject or the problem in the particular session he begins to direct, he is in a natural fashion the "most qualified" session leader for that time and place. In short, the expert of the moment may be emotionally crippled in many personal areas, but in the session where he is permitted by the group to take therapeutic command, he may be the most qualified therapeutic agent.

Synanon, as a side effect, trains persons to become a new brand of therapeutic agent in the correctional field. The system provides the opportunity for offenders to modify their own deviant behavior and then work with other offenders. In this context I view the phenomenon of Synanon at Terminal Island as a major break-through in the field of correction.

Although ex-offenders have been randomly used over the years in the processes of correction, Synanon provides a unique contribution. One can view the seven 2-year-clean Synanon participants in the Terminal Island project as a new type of "therapeutic agent" for dealing with the crime problem. Unlike most professional or ex-offender workers in the field the trained synanist has three levels of experience which uniquely qualify him for work with other offenders.

1. He has a lengthy history of criminal experience. He himself has made the "scene." He knows the crime problem in its many dimensions—at first hand.

2. At Synanon, this individual has deeply experienced the emotional upheaval of rejecting one way of life for another. He has "in his gut" gone through a resocialization process and knows something about the set of experiences and the pain involved in the transition.

3. He knows the Synanon social system. He has a subconscious conception of the processes at work for helping others and he is himself a functional part of this organization. He has been trained at "the Synanon College" for working with recalcitrant offenders.

This triad of experiences qualified the Synanist uniquely for the task at hand. Terminal Island inmates in the Synanon project know they are encountering in the Synanist a new breed of "treatment man." The Synanist is difficult to con or juggle out of position. The Synanist cannot easily be out-maneuvered from his zeal to point up a new direction in life to replace the roles of crime and addiction which he now views as wasteful and stupid behavior. This point of view of the Synanist seems to get across to the inmate seeking a noncriminal mode of existence.

Although the synanon form of group therapy is an important aspect of the method, the basic therapeutic force is the overall synanon social system. The best way to reveal this overall dynamic is to examine its impact on one successful resident.

FRANKIE: A CASE STUDY OF THE SYNANON SYSTEM[5]

FRANKIE, a 2-year-clean Synanon resident, first came to the author's attention in an unusual fashion. While listening to some tapes being played on the Egyptian King gang killing (an incident studied intensively by the author), Dederich detected a familiar voice. Hearing one King comment, "I kicked him in the head, it was the least I could do," Dederich remarked, "That sounds like Frankie." It was later confirmed that Frankie was this Egyptian King gang member's older brother. It was also determined that Frankie's early case history and violent gang life pattern paralleled his younger brother's. Frankie later turned to using and pushing drugs, a criminal career, which carried him to the Federal Correctional Institution at Danbury, Conn., New York City's Riker's Island Penitentiary, and finally Bellevue Hospital in New York City. As a result of his experience at Synanon, Frankie was at the time free and clear of drugs and violence for over 2 years.

"Frankie would never use a knife; unless he had to. Mostly with his fists he would beat a guy down and try to kill him right there. They pulled him off this big guy one time—he wouldn't stop punching him in the face." This was a casual observation made by Frankie's ex-"crime partner," the girl with whom he had lived for 5 years in New York. (She is also currently a successful resident at Synanon.)

Frankie's first reaction to Synanon was confusion. "The first thing they hit me with flipped me. This tough looking cat says to me—'there are two things you can't do here, shoot drugs or fight.'" Frankie said, scratching his head, "I was all mixed up—these were the only two things I knew how to do."

Frankie first came West at the insistence of his parents "to try a new way of life." "The family chipped in, gave me a plane ticket, and told me to straighten out or drop dead." He accepted the plane ticket they gave him and came West under the assumption of continuing his old way of life. In the Los Angeles situation he had trouble getting a good drug connection and stealing enough money to supply his habit. He heard about Synanon, and decided to try it. His initial motives were not pure. His thought was "to get cleaned up a little" and either get organized for a new onslaught on Los Angeles or steal enough to return to New York and his old criminal pattern. Something happened at Synanon to make Frankie stay "clean" for 2 years and later assume the administrative role of "coordinator" at Synanon.[6]

The Synanon environment was interesting and exciting for Frankie. There were, in the addicts' jargon, "lots of hip people." Jimmy the Greek, who at 48 had been an addict for 20 years and a criminal and con-man for over 30 years[7] and Jimmy Middleton who now ran the kitchen at Synanon. In the kitchen Frankie received his first job scouring pots and pans and mopping floors. According to Frankie, Jimmy M. could not be conned or manipulated out of position like the therapist Frankie had encountered at Riker's Island Prison. Jimmy M., of course, knew the score and to him Frankie with all his exploits was a "young punk," who could give him no trouble. "I've met kids like this all my life—in and out of the joint."

According to Frankie, "I hated this '. . . .' for no good reason. I used to sometimes sit and plan ways to kill him." When Frankie wanted to fight Jimmy over a disagreement about work (no fighting allowed at Synanon) Jimmy laughed and told him if he wanted to fight he would be thrown out of Synanon.

The usual prison situation was reversed and confusing to Frankie. In the "joint" (prison) if Frankie got in trouble confinement became increasingly severe with the "hole" (solitary confinement) as an end point. At the Bellevue Hospital psychiatric ward where Frankie had also "done time" it was a straight-jacket. What made Frankie remain, even behave in order to stay at Synanon with its open door?

The fact that Frankie was exported from New York to Los Angeles was a significant force initially in keeping him at Synanon, as he stated it: "At times I felt like splitting (leaving), then I thought it will be hard to make it back to New York. I didn't know Los Angeles and I was afraid to make it out there—cause I didn't know the people. Synanon was better than anything else I could do—at the time."

Also, Synanon House was on the beach. The meals were good. In the evening many ex-addict top musicians would play cool jazz.[8] Also there were, according to Frankie, "broads to dance with and get to know." But highly important in this antiaddiction, antidelinquency society there were others who understood him, had made the same "scenes" and intuitively knew his problems and how to handle him. He respected people he could not con. He belonged and was now part of a "family" he could accept.

At Synanon Frankie could also make a "rep" without getting punished or locked up. In prison, the highest he could achieve in terms of the values of "his people" was to become "King" of the sociopathic inmate system, acquire a "stash" of cigarettes, obtain some unsatisfactory homosexual favors, and land in the "hole." In the "inmate system" of Synanon he could achieve any role he was "big enough of a man" to acquire and this carried the highest approval of his fellows. He could actually become a *director* in this organization—which was now in the national spotlight.[9] Articles on Synanon had been published in national magazines like *Time, Life,* and *Nation,* and were coming out daily in the press. For the first time in his life, Frankie was receiving status for being clean and nondelinquent.

Of course, when he first arrived at Synanon, Frankie attempted to gain a "rep" by conniving and making deals in accord with his old mode of relating. He was laughed at, ridiculed and given a "hair-cut" (a verbal dressing down) by other "old-time con men" members of the organization. He was accused of "shucking and sliding" (simply not performing adequately). The old-time Synanists were ferocious about keeping the organization, which had literally saved their lives and given them a new life status, operating smoothly.

Frankie found that "rep" was acquired in this social system (unlike ones he had known) by truth, honesty, and industry. The values of his other life required reversal if he was to gain a "rep" at Synanon. These values were not goals *per se* which someone moralized about in a meaningless vacuum; they were means to the end of acquiring prestige in this tough social system with which he now intensely identified.

In the small *s* synanons, three nights a week Frankie participated in a form of leaderless group psychotherapy. In these synanons the truth was viciously demanded. Any system of rationalizations about past or current experience were brutally demolished by the group. There was an intensive search for self-identity.

In the process the individual attempted to learn what goes on beneath the surface of his thoughts. For Frankie this was the first time in his life that he discovered others had some idea about what he was thinking underneath. He had individual group therapy in prison—but there he could "con" the therapist and most important, "I said what I thought they wanted to hear so I could hit the street sooner."

Most important Frankie began to get some comprehension of what others thought in a social situation. The fact of empathy or identifying with the thoughts and feelings of others became a significant reality.

Frankie was at first empathic in his usual pattern of sociopathic self-centered manipulation. However, a new force was introduced into the situation—he began to care about what happened to others at Synanon. This was at first selfish. Synanon was for him a good interesting way of life. He had identified with the system and learned "gut level" that if any Synanon member failed, he too was diminished and failed. In Cressey's words which Frankie learned to quote (since after all Professor Cressey was a friend of his) "When I help another guy, it helps me personally."

In the status system, Frankie's rise to the role of coordinator was not quick nor easy. He moved from the "dishpan" to serving food at the kitchen counter.

After several months he was allowed to work outside on a pickup truck which acquired food and other donations. With two other individuals who worked with him on the truck a group decision was made one day "that one shot wouldn't hurt." One individual knew a "connection" on the route. They went to his home. All they could get were some pills.

When they arrived back at Synanon their slightly "loaded" appearance immediately became apparent to the group ("they spotted us right away") and they were hauled into the main office and viciously (verbally) attacked to tell all ("cop-out") or get out of the building. A general meeting was called and they were forced to reveal "all" before the entire group.[10] Frankie was back at work on the dishpan that evening.

Such "slips" often come out in the synanon. In a sense, in addition to other forces of growth from the synanon it serves as a form of "first-aid" therapy. If anyone reveals a minor "slip," the personal wound is examined and cleaned up by the group before a serious act of misbehavior occurs. (The synanon situation has some of the characteristics of an underground organization operating during wartime. If any member "falls," it may entail the destruction of the entire organization.)

The norms of synanon society are the reverse of the criminal code. On one occasion Frankie, with two other members of Synanon, went for a walk into town. One individual suggested buying a bottle of wine. (No drinking is permitted). The other two (including Frankie) smashed the idea. However, no one revealed the incident until 2 days later it came up in a synanon. The group jumped hardest on Frankie and the other individual who did not reveal the potential "slip," rather than on the transgressor who had suggested the wine. Frankie and the other "witness" were expected to report such "slips" immediately, since the group's life depended on keeping each other "straight." For the first time in his life Frankie was censured for *not squealing.* The maxim "thou shalt not squeal" basic to the existence of the usual underworld criminal culture was reversed at Synanon and just as ferociously sanctioned. An individual could get "kicked out" of Synanon for *not* being a "stoolie."

The rule of no physical violence was at first extremely difficult for Frankie to grasp and believe, since his usual response to a difficult situation would be to leap fists-first past verbal means of communication into assault. As a result of the synanons and other new patterns of interaction, Frankie's social ability for communication increasingly minimized his assaultive impulse. Although at first he was controlled from committing violence by the fear of ostracism, he later no longer had a need to use violence since he now had some ability to interact effectively. He could express himself with a new form of communication on a nonviolent, verbal level.

On occasion Frankie would regress and have the motivation for assault —but the system had taken hold. In one synanon session I heard him say, "I was so . . . . mad yesterday, I wished I was back at Rikers (prison). I really wanted to hit that bastard Jimmy in the mouth."

Frankie had a sketchy work record prior to Synanon. Other than gang fighting, "pimping," armed robbery, pushing heroin, and some forced work in prison, he seldom acted in any role resembling formal work. His theme had been "work was for squares." He learned how to work at Synanon automatically as a side effect of his desire to rise in the status system. He also learned as a side effect of the work process, the startling fact "that talking to someone in the right way made them do more things than belting them."

Frankie's most recent position involves the overall supervision of Synanon's number two building. Here 12 mothers (ex-addicts) in residence at Synanon live with their children. Frankie supervises a budget, the care and feeding of the establishment and the inevitable daily counseling of his "wards." Although it is not apparent on the surface of his efficient administration, Frankie beneath maintains a state of personal amazement about his new social role in society.

As a consequence of living in the Synanon social system, Frankie developed an increasing residual of social learning and ability. His destructive pattern of relating to others withered away because it was no longer functional for him within this new way of life. Synanon developed his empathic ability, produced an attachment to different, more socially acceptable values, and reconnected him adequately to the larger society within which Synanon functioned as a valid organization.

PRINCIPAL FORCES AT WORK IN THE SYNANON SOCIETY

Involvement. Initially, Synanon society is able to involve and control the offender. This is accomplished through providing an interesting social setting comprised of associates who understand him and will not be out-maneuvered by his manipulative behavior.

An Achievable Status System. Within the context of this system he can (perhaps, for the first time) see a realistic possibility for legitimate achievement and prestige. Synanon provides a rational and attainable opportunity structure for the success-oriented individual. He is no longer restricted to inmate status; since there is no inmate-staff division. All residents are staff.

New Social Role. Synanon creates a new social role which can be temporarily or indefinitely occupied in the process of social growth and development. (Some residents have made the decision to make Synanon their life's work.) This new role is a legitimate one supported by the ex-offender's own community as well as the inclusive society. With the opening of new Synanons and increasing development of projects like the one at Terminal Island, Synanon trained persons are increasingly in demand. Since the Synanon organization is not a hospital or an institution, there is no compulsion to move out of this satisfying community.

Social Growth. In the process of acquiring legitimate social status in Synanon the offender necessarily, as a side effect, develops the ability to relate, communicate and work with others. The values of truth, honesty, and industry become necessary means to this goal of status achievement. After a sufficient amount of practice and time, the individual socialized in this way in a natural fashion develops the capability for behaving adequately with reference to these values.

Social Control. The control of deviance is a by-product of the individual's status-seeking. Conformity to the norms is necessary in order to achieve. Anomie, the dislocation of goals and means, becomes a minimal condition. The norms are valid and adhered to within this social system since means are available for legitimate goal attainment.

Another form of control is embodied in the threat of ostracism which becomes a binding force. After being initially involved in Synanon, the individual does not at the time feel adequate for participation in the larger society. After a sufficient residue of Synanon social living has been acquired the individual no longer fears banishment; however, at the same time he is then better prepared for life on the outside (if this is his choice). He no longer fears ostracism and may remain voluntarily because he feels Synanon is a valid way of life for him. In Synanon he has learned and acquired a gratifying social role which enables him as a "coordinator" or a "director" to help others who can benefit from Synanon treatment.

Other forms of immediate social control include ridicule ("hair-cuts," the "fireplace") and the synanon sessions. The individual is required to tell the truth in the synanon. This also regulates his behavior. Real life transgressions are often prevented by the knowledge that the individual's deviance will automatically, rapidly, and necessarily be brought to the attention of his community within the synanon session. He is living within a community where others know about and, most important, are concerned with his behavior.

Empathy and Self-Identity. The constant self-assessment required in his daily life and in the synanon sessions fosters the consolidation of self-identity and empathy. His self-estimation is under constant assessment and attack by relevant others, who become sensitive to and concerned about him. The process provides the opportunity for the individual almost literally "to see himself as others do." He is also compelled as part of this process to develop the ability to identify with and understand others. A side consequence is the development of self-growth, social awareness, the ability to communicate and empathic effectiveness. When these socialization processes are at work and take hold the youth becomes reconnected with the legitimate society and no longer finds it necessary to use drugs or assume a deviant role.

SYNANON'S FUTURE

FROM its unusual beginnings the Synanon Foundation has emerged as a highly efficient organization. The Foundation has federal tax exempt status and is a corporate entity in the State of California. The State Legislature passed and the Governor signed into law The Petris Bill on June 15, 1961, officially sanctioning Synanon as a "Place" for rehabilitating drug addicts.[11]

Synanon, over the past year, as a partial consequence of donations and the earning power of its residents, has rented four buildings with a total rental of over $1500 a month. Although its budgeting is tight, comparable to other nonprofit organizations, it has met all of its financial obligations as a result of community support. The organization over the past year has sustained approximately 85 residents in food and clothing, and has entertained approximately 19,000 guests (mostly professional visitors). In addition to the Terminal Island project a Synanon educational and addiction-prevention program has involved most of the 100 Synanon members in over 400 speaking engagements delivered to business, professional, religious, youth, and college and university groups. One evening a week about 40 nonaddicts from all segments of society participate in the so-called "Square Synanons." Here the variety of human problems are examined through utilization of the Synanon method involving Synanon residents mixed with "squares." This interaction and cross-fertilization of ideas and insights appear to be of benefit to all.

As a social science research center Synanon is unique. In this open-door environment run by ex-offenders themselves, persons with long addiction and criminal background freely provide important data unavailable in the usual custodial setting. Synanon thus enables the systematic gathering of much useful information about crime, addiction, and the solution of these problems.

The Synanon approach which has emerged under the creative and capable leadership of Dederich and his uniquely trained staff of directors as an effective anticriminal and antiaddiction society, also involves an organization of distinguished citizens from all walks of life called "S.O.S." or Sponsors of Synanon. This supportive organization has a national membership of over 600 persons who donate money, goods, and services. They are currently launching a building program for an ideal Synanon community.

The organization is naturally committed to expansion. Synanon-trained personnel of the type carrying out the program at Terminal Island will no doubt shortly be utilized as the core staff for Synanon Houses planned for other communities. Each new establishment has the potential for "cleaning-up" another hundred offenders.

As viewed by its founder, Charles Dederich, Synanon is still in its infancy. The fact of 100 individuals with long addiction and criminal histories currently clean attests to its effectiveness. However, Synanon, as a social movement or community way of life, appears to have possibilities beyond exclusive application to the addiction problem. As Middleton commented at the outset: "It is conceivable to me as an ex-inmate myself that someday Synanon could become an established part of the prison program throughout the United States."

NOTES TO CHAPTER 52

1. The name Synanon was derived from the slip-of-the-tongue of a confused addict attempting to say seminar. It was adopted because it is a new word for describing a new phenomenon.
2. Donald R. Cressey, "Changing Criminals: The Application of the Theory of Differential Association," *American Journal of Sociology*, September 1955, pp. 116-120.
3. *Ibid.*, p. 117.
4. *Ibid.*, p. 118.
5. This section is partially derived from a recent volume by the author, *The Violent Gang* (New York: The Macmillan Company, 1962).
6. A coordinator works a 4-hour shift, answering phones, catering to visitors and generally handling the House's business as it emerges. It requires some ingenuity and administrative ability.
7. Jimmy's personal statement in the *Synanon Issue* of the *Terminal Island News* further reveals his criminal background and current view of life: "My addiction history goes back to when I was 12 years old (I am close to 50) but up until the time I came to Synanon, 31 months ago, I never knew what it was to be "clean" on the streets. I have done just about everything illegal to obtain money; work was not a part of this life, for I could not

support a habit working. I have spent almost 10 years in county jails, the Lewisburg federal penitentiary, and chain-gangs. I can go so far as to say that I had never met a 'clean' dope-fiend until I came to Synanon. . . .

"I have been a resident of Synanon for 31 months. I plan on staying for some time to come. For the first time in my life I like what I am doing—Synanon is growing and I am part of it. There is a group from Synanon attending meetings at Terminal Island every week, for the past 4½ months; I am project director of this group. There are plans in the making to start Synanon meetings on the women's side at Terminal Island—and eventually, men and women together. I am sure with the cooperation we have been getting this plan will come about in the near future."—James (Greek) Georgelas.

8. The Synanon Band recently produced a widely acclaimed professional record album, appropriately called: *Sounds of Synanon*.

9. There are currently 8 directors of the Synanon Foundation. This is the highest and most respected status level of achievement in the organization.

10. This process known as a "fireplace" may be called at anytime, day or night. The "transgressor" is placed at the fireplace in the main living room in front of all other residents. They are ridiculed into an open-honest revelation of their "offense." The group may then decide to evict or give the individual another chance.

11. The Petris Bill especially passed for Synanon is here presented in full:

Assembly Bill No. 2626 (State of California). An act to amend Section 11391 of the Health and Safety Code, relating to narcotic addiction.

The people of the State of California do enact as follows:

Section 1. Section 11391 of the Health and Safety Code is amended to read:

11391. No person shall treat an addict for addiction except in one of the following:

(a) An institution approved by the Board of Medical Examiners, and where the patient is at all times kept under restraint and control.

(b) A city or county jail.

(c) A state prison.

(d) A state narcotic hospital.

(e) A state hospital.

(f) A county hospital.

This section does not apply during emergency treatment or where the patient's addiction is complicated by the presence of incurable disease, serious accident, or injury, or the infirmities of old age.

Neither this section nor any other provision of this division shall be construed to prohibit the maintenance of a place [Synanon] in which persons seeking to recover from narcotic addiction reside and endeavor to aid one another and receive aid from others in recovering from such addiction, nor does this section or such division prohibit such aid, provided that no person is treated for addiction in such place [Synanon] by means of administering, furnishing, or prescribing of narcotics. The preceding sentence is declaratory of pre-existing law. Every such place [Synanon] shall register with and be approved by the Board of Medical Examiners.

The board may inspect such places [Synanons] at reasonable times and, if it concludes that the conditions necessary for approval no longer exist, it may withdraw approval. Every person admitted to such a place [Synanon] shall register with the police department of the city in which it is located or, if it is outside of the city limits, with the sheriff's office. The place [Synanon] shall maintain its own register of all residents. It shall require all its residents to register with said police department or sheriff's office and, upon termination of the residence of any person in said place [Synanon], it shall report the name of the person terminating residence to said police department or sheriff's office.

CHAPTER 53   The Interpersonal Behavior
of Children in Residential Treatment[*]

HAROLD L. RAUSH, ALLEN T. DITTMANN
AND THADDEUS J. TAYLOR [1]

THIS report is concerned with the interpersonal behavior of a small
group of disturbed children and with changes in their behavior over
a period of a year and a half in a residential treatment program. In
general, the study was exploratory, oriented toward description and a
search for order in complex behavioral events, toward the evaluation of
behavioral change in treatment, and toward the evaluation of a method
for observing and coding interpersonal behavior.

TOWARD DESCRIPTION

THE source of data was spontaneous behavior as it appeared in the daily
activities of six "hyperaggressive" or "acting-out" boys. To some extent,
then, the paper presents a naturalistic study of the social behavior of a
small group of children. Studies of small groups have mostly centered on
the social interactions of adults in task-oriented situations (Bales, 1950;
Hare, Borgatta, & Bales, 1955), whereas interest in the social behavior of
children has generally focused on specific variables in relation to more or
less specific hypotheses (Baldwin, 1955). The work of Barker and Wright
(1954) on the ecology of children's behavior in a small Midwestern town
is an exception to the trend. The methods of the present study differ from
those of Barker and Wright—a difference in part guided by doubts about
the usefulness of a level of approach that is so strictly phenomenological.
But there is a major shared value orientation: that it would be useful to
have objective and manageable descriptions of the quality, frequency, and

[*] Reprinted from the *Journal of Abnormal and Social Psychology*, 58 (1959), 9–26,
by permission of the authors and the *Journal*.

[772]

intensity of everyday behavior for all sorts of groups and for all sorts of situations. Such a statement is not an exhortation to random empiricism. Description is not necessarily atheoretical, and an interest in descriptive patterns of everyday behavior is not necessarily antithetical to the testing of hypotheses about specific variables. To some extent, there is, however, a question of order. Anthropologists, for example, have learned that one cannot legitimately interpret specific actions in isolation from other actions or in isolation from patterns within a culture, and they have learned how misleading isolated hypotheses may prove when contextual information is lacking. Adequate psychological descriptions of the everyday behavior of various subgroups, theoretically or pragmatically defined, would constitute a step toward the formulation of specific hypotheses. Such descriptions would also constitute a step toward a general ethology of human behavior.

The group under study was small, and it was a rather special one in the sense that it was selected for a particular syndrome to which considerable social interest accrues in relation to delinquency and which is recognized as difficult to treat clinically. As a group, it was not task-oriented, nor had it come together through the common interests of its members. The environment was also a special one—even if only because psychiatric institutions are not typical of children's living arrangements. Because of the selection process, the children were rather homogeneous, and they lived together under the protection, supervision, and control of a professional staff in the rather homogeneous environment of the institution. The limitations of the present study are, however, perhaps not so much in the special characteristics of the subjects or of their environment, but rather in the lack of comparative data.

TOWARD EVALUATION OF CHANGE

THE second aim is toward the evaluation of treatment change, not as measured by ratings or by tests, but rather as manifested in the interactions of everyday life. It was, of course, expected that the children would show some improvement in their overt interpersonal relations. Findings of improvement would be consistent with clinical impressions about most of the children. But long-term clinical work has its hazards, one of which is that changes, if and when they occur, are often so gradual that an awareness of the similarities and contrasts between the then and the now is easily lost or distorted. A more formal method would exercise a discipline on both clinical wishes and clinical doubts, while perhaps also pointing to areas and problems which were less clinically obvious.

Clearly, the study is not definitive in relation to treatment of the "acting-out" child or in relation to any of the specific variables that enter into the residential treatment situation. Critical tests of treatment benefits can most relevantly be made outside the framework of a therapeutically focused environment; critical tests would involve variables in addition to those overt aspects of interpersonal behavior which are investigated here; and finally, critical tests would involve adequate controls. What can be fruitfully investigated is whether a group of children change systematically in their ordinary interactions. Given evidence of such changes, examination may be made of their relevance to treatment aims. From the viewpoint of therapeutic concerns, the possibilities of favorable modification in the behavior of a clinically difficult subgroup might be shown, and perhaps the clinical worker may be encouraged in his efforts.

TOWARD EVALUATION OF THE METHOD

At the least, a method for evaluating interpersonal behavior and behavioral change was studied. The method involved multiple observations of children in naturalistic settings and the coding of these observations by a scheme which was originally devised for studying the group behavior of adults (Freedman, Leary, Ossorio, & Coffey, 1951; Leary, 1957). A partial proof of the method lies in its success or failure in demonstrating expected phenomena. That is, one aspect of the study is related to a question of construct validity (Cronbach & Meehl, 1955). To the extent that the approach achieves the differentiations that might reasonably be expected of it, the method offers promise for investigations of other groups in other environments.

METHOD

THE CHILDREN AND THE INSTITUTION

The six boys were the total patient population of a hospital ward which they entered when they were from 8 to about 10 years old. There was—and still is—no diagnostic category into which they fit easily. In general, their pathology and their actions were beyond the realm of the typical childhood neuroses, yet at the same time they did not represent childhood psychoses. The behavior of the children was characterized by such overwhelming aggressiveness that they could not be tolerated by community, schools, foster parents, or parents. Four boys had been referred to courts for destructive behavior, and three of these had been sent to a reformatory shortly before their admission. The two children who had not come to the attention of the courts had been excluded from several schools because of their antisocial actions. There was usually a history of multiple contacts with social agencies, but outpatient clinical treatment and special school programs seemed to be of little use, at least in the long run, in these cases. None of the boys were "gang" delinquents. Their problems seemed rather a function of intense personality disturbances with a marked deficiency in ego controls, particularly where aggression was concerned. They were children such as Redl and Wineman (1957) have described, children often called hyperaggressive or "acting-out," although neither of these terms is ideal. All six were physically healthy, and so far as could be judged from psychological and psychiatric examinations, they were of normal intelligence and showed no evidence of gross brain damage. They came from socioeconomic milieux ranging from lower-lower through lower-middle class, with two children from lower-middle class homes and the rest lower in socioeconomic status.

Throughout the time of these investigations, the children lived on the ward. Their program was planned intensively and minutely. All were seen approximately four hours weekly in psychotherapy; their schooling, which took place adjacent to the ward, was with specially trained and experienced teachers and clinicians; ward programing and the handling of clinical problems of daily living were closely planned and organized, again by people with considerable experience with disturbed children. Most of all, considerable time and effort were devoted to the coordination and integration of the various levels of treatment. This brief description, though markedly oversimplified, is relevant for interpreting the results of the study.

The present report examines the interpersonal behavior of the children at two phases. When the initial series of observations was made, two of the children had been at the institution between three and four months, and the other four had been there nine or ten months. One may suppose, then, that they knew each other fairly well and that they were familiar with the general pattern of living within the ward. Their ages, at the start of the study, ranged from 8 years, 11 months, to 10 years, 11 months, with the median age at 10 years. The second series of observations was made some 18 months later.[2]

THE OBSERVATIONS

IN EACH phase of the study, each of the six children was observed twice in each of six settings. There were, thus, a total of 144 observations, 72 in each phase. A number of observers were involved, but each single observation was made by a single observer.[3] The observer would go over to the ward or to the gym or to the outdoor play area, for example, to observe a particular child according to his assignment of children and settings. He would concentrate on that particular child, trying to follow as much as was possible the transactions between this child and other children or adults. But he would also try to note what went on among the other children within the locus of observation. The observer did not take notes; he would gauge the length of his observation to the amount of the specific activity that he could remember. This meant that the time period of observation was highly variable. If there was, for example, an extremely rapid interplay of behavior, the observation time might be as brief as several minutes; on the other hand, it might extend, if the interchanges were few and far between, to as much as 20 minutes or a half hour. The mean time for an observation was about 8 minutes. An analysis of variance indicated that differences in observation time allotted to either individual children or to different settings were not significant.

After leaving the setting, the observer would immediately dictate onto tapes or Audograph discs a factual, descriptive report of his observation. Observers were cautioned to focus on interaction, to be as specific and concrete as possible, and to avoid psychological terms and inferential conclusions. In general, observer training required only several practice trials.[4] The protocols of the observations resemble those obtained by Barker and Wright (1954), though their descriptions were undoubtedly more fully detailed.

THE SETTINGS

DIFFERENT situations—for example, even different games—exert a pull for different behaviors, and they differ in the kinds of behavior they sanction, positively encourage, or inhibit (Redl & Wineman, 1957). The opportunity rarely exists to study behavior in a representative variety of settings, to relate behavior to what Brunswik (1947) has called "the ecology of environmental events." A residential treatment center provides such an opportunity. The design of the study utilized a *somewhat* representative sampling of the kinds of activities around which the children lived their lives so as to allow investigation of the relevance of different settings for interactive behaviors. This aspect of the study will not be discussed here, but the settings should be noted: (*a*) breakfast—an early morning observation; (*b*) snacks in the period just before the children went to bed at night; (*c*) other mealtimes; (*d*) structured game activities, ranging from cards to basketball;[5] (*e*) unstructured group activities where the specific external task structure was minimal—for example, social conversations; and (*f*) an arts-and-crafts period. Since one phase of the study occurred during the summer, when school was not in session, this last setting was utilized as an approximation to an instructional situation. Since selection was in terms of kind of activity, the data are not representative of time as a time sample would be; the nature of the settings did, however, insure that various times of the day were included. Relevant settings omitted from the study were psychotherapy, other two-person group situations, where the presence of an observer might be intrusive, and school situations other than arts and crafts.

THE CODING SCHEME

THE search for methods for describing human interactions and the problems involved in extant approaches have been reviewed by Heyns and

Lippitt (1954). The present need was for a scheme (*a*) applicable to a wide variety of situations, (*b*) relevant for the study of personality and individual behavior patterns, (*c*) suitable for dealing with the behavior of both children and adults, and (*d*) relatively comprehensive. The approach initially described by Freedman et al. (1951), and discussed in detail by Leary (1957), was used.

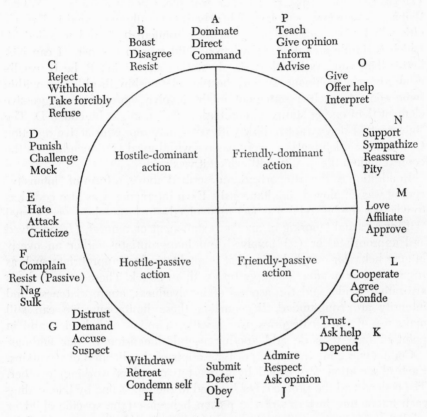

FIG. 1. CATEGORIES OF INTERPERSONAL BEHAVIOR
Modified from Freedman et al. (1951) and Leary (1957, p. 65)

The scheme (Fig. 1) is based on two polar coordinates. One is along the dimension of affection: love (affiliate, act friendly) to hate (attack, act unfriendly). The other axis is concerned with status: dominate (command, high status action) to submit (obey, low status action). Each action of one person toward another is coded by letter into one of 16 categories along the periphery of the circle in accordance with its blending of the two coordinates. The words below the letters are simply examples of the kinds of actions that might be coded at that position. In practice, coding was generally a compromise between the words representing the categories and the position relative to the two axes, but in cases of doubt the position was utilized rather than the words.[6]

As in the Bales scheme (1950), the attitude taken by the coder is that of the "generalized other." The question he attempts to answer via his categorization is, "What is this person doing to the other? What kind of relationship is he attempting to establish through this particular behavior?" (Heyns & Lippitt, 1954, p. 91). For example, when a child says, "Wasn't that a good movie we saw last night?" he is generally not coded J (Fig. 1), although J can include asking someone's opinion; he is rather coded M, which is simple affiliation. Or when a child says to another, "I can kick better than you," rather than simply stating an opinion P, he is usually establishing a dominant, slightly hostile relationship B, although within some contexts such a statement might involve more of an aggressive element than one of status differentiation and so might be coded D. The statement, "I don't want to play with you," may represent active rejection C, whiny complaining F, or very passive withdrawal H, depending on the context and on the quality with which it was said.

In addition to the categorization described above, a form of "intensity" coding was employed simultaneously. Each interaction was also coded as to whether the behavior was (a) uninvolved—for example, a very casual "Hi" or a casual ignoring of another's statement or request, (b) involved and appropriate, or (c) involved and inappropriate—either an overly intense behavior or a behavior that is qualitatively inappropriate such as responding to an affectionate gesture with an attack. These latter codings are rather crude, and the aspects of involvedness, appropriateness, and intensity are confounded. Recognizing these limitations, we can still make use of these categories over a wide sampling of behavior, and in point of fact, they do add another useful dimension to our findings.

Coding was done from tapes or typescripts of the dictated observations. Each observation was coded by at least two coders working together. The coders read the protocol (or listened to the tape) line by line, coding each interaction in terms of the person behaving (the specific child or adult), the interpersonal quality and "intensity" of the behavior, and the person toward whom the behavior was directed. Thus, one may obtain in chronological sequence the interactions of any given child toward any other child or adult, and also the behavior of others, children or adults, towards him.[7]

RESULTS AND DISCUSSION

IN THE discussion that follows, the basic source of material was, for each child, the 24 protocols—12 in each phase—in which he served as the central focus for observation. For analyzing qualitative changes, the interactions of individual children were distributed into the four quadrants of the circle (Fig. 1); frequencies at the midpoints (M, I, E, and A) were divided evenly between the two adjacent quadrants with any remaining odd entry randomly assigned.[8] Further data from individual segments of the 16-category scheme are noted occasionally, where this would seem to provide clarification. The approach to analyzing the reaction of others to individual children is commented on later.

The statistical method employed was chi square which, though it fails to take into account the continuity postulated in the circle scheme, involves few assumptions as to the nature of the data. The indices suggested by Leary (1957, pp. 68-71), while mathematically more elegant, would seem to require assumptions even beyond those of ordinal classification. The data for each child were analyzed independently in order to avoid confounding. Where individual chi squares for each child are summed to yield a total estimate of group change, the formula is the sum of chi squares in one direction minus the sum of chi squares in the other direction. Since there are no rational bases for expected distributions of behavior—any assumption that behavior should be distributed equally into each category is obviously untenable—total marginal distributions for individual children were used in obtaining theoretical values. Significance tests are reported for two-tailed distributions, for although some expectations are rather obviously directional in studying behavior change for this group of children, we were at this stage interested in exploring both sides of any coins which seemed worth examining.

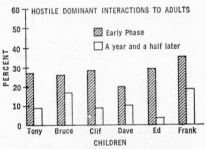

FIG. 2. CHANGES IN PROPORTIONS OF
HOSTILE-DOMINANT INTERACTIONS
BY CHILDREN TO ADULTS

CHANGES IN INTERACTIONS TOWARD ADULTS

Hostile-dominant interactions. Figure 2 presents for each of the children the percentage of his total responses toward adults which were coded as hostile-dominant at each of the two phases. The category represents active forms of aggressive behavior. Included are such interactions as actively refusing to comply with adult requests, making boastful demands on adults, threatening or challenging adults, attempting to "argue down" an adult, poking unfriendly fun at an adult, ordering adults around in a boastful or unfriendly manner, and any attack on the adult in his role of authority with the attempt to negate or degrade the authority component. Difficulties in authority relationships were prominent in the case records of all six boys prior to their admission. In one sense, the chief symptoms which entered into their selection were their consistent failure to accept the roles that adults define for children and their active rebellion against adult authority.

In the early phase, the mean percentage of hostile-dominant interactions toward adults was 28. This proportion is, of course, difficult to evaluate without control studies of more normal pre-adolescents in a comparable environment. For the clinical staff, however, it is a patent understatement to say that the amount of active hostility shown by these children was high.[9] In the later phase, the mean percentage of hostile-dominant responses toward adults dropped to 11. Over the year and a half between the two phases, each of the children changed in the expected direction. The shift was examined for each child separately by chi square—comparing frequencies of hostile-dominant vs. all other behavior toward adults over the two phases. The changes were significant for one child at $p < .001$, for two children at $p < .01$, for one child at $p < .02$, and for two children at $p < .20$. The sum of the individual chi squares was 44.23, which with 6 df (one for each two-by-two table) indicates a change at a level of confidence well beyond .001.

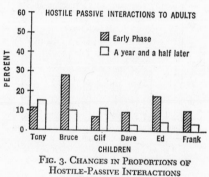

FIG. 3. CHANGES IN PROPORTIONS OF
HOSTILE-PASSIVE INTERACTIONS
BY CHILDREN TO ADULTS

Hostile-passive interactions. Hostile-passive modes of expressing hostility were, in general, less prominent in the relations of the children with adults than were the more dominant forms of aggression discussed above. Such behaviors as whining and complaining in relation to adults, accusing adults of punitive behavior or attitudes, demanding something of an adult in such a way as to imply that the adult is an ungiving monster, sulky withdrawal from interaction, tearful refusals—these constituted a mean of 14% of the behavior toward adults in the earlier phase (Fig. 3). A year and a half later, the mean percentage had dropped to 8. Four of the six children showed a decrease in passive expressions of aggression—one at $p < .01$, one at $p < .02$, one at $p < .10$, and one at $p < .20$; two children showed an insignificant increase ($p < .50$ in both cases). The sum of the four chi squares in the expected direction minus the two chi squares in the contrary direction is 17.62, which with 6 *df* is significant at a confidence level beyond .01. Thus, it would seem that while the magnitude of decrease in passively hostile interactions toward adults was significant, the change was not nearly as great as in the case of dominant expressions of hostility.

Friendly-passive interactions. It is interesting that despite the fact that these were hyperaggressive children, selected because of their unmanageability, the modal response toward adults was in the friendly-passive category (Fig. 4). Even in the earlier phase, friendly-passive behaviors

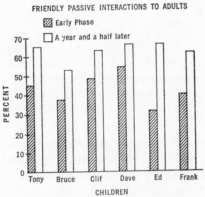

FIG. 4. CHANGES IN PROPORTIONS OF
FRIENDLY-PASSIVE INTERACTIONS
BY CHILDREN TO ADULTS

made up the greatest proportion of interactions with adults for each of the children with a mean of 43%. Examination of the total interactions toward adults of all six children when each was in the primary focus of observation indicates that in the earlier phase the three highest ranking of the 16 categories (Fig. 1) were affiliative behaviors (M), cooperative behaviors (L), and help-seeking behaviors (K), which produced respectively 15, 14, and 12% of all interactions toward adults.[10] This phenomenon, rather than indicating that the children were not "really" hyperaggressive, would seem to point in two directions. First, these are children and their behavior in many ways must resemble that of other children of their age. Second, each interaction in these analyses carries a single weight, and while this arrangement serves its purposes, it is unlikely that the recipient, for example, is equally impressed by one friendly "hello" as by a single attack of murderous rage. The relatively high frequencies of friendly-passive behaviors do not negate the difficulties in living with these children. The problem is that there are no units for effectively gauging the psychological impact of an action on the recipient.

By the time of the later period, the percentage of friendly-passive interactions with adults had risen to a mean of 63%. Each of the children showed an increase in such responses—one at $p < .001$, two at $p < .01$, one at $p < .05$, one at $p < .10$, and one at $p < .30$. The sum of the chi squares is 45.37, which with 6 df is significant at a confidence level well beyond .001. Further consideration of the specific nature of the changes appears below.

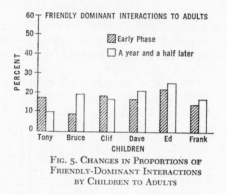

FIG. 5. CHANGES IN PROPORTIONS OF
FRIENDLY-DOMINANT INTERACTIONS
BY CHILDREN TO ADULTS

Friendly-dominant interactions. It is difficult to know what to expect in the friendly-dominant area, both in proportions and in actual changes. In contrast with the situation for aggression and dependency, there has been little theoretical or research interest in such children's behaviors as sympathizing with or reassuring adults, offering help to adults, and teaching or advising adults. One might guess that such actions are perhaps not very appropriate as a major aspect of the relations of pre-adolescent boys with adults. For the present group, friendly-dominant responses constituted a rather small proportion of behaviors toward adults. The values in Fig. 5 and the mean values—16% in the early and 18% in the later phase—are somewhat spuriously high because the major contributory entry was from affiliative responses (M), which in the analyses were distributed equally between friendly-dominant and friendly-passive interactions.[11] Only for one child, Bruce, did the change between the two phases approach significance ($p < .10$), and here it was almost wholly a function of the increase in affiliative responses (M). The sum of the four chi squares showing increase minus the two showing decrease was 2.95, which is not significant ($p < .90$).

The "intensity" dimension. Most of the children's behavior was considered by the coders to be appropriate and involved. In the early phase, this "intensity" category comprised a mean of 75% of the children's action toward adults (Fig. 6). Only 9% of the behavior in this period—a mean for the six children—was coded as inappropriate and involved, that is, as being overly intense or qualitatively inappropriate to the circumstances. Uninvolved interactions yielded a mean of 16% of the behaviors in this phase; these included such actions as silent rejections of adult requests, subtle provocations, as well as token gestures of acceptance or affiliation, and the term *uninvolved* is not very adequate.

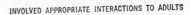

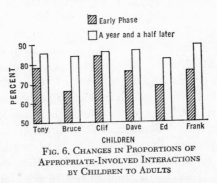

FIG. 6. CHANGES IN PROPORTIONS OF
APPROPRIATE-INVOLVED INTERACTIONS
BY CHILDREN TO ADULTS

In any case, the proportions of appropriate-involved interactions increased in the later phase from a mean of 75% to a mean of 86%. Each of the children changed in the expected direction. Comparing the frequencies of appropriate-involved behaviors with the summed frequencies of the other two categories over the two phases yielded chi squares at confidence levels of $p < .01$ for one child, $p < .05$ for two children, $p < .20$ for two children, and $p < .90$ for the sixth child (two-tailed tests). The sum of the chi squares was 21.19, which with 6 df is significant at $p < .01$. Five children showed a decrease in inappropriate-involved behavior; the means went from 9% to 4%. All six children showed a decrease in uninvolved actions toward adults, the means dropping from 16% to 10%. The raw frequencies are in some cases too small to warrant statistical analysis, but the trends seem obvious.

Summary comments on changes in interactions with adults. Over the year and a half the children changed considerably in their behavior toward adults. Primarily, they lessened their attempts to dominate adults aggressively, and they increased their friendly and compliant associations with adults. Passive expressions of hostility also decreased, and in general, behavior became more appropriate, but these latter changes, while statistically significant, were less striking.

It is obvious that improvement occurred in overt behavior toward adults. During the period of the study, however, the boys had not only been under an intensive residential treatment program, but they had also grown older. Where so little is known in any systematic way about the interpersonal behavior of normal children and about developmental changes in such behavior, there is the perplexing question that is often put as an issue between maturation and learning (or treatment). The question is a complex one, since social maturation can never be divorced from considerations of the particular environment involved and its indulgences, tolerances, and demands. For example, the treatment of children, in order to be adequate, must take growth and development into account. Conversely, maturational phenomena will be influenced by the environmental medium in which they occur. In the present situation, one may legitimately ask: Are the changes necessarily to be attributed to the treatment program together with growth and development or are they, perhaps, primarily a function of normal development within a *somewhat* benign environment? No definitive answer can be given without control studies, and there are manifold problems even so. There are, however, some partial cues in the data which indicate that the treatment, in a broad sense, is a critical factor. Thus, while one might *possibly* expect decreased aggression and decreased dominance in relation to adults as part of a "normal" growth process, though the argument would be tenuous, one would not expect to find much increase in trusting, dependent relations with adults. It is interesting that out of the 16 possibilities (Fig. 1), the category that showed the greatest shift was K, which deals with requesting, depending, and asking-help behavior, and that the percentage of responses in this category went from 12% of all behaviors toward adults in the early phase to 24% in the later phase. In frequency of responses, K shifted from third to first rank. It would seem that this was not a maturation phenomenon—that is, it is unlikely that children either become increasingly dependent or increasingly admit their dependency on adults with age. One may speculate that the evidence points to the dissolution of a defensive layer so that dependency emerges; such a speculation dovetails with the impressions of the psychotherapists that oral themes became very prominent in the later phases of psychotherapy with these children. The critical question about what factors in the treatment program contributed to change can unfortunately not be answered by a study such as this, but some further issues in the process of change will be considered below in the discussion of behaviors directed toward each of the children.

CHANGES IN INTERACTIONS TOWARD PEERS

WE TURN to the behavior of the children toward their peers, again considering each child when he was the focal subject for observation, but now investigating changes in the behavior that he directed toward other children. The discussion can be briefer in this section because some of the contextual material has already been presented.

Hostile-dominant interactions. Figure 7 presents for each child at the two phases the percentage of his actions which were hostile-dominant in

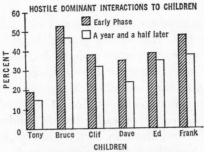

FIG. 7. CHANGES IN PROPORTIONS OF
HOSTILE-DOMINANT INTERACTIONS
BY CHILDREN TO PEERS

orientation toward other children. In both phases the means are higher than was the case for behavior toward adults—39% as compared to 28% in the early phase, and 32% as compared to 11% in the later phase. Five of the six boys were in the early period more dominantly aggressive toward their peers than toward adults, and all six showed this trend in the later period. That is, aggressive attempts at dominance were, as might be expected, more readily expressed toward peers than toward the higher status adults.

All six of the children showed expected decremental changes over the 18 months. While this directional consistency for six cases is significant at a confidence level of $p = .03$ by a simple two-tailed binomial test, none of the individual changes reached statistical significance, and the sum of the individual chi squares was also nonsignificant. Thus, in contrast to the marked shifts between the two phases in proportions of hostile-dominant interactions toward adults, the changes in interactions with peers were, at the most, slight.

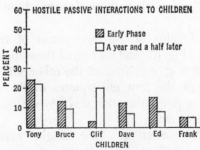

FIG. 8. CHANGES IN PROPORTIONS OF
HOSTILE-PASSIVE INTERACTIONS
BY CHILDREN TO PEERS

Hostile-passive interactions. Although four of the six children showed a decrease in hostile-passive behaviors (Fig. 8), in no case was the change significant. One child, Clif, increased in passive expressions of aggression toward the others, and the shift was significant by chi square at $p < .001$. For this child, both passive resistance (F) and withdrawal (H) increased over the year and a half. His over-all proportion of hostility rose somewhat, though not significantly, since a slight decline in hostile-dominant interactions did not compensate for the increased passive hostility. The situation thus points to the possibility of a slight deterioration in peer relationships for this child over the period of the study. The mean percentages of hostile-passive responses for the six children are the same in the two phases, 12%, and the sum of the chi squares for the positive change direction minus those in the negative direction is, although opposite to the direction of improvement because of Clif's contribution, not significant.

Friendly-passive interactions. Just as active aggression was more characteristic in response to peers than to adults, so friendly-passive interactions, at the opposite side of the circle, were less characteristic in peer relationships than in relationships with adults. In the early phase, friendly-passive actions made up 43% of the responses to adults and 24% of the responses to other children; in the later period, the respective percentages were 63 and 29. In behavior toward adults, Categories M, L, and K (Fig. 1) held the three highest ranks for response frequencies in each of the two phases, based on the total number of responses of all children in each phase. In behaviors toward peers, M (affiliative responses) and L (cooperative responses) were at Ranks 1 and 4.5 in the early phase and at Ranks 1 and 2.5 in the later phase. But the position of K (trusting, dependent, help-seeking responses) was quite different in relations with peers. In the early phase, only 2% of all responses were coded K, a ranking of 14 in a triple tie; in the later phase, only 3% of all responses was coded K, a ranking of 11.5 in a quadruple tie. Thus, unlike the case in relation to adults, dependency responses among the children occurred relatively infrequently, and they showed rather little shift between the two times of study.

Four boys showed gains in the proportions of friendly-passive behaviors toward peers (Fig. 9), and for two of them the change was significant by chi square at $p < .05$. None of the other shifts were statistically significant; the sum of the four chi squares in the expected direction minus the two in the opposite direction was 8.87 which, with 6 *df*, yields a confidence level of $p < .20$.

Friendly-dominant interactions. One might expect the friendly-dominant mode of interaction to be more characteristic of relations among children than from children to adults, and such an expectation appears to be legitimate. In the early phase, an average of 26% of the children's responses to peers were friendly-dominant in orientation in contrast to the average of 16% in responses to adults; in the later phase, the two averages were 28% and 18%, respectively. The category M again consti-

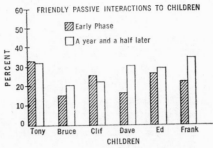

FIG. 9. CHANGES IN PROPORTIONS OF
FRIENDLY-PASSIVE INTERACTIONS
BY CHILDREN TO PEERS

tuted a major source of data for the quadrant, and that the values are not deceiving is shown by the fact that Categories N, O, and P yielded 15% of all responses toward children in each of the two phases and 7% of all responses toward adults in each of the two phases.

Figure 10 shows four of the six changes to be in the direction of an increase in friendly-dominant behaviors toward peers, but none of the changes in either direction is significant; neither is the sum of the chi squares.

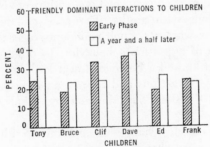

FIG. 10. CHANGES IN PROPORTIONS OF
FRIENDLY-DOMINANT INTERACTIONS
BY CHILDREN TO PEERS

The "intensity" dimension. The distributions of responses toward peers are strikingly similar to the distributions of responses toward adults in the three-category "intensity" classification. In the early phase, the mean proportions of interactions toward children were 74% appropriate-involved (as compared to 75% for behavior toward adults), 16% uninvolved interactions (as compared to 16% for behavior toward adults), and 9% inappropriate-involved interactions (as compared to 9% for behavior toward adults). In the later phase, the three means are, respectively, 84%, 11%, and 5% as compared to 86%, 10%, and 4% in behavior toward adults.

INVOLVED APPROPRIATE INTERACTIONS TO CHILDREN

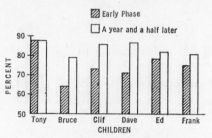

FIG. 11. CHANGES IN PROPORTIONS OF
APPROPRIATE-INVOLVED INTERACTIONS
BY CHILDREN TO PEERS

Figure 11 shows the shifts in the proportions of appropriate-involved behaviors for each of the children. All changes were in the expected direction of increase. For one child the change was significant at $p < .02$, for another at $p < .05$, and for a third at $p < .10$; for the other three children there is less conclusive evidence of change. The sum of the chi squares is 15.85, which, with 6 df, is significant at a level of $p < .02$. Decreases in inappropriate-involved and in uninvolved actions toward peers seem by inspection to be less consistent than they were in behavior toward adults.

Summary comments on changes in interactions toward peers. Certainly, the evidence of change in relations with peers is much less than in the case of relations with adults. The only general change in peer directed action that warrants much confidence was the increase in the relative proportion of appropriate behavior. In other aspects, the directions were similar to those for behavior toward adults—toward a decrease in dominant aggressive actions and toward an increase in friendly compliant actions—but the shifts over the year and a half were, for the most part, unimpressive.

To the question of why changes in relations to adults were so much more striking than were changes in peer relations, no clear answer can be given. There is the possibility that interpersonal behavior with peers was less disturbed than that with adults. Control studies would be required to confirm or disaffirm this statement. There is also the possibility that changes occur earlier in the treatment process in relation to adults than in relation to peers. Such an hypothesis would be reasonable though not necessary on the basis of clinical evidence that the difficulties of these boys developed out of primary relationships with parental figures. Perhaps, with these primitive children, some resolution of earlier relationship problems must occur before the genetically more advanced problems of peer relationships can be met. Follow-up studies and studies of other clinical groups would be useful here. There is also a possibility that the observation method and the instrument are less potent for gauging peer interactions than for interactions of children toward adults. Some light is cast on this latter issue in the discussions that follow.

FURTHER EXPLORATIONS

THE aim in the following sections is to explore some phenomena of group and individual interpersonal behavior. Such exploration can perhaps illuminate some of the findings already referred to. It can point to further potentialities or limitations of the methods. Most important, it can probe toward the formulation of general principles.

GROUP SIMILARITIES

THE selection of the children and their environmental homogeneity within the institution should make for behavioral similarities in their interactions. That the children did resemble one another in interpersonal behavior is shown as follows: When the 16 categories were ranked for each child in accordance with the frequencies of his interactions, Kendall Ws, computed for the six children and corrected for ties, were .61 for interactions toward peers and .59 for interactions toward adults in the early phase; in the later phase, the corresponding Ws were .61 and .76. All Ws are significant at levels of $p < .001$. Furthermore, behavior between the two phases correlated significantly. When the interactions for the group taken as a whole in the 16 categories were ranked for each phase, the Spearman rho corrected for ties, for behavior toward peers was .79. Even in the case of interactions toward adults, where the differences between phases were highly significant, the rank orders of interaction categories were similar between the two periods a year and a half apart. The rho, corrected for ties, was .75.[12] Thus, although interpersonal behavior may change over time, it also seems to maintain a certain consistency.

The concordances among individuals and the consistencies in group behavior raise a number of questions. We do not know to what extent correspondences are a function of the homogeneity of the group and of the environmental milieu, or, on the other hand, to what extent they are related to the facts that the subjects are children of a given age, or children in a specific culture, or that they are simply children. Speculations here would perhaps be promiscuous. There are, however, some data presented by Barker and Wright (1954, Ch. 12) which offer possibilities for very crude comparison. These authors show rankings of interactive categories for the behavior of eight "normal" children, each of whom was observed individually for a day in the small Midwestern town in which the children lived. All interactive behavior was noted and later coded. Four of the children were boys and four were girls; ages range from 1 year, 10 months through 10 years, 9 months, with a median age of 5 years, 10 months. Thus, the children and their environments were very different from those of the present study. The behavioral categories employed in the two studies also differed, but on an a priori, face-validity basis, it was decided which categories were comparable in the two schemes.[13] The rank orders of interactive behavior for these two different samples of children in different environments were correlated. Behavior toward adults yielded rhos of .24 and .31 between the Barker and Wright data (1954, p. 429) and the present study's early and late phases, respectively; behavior toward children yielded rhos of .43 and .29. Although none of the rhos is significant with eight sets of ranks, all are positive.

By themselves, positive correlation coefficients can be artifacts of the categories employed; for example, by choosing walking and flying as categories for classification, it can be shown—not wholly illegitimately— that people are all alike. The matter is, however, not so readily dismissed. In the course of the day, the Barker and Wright children had transactions with adults; the same was true for the six boys in the present study. When the total adult behaviors toward the Barker and Wright children (1954, p. 425) were compared in rankings with the total adult behaviors directed toward the six hyperaggressive boys, the rhos were .93 ($p < .01$) for the early phase and .79 ($p < .05$) for the later phase. That is, despite the differences in children in age and psychological status, despite the differences in environments (home, school, and neighborhood versus a psychiatric milieu), despite the differences in adults (parents, neighbors, and teachers as against counselors, nurses, physicians, and teachers), and despite differences in methods of study, patterns of behavior of adults toward children apparently have much in common. The patterns of behavior of the very different samples of children would seem to have less— though still something—in common. In isolation, such findings are difficult to evaluate. They do, however, point to the desirability of investigating commonalities and differences in interpersonal patterns in relation to maturational factors and in relation to cultural and subcultural variations.

INDIVIDUAL DIFFERENCES

ANOTHER side of the coin is the matter of individual differences. The side one emphasizes, resemblances or differences, depends on what one wishes to talk about. General arguments as to which are greater are specious, a pitfall researchers have not always avoided. For a scheme to be maximally useful, it should be capable both of abstracting general phenomena and of demonstrating differentiations, and, all other things being equal, the finer its discriminations, the greater its potential. An initial and minimal test of the clinical utility of an instrument is its capacity for showing individual differences. Considering the earlier observations by quadrants, the six children differed among themselves in both interactions toward each other (Table 1, $p < .001$) and in interactions toward adults (Table 2, $p < .01$). The "intensity" codings seemed less sensitive to individual factors (Table 3, $p < .01$ in interactions with children; Table 4, $p < .10$ in interactions with adults). Individual differences among the children

TABLE 1.

Individual Differences in Modes of Interaction Toward Peers—Early Phase
(N = 568)

	HOSTILE-DOMINANT ACTIONS	HOSTILE-PASSIVE ACTIONS	FRIENDLY-PASSIVE ACTIONS	FRIENDLY-DOMINANT ACTIONS
Tony	19 (38.97)[a]	24 (11.49)	35 (24.78)	24 (26.76)
Bruce	33 (23.69)	8 (6.99)	10 (15.06)	11 (16.26)
Clif	37 (37.44)	3 (11.04)	26 (23.81)	32 (25.71)
Dave	34 (37.44)	12 (11.04)	17 (23.81)	35 (25.71)
Ed	26 (25.60)	10 (7.55)	18 (16.28)	13 (17.58)
Frank	68 (53.87)	7 (15.89)	32 (34.26)	34 (36.99)

[a] Expected values based on marginal distributions are in parentheses. $\chi^2 = 60.13$, $df = 15$, $p < .001$.

TABLE 2.

Individual Differences in Modes of Interaction Toward Adults—Early Phase
(N = 542)

	HOSTILE-DOMINANT ACTIONS	HOSTILE-PASSIVE ACTIONS	FRIENDLY-PASSIVE ACTIONS	FRIENDLY-DOMINANT ACTIONS
Tony	24 (24.96)[a]	10 (12.97)	40 (36.29)	15 (14.78)
Bruce	23 (24.96)	25 (12.97)	33 (36.29)	8 (14.78)
Clif	15 (15.70)	4 (8.16)	27 (22.83)	10 (9.30)
Dave	13 (18.51)	6 (9.62)	36 (26.91)	11 (10.96)
Ed	42 (40.10)	24 (20.84)	45 (58.31)	32 (23.75)
Frank	35 (27.76)	10 (14.43)	40 (40.37)	14 (16.44)

[a] Expected values based on marginal distributions are in parentheses. $\chi^2 = 34.94$, $df = 15$, $p < .01$.

TABLE 3.

Individual Differences in "Intensity" of Interaction Toward Peers—Early Phase
(N = 568)

	UNINVOLVED ACTIONS	INVOLVED-APPROPRIATE ACTIONS	INVOLVED-INAPPROPRIATE ACTIONS
Tony	12 (16.34)[a]	86 (76.50)	4 (9.16)
Bruce	14 (9.93)	40 (46.50)	8 (5.57)
Clif	24 (15.70)	72 (73.50)	2 (8.80)
Dave	14 (15.70)	70 (73.50)	14 (8.80)
Ed	7 (10.73)	52 (50.25)	8 (6.02)
Frank	20 (22.59)	106 (105.75)	15 (12.66)

[a] Expected values based on marginal distributions are in parentheses. $\chi^2 = 24.71$, $df = 10$, $p < .01$.

TABLE 4.

Individual Differences in "Intensity" of Interaction Toward Adults—Early Phase
(N = 542)

	UNINVOLVED ACTIONS	INVOLVED-APPROPRIATE ACTIONS	INVOLVED-INAPPROPRIATE ACTIONS
Tony	14 (14.61)[a]	69 (65.19)	6 (9.20)
Bruce	18 (14.61)	59 (65.19)	12 (9.20)
Clif	5 (9.20)	47 (41.02)	4 (5.79)
Dave	14 (10.84)	50 (48.34)	2 (6.82)
Ed	23 (23.48)	97 (104.74)	23 (14.77)
Frank	15 (16.26)	75 (72.51)	9 (10.23)

[a] Expected values based on marginal distributions are in parentheses. $\chi^2 = 16.83$, $df = 10$, $p < .10$.

TABLE 5.

Individual Differences in Modes of Interaction Toward Peers—Later Phase
(N = 430)

	HOSTILE-DOMINANT ACTIONS	HOSTILE-PASSIVE ACTIONS	FRIENDLY-PASSIVE ACTIONS	FRIENDLY-DOMINANT ACTIONS
Tony	9 (18.98)[a]	13 (6.84)	20 (17.58)	18 (16.60)
Bruce	25 (16.76)	5 (6.04)	11 (15.53)	12 (14.67)
Clif	24 (23.40)	15 (8.43)	17 (21.68)	18 (20.48)
Dave	20 (26.57)	6 (9.57)	26 (24.61)	32 (23.25)
Ed	28 (24.99)	6 (9.00)	24 (23.15)	21 (21.86)
Frank	30 (25.30)	4 (9.12)	28 (23.44)	18 (22.14)

[a] Expected values based on marginal distributions are in parentheses. $\chi^2 = 36.88$, $df = 15$, $p < .01$.

TABLE 6.

Individual Differences in Modes of Interaction Toward Adults—Later Phase
(N = 438)

	HOSTILE-DOMINANT ACTIONS	HOSTILE-PASSIVE ACTIONS	FRIENDLY-PASSIVE ACTIONS	FRIENDLY-DOMINANT ACTIONS
Tony	9 (10.96)[a]	15 (8.50)	64 (61.08)	10 (17.45)
Bruce	13 (8.61)	8 (6.68)	41 (47.99)	15 (13.71)
Clif	6 (7.83)	8 (6.07)	44 (43.63)	12 (12.47)
Dave	6 (6.82)	2 (5.29)	40 (38.02)	13 (10.86)
Ed	3 (7.50)	3 (5.81)	44 (41.76)	17 (11.93)
Frank	12 (7.27)	2 (5.64)	40 (40.51)	11 (11.58)

[a] Expected values based on marginal distributions are in parentheses. $\chi^2 = 27.81$, $df = 15$, $p < .05$.

TABLE 7.

Individual Differences in "Intensity" of Interaction Toward Peers—Later Phase
(N = 430)

	UNINVOLVED ACTIONS	INVOLVED-APPROPRIATE ACTIONS	INVOLVED-INAPPROPRIATE ACTIONS
Tony	2 (6.84)[a]	53 (50.51)	5 (2.65)
Bruce	4 (6.04)	42 (44.62)	7 (2.34)
Clif	8 (8.43)	64 (62.30)	2 (3.27)
Dave	11 (9.57)	73 (70.72)	0 (3.71)
Ed	13 (9.00)	65 (66.51)	1 (3.49)
Frank	11 (9.12)	65 (67.35)	4 (3.53)

[a] Expected values based on marginal distributions are in parentheses. $\chi^2 = 24.41$, $df = 10$, $p < .01$.

TABLE 8.

Individual Differences in "Intensity" of Interaction Toward Adults—Later Phase
(N = 438)

	UNINVOLVED ACTIONS	INVOLVED-APPROPRIATE ACTIONS	INVOLVED-INAPPROPRIATE ACTIONS
Tony	10 (9.84)[a]	84 (83.90)	4 (4.25)
Bruce	7 (7.74)	65 (65.92)	5 (3.34)
Clif	4 (7.03)	60 (59.93)	6 (3.04)
Dave	7 (6.13)	53 (52.23)	1 (2.65)
Ed	10 (6.73)	55 (57.36)	2 (2.91)
Frank	6 (6.53)	58 (55.65)	1 (2.82)

[a] Expected values based on marginal distributions are in parentheses. $\chi^2 = 9.55$, $df = 10$, $p < .50$.

also appeared in the later phase in interactions toward peers (Table 5, $p < .01$) and in interactions toward adults (Table 6, $p < .05$), but they seemed somewhat attenuated, perhaps by the long period of close communal living. The "intensity" codings yielded results similar to the earlier phase (Table 7, $p < .01$ for interactions with peers; Table 8, $p < .50$ for interactions with adults), but again perhaps somewhat attenuated.

In all these analyses, individual differences in behaviors toward children seem greater than do individual differences in behaviors toward adults. This trend would indicate that those failures to find significant differences in peer relations between the two phases, as compared to the significant phase differences in relations with adults, were not a function of the lack of sensitivity of the method to peer interactions. On a theoretical level, the trend may point to a more general issue of role relationships. We may speculate that people will tend to act in a more individualized fashion toward those in their own status group than they do toward groups of rather different statuses. That is, not only may there be a cognitive tendency for one group to stereotype another group of very different status, but patterns of behavior in a group may be less variable in relations to other groups than in relations to peers. To the other-status recipient of behavior, the behavioral cohesiveness of a group may then appear to be greater than it actually does to the within-group members.

SOME DYNAMIC ASPECTS OF INTERPERSONAL PROCESSES

In all the foregoing discussion, it is as though each child were an independent, self-determined unit. Yet one of the basic facts of interpersonal processes is the interdependence and continuity of behavior. One's actions evoke actions by others, and the actions of others, in turn, stimulate one's own behavior. Leary (1957, Ch. 7) has commented on and given some examples of reciprocality in interpersonal behavior among adults. For cues as to this issue, the behavior that each child received from his peers and from adults was examined. Tables 9 through 12 present the frequencies of interactions and percentages in the four categories of response for behavior each child received from others.[14]

Reciprocality in adult behavior toward children. The behavior of the adults contrasted sharply with that of the children. The majority of the adult interactions—a mean over the six children of 58% in the early phase and 72 in the later—were in the friendly-dominant category, composed of friendly, nurturant, supporting, giving, and guiding activities. A further demonstration of the contrast lies in the comparison between behavior "sent" by the children and the behavior they "received." In the early phase, a mean of 51% of the responses which individual children "sent" toward each other were hostile in orientation (Table 1); they "received" a mean of 51% hostile actions from each other (Table 9). For the later phase, the values were 44% hostile responses "sent" and 43% "received"

(Tables 5 and 11). In contrast was the situation with adults. Whereas the children in the early phase "sent" a mean of 42% hostile actions to adults, they "received" a mean of only 25% hostile actions in return (Tables 2 and 10). For the later phase, the values were 19% "sent" and 15 "received" (Tables 6 and 12). Although the data are, of course, not definitive, they hint that processes of interpersonal change, insofar as change occurred, were adult rather than child initiated. It would seem reasonable that if interaction were purely reciprocal—an eye for an eye—one could not expect changes in the direction of the participants' actions, at least after a stable status order had been established. It is probably at the interruptions in patterns of reciprocality that the potential for interpersonal change arises. This is not to say that such interruptions are sufficient requirements for change, although they may be necessary ones.

Nor does the foregoing discussion imply that the adults did not, in some measure, respond reciprocally to the children. Although the adults may have initiated the process of change, they, like the children, showed systematic shifts in behavior between the two phases. The proportions of aggression expressed by adults decreased in relation to each of the six boys.[15] Noted previously was the fact that the major single shift in the 16 categories on the part of the children in their behavior toward adults was the increase in help-requesting, dependent actions (K); it is interesting that the major single category of change in adult responses over the two phases was the increase in giving and help-offering responses (O) from 23 to 34% of the total adult behaviors. The adults also changed in the "intensity" of behavior toward the children. The proportions of appropriate-involved behaviors as compared to uninvolved and inappropriate-involved behaviors increased in relation to each child, the means going from 82 to 90%.

Reciprocality in peer behavior. Changes in actions "received" from peers also, in general, paralleled the previously noted changes in actions "sent" toward peers. The evidence for a general systematic change in the quality of interactions toward peers was noted as slight. Similarly, there appears to be little over-all change in the quality of interactions received from peers (Tables 9 and 11). Dave was the child who changed most in the direction of decreased aggression toward peers. Other children changed similarly in their behavior toward him. A further parallel appears in the case of Clif, who, as mentioned previously, was unusual in that while he decreased in dominant forms of aggression toward peers, he showed significantly more passively hostile actions in the later phase. In the later as compared to the earlier period, Clif received more dominantly hostile but fewer passively hostile actions from peers—the only instance where this occurred. "Intensity" changes in "received" behavior parallel "intensity" changes in "sent" behavior. In all six cases the proportions of appropriate-involved actions increased. But there are deviations from

TABLE 9.

Actions by Peers Toward Each Child—Early Phase
(N = 1034)

	HOSTILE-DOMINANT ACTIONS		HOSTILE-PASSIVE ACTIONS		FRIENDLY-PASSIVE ACTIONS		FRIENDLY-DOMINANT ACTIONS	
	FREQ.	%	FREQ.	%	FREQ.	%	FREQ.	%
Tony	74	46	9	6	33	21	44	27
Bruce	51	37	16	12	38	28	31	23
Clif	65	35	18	10	57	31	44	24
Dave	96	42	29	13	54	24	48	21
Ed	50	40	11	8	27	22	37	30
Frank	78	39	31	15	56	28	37	18

parallelism. For example, there is little evidence that Bruce changed much in his actions toward peers. They, however, seemed to change toward him. He received less aggression and less inappropriate behavior in the later phase.

In general, then, there is a mutuality in interpersonal processes of change. As interpersonal behavior changes, new equilibrium relations tend to form between the person and others. Unfortunately, the study can say all too little about the circumstances under which changes in equilibria occur, or about such problems as lags in mutual rearrangements. It would also seem that realignments may occur on bases which this study missed. One would guess that such factors as interpersonal skills and sensitivities, special cognitive abilities, stability or erraticness of behavior, special friendship and leadership patterns all play a part.

What can be said about the specific nature of reciprocal action? Ob-

TABLE 10.

Actions by Adults Toward Each Child—Early Phase
(N = 557)

	HOSTILE-DOMINANT ACTIONS		HOSTILE-PASSIVE ACTIONS		FRIENDLY-PASSIVE ACTIONS		FRIENDLY-DOMINANT ACTIONS	
	FREQ.	%	FREQ.	%	FREQ.	%	FREQ.	%
Tony	16	18	1	1	8	9	65	72
Bruce	19	23	0	0	13	15	52	62
Clif	24	33	1	1	12	17	35	48
Dave	20	20	2	2	12	12	66	66
Ed	16	16	5	5	28	27	54	52
Frank	26	24	6	6	23	21	53	49

TABLE 11.

Actions by Peers Toward Each Child—Later Phase
(N = 920)

	HOSTILE-DOMINANT ACTIONS		HOSTILE-PASSIVE ACTIONS		FRIENDLY-PASSIVE ACTIONS		FRIENDLY-DOMINANT ACTIONS	
	FREQ.	%	FREQ.	%	FREQ.	%	FREQ.	%
Tony	37	42	6	7	20	23	25	28
Bruce	37	26	7	5	51	37	44	32
Clif	91	41	11	5	58	27	58	27
Dave	36	23	15	9	61	38	47	30
Ed	56	40	19	13	31	22	35	25
Frank	59	34	22	12	54	31	40	23

viously, nothing definitive, but there are some cues. Let us look, for example, at Tony's relations with the other boys during the early phase. Tony was the least dominantly aggressive and the most passively aggressive of the children. Complementarily, Tony received the greatest proportion of dominant aggression and the lowest proportion of passive aggression from his peers.[16] While Tony initiated the highest proportion of friendly-passive responses to other children, he received the lowest proportion of such responses from peers but the second highest proportion of friendly-dominant behaviors. In contrast to Tony, Frank "sent" a high proportion of dominantly aggressive and a low proportion of passively aggressive behaviors toward the other boys and received from them a high proportion of passive-hostile and a relatively low proportion of dominant-hostile responses. But, as seems true for reciprocality in change, patterns of complementariness in action are not equally clear for all children.

TABLE 12.

Actions by Adults Toward Each Child—Later Phase
(N = 658)

	HOSTILE-DOMINANT ACTIONS		HOSTILE-PASSIVE ACTIONS		FRIENDLY-PASSIVE ACTIONS		FRIENDLY-DOMINANT ACTIONS	
	FREQ.	%	FREQ.	%	FREQ.	%	FREQ.	%
Tony	19	16	0	0	10	8	91	76
Bruce	18	15	2	2	16	13	83	70
Clif	20	19	0	0	8	7	78	74
Dave	6	8	0	0	13	18	55	74
Ed	8	7	5	4	22	19	82	70
Frank	22	18	1	1	17	14	82	67

That passive aggression evokes dominant aggression and that dominant aggression evokes passive aggression is not unexpected. What is more interesting is a tendency in the data for passive aggression to evoke friendly-dominant behavior, and for dominant aggression to evoke friendly-passive behavior. The evidence is obviously meagre and the indications are not wholly consistent, but it would seem that hostile oriented actions were not always met with counterhostility. Do "successes" maintain the behaviors? If so, how is the alternative cycle of reciprocal aggression to be counteracted?

SUMMARY

AN EXPLORATORY study was made of the interpersonal behavior of six hyperaggressive boys in residential treatment. Each child was observed twice in six life settings and his interactions with both peers and adults were noted. The observations were repeated after a year and a half in the treatment program.

Over the year and a half the interpersonal behavior of the children shifted considerably. The major changes were in the relations of the children with adults. Here, there was primarily a decrease in hostile-dominant behavior and an increase in friendly-passive behavior. The appropriateness of behavior increased both in relations with children and with adults. The patterns of change were consistent with treatment aims, and they seemed, at least in part, a function of the treatment program.

Group similarities and individual differences among the children were noted, and patterns of reciprocality in behavior between children and adults and among children were explored. In relations with peers, the children received about the same amount of aggression as they expressed. They received less aggression from adults than they expressed toward them. Changes in patterns of behavior toward others were accompanied, in general, by reciprocal changes in the behaviors of others, both adults and children.

The study demonstrates (*a*) that systematic observation and coding of the interpersonal behavior of a small group of children in naturalistic settings can yield tenable descriptions, orderly relationships, and some tentative hypotheses about interpersonal processes, (*b*) that hyperaggressive children can change in residential treatment in a direction consistent with therapeutic aims, and (*c*) that the mode of observation described here, together with the scheme for coding interpersonal behavior (Freedman et al., 1951; Leary, 1957), has some measure of utility.

NOTES TO CHAPTER 53

1. Among the people, other than the authors, who have been involved in this study at one time or another, special note should be made of the contribu-

tions of Donald S. Boomer and D. Wells Goodrich. They were not only contributors to the observation and coding processes, but the procedures and methodology used here owe much to them. Fritz Redl, Chief of the Child Research Branch, and the Child Care Staff made the study possible by their cooperation.

2. The first series was completed within a month; the second series took some five months to complete.

3. In addition to the authors and others already mentioned, Joseph H. Handlon and Jeston Hamer served as observers.

4. The problems of making formal observations in an on-going clinical operation and the methodological issues in pretesting the approach are complex matters. Discussions of these questions by A. T. Dittmann and by D. W. Goodrich are in preparation.

5. Behaviors specific to the game itself—for example, passing a ball, playing a card, or claiming one's turn—were not coded or considered in the analyses to follow.

6. Practical coding problems were sometimes resolved by double codings, but such solutions are not wholly adequate.

7. Freedman et al. (1951, p. 155) present some data on interrater agreement in coding verbal behavior of adults. Adequate assessment of reliability is made difficult by the fact that there is no baseline for evaluating correlational indices with data scored in this fashion. Rank order correlations between codings from protocols of independent observers of the same events and between pairs of coders of the same protocols are invariably high, but they are likely to be somewhat spurious, since there is some doubt that correlations between random protocols are of zero order. Dittmann (in press) discusses a number of aspects of the reliability of the system. Considering agreement between two pairs of coders working with the same material, Dittmann notes that item-by-item agreement, analogous to test item reliability, is far greater than chance expectancy, but he also notes that there remain appreciable discrepancies. When, however, the single interactions are grouped to form a profile for an observation, a situation analogous to test reliability, discrepancies between independent pairs of coders are far smaller than could be expected by chance. Similarly, the protocols from independent observers of the same events yield smaller differences than could be expected by chance. A recent check by the present authors compared different observers who observed the same children in matched, rather than identical, settings—a situation analogous to alternate forms. Differences, which might have resulted from observer variations or from lack of equivalence in the matched settings or from both, were well within chance limits. Furthermore, a series of observations made approximately two months apart with the same children also failed to yield significant differences.

Clearly, none of these results allows a statement about level of reliability comparable to the usual Pearson *r*. The significant item-by-item agreement, together with the failure to find evidence of bias in the sources tested, and together with the finding of consistent individual differences, discussed below, would, however, seem to warrant the conclusion reached by Dittmann

(1958). The conclusion is that reliability is adequate for grouped data—such as the individual profiles considered in the present study—although it may not be adequate for the analysis of single sequences.

There remains a question of possible bias occurring between the two phases of the study, and the only answers at present are indirect ones. First, the scheme seems fairly objective; second, raters have been aware of the problem, and their continued sensitivity to the possibility of bias has probably served to reduce that possibility; third, the data yield negative as well as positive results, whereas a bias would be likely to operate more consistently. It is recognized that such answers are incomplete. A more definitive check, which has awaited the presence of uncontaminated raters for whom protocols can be adequately disguised, is currently in process.

8. For the early phase observations, the median was 98 interactions for a child toward other children (range 62 to 141), and the median was 89 interactions toward adults (range 66 to 143). In the observations made 18 months later, the median number of interactions toward children was 77 (range 53 to 89); toward adults, it was 69 (range 61 to 98).

9. Preliminary data from control studies confirm staff impressions.

10. Active resistance or disagreement (B) was next with 10%.

11. The total of the three categories, N, O, and P, contributed 7% to the total number of interactions in each of the two phases, whereas M contributed 15% and 21% to the early and late phase, respectively.

12. The critical value for significance at $p = .01$ (one-tailed test) is a rho of .60.

13. Dominance in the Barker and Wright scheme was considered equal to the sum of A and P (Fig. 1), Appeal = K and J, Resistance = B, C, and F, Nurturance = N and O, Aggression = D and E, Submission = I, Compliance = L, and Avoidance = G and H. Affiliative responses, M, were ignored, since affection is treated under a different coding system by Barker and Wright (1954, Ch. 10).

14. These tables were constructed using the interactions of the children when they were *not* in the central focus of observation. That is, in tabulating, the interactions of the central subject were ignored; the interactions of all other persons, children and adults, were tabulated according to whom they were directed toward. This arbitrary rule insures that the same data which entered into the previous tables (1 through 8) do not enter into these tables. At the same time, it should be noted that the entries in any cell do not necessarily represent the equal contribution of all participants to the behavior directed toward a given child. For example, Tony may have received 10 hostile-dominant actions from Bruce and 5 hostile-dominant actions from Frank. Because of such possibilities of confounding, these data are not analyzed by chi square. The discussion that follows is based on visual inspection of the data.

15. The mutual changes raise the possibility of an interesting counter-argument that the children do not "really" change at all; rather, they simply respond reciprocally to "improvement" in the adults brought about through training and experience. An adequate refutation of this view as a complete explanation of the changes in the children's relations with adults would probably require data extraneous to the present study, although study of the se-

quences of interactions would provide some cues. Note that such a counter-
argument can only arise when there is actual information about the behavior of the "others." The usual assumption in studies of change is of a
constant or randomly fluctuating environment. The data put into question
the tenability of such an assumption.

16. Information for these and the following comments may be reconstructed
from the tables presented.

REFERENCES

Baldwin, A. L. *Behavior and development in childhood.* New York: Dryden,
1955.

Bales, R. F. *Interaction process analysis: A method for the study of small groups.*
Cambridge, Mass.: Addison-Wesley, 1950.

Barker, R. G., & Wright, H. F. *Midwest and its children.* Evanston, Ill.: Row,
Peterson, 1954.

Brunswik, E. *Systematic and representative design of psychological experiments.*
Berkeley, Calif.: Univer. Calif. Press, 1947.

Cronbach, L. J., & Meehl, P. E. Construct validity in psychological tests.
Psychol. Bull., 1955, 52, 281-302.

Dittmann, A. T. Problems of reliability in observing and coding social interactions. *J. consult. Psychol.,* 1958, 22, 430.

Freedman, M. B., Leary, T. F., Ossorio, A. G., & Coffey, H. S. The interpersonal
dimension of personality. *J. Pers.,* 1951, 20, 143-161.

Hare, A. P., Borgatta, E. F., & Bales, R. F. (Eds.) *Small groups—Studies in
social interaction.* New York: Knopf, 1955.

Heyns, R. W., & Lippitt, R. Systematic observational techniques. In G. Lindzey
(Ed.), *Handbook of social psychology.* Cambridge: Addison-Wesley,
1954. Pp. 370-404.

Leary, T. *Interpersonal diagnosis of personality.* New York: Ronald Press, 1957.

Redl, F., & Wineman, D. *The aggressive child.* Glencoe, Ill.: Free Press, 1957.